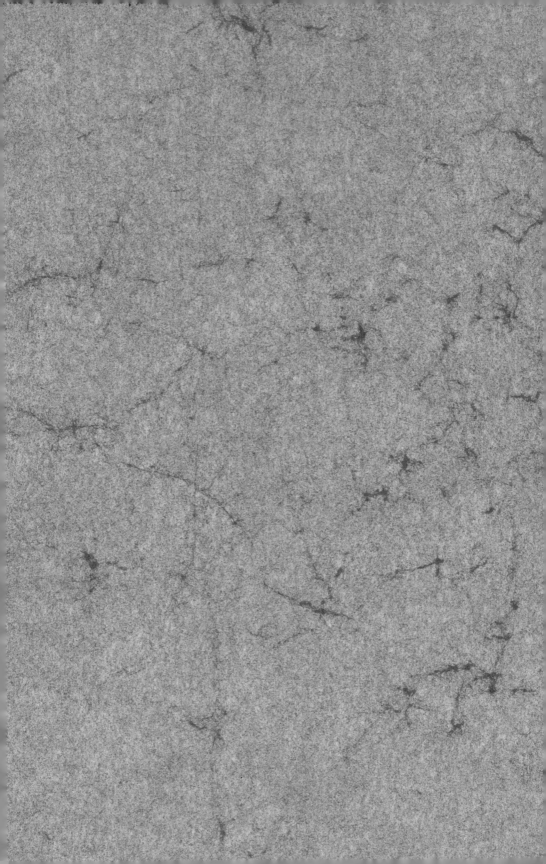

HANDBOOK OF PSYCHIATRIC THERAPIES

Handbook of Psychiatric Therapies

edited by
Jules H. Masserman, M.D.
Professor and Co-chairman of Psychiatry,
Northwestern University

JASON ARONSON

TO CHRISTINE

TABLE OF CONTENTS

ACKNOWLEDGEMENTS

The following have been reprinted from *Current Psychiatric Therapies* by permission of Grune and Stratton, Inc.:

Genetic Counseling in a Psychiatric Setting, by John D. Rainer, M.D., Volume VII, pp. 82-91

Child Psychotherapy, by Frederick H. Allen, M.D., Volume VII, pp. 48-54

Pharmacotherapy in Children's Behavior Disorders, by Barbara Fish, M.D., Volume III, pp. 82-90

Therapy of Childhood Seizures, by Herbert Grossman, M.D., Volume X, pp. 11-24

Therapy of Autistic Children, by Charles Wenar, Ph.D. and Bertram Ruttenberg, M.D., Volume IX, pp. 32-42

Adolescent Psychiatry, by William Schonfeld, M.D., Volume IX, pp. 52-60

Therapy of the Alienated College Student, by Seymour Halleck, M.D., Volume X, pp. 76-82

Youthful Offenders in Psychotherapy, by Herman P. Gladstone, M.D., Volume IV, pp. 83-91

Present Trends in Psychoanalytic Therapy, by Sandor Lorand, M.D., Volume III, pp. 68-73

Freedom in Analytic Therapy, by Ian Alger, M.D., Volume IX, pp. 73-78

Direct Psychoanalysis, by John N. Rosin, M.D., Volume IV, pp. 101-107

Existential Theory and Therapy, by Rollo May, M.D. and Adrian Van Kaam, Ph.D., Volume III, pp. 74-81

Reality Therapy, by William Glasser, M.D. and Leonard M. Zunin, M.D., Volume XII, pp. 58-61

Behavior Therapy, by Edward Dengrove, M.D., Volume XI, pp. 33-44

Art Therapy, by Mardi J. Horowitz, M.D., Volume XI, pp. 61-67

Contributions of Hypnosis to Psychotherapy, by Lewis R. Wolberg, M.D., Volume XII, pp. 48-57

Practical Pastoral Counseling, by Calvert Stein, M.D., Volume XII, pp. 62-69

Aversion Therapy of Homosexuality, by N. McConaghy, D.P.M., Volume XII, pp. 38-47

Group Psychotherapy for Male Homosexuals, by Samuel B. Hadden, M.D., Volume VI, pp. 177-186

Therapy of Transvestism and Transsexualism, by Robert J. Stoller, M.D., Volume VI, pp. 92-103

Treatment of Sex Offenders, by Asher R. Paught, Ph.D., Seymour L. Halleck, M.D. and John C. Ehrmann, Ph.D., Volume II, pp. 173-179

Therapy of Psychopaths, by Melitta Schmiedeberg, M.D., Volume II, pp. 180-184

Treatment of Depressions, by Paul Huston, M.D., Volume XI, pp. 73-85

Outpatient Therapy of Chronic Schizophrenia, by Werner M. Mendel, M.D., Volume IV, pp. 121-126

Comprehensive Therapy of Schizophrenia, by Elvin V. Semrad, M.D., Volume VII, pp. 77-81

PREFACE

Every discipline, particularly those intimately concerned with human welfare, should review its basic tenets and techniques at least every dozen years. This is especially true for psychiatry, which owes a clear explication of the developing theories and modalities in its interrelated fields to psychiatrists who may find it difficult to cover the immense literature in their various subspecialties. Such a review is also recommended for allies in social work, nursing, psychology, jurisprudence, urban organization, penology, and other professions who are necessarily and increasingly involved in individual, group, family, and community therapy of behavior disorders. This *Handbook*, a compilation of the most clinically useful chapters from the twelve volumes of *Current Psychiatric Therapies*, is designed to present just such a clear, specific, comprehensive, and integrated overview of progress in various modalities of psychiatric therapy.

For the past twelve years, scores of authorities in various modes of psychiatric therapy have been invited to submit brief reviews of the latest developments in their respective fields, with a reprise of their own significant contributions. The manuscripts accepted for publication were a perennial joy. They furnished rational and specific clinical directives of progress in the fields of psychiatric therapy from which they had been solicited. A retrospective glance at these works reflects certain important shifting emphases over the years, notably the following:

A marked increase in concern about "primary prevention"—the amelioration of poverty, overcrowding, ignorance, physical disease, and other presumed direct or indirect causes of disorders of behavior.

A concentration on problems of childhood and adolescence.

A diversification of adult dyadic therapies, with stereotyped psychoanalytic techniques giving place to more directly goal-oriented, versatile, briefer, and operationally effective methods.

An increasing emphasis on group dynamics, ranging in focus from nuclear families to wider "systems approaches" comprising extensive kinship, educational, neighborhood, industrial, and other transactional relationships.

An exploration of new and sometimes daring procedures in group therapies, from brief "training" episodes through cathartic "sensitivity" sessions to prolonged and searchingly protracted "marathons."

A peaking of interest in psychopharmacology succeeded by the advocation of greater restraint in the use of medication and more conservative expectations as to lasting therapeutic effects.

Reevaluations of "community psychiatry," with growing reservations as to the usefulness of many "mental health centers" unless they developed special programs for limited objectives such as help for unwed mothers, the legalized supervision and therapy of alcohol and drug addictions, the rehabilitation of patients discharged from psychiatric hospitals, and other such target endeavors.

A growing appreciation of relevant progress in other countries, including those with contrasting economic and political systems.

A concurrent rejection of doctrinaire rigidity in psychiatric theory and practice; a salutary tendency toward more culturally, biologically, and experientially contingent formulations of human behavior and its vicissitudes; and a concern that, accordingly, young psychiatrists be more broadly and comprehensively trained.

Finally, a growing, editorially welcome aversion to jargon, ambiguity, and prolixity in favor of greater brevity, clarity, and style in psychiatric writing.

This *Handbook* is a reflection of this progress, an integrated compendium of the most cogent chapters, republished with the kind permission of Grune and Stratton, from the twelve annual issues of *Current Psychiatric Therapies*. May it receive the recognition due the theoretical sophistication, the therapeutic expertise, and the expository skills of its distinguished contributors.

Jules H. Masserman, Editor
Northwestern University

HANDBOOK
OF
PSYCHIATRIC
THERAPIES

PART I

GENETICS

Genetic Counseling in a Psychiatric Setting

by JOHN D. RAINER, M.D.

D URING the past 20 years, the Department of Medical Genetics of the
New York State Psychiatric Institute has made genetic counseling
services available on a modest scale as part of its research and teaching
program. Two corollaries may be expected from the association of a genetic
counseling center with a psychiatric institute: (1) That many of the
familial conditions for which advice has been sought are in the psychiatric
or neurological area and (2) that the spirit in which the counseling is
provided has been psychiatrically guided and indeed psychotherapeutically
oriented. With both of these distinctive features present, it is the purpose
of this chapter to describe something of the background and techniques,
the teaching, the philosophy, and the results of the genetic counseling so
developed.

BACKGROUND

The Department of Medical Genetics was organized over 30 years ago
by the late Franz J. Kallmann, who already had an extensive background
in clinical psychiatry and genetic family research abroad. His dedication to
the highest principles of medical ethics and his affirmation of "the liberty
of the individual to determine his own fate within the limits of his natural
sovereign rights" were totally at odds with the developing philosophy in his
native land and had much to do with his coming to New York. The
Department itself grew steadily and by the beginning of its second decade
represented an interdisciplinary research group which undertook as one of
its regular activities the provision of genetic counseling to properly referred
individuals, couples, and families. As Table 1 indicates, during the next 20
years 355 persons or couples came for marriage or parenthood counseling.
Couples seeking advice on whether or not to marry accounted for about

TABLE 1

Applicants for Genetic Counseling Seen at the New York State Psychiatric Institute
1947-1966

Total number of applicants	355
1st decade	110
2nd decade	245
Questions of marriage	82
Questions of parenthood	217
Other questions (e.g., prognosis, adoption)	56

one-third of this number, and parents with a genetic or suspected genetic condition in their first child or in other family members accounted for the balance. During the decade 1946-1956, 110 requests for counseling were received, while in the following decade, 1956-1966, the number increased to 245.

In Table 2 is represented the variety of conditions or questions with which the persons came for help. The largest number of problems have indeed involved mental illness, neurological disease, or mental deficiency. A large-scale demographic, psychiatric, and genetic study of early total deafness conducted by the Department since 1955 is reflected in the sizable number of cases in which deafness is the major factor.

Other syndromes—some clearly defined, others less specific—together with a large group of birth anomalies, account for the remaining referrals, while the problem of cousin marriage has been a major and perennial source of anxiety for young couples throughout the years.

TECHNIQUES

This discussion of the technique of genetic counseling as conducted in a psychiatric setting may be divided into two sections: (1) The description of some procedures and principles of genetic investigation basic to genetic counseling and (2) an account of some of the important psychiatric and psychological aspects.

Data Collection

Genetic counseling, like any clinical procedure, draws upon a combination of scientific knowledge and humane understanding. The gathering of data needed for thoughtful genetic counseling has to begin with an ac-

TABLE 2

Specific Areas of Inquiry in 355 Applicants for Genetic Counseling

Mental Illness	
Schizophrenia	37
Manic Depressive Psychosis	6
Other mental illness or undefined	19
Mental Deficiency	
Down's syndrome	27
Other chromosomal anomalies	4
Undefined	36
Neurological Illness	
Huntington's Chorea	33
Epilepsy	23
Spina Bifida	4
Other (e.g., Friedreich's ataxia, amyotonia, neurofibromatosis)	15
Sensory Defect	
Deafness (including retinitis pigmentosa)	15
Opthalmological	7
Birth Anomalies	
Cleft palate, microcephaly, syndactyly, etc.	40
Other Syndromes	
Tay Sachs disease	6
Muscular dystrophy	5
Hemophilia	5
Achondroplasia	4
Osteogenesis imperfecta	2
Cystic fibrosis	2
Von Gierke's disease	1
Gargoylism	1
Cancer	1
Cerebral palsy	1
Albinism	1
Arthritis	1
Miscellaneous orthopedic	10
Miscellaneous cardiac	3
Other Problems	
Cousin marriage	33
Suicide	4
Adoption	4
Skin color	2
Geneology	2
Homosexuality	1

curate diagnosis of the condition about which the person is troubled. In the case of psychiatric illness, this diagnosis will depend upon accurate histories, hospital records, and direct observation and interview of affected family members. Often, the person seeking counseling will himself be an affected individual. If the counselor is a psychiatrist, he may form a direct diagnostic impression and take steps to substantiate it. Roberts actually believes that "genetic advice on mental diseases must be left to psychiatrists. Some of those interviewed, and the histories they give, need psychiatric appraisal. What is even more important is the difficulty to anyone not a psychiatrist of interpreting and assessing psychiatric reports."

In mental deficiency, accurate psychological testing, histories of school and hospital stays, and often cytogenetic analysis are necessary to confirm both the nature and the extent of the retardation. With neurological illness, careful and detailed neurological examinations are required; electroencephalograms in cases of convulsive disorder are essential, and actual family histories themselves may be needed to confirm the presence of a dominant genetic disease such as Huntington's Chorea.

For sensory defects, audiograms or accurate eye examinations, including visual fields, are needed, while the appropriate specialist may be asked to provide differential diagnoses in the case of metabolic, cardiac, orthopedic, or hematological syndromes. In all cases physical examinations have to be made available.

After proper diagnosis, an accurate family pedigree is essential. In obtaining this, it is desirable to question those seeking assistance about every family member: children, brothers, sisters, parents, uncles, aunts, cousins, grandparents, and, if possible, great-uncles and great-aunts. The informants must be asked to train their attention in succession upon each family member and to provide what pertinent information they can. If this is not done, some very important data may be conveniently forgotten. Information on miscarriages and stillbirths must be specifically sought, and instances of consanguineous marriage noted. Careful inquiry must be made about specific environmental factors such as drug ingestion, virus disease, nutrition, and radiation exposure of parents, especially of mothers during pregnancy. After this procedure, certain laboratory tests will often be suggested. These tests may include biochemical measurements of hormones or intermediary metabolites, or cytological studies such as chromosome counts or buccal smears.

Genetic Risks

Having determined the nature of the condition and its distribution throughout the given family, the genetic counselor must now draw upon his knowl-

30

edge of the genetic syndromes and their transmission and must give himself time to search the literature for pertinent observations, recent studies, and clinical variations. Established genetic syndromes may be inherited in a dominant pattern, a recessive pattern, a sex-linked pattern, or in variations and modifications of these; in some cases more than one form of inheritance is described for a given clinical picture.

In *dominant* inheritance, it is sufficient for a child to receive one gene from one parent in order to manifest the condition. It follows that the genetic risk for the child of a parent with a dominant condition is 50 per cent, and that if a child does not have the condition his offspring will usually be free of it forever. An example of dominant inheritance in the neurological field is Huntington's Chorea. Barring relatively rare cases of new mutations, an individual with Huntington's Chorea will be the son or daughter of a parent with the same condition. In many instances, however, old records are poor, and the parent in question may have been diagnosed as schizophrenic or alcoholic, or may have died before manifesting the illness clinically. It is a peculiarity of this disease that it develops late in life, often in the fourth or fifth decade. Therefore, while the pattern of genetic transmission is relatively simple, the counseling problem is a very difficult one. An adult who seeks to marry or have children and who is the son or daughter of a patient with Huntington's Chorea may have no way of knowing whether he himself will be affected until he is past the age in which he would ordinarily reproduce. Methods of early detection would be a great boon; at present the counselor must offer not only the stark facts but careful and empathic discussion.

In a *recessive* condition two genes are required to determine its clinical manifestation, one passed on from each parent. An example of such a syndrome is phenylketonuria. In this condition, the parents themselves, each carrying only one gene for the condition, are *heterozygotes* and are usually clinically free, although their genetic state (genotype) may sometimes be ascertained by special tolerance tests after heavy phenylalanine intake. The presence of a recessive gene in a family may often not become evident until one affected child has been born, whereupon the risk for each subsequent child will be 25 per cent. Sometimes, however, a person may know of such recessive genes in his own family as a result of having affected brothers, sisters, uncles, or aunts, and may come for advice about marrying. In that case, the family of the prospective spouse must be carefully investigated to see if the same condition exists in an equally close relative. The risk of both members of the couple being heterozygotes and of any child being affected may then be calculated and discussed with them. In such families, first cousin marriages carry a particularly high risk.

31

Sex-linked inheritance shows various forms. The particular recessive form of X-linked inheritance exemplified by hemophilia or the Duchenne form of muscular dystrophy is marked by affected males passing the gene on to their daughters who are not themselves affected because they have a second X-chromosome carrying a normal gene. The daughters however will subsequently transmit the gene and the condition to their sons with a 50 per cent risk in each case. In this type of inheritance, therefore, pedigrees going back at least two generations are important.

Cytogenetics

Aside from the classical patterns of gene transmission, a great deal of attention has recently been focused on disarranged chromosomes as observed in cytogenetic studies. With the establishment of 46 as the correct number of chromosomes in man in 1956, a productive decade of research has uncovered the chromosomal basis for a number of important genetic conditions. In 1959, for example, mongolism or Down's syndrome was found to be characterized in most cases by possession of an additional small (Group G) chromosome, making 47 in all. This *trisomic* condition originates as a result of *nondisjunction* or asymetrical separation in the formation of the ovum.

In a second mechanism involved in the etiology of mongolism the extra chromosome is attached to one of the others, so that the total count is still 46. Not as common as the usual trisomy, this phenomenon, known as *translocation,* may sometimes indicate a similar phenomenon (balanced translocation) in the mother or father, who however is unaffected through having one less free chromosome.

Of course very few mongoloid mothers themselves reproduce or seek genetic counseling. (About ten children have been reported born to mongoloid women; as would be expected, roughly half of the children are themselves mongoloid.) A common cause for referral, however, is the production of one mongoloid child by a mother who is now concerned about future children. In order to establish the etiology of the mongolism in the child, a karyotype or cytogenetic study must be performed. These studies still require a good deal of time and effort, approximately 25 man-hours apiece. If the child is trisomic, the risk of the same event occurring in a subsequent pregnancy is actually very little greater than that for any mother of the same age. The overall risk is about one in 650, although it is higher for older mothers, as great as one in 50 for mothers over the age of 45. However, if cytological study shows a translocation, the chromosomes of the parents must be studied, since a balanced translocation in the parent carries a risk for future children as great as one in three.

Empirical Risk

In many conditions simple ratios are not available for determining the genetic risk. These conditions include certain birth anomalies (e.g., harelip, cleft palate, spina bifida) and other characteristics which are probably transmitted by the combined action of many genes. For these cases the genetic counselor must rely on empirical risk data which distill the results of the observations of large series of families. Such data may serve as the basis for counseling discussions, though they are admittedly tentative and subject to revision in the light of future research into the precise etiology and mechanism.

In some of the major psychiatric conditions, complex interaction with environmental circumstances, as well as other aspects of variable expressivity, make it particularly difficult to discuss precise genetic ratios. Here again large-scale family studies have provided useful empirical risk figures. In schizophrenia, for example, it has been found that the risk for individuals with two affected parents is 40 to 70 per cent; with one affected parent, 9 to 16 per cent; and with an affected sibling, 11 to 14 per cent.

Psychiatric Implications of Counseling Procedures

In addition to developing appropriate methods of data gathering and genetic risk determination, psychiatry has contributed much insight to the field of genetic counseling concerning ways of presenting material and discussing it with persons who seek help. In actual practice persons come for genetic counseling on their own or are referred by their physician. While the latter is preferable, persons who write or call are invited to come for consultation but are asked to provide in advance whatever medical data their physician can supply. It is implicit in the approach to genetic counseling presented here that counseling over the telephone or by mail is not generally satisfactory. At best, such procedures can provide only sketchy information; and at worst, they may do great harm. If couples are seen together in person and under the strictest codes of medical ethics, and if they are made to feel comfortable, they will express their motives and feelings and tell a great deal about themselves to a trained interviewer.

Clientele

Aside from general information seekers, persons coming for help fall into two groups—those contemplating marriage and married persons contemplating parenthood, with or without one defective child already born. While some persons who come have read widely and are quite sophisticated, most have been filled with misinformation, superstition, and emotionally tinged attitudes. One of the first interests of the psychiatrist is to probe the motives of the applicant. Some prospective couples who come for genetic advice are really seeking to rationalize an attempt to avoid a marriage sanctioned either by parents or by their social group. On the other hand, particularly poignant are the many young people related as first or second cousins who are on the brink of marriage but are concerned with social pressure, their incestuous fears, and some of the more lurid old wives' tales that persist about weak children born to such marriages. The facts about cousin marriage are simple enough to convey. If there are clear-cut recessive genetic conditions in the close family, parenthood is contraindicated. Otherwise, while such marriages are less desirable in theory, they need not be discouraged in any particular case; and indeed positive genetic qualities, general constitutional health, intelligence and so on may well be transmitted to the offspring.

If parents have already had a defective child, the profound impact of this event upon the couple must be considered: the tendency of each parent to blame the other and project his or her guilt, the shame and the sense of worthlessness in having produced a defective child, and, on the other hand, the desire to overcompensate by producing healthy offspring. All parents want perfect children, and defects are often seen as some kind of punishment. Many marital problems may arise—anxiety, hostility, impotence and frigidity. The counselor may help greatly in a variety of practical matters, such as the prognosis for a defective child, problems of raising one or more healthy children with the added burden of the defective child, adoption, institutionalization, finances and sources of aid, abortion, sterilization, and artificial insemination. All the facets of individual and family dynamics will come into view during genetic counseling.

In dealing with considerations of risk, many people may be familiar with odds on the gambling table, but the emotional valence is quite different when it comes to having children. Helpful discussions of the meaning of risks, how other people have interpreted risks, the desire of the couple to have children, and their specific fears must all be included in any final synthesis. It is not generally known that the risk of serious malformations apparent at birth or becoming manifest in early life has been variously estimated at from 1/40 to 1/100 in any random pregnancy. Some stoic couples will accept a $\frac{1}{4}$ risk and even go through one or more painful experiences in order to have a healthy child, if the recessive condition is an early lethal one such as Tay Sachs disease and does not lead to prolonged dependency. On the other hand others, because of neurotic fears or a compelling desire to avoid having an affected child at all costs, will shy away from a very small risk. The weight given to emotional factors will vary with every case.

34

In the last analysis, genetic counseling is a clinical procedure which serves as the final common pathway of the rapidly developing sciences of family dynamics and genetics. There are few decisions in a person's life more emotion laden or fateful than the one to marry and the one to assume parenthood. Both are so consequential for the prospective parents and their future children that competent and thoughtful counsel must be available in the presence of any uncertainty or doubt. It is rare that the process of genetic counseling can be completed in one or two interviews; rather the process must resemble a brief psychotherapeutic program. Neither advice nor data are usable if their impact is ignored.

Eugenics

It will be noted in this discussion that the eugenic aspect of genetic counseling has been placed in the background in favor of immediate value to the family. This does not minimize the important demographic and social importance of family planning or the long-run population-genetic and evolutionary significance of deliberately chosen trends in assortative mating patterns and fertility. However, the most immediate and most cogent considerations in the counseling room relate to the well-being and happiness of the parents themselves. The therapeutic sessions before anything else ought to develop insight into the effect of any new child upon the mental or physical well-being of the mother or father, upon the stability of the marriage, and upon other children in the family. Healthy children, in terms of genetic endowment, developmental circumstances, and emotional climate in the home are both the product and the source of health in the parents.

Training and Organization of Services

From what has been said it would seem that the ideal genetic counselor should be a person who is trained in many areas—e.g., in genetics; in clinical medicine, including medical specialties; and in psychology, psychodynamics, and the art of human understanding. Since few people have formal training in even two of these fields, the teaching of genetic counseling must essentially fill in the gaps. On the postdoctoral level, for example, a training course may be open to individuals of personal integrity, with a background in either genetics, clinical medicine, or psychiatry or psychology. It should include adequate and lengthy preparation in the principles of genetics and in the principles of counseling; exposure to laboratory procedures, statistical methods, and the vast and growing literature on the subject; and a great deal of supervised experience. Genetic counseling

35

services are best provided in a university, hospital, or clinic setting, where the ancillary disciplines and specialties are available.

RESULTS

At present it is difficult to find quantitative measures of the benefits derived from genetic counseling programs. There is insufficient follow-up of families who have received help, partly due to the administrative problems involved but also because many counselors are still uncertain of their role and are hesitant to find out what might have happened. The families themselves are often in inadequate rapport with the counselor to come back to him with this information. Better attention to the psychiatric and emotional aspects of counseling would lay the groundwork for more intensive follow-up studies. Nevertheless, there are many individual gratifying cases to cite. Since the decisions reached are as often affirmative as negative, people have been helped to become parents who might otherwise have refrained. The positive happiness thus achieved is not the least of the fruits of responsible effort in this field.

REFERENCES

1. HAMMONS, H. G. (Ed.): Heredity Counseling. New York, Hoeber (Harper & Row), 1959.
2. KALLMANN, F. J.: Psychiatric aspects of genetic counseling. Amer. J. Hum. Genet. 8:97-101, 1956.
3. KALLMANN, F. J., AND RAINER, J. D.: Psychotherapeutically oriented counseling techniques in the setting of a medical genetics department. In: Topical Problems of Psychotherapy. B. Stokvis, Ed. Basel, S. Karger, 1963.
4. KALLMANN, F. J., AND RAINER, J. D.: The genetic approach to schizophrenia: clinical, demographic, and family guidance problems. In: Schizophrenia. L. C. Kolb, F. J. Kallmann, P. Polatin, Eds. Boston, Little, Brown & Co., 1964.
5. KALLMANN, F. J.: Some aspects of genetic counseling. In: Genetics and the Epidemiology of Chronic Diseases. J. V. Neel, M. W. Shaw, W. J. Schull, Eds. Washington, D. C., U.S. Dept. of Health, Education, and Welfare, 1965.
6. RAINER, J. D., ALTSHULER, K. Z., AND KALLMANN, F. J. (Eds.): Family and Mental Health Problems in a Deaf Population. New York, New York State Psychiatric Institute, 1963.
7. ROBERTS, J. A. F.: An Introduction to Medical Genetics. London, Oxford University Press, 1963.

PART II

THE CHILD

Child Psychotherapy

by Frederick H. Allen, M.D.

T HE BASIC characteristic of childhood is the dependency upon the parental figures from whom the child differentiates himself and emerges as a separate but related human being. Emotional problems emerge out of this growth process, even where the child has been organically damaged. Therapeutic efforts will be built on this foundation and our knowledge of the nature of the psychologic growth process will be incorporated into it.

Adult and child, acting on and reacting to each other, giving a living quality to this universal relation wherever the human drama unfolds. In its early phases the parent, usually the mother, is the giver, the child the taker. This is the dependency feature from which emerges the normal shifts as the child, who in using what is given, starts on the road to self development. This individuating process is always one of differentiation with other living or human beings. The *I* and the *You*, always separate and different, come into a functioning relation to each other.

Three basic movements emerge as parent and child interact on each other in this process: The first is the movement away from the maternal figure. Birth with biologic separation is a total separating event. Following this, the psychologic reunion with the maternal figure occurs as it is clear the child cannot live as a separate person. But the early moving away occurs as he becomes aware of being a person apart from the mothering figure. He can move about, he can manipulate objects, he can perceive the presence and absence of the giving person. He can do things on his own as he reaches out to satisfy his basic needs.

From this first movement emerges the second—the moving toward or the reuniting process—so essential because of the dependency element. The separating movement arouses anxiety in some degree. The child feels alone and the positive values of this feeling is that it motivates the

39

second movement toward the object from which he feels separated. He discovers he is a separate person but wishes to reunite himself with the those upon whom he is dependent. This is beginning of the balance so essential in these two primary movements.

Early in this process emerges the third movement—the oppositional or the anti-movement. The child is not a passive organism and reacts against restrictions of his body movements, against delays which leave him hungry, etc. In fact, he reacts in varying degrees against the necessary organizational efforts of the adult. He learns also to yield and gradually balance is established.

So many if not all the behavioral problems, which necessitate therapeutic intervention, emerge as these three movements get out of balance and dilute the normal values of each in relation to the others. The unseparated child clinging to the mother, the remote and isolated child who has few rewards from his affectional relation to the parent, the rebel who asserts against the outer world—all represent an imbalance and a hiatus in the normal growth process. Anxieties beyond the capacity of the child to master becomes the dominant, emotional tone.

This preamble to a discussion of psychotherapy with children lays the foundation for a new and unique growth experience which therapy should provide. Building the structure on this sound understanding is essential. Child psychiatry, as this specialty has evolved, has become family centered with the focus of concern on an emotionally disturbed child. This has happened because the structure has been built both on understanding the nature of childhood and the dynamics of family interaction. The child is a dependent organism and needs the support of the adult figures as he moves in an unsteady way to becoming a person. He is vulnerable to stress, to parental uncertainties and anxiety. He is responding to his own internal needs. While striving for individuality the child at the same time discovers he is awakening in a world of other people who guide and influence the kind of individual he becomes. Here is the universal conflict between the need to maintain individuality and the need to become a related and social being. From this basic conflict arise many of the problems in the parent/child interaction that opens the need for psychotherapeutic intervention.

Psychotherapy with children has many unique characteristics. An important one is that a child does not initiate the process. He is impelled into this by significant adults, usually the parents, who are concerned about the child and who seek help. They open the therapeutic door and in doing so, discover the part they will need to play in sustaining what they have started.

Every parent, in making a tentative move to seek psychiatric help

40

for a child, has some anxiety and doubt about this decision. In this first phase, they need help to bring their feelings into the period of planning with those who are providing help. This is the parent-centered phase and is designed to help the parents test out the validity of their first move. They must be aided to bring into the open their doubts and misgivings and to feel that the problem they describe in their child warrants going ahead with this plan. They learn the part they will need to take after the child is included and to discuss how they can prepare the child. The decision to go ahead may be made in this first interview, but in most instances the parents need time to digest what took place and to return for a second conference before the child is included.

Where the child lives with both father and mother, it is important that both participate in this first phase. The therapeutic process is then geared to the family realities and the role distortions among father, mother and child are more clearly defined and brought into the open. Fragmentation, so commonly found in families with an emotionally disturbed child, can be accentuated if the planning involves only one parent. For example, the mother may take the full responsibility for initiating the helping process on the assumption that the father has no interest or is even opposed to seeking psychiatric help. To proceed on such a basis can distort further the family drama and isolate the father from an experience which aims not just to help the child but to restore a balance in the family reality with the father, mother, and child finding new values in their interacting roles. Achieving this is the ultimate goal of psychotherapy with children.

An essential element in enlisting parents in a therapeutic program for a child must be based upon a positive foundation. Their participation in this program is needed not just because of their involvement in the child's emotional problem, but more because they are so important in helping the child to gain a new balance, both in himself and in his relation to them. They are the important persons in a child's world and need to feel this in a therapeutic program. While many may feel their job is completed by turning the child over to a psychiatrist, they must realize that they are needed to nourish what gains the therapist can bring about in the child. To isolate the child's experience from the day-to-day realities they provide would be a fairly sure way of minimizing those values and defeat the basic purpose of the experience to bring about a new family climate in which the child could grow.

This is the essence of the more positive approach to the parents. They come expecting to be blamed and are ready to defend themselves in one way or another. Many fathers stay away because this is their concept of clinical help. However, so many fathers enter the clinical program

41

when they can feel they are needed. For many fathers this is a new concept, particularly in the many families where they have been kept on the side lines and allowed a minimal participation in the growing up of the child.

The fact that parents have asked for help is in itself evidence of some strength and responsibility, although this may be disguised by the many conflicted feelings parents have toward themselves and toward the child. The swirl of these feelings become focused around the fact that they are concerned enough about the child to ask for help. This is the starting point, and those who work with the parents must never lose sight of this fundamental fact.

Just as the growth process is one of differentiation with the emergence of the self pattern of the child, so the therapeutic process provides an unique growth experience for the child. In this unique setting, the child participates in a variety of ways: sometimes in silence, other times through verbal communication or through acting out his disturbed feelings. He may use available material to dramatize the nature of his emotional problems while, at the same time, telling his therapist how he feels about this new relation into which he has been impelled. Important content is brought out by the child as he begins to communicate. He reveals the nature of his anxiety and fears, his hostile feelings toward significant adults, his negative feelings, etc. Content and process come into a new relation to each other. The dichotomy between fact and feeling is also partially bridged in these early hours. For example, a fearful child may verbalize what he is afraid of—this is fact—but in the process of revealing, he is being helped to have a beginning experience in mastering the fear engendered by being propelled in a new experience. What he reveals and the new opportunity provided by the therapist, provide the dynamic that gives the therapeutic potential.

Throughout, a child creates its own realities not unlike those of everyday life against which he may be reacting. He has his regular time with the same psychiatrist, limited to an hour and adhered to. The child may seek to control these boundaries and his aggressive reactions bring out both feelings and action. He meets limits on action but has complete freedom to express his feelings. He can use available material but he is not allowed to destroy it. These limits are not for restrictive purposes but more to define the boundaries. They have dynamic values in that the child's efforts to control bring out much of this feeling. He has the opportunity both to assert and yield, and to use and feel the strength of his therapist who stands steady in face of the child's swirling conflicts.

42

Psychotherapy with a child has three phases, all interwoven but having fairly well defined characteristics: the beginning phase, the reorganizational phase, and the ending phase. Throughout each, the three basic movements described earlier are in evidence in this new and unique experience. These are the toward, the away, and the against directions. The differentiating process involved in each contains the dynamic and the impact of this new experience modifies the ongoing reality of the child in his family.

The Beginning Phase

Introducing the child into the plan is a recognition by all concerned that he has a part in creating his emotional disturbances. He is not regarded as a nonparticipating victim of external influences. He is not a pawn but a reactor, and can bring about change.

Children are prepared for this first visit in a variety of ways. With many, this is done sensitively and realistically by the parents; others come with inadequate or confused preparation. Irrespective of how this has been explained to the child, one element always is present: he is being exposed to a person who is going to help him. Every child organizes himself against being changed, although the oppositional direction is overtly acted out with some, and well disguised with others. He may move in almost totally, and thus neutralize the assumed power of this new force; or move away into a corner and refuse to communicate, or be openly hostile thus disguising his anxiety. He may state his problem with the assumption that this person will take over and correct the situation, or he may deny having any difficulty. In a variety of ways he reacts with his own feeling to this new experience and in reacting he is engaged in a beginning relation that has a potential for being helpful.

In this beginning phase important things happen both for the child and for the therapist. For the child, he finds a person interested in the way he feels, who helps him to express being afraid, hostile, withdrawn, etc. For the therapist, this beginning phase provides an important diagnostic opportunity. He sees the child as he is and not just the person described in a variety of ways by the parents. Here is a living entity. The therapist is able to get impressions about the degree of accessibility, what the child presents as his own problem, and the way he can express feeling engendered by this new experience. The therapist observes how the child leaves the parent to come with him and how he returns to the parent at the end of each session. In a variety of ways, the therapist gets a tentative diagnostic picture, while opening the door to a therapeutic journey which may follow.

In the early phases of the process, the child will perceive the therapist as he has other adults in his life—hostile, possessive, benevolent, etc. He will project on the therapist both what he expects, what he wishes, and what he fears him to be. The child will invest him with the magic to cure without having to do anything himself. The therapist will both allow and help the child to test out these preconceptions, but will maintain his own integrity and not become the projection. While the child tries to make him be the good or the bad parent, the therapist remains himself and thus provides a new, differentiating experience for the child.

From the beginning phase, with its diagnostic and therapeutic values, emerges a plan for sustaining what opens up in this period. This plan is based upon the physical condition of the child, the evaluative studies by the psychologist, the child's capacity to form a relation to the psychiatrist, and the parents' commitment to go ahead. All are factors in determining both the nature of the child's problem and the mode of proceeding. Important shifts in the family and in the child can be evaluated at this point and, in many instances, new directions are noted which are important determinants. In less severe cases, they acquire a new grip on the situation and decide to go on their own. But here we are concerned with the clearer indications that a more sustained process is needed and agreed upon.

The tempo of that which follows is geared both to the severity of the problem and what is realistically possible. In clinic practice, it is common to set up a plan for weekly appointments. More frequent interviews may be needed, but it is important that a definite schedule be agreed upon, with child and parents having separate and wherever possible concurrent appointments, since much of the family-centered emphasis gets clouded when the child comes at one time and the parents at a different time. The integrated plan of concurrent but separate interviews is more feasible in clinic practice where the team plan allows the parents to work with one staff person, usually the social worker, and the child with his therapist, usually the psychiatrist.

The primary emphasis throughout is on the experiential values of the relationships that unfold for the child and his parents. All three reveal a great deal of their troubled past but the process of revealing to those who symbolize a new direction, is the important element that brings them into the new and present. The therapist who is sensitive to the uses the child makes of him will be aware of signals that indicate the child is moving out and is approaching the final and in many ways the most important phase, the one of ending.

As indicated earlier, the uniqueness of this relationship is that it is begun with the goal of ending it. In the beginning, the child experiences anxiety about leaving the parent and embarking on a new and unknown course. In the final phases he frequently feels anxiety about leaving his therapist. Just as he struggles in one way or another the impact of the new experience, he will struggle in a variety of ways against its termination and resuming his day-to-day living without this specialized help. In the beginning, he has the experience of mastering this anxiety; in the end phase he has the same experience but with a new sense of values about himself. He learns that a change has taken place within himself and that he has been a participant in bringing this about. At the beginning, he projects on the therapist the power to change him. In the end phase, he has the opportunity to own his part in bringing about the change. As one ten year old girl said in her end phase, "At first, I thought you were going to cure me of my fears. Then I discovered I had to do something myself." She did.

Therapy for a child and his parents helps them to move away from a troubled past in which all have been caught. It can open the door to new values in which the important roles each must fulfill are more clearly interwoven. Where therapy has achieved this, the family becomes one in which each member has gained a new sense of individual values.

If therapy ends with this real quality, it has achieved its real. It will have been more than digging into the past, revealing the pains and struggles of a child's life. It will have been more than a mechanistic experience with emphasis on what was wrong. It will have been what all therapy should be: a meaningful human experience with a person who, from the beginning, was concerned with postive values and with providing an opportunity for a child and his parents to affirm them.

Pharmacotherapy in Children's Behavior Disorders

by Barbara Fish, M.D.

Since 1940, amphetamines, anticonvulsants and antihistamines have been used to treat children with behavior disorders. The introduction of chlorpromazine and reserpine enlarged the scope of pharmacotherapy, but it also heightened the controversy about the role of drugs. Glib claims of "improvement" were countered by dire warnings about the effect of drugs on learning and the psychotherapeutic relationship.[1] Controlled studies are needed to establish specific indications and contraindications, using criteria that can be compared in different centers. Pending such definitive studies, one must draw upon the accumulated clinical experience of the past twenty years to establish a practical modus operandi.

What Drugs Can and Cannot Do

Drugs are most effective in reducing psychomotor excitement. Optimally the reduction of impulsivity and irritability is accompanied by lessened anxiety and improved attention-span. To a lesser extent drugs can increase spontaneous activity and affective responsiveness in states of apathy and inertia.

The response of complex behavior patterns to physiological treatment is far less predictable. Hallucinations, perceptual distortions and thought disorders subside in some children with the lessening of psychomotor excitement; other children retain residual defects. Whether drugs can improve intellectual functioning has still to be determined. Children with severe mental retardation, associated with organic brain disease or schizophrenia show the least response to drugs. The more severe, unchanging

46

deficits in function appear to have the same prognostic significance in children as do long duration and chronicity of symptoms in adults.[2]

Drugs may modify a child's responsiveness to current and past experiences but chemicals alone cannot undo previously learned behavior, alter character patterns or neurotic attitudes. Thus aggressive behavior may respond to drugs only if it is associated with gross psychomotor disturbance. Less disturbed children frequently resent the physiological changes produced by drugs and the threat to their autonomy which such manipulations represent.

If drugs cannot alter established patterns in the most severe psychoses or the mildest conduct disorders, they can modify appropriate target symptoms in moderately severe schizophrenia and chronic brain syndromes, or in severe behavior disorders. In addition some neurotic children with persistent anxiety, inhibitions and phobias become more spontaneous and increase their adaptive functioning if given drugs. The younger the child, the more is psychiatric disturbance of any type expressed in hyperexcitability, hyperactivity, and disorganized behavior which can respond to medication. Symptomatic pharmacotherapy may enable severely disturbed children to participate in group activities and special classes; it helps others to become amenable to psychotherapy and education which would otherwise be impossible; it can accelerate the therapy of less disturbed children.[3,4]

WHEN TO INTRODUCE DRUGS INTO TREATMENT

Good medicine dictates that one must first evaluate the child's psychopathology and the relation of his symptoms to his family and environment before introducing any foreign agent into this complex situation. The child's ability to change in the new setting of ambulatory or institutional psychiatric treatment should be observed for two to four weeks before starting a trial of drug therapy. If an acute crisis demands immediate medication, drugs can be withheld later, to evaluate the child's own capacity for reintegration.

If symptoms disappear completely, in the child's usual environment, with full resumption of social and academic activities, using social manipulation and psychotherapy alone, obviously no additional treatment is indicated. However, if considerable anxiety or a limitation in function persists after four weeks, one should not withhold drugs which could accelerate recovery, even if the child is responding slowly to other measures. Medical judgment must weigh the slight chance of harm from drugs against the limitation in the child's function and the strain imposed on his family if drugs are withheld. A potentially useful treatment may be withheld in a controlled experiment comparing different treatments; it should not be postponed merely to satisfy the therapist's desire for psychotherapeutic omnipotence.

DRUGS AND PSYCHOTHERAPY

Pharmacotherapy need not interfere with the subtler interpersonal operations of psychotherapy if the physician has a constructive and common sense attitude toward drugs and is alert to the transference problems which may arise. The therapeutic meaning of biologic measures, verbal interpretations or environmental restrictions depends upon the conscious and unconscious attitudes of all the participants. Drugs would destroy therapy if the doctor used them as a quick expedient to avoid responsibility for the child's complex problems in living, or if he saw drugs as the ultimate weapon of authority to enforce compliance on a problem child, or if he felt drugs were a measure of desperation to be used only after all other measures failed.

If drug therapy is put into its proper perspective by the physician, the auxiliary use of drugs does not permit parents to minimize the child's problems. Parents should be told that at best drugs produce only quantitative changes and the child will not be cured or "made over." Discussions of all the other measures needed to help the child emphasize this point. Even very young children can understand that medicine just "helps the way your stomach feels when you're scared," or "angry," or "jumpy" and that once they feel better it is easier to do something about these other problems.

The use of drugs will not alarm parents about the seriousness of the child's disturbance, if the doctor does not wait for a desperate or hopeless situation to force his hand, but uses drugs for specific indications of varying severity. The physician must relieve parents' anxieties by explaining the effects of drugs and by being available between appointments to discuss any questionable side effects. Children are usually reassured by the information that their "funny feelings" are not unique, and by finding out that these feelings can be helped by medication. Seriously disturbed children who need maintenance drug therapy need to understand that this is to help their "over-sensitivity" at the times in their life when this is necessary.

The child does not experience medication as a weapon of authority when his own distress is made the mutual concern of himself and the therapist, and he is given the responsibility to report which medicine makes him feel better, or sleepy or jumpy. The management of medication between child and doctor can become part of a new and constructive experience for a child who is not used to being listened to or taken seriously by an adult.

48

When parents are helped to understand the child's symptoms in terms of anxiety or disturbances in development, the emphasis of treatment is shifted away from blaming the child for being "bad," or the parent for being inadequate. Specific goals should be set for increasing the child's function so that medication becomes a positive tool and not a way to make the child "behave." Additional precautions must be taken to prevent the actual giving of medication from becoming an issue between mother and child. First, medicine is given regularly at specific times; the mother is not to offer it to the child just when he becomes upset, or if he happens to annoy her. Second, the mother does not adjust the dose herself for what might be subjective reasons. Finally, if a child objects to drugs, the mother should not force the issue. The child's feelings about pills, as about any other aspect of treatment, are a matter for him to discuss with his doctor.

Children typically tend to deny physical and psychological difficulties, and are all too ready to terminate medication as soon as their distress is lessened. Rarely, an older neurotic child may use medication in the interest of his hypochondriasis or secondary gain. If the physician himself is sceptical about the effects of medication and is alert to these transference complications, they can be readily resolved.

The regulation of medication creates transference complications, but these can be handled just like the similar problems encountered in the absence of drugs. Medication itself can be readily accepted by parent and child as simply another way in which the doctor tries to help the child. In the interest of good medical and psychotherapeutic management, the psychological and pharmacological aspects of treatment should not be split between two therapists.

INDICATIONS FOR SPECIFIC DRUGS

In general the more severe the disorder the more potent is the drug required to produce a response. The standard diagnostic categories serve as a gross guide to severity. Within a diagnostic group, severity increases with greater intellectual, perceptual, and neurological impairment, and with greater affective and motoric disturbance.[2] Hyperactive and hypoactive children may react differently to drugs and there are also individual differences in response to the sedative and stimulating properties of medications.

The clinician should become familiar with a few representative minor and major tranquilizers and stimulants which span the spectrum of potency and differential effects. Additional drugs may be used if sensitivity to previous drugs makes substitution necessary.

The following discussion is limited to children's behavioral and central

49

nervous system responses. The clinician should be familiar with the possible systemic, allergic and other toxic effects, and should observe all the precautions which are taken with adults.[5,6] Any of these drugs may also produce undesirable exaggerations of their therapeutic effects on the nervous system, if the dose is too high for the particular child. However, excessive sedation or irritability readily subside if the dose is reduced.

MINOR TRANQUILIZERS

These drugs are primarily useful in mild to moderately severe neurotic and "primary" behavior disorders, comparable to their use in adult patients. Unlike adults and adolescents, prepuberty children do not tend to become addicted to medication. Children with moderately severe organic and schizophrenic reactions are frequently helped by certain of the mild medications, as if their patterns were more malleable than adults', or the immature nervous system reacted differently to drugs.[2,3]

Diphenylmethane Derivatives

Diphenhydramine (Benadryl) has been used for over ten years to treat disturbed children.[3,7,8] It is most effective in behavior disorders associated with hyperactivity, but it also reduces anxiety in very young children who are not hyperactive and may be helpful in moderately severe organic or schizophrenic disorders. Unlike the other drugs, diphenhydramine drops in effectiveness at puberty. In young children it reduces anxiety without producing drowsiness or lethargy; after ten years of age children respond like adults: the drug frequently produces fatigue or drowsiness and is most useful as a bedtime sedative.[3] Hydroxyzine (Atarax) and Azacyclonol (Frenquel) appear to be weaker and more variable in their action than diphenhydramine. Captodiamine (Suvren) is similar chemically to diphenhydramine, and has been reported to be effective in organic brain disorders.[9]

Substituted Diols

Meprobamate (Equanil, Miltown) is effective in neurotic and behavior disorders including those associated with mild organic brain disease.[8] I found it less effective for hyperactivity than diphenhydramine in the same subjects, but unlike diphenhydramine it continues to be effective in neurotic children into adolescence.

Miscellaneous

Promethazine (Phenergan) is structurally related to the phenothiazines but acts as a mild tranquilizer. It has been reported to be effective in

50

severely disturbed children,[7] but I found it less effective than diphenhydramine in the same subjects. *Chlordiazepoxide* (*Librium*) is apparently comparable in potency to the most effective minor tranquilizers, but preliminary work suggests that it may also have excitatory effects which require further exploration.[10]

ANTICONVULSANTS

Early studies reported encouraging results in the use of hydantoin compounds in the treatment of children whose behavior disorders were associated with non-specific EEG abnormalities.[11,12] Later reports failed to confirm these findings,[8,13] and my own experience agrees with this latter impression.

HYPNOTICS

These drugs have not been demonstrated to be effective in psychiatric disorders of prepuberty children. Barbiturates may actually increase anxiety and disorganization in severely disturbed children. When night-time sedation is needed, chloral hydrate or the more effective mild tranquilizers usually suffice.

MAJOR TRANQUILIZERS

Phenothiazines

Extensive experience has demonstrated that these compounds are highly effective in severely disturbed children with "primary" behavior disorders, schizophrenia, or organic brain disease. Used with the proper precautions,[6] these drugs are safe enough to warrant use in disorders which resist milder therapies.

Dimethylamine Series

These drugs are relatively less potent than the piperazine series. They show a predominance of sedative over stimulating effects, are very effective against psychomotor excitement, but small doses may depress less agitated children. Extra-pyramidal reactions are rare in disturbed children and can be terminated promptly by reducing the dose.

Chlorpromazine (*Thorazine*) serves as the standard of comparison for the others. *Promazine* (*Sparine*) is about half as potent as chlorpromazine and intermediate in action between the major and minor tranquilizers. *Triflupromazine* (*Vesprin*) is two to three times as potent as chlorpromazine.

Piperidine Series

Thioridazine (*Mellaril*) has not yet been shown to have any advantage over chlorpromazine for children that outweighs the possible complication of toxic retinitis. It has a low incidence of extra-pyramidal symptoms in adults, but this is not a problem in children. *Mepazine (Pacatal)* has a relatively high incidence of severe toxicity in adults.[6]

Piperazine Series

These drugs are useful especially in hypoactive schizophrenic or severely neurotic children and children who tend to be depressed by the administration of chlorpromazine. Severely apathetic schizophrenic children with IQ's under 70 may require relatively large doses by body weight. However, most children tend to be more sensitive than adults to the stimulating effects of these drugs and may show irritability, agitation and then dyskinesia with small doses. The adult dose adjusted strictly for body weight, may be two to five times too high for a child.[3] This may well account for the high incidence of dystonic effects reported.

Trifluoperazine (Stelazine) may be 20 to 100 times as potent as chlorpromazine in the same child. Its stimulating effects are especially indicated to increase alertness and motor drive in severely apathetic, withdrawn, schizophrenic children. If these children are very young the drug may even increase motor skills, social responsiveness, and language. *Fluphenazine (Permitil, Prolixin)* has effects similar to trifluoperazine but is more potent. *Prochlorperazine (Compazine), Perphenazine (Trilafon), and Thiopropazate (Dartal)* are about five to ten times as potent as chlorpromazine in the same child. Their sedative and stimulating properties are intermediate between the dimethylamine group and trifluoperazine.

Rauwolfia Alkaloids

These drugs have a less reliable action than the phenothiazines and are now generally reserved for severe schizophrenics who have not responded to phenothiazines.

MINOR STIMULANTS

Amphetamines have been used for over twenty years to treat children with behavior disorders. They stimulate overly inhibited neurotic children and are especially useful in prepuberty children with school phobias and those who are disturbed by sexual preoccupations and fantasies. Many workers report that doses up to 40 mg. per day also quieted hyperactive children including those with organic brain disorders.[14,15] Others have not confirmed this effect using a maximum, however, of 20 mg. per day.[3,7,8] In my own experience, children complained of uncomfortable

52

side effects if given more than 20 mg. *Methylphenidate* (*Ritalin*) and *Pipradol* (*Meratran*) have not yet been demonstrated to have any advantages in children over the amphetamines.

MAJOR STIMULANTS AND ANTIDEPRESSANTS

Since psychotic retarded depressions are rare before midadolescence, these drugs are being tested primarily in apathetic schizophrenic children, but effectiveness and safety have not yet been established.

TABLE 1.—*Suggested Dosages for Children's Psychiatric Disorders**

Name of Drug	Dose Range (mg./Kg./day)	Average Dose (mg./Kg./day)
Amphetamine	0.15- 0.80	0.2
Diphenhydramine (Benadryl)	2.0 -10.0	4.0
Meprobamate (Equanil, Miltown)	4.0 -30.0	15.0
Chlorpromazine (Thorazine)	1.0 - 8.0	2.0
Trifluoperazine (Stelazine)		
a) hypoactive schizophrenic children	.1 - 1.0	0.5
b) all others	.02- 0.2	0.1

An Approach to Regulating Medication

Pharmacotherapy should start with the mildest drug which might be effective for a particular child. The dose is gradually increased until symptoms disappear or the first signs of excess dose appear (mild headache, fatigue, irritability, etc.), to make certain that the useful dose range has been fully explored. The child's response may indicate that a more sedative or more stimulating agent is required. If drug-susceptible symptoms persist with the highest tolerated dose of a mild drug, more potent drugs should be explored in the same way. The optimal dose is the level which reduces symptoms and increases function without causing discomfort. In disturbed children with severe impairment of function, one must carefully weigh the positive and negative effects of increasing dosage.

In mild disorders where symptoms disappear with mild medication, drugs need only be continued for a brief period, to give the child and his family sufficient time to establish a new level of adaptation in the

---

*Physicians who plan to use these drugs should consult the recommendation on dosage provided by the manufacturers. The dosages presented above are used by the author in in-patient and out-patient psychiatric treatment with children but they are intended only as a general guide, to indicate the relationship of children's doses to adults'. *See text also.*

absence of symptoms. In severely disturbed children who do not get complete relief of symptoms even with potent medication, pharmacotherapy must be maintained just as it is in chronic adult patients, readjusting the medication as indicated. There have been no reports to date that maintenance medication of the phenothiazines continued for five to six years leads to any disturbance of growth or endocrine development in adolescence.

Until much more is known about the mechanism of action of these drugs, and the physiological and psychological factors that make up individual differences in responsiveness, pharmacotherapy will continue to be on an empirical basis. But even so, it provides an invaluable adjunct to the total psychiatric treatment of the disturbed child.

REFERENCES

1. FISHER, S., (Ed.): Child Research in Psychopharmacology. Springfield, Illinois, Charles C Thomas, 1959.
2. FISH, B.: Evaluation of psychiatric therapies in children. Delivered at the American Psychopathologic Assn. Meeting, February 1962.
3. ———: Drug therapy in child psychiatry: pharmacological aspects. Comprehensive Psychiatry, 1:212-227, 1960.
4. ———: Drug therapy in child psychiatry: psychological aspects. Comprehensive Psychiatry, 1:55-61, 1960.
5. NYHAN, W. L.: Toxicity of drugs in the neonatal period. J. Pediat., 59:1-20, 1961.
6. SCHIELE, B. C., AND BENSON, W. M.: Tranquilizing and Antidepressive Drugs. Springfield, Illinois, Charles C Thomas, 1962.
7. BENDER, L., AND NICHTERN, S.: Chemotherapy in child psychiatry. New York State J. Med., 56:2791-2796, 1956.
8. FREEDMAN, A. M.: Drug therapy in behavior disorders. Pediatric Clinics of North America. Baltimore, W. B. Saunders Company, 1958.
9. LOW, N. L., AND MYERS, G. G.: Suvren in brain-injured children. J. Pediat., 3:259-263, 1958.
10. KRAFT, I. A.: Personal communications, September 1962.
11. LINDSLEY, D. B., AND HENRY, C. E.: Effect of drugs on behavior and electro-encephalograms of children with behavior disorders. Psychosomatic Med., 4:140-149, 1942.
12. WALKER, C. F., AND KIRKPATRICK, B. B.: Dilantin treatment of behavior problem children with abnormal E.E.G.'s. Am. J. Psychiat., 103:484-492, 1947.
13. PASAMANICK, B.: Anticonvulsant drug therapy of behavior problem children with abnormal encephalograms. Arch. Neurol. & Psychiat., 65:752, 1951.
14. BRADLEY, C.: Benzedrine and dexedrine in the treatment of children's behavior disorders. Pediatrics, 5:24-37, 1950.
15. LAUFER, M. W., DENHOFF, E., AND SOLOMONS, G.: Hyperkinetic impulse disorder in children's behavior problems. Psychosomatic Med., 19:38-49, 1957.

Therapy of Childhood Seizures

by HERBERT J. GROSSMAN, M.D.

IN RECENT YEARS, considerable progress has been made in delineating various facets of the complex medical disorder called epilepsy. Recent longitudinal studies correlating clinical data, pathological determinations, EEG, and other laboratory findings have provided greater understanding of convulsive disorders. This increased knowledge has enabled us to refine our diagnostic categories with more precision, leading to more effective management. Newer anticonvulsant drugs have provided more effective control of seizures. However, the specific mechanisms by which certain biochemical and physiological factors can precipitate a seizure attack remain ill-defined.

Treatment of epilepsy will require a continuous relationship between the patient and physician as well as the patient's thorough understanding of the clinical problem and the efforts necessary to cope with it. Such understanding includes basic information about the disorder, factors that may precipitate or aggravate attacks, and the reasons for regular, daily administration of medication. Most patients will require anticonvulsant medications over a long period of time, many for a lifetime. It is also important for the patient and the parents to understand that although epilepsy may be a chronic disorder, it is not necessarily a handicapping condition. When control of the seizures is achieved, the child should be encouraged to return to school and engage in normal physical and social activities. Patients and parents can be helped by the physician to express their feelings about the disease. Feelings of fear and anger, concern, and embarrassment are inevitable. The physician's understanding and empathic approach to the patient and his family are most important for the long-term management of the disease and the development of the individual.

During a generalized convulsion, management should be primarily directed toward preventing secondary complications from respiratory interference or injury, or both. Parents, teachers, and other adults who have close contact with children should be instructed in the simplest and most ef-

55

fective method to provide an adequate airway during a seizure. The most important step is to place the patient in a horizontal position, preferably on his side or in a prone position with the head to one side. The nose and mouth should remain unobstructed. This position tilts the tongue forward and minimizes the possibility of occlusion of the airway, which might occur if the patient were in the supine position. The side or prone position decreases the danger of aspiration of oral, pharyngeal secretions, or emesis if this presents a problem. Such placement also precludes falling and sustaining secondary injuries. If it is available and convenient, a throat stick padded with gauze should be placed between the teeth to prevent biting of the tongue. However, it is unwise to expend an excessive amount of time, effort, and energy to insert the throat stick.

ANTICONVULSANT THERAPY—GENERAL PRINCIPLES

For the purposes of this presentation we shall concentrate on the management of seizures for which there is no correctible cause. In cases where a specific, remediable etiology can be established, it should be treated appropriately, either medically or surgically or both. In cases where a remediable cause cannot be discerned, treatment should be initiated after the first convulsion, regardless of the type of seizure.

The control of seizures in most patients with epilepsy is based upon the regular administration of anticonvulsant medication. Although there are many available preparations, only a few meet two essential requirements: effective seizure control and freedom from undesirable side effects. None of the pharmacological agents "cures" the epilepsy; drug action limits the initiation or propagation of seizure activity in the brain. Choice of drug will depend primarily upon the type of seizure. A list of suggested medications appropriate for various types of seizures is presented in Tables 1, 2, and 3.

The ketogenic diet has a limited role in the treatment of intractable cases of grand mal, petit mal, akinetic, and myoclonic seizures that do not respond to anticonvulsant medication. The diet is extremely difficult to administer to older children.

Clinical management of epilepsy is a dynamic process. Drugs are given initially in arbitrary, minimum doses. Dosages are increased until the seizures are controlled or toxic side effects develop. If intoxication appears before control of seizures is achieved, the drug dosage is reduced and a second drug is added. Changes in therapy should be introduced in orderly sequence, limited to one drug at a time in order to assess the clinical results. Changes should be gradual except when a serious untoward reaction develops.

Medication must be appropriately spaced to provide adequate blood levels

56

of the drug at all times. This is usually obtained by administering the medication in two to four divided doses throughout the waking day. The total dosage of a drug is apparently more important for seizure control than the precise intervals between the individual doses. Thus it is usually possible for the patient to take his medication while he is at home: morning, noon, after school, and bedtime.

Since drowsiness is a common side effect, every effort should be made to avoid oversedation during waking hours. If drowsiness is an initial problem even with minimum dosage, a larger amount of the drug can be administered at bedtime, with lesser amounts during the day. When the symptom of initial drowsiness subsides, the various divided dosages can be equalized. Administration of anticonvulsant agents should be adjusted so that there will be minimum interference with the child's normal activities.

Anticonvulsant drugs as a group produce considerable toxic and sensitivity reactions. The toxic reactions, related to dosage, are usually reversible. The sensitivity phenomena are less common, often severe, and may be fatal. The hematopoietic, hepatic, and renal systems are of particular concern. Skin rashes are common. Nausea, vomiting, drowsiness, diplopia, ataxia, lymphadenopathy—lymphosarcoma-like phenomena—and lupus erythematosus have been seen, and psychotic states may develop. Patients should be alert to possible problems and should be observed regularly by a physician. Periodic blood and urine examinations should be made. When indicated, further laboratory tests should be done, including those for liver function.

Common mistakes in drug therapy are (1) insufficient trial period, (2) reluctance to increase drug dosage because of fear of toxicity, (3) the sudden withdrawal of a drug when a new medication is added, and (4) the abrupt discontinuation of anticonvulsant medication. It is sometimes incorrectly assumed that medication should be withdrawn prior to a diagnostic electroencephalogram. Any sudden withdrawal may precipitate convulsions or status epilepticus.

DISCONTINUANCE OF MEDICATION

An effective therapeutic program should be continued for an indefinite period of time, or at least until the child is free of seizures for a minimum period of two to three years. If the clinical state and EEG are normal at this time, medication may be gradually withdrawn over a period of several months.

TYPES OF SEIZURES

Seizure activity in children is different in many respects from the convulsions seen in adult patients. Clinical manifestations of the convulsive disorder may change as a reflection of age and maturation. Although seizure patterns are often associated with characteristic EEG findings, treatment should be based upon clinical assessment rather than the EEG interpretation alone. EEG findings are not always specifically related to individual seizure patterns, nor do all patients with seizures have EEG abnormalities. An accurate, detailed history, a thorough neurological evaluation, and an EEG are all essential for diagnosis.

The seizure patterns described below are frequently encountered in infants and children. The classifications have implication for treatment, management, and prognosis.

Infantile Spasms

Infantile myoclonic seizures (infantile spasms) are lightning-quick seizures which may resemble a startle reflex. Frequency varies considerably, from several times a day to several hundred each day. Five to six months is the usual age of onset. Severe developmental retardation is usually a concomitant problem.

The EEG on these patients shows a characteristic pattern called hypsarrhythmia. There is a poorly organized high-voltage spike and slow-wave activity in all leads, resulting in an extremely abnormal EEG.

Causes of infantile spasms include metabolic derangements such as phenylketonuria, pyridoxine deficiency, structural abnormalities, degenerative nervous system disorders, and infectious diseases such as toxoplasmosis and encephalitis. However, the etiology for most cases of infantile spasms remains obscure, despite extensive clinical investigation.

ACTH or steroids, or both, have proved valuable in controlling seizures. Corticosteroid therapy can be administered using prednisone 2.2 mg/Kg per day in divided doses. Benefits, when seen, usually appear within 10 to 14 days. If no improvement is noted, the dose is gradually tapered to discontinuance over one to two weeks. Treatment may be continued for weeks or months, but then signs of hyperadrenocorticism appear. Recent studies suggest that infants having primary idiopathic or cryptogenic infantile spasms respond somewhat better than those with symptomatic spasms. ACTH does not appear to have any advantage over prednisone. With treatment, the EEG will often revert to a normal pattern, even though seizures may not be completely controlled. Other anticonvulsant drugs, used to treat grand mal seizures, are usually necessary. Clinical seizures and the typical hypsarrhythmia sometimes subside when the patient is between two and five years old. However, other types of seizures with abnormal EEG patterns may persist. Brain damage is irreversible in most cases and mental development will be severely retarded.

Febrile Convulsions

Febrile convulsions are the most common type of seizure in infants and young children, occurring most frequently between six months and three years of age. Febrile convulsions occur as a complication of infection and fever even though the disease process does not directly involve the central nervous system. Very high fevers are not necessary; susceptible children may have a seizure with a temperature of 102° to 104° F. The particular infectious process *per se* is not relevant in a febrile convulsion, nor is the rate of the rise of the fever. Neurological examination and EEG are usually normal.

Febrile convulsions are treated initially by aspirin intravenously to reduce fever, and by diazepam or phenobarbital, or both, to control the seizure. Prevention of further seizures is most important. Febrile convulsions are managed the same as those occurring without fever. Anticonvulsant medication should be initiated immediately after the first seizure and continued on a prophylactic basis until the child has been free of seizures at least two years and the EEG is normal. Medication should be withdrawn slowly.

Breath-Holding Seizures

Breath-holding seizures, or apneic spells, have a period of onset similar to febrile seizures, roughly between six months through three years of age. These seizures are precipitated by frustration or minor trauma. The susceptible child begins to cry, building up to the point of breath holding, followed by apnea. During this episode, the child may become cyanotic, and lose consciousness and postural control. The episode generally does not last very long. In some instances a generalized seizure is associated with the breath holding. The EEG in these patients is almost always normal. Studies have indicated that the prognosis is good and that breath-holding does not seem to fall into a category of a true epileptic disorder. Anticonvulsant medication is indicated only in those cases that have associated convulsive manifestations.

PETIT-MAL-VARIANT SEIZURES

Petit-mal-variant seizures (akinetic, minor-motor, salaam, jack-knife, etc.) usually begin during the preschool period and persist through the school-age years. These seizures are characterized by sudden nodding of the head, a jack-knifing of the body, and loss of postural control. The frequency of these seizures varies considerably from once or twice a day up to several dozen times daily. These seizures may be associated with generalized convulsions. Many of these patients have the concomitant problem of mental retardation. In addition, a large percentage have other evidence of nervous

59

system disease with clear-cut neurological findings. The EEG abnormality usually is one of a spike and a ½ to 2 cycle per second wave activity that often has some polyphasic spike discharges intermixed. The pattern, although a spike and wave phenomenon, is significantly different from that seen in true petit mal. These seizures are generally very difficult to control and usually require more than one anticonvulsant agent. Treatment is best attempted by utilizing drugs used for grand mal seizures. These patients may have grand mal seizures in later life.

Myoclonic Seizures

Myoclonic seizures consist of sudden, momentary, jerking movements of the extremities. There may be a single jerk or repetitive jerks. They are not associated with loss of consciousness. Myoclonic jerks may precede a generalized convulsion. Irregular myoclonus is seen with diffuse neuronal disease. An early onset of myoclonic seizures suggests a poor prognosis, particularly impaired mental development. Myoclonic seizures respond poorly to anticonvulsant therapy and all drugs have been used with varying degrees of effectiveness.

Petit Mal Seizures

Petit mal seizures ("absence attacks") are sudden, brief episodes of lapses of consciousness with staring, often accompanied by rhythmic blinking. There is usually no loss of postural control and the child resumes his previous activity. Petit mal occurs primarily in children of school age. Generally, children having petit mal seizures do not have any abnormal neurological findings, nor do they have significant impairment of intellectual abilities. Recent studies indicate that a considerable number of these patients have borderline or lower than normal intelligence. EEG usually shows a typical spike and 3 cycle per second wave activity. Petit mal seizures may be precipitated by hyperventilation, a fact very practical in making a diagnosis during the clinical examination or the EEG. Flickering light may also trigger these seizures in susceptible individuals.

Approximately one half of these youngsters will have grand mal seizures before the age of 16 years. Grand mal seizures are more likely to occur when there is poor control of the petit mal seizures, positive family history, subnormal intelligence, abnormal EEG activity (in addition to typical petit mal pattern), and in those patients whose petit mal seizures persist into adolescence.

When petit mal seizures are associated with grand mal convulsions, control is often quite difficult, requiring combinations of anticonvulsant agents. Because of the frequency of grand mal seizures, phenobarbital is often prescribed in addition to the drugs more specific for petit mal. All other drugs used in the control of petit mal have a greater incidence of toxicity than does phenobarbital. Ethosuximide (Zarontin) and methsuximide (Celontin) are of particular value in treating mixed seizure patterns. Both have caused severe toxic reactions, including bone marrow depression. Phensuximide (Milontin) is less toxic, but also less effective in controlling seizures, and has limited value.

Trimethadione (Tridione) has been widely used in controlling petit mal seizures. However, it may precipitate grand mal seizures. Severe toxic reactions including bone marrow depression and nephrosis have been noted. Paramethadione has similar side effects, although they are less frequent. It is also less effective.

Acetazoleamide (Diamox), a carbonic anhydrase inhibitor, is not a particularly effective drug in the control of petit mal, although it is valuable as an adjunct for some patients.

Epileptic Equivalents

An "epileptic equivalent" seizure is defined by a common clustering of clinical manifestations. Among these are diencephalic epilepsy, autonomic epilepsy, abdominal epilepsy, and the 14 and 6 per second positive-spike phenomenon. Although symptoms vary widely, they seem to be specific for the individual patient. There is usually a paroxysmal onset, with or without an aura. An aura may be perceived by the patient without further seizure manifestations. Symptoms may include headache, syncope, nausea, vomiting, or abdominal pain. Flushing, circumoral pallor, sweating, and changes in pulse and respiration may be noted. Patients may lose consciousness. Seizures may be followed by weakness, lethargy or sleep, or both, suggesting a postictal phenomenon. Paroxysmal aggressive behavior has sometimes been described as an "epileptic equivalent," but studies generally do not confirm this.

In some patients with "epileptic equivalent" seizures, the EEG has shown 14 and 6 per second positive spikes during drowsiness or light sleep. However, diagnosis must be made by a clinical assessment and not by EEG findings alone. Aggressive behavior as an isolated symptom is not a clear indication of a convulsive disorder. Recent investigations have shown that the 14 and 6 per second positive spikes are found in the EEGs of the majority of normal children. These "epileptic equivalent" seizures respond to drugs used for grand mal seizures.

Grand Mal Seizures

Grand mal seizures may begin with an aura that may be unrecognized because of the extreme rapidity of onset of the seizure. The typical seizures

61

begin with a strong state of tonus followed by a clonic phase with generalized rhythmic twitching, most evident in the extremities and face. There is loss of consciousness during the seizure; bladder and bowel incontinence may occur. The actual convulsion is usually followed by the postictal period during which the patient may suffer headaches, extreme lethargy, or even a profound coma of varying duration.

Diphenylhydantoin, phenobarbital, and primidone are the most useful drugs for the treatment of grand mal and focal attacks. Diphenylhydantoin may be useful in combination with either phenobarbital or primidone. A significant proportion of primidone is converted to phenobarbital endogenously, causing severe drowsiness; therefore these two drugs should not be used in combination.

Initial treatment may consist of (1) phenobarbital or diphenylhydantoin alone, (2) a combination of the two, (3) primidone alone, and (4) primidone plus diphenylhydantoin.

The somnolence initially seen with phenobarbital or primidone may be minimized by introducing small amounts of these drugs, gradually increasing the dosage over a period of weeks to a more effective level. Occasionally the concomitant use of dextroamphetamine, methylphenidate, or methamphetamine may be effective in combating drowsiness.

Psychomotor Seizures

Psychomotor seizures are usually characterized by gustatory phenomena (sucking, chewing, or swallowing movements), body movements, and stereotyped automatisms. Motions such as fidgeting, picking, shuffling, or walking around aimlessly are frequent. Inappropriate behavior and irrelevant speech are often seen. Disturbances of mental functioning may include alterations of consciousness, fears, derangement of thought, and hallucinations. These seizures may be preceded by an aura of varied sensory phenomena and a feeling of anxiety. Psychomotor seizures are usually brief, followed by postictal confusion, lethargy or sleep, or both. Many of these patients have behavioral difficulties between seizures.

The EEG reflects a focal abnormality in the anterior part of the temporal lobe. Psychomotor seizures are treated with the same drugs used in the management of grand mal seizures. Phenobarbital, diphenylhydantoin, or primidone may be effective in about one half of the cases.

Status Epilepticus

Status epilepticus is assumed when the patient has a series of recurrent convulsions without recovering consciousness between episodes. It can occur

62

with any type of seizure, but is of prime concern with generalized or focal motor seizures.

Status epilepticus requires immediate and continued medical management. Unless the seizures can be controlled, death or permanent neuronal damage can result. Death occurs in approximately 15 per cent of the patients with status. Mortality may be related directly to status epilepticus or result from negative effects of sedatives or hypnotic compounds on the already depressed medullary centers.

The specific etiologic factors leading to status epilepticus are not clearly understood. The condition is more common in individuals with symptomatic epilepsy. Rapid or sudden withdrawal of anticonvulsant medication or intercurrent infections, or both, are common precipitating factors.

The most important considerations in the management of status epilepticus are (1) maintenance of an adequate airway, and (2) suppression of the seizures as rapidly as possible. Subsequently, general supportive measures should be introduced, followed by initiation of a maintenance dose of anticonvulsant medication. Etiologic factors should always be explored, including appropriate examination of blood, urine, and spinal fluid. Electroencephalography is not essential in the management of status epilepticus. Subsequent specialized diagnostic studies are dependent on the clinical course. These may include skull x-rays, electroencephalograph, brain scans, and (on rare occasions) contrast studies.

Suppression of the convulsions is of primary concern and requires the immediate use of intravenous anticonvulsant drugs in dosages adequate to arrest all seizure activity. Two potential dangers may be cited: (1) administration of the drug intramuscularly, and (2) the use of inadequate dosages, with resultant toxicity and continued status. In the rare situation when the intravenous route cannot be achieved, intramuscular injection may be necessary. Currently the drug of choice in the treatment of status epilepticus is diazepam (Valium). Seizure activity is suppressed within minutes and adverse reactions such as respiratory depression and hypotension are rare in children, although they have been reported in adults. The dosage of 0.3 mg/Kg of diazepam, with a maximum dose of 10 mg, is both safe and effective when administered by slow intravenous injection over a period of one to two minutes. If seizures persist, the same dose should be administered in similar fashion after a 30-min. wait.

When diazepam is not effective, sodium phenobarbital should be tried. The usual dose is 10 mg/Kg administered intravenously. Small doses of phenobarbital (2 to 3 mg/Kg) should be avoided. Such doses are usually inadequate in controlling status. Paraldehyde solution (4 per cent) is sometimes effective in controlling status epilepticus. The recommended

TABLE 1

Drugs Used in the Treatment of Grand Mal and Focal Seizures

Drugs	Preparations	Dose/24 hr Divided 3-4 x/day	Toxicity	Indications for Immediate Discontinuance of Drug, Hypersensitivity	Comments
FIRST-ORDER DRUGS					
Phenobarbital	15, 30, 60, 100 mg tabs; Elixir 15 mg/tsp	1-5 mg/Kg/day; 7-15 mg t.i.d. infants	Drowsiness, irritability	Rash (rare)	
Diphenylhydantoin (Dilantin) Parke Davis	50 mg tabs, 30, 100 mg capsules, suspension 100 mg/tsp, 100 mg delayed-absorption capsule	3-8 mg/Kg/day	Gingival hyperplasia, ataxia, nystagmus, tremor, diplopia, hypertrichosis, nausea, vomiting, anorexia, periph. neuropathy	Rash, aplastic anemia, neutropenia, hepatitis, megaloblastic anemia, lymphosarcoma-like syndrome, lymphadenopathy	
Primidone (Mysoline) Ayerst	50, 250 mg tablets, suspension 250 mg/tsp	12-25 mg/Kg/day	Nausea, vomiting, vertigo, *drowsiness*, ataxia, irritability	Rash, Megaloblastic anemia	Begin with small doses gradually increasing over a period of weeks to minimize drowsiness

SECOND-ORDER
DRUGS

Mephobarbital (Mebaral) Winthrop	32, 50, 100, 200 mg tablets	2-8 mg/Kg/day	Drowsiness, ataxia	Rash	
Metharbital (Gemonil) Abbott	100 mg tablets	5-15 mg/Kg/day	Drowsiness, Nausea	Rash	
Mephenytoin (Mesantoin) Sandoz	100 mg tablets	3-10 mg/Kg/day	Drowsiness, ataxia	Aplastic anemia, rash and fever, neutropenia	Extremely toxic. Not recommended for children
Ethotoin (Peganone) Abbott	250 and 500 mg tablets	80 mg/Kg/day	Drowsiness, ataxia, nausea, diplopia	Rash lymphadeno-pathy	Of little value
Phenacemide (Phenurone) Abbott	500 mg tablet		Drowsiness, psychosis	Aplastic anemia, neutropenia, hepatitis	Extremely toxic. Not recommended for children

TABLE 2

Drugs Used in the Treatment of Petit Mal Seizures

Drug	Preparations	Dose/24 hr.	Toxicity	Indications for Immediate Discontinuance of Drug, Hypersensitivity	Comments
FIRST-ORDER DRUGS					
Ethosuximide (Zarontin) Parke Davis	250 mg capsules	Infants up to 6 years: 250 mg/ day; children: 500-1000 mg/day	Nausea, vomiting, drowsiness	Rash, aplastic anemia, leuko-penia, agranulo-cytosis	
Trimethadione (Tridione) Abbott	150, 300 mg cap-sules, 150 mg chewable tablets, solution 150 mg/ tsp	20-50 mg/Kg/day	Drowsiness, hemeralopia	Nephrosis, aplastic anemia, lupus erythematosus, lymphadeno-pathy, nephrosis, neutropenia, aplastic anemia, rash, hepatitis	
Paramethadione (Paradione) Abbott	150, 300 mg cap-sules, solution 300 mg/cc in 50-ml bottles with graduated droppers	20-50 mg/Kg/day	Drowsiness, hemeralopia (blurring of vi-sion in bright light)		May precipitate grand mal seizure
SECOND-ORDER DRUGS					
Methsuximide (Celontin) Parke Davis	150, 300 mg cap-sules	5-20 mg/Kg/day	Drowsiness, ataxia, irritability, head-ache, nausea, vomiting, dizzi-ness	Rash, aplastic anemia	
Acetazoleamide (Diamox) Lederle	125, 250 mg tablets	8-30 mg/Kg/day	Anorexia	Leukopenia, rash, urticaria, fever	
Phensuximide (Milontin) Parke Davis	250, 500 mg cap-sules, suspension 250 mg/tsp	20-40 mg/Kg/day	Drowsiness, nausea, vomiting,	Granulocytopenia, leukopenia, aplastic anemia,	

TABLE 3

Other Drugs Used in the Treatment of Seizures

Drug	Preparation	Dose/24 hr divided 3-4 x	Toxicity	Indications
ACTH Gel	20, 40, 80 units/ml vials, 40 units/ml cartridge	0.8 units/Kg/day in single dose IM	Hyperadrenocorticism	Infantile spasms
Prednisolone	1, 2.5, 5 mg tablets	2.2 mg/Kg/day, 4 divided doses	Hyperadrenocorticism	Infantile spasms
Dextroamphetamine (Dexedrine) Smith, Kline & French	5 mg tablets; 5, 10, 15 mg time-release capsules; Elixir 5 mg/tsp	0.2-0.3 mg/Kg/day	Irritability, anorexia, weight loss, headache, tachycardia, flushing, skin rash	Adjunct in petit mal seizures. Antisoporific to counteract effect of other drugs
Methylphenidate (Ritalin) Ciba	5, 10, 20 mg tablets	0.75 mg/Kg/dose 20 mg/M²/dose		
Bromides				Toxic. Not recommended for children
Phenacemide (Phenurone) Abbott	0.5 Gm tablets	20-35 mg/Kg/day	Severe toxic hepatitis, aplastic anemia	Too toxic to use.
Diazepam (Valium) Roche	2, 5, 10 mg tablets 2 ml. ampul (5 mg./ml)	0.15-2 mg/Kg/day. For status epilepticus (see text): 0.3 mg/Kg/ I V with maximum dose of 10 mg	Drowsiness, ataxia, nausea, dizziness	Questionable value as adjunct in management of petit mal. Drug of choice in status epilepticus
Paraldehyde	4 per cent solution	0.5 ml/Kg I V slowly, with a maximum total dosage not to exceed 6-8 ml	Pulmonary edema hemorrhage	Status epilepticus. Avoid in hepatic or pulmonary disease. Avoid plastic syringes (use glass). Overrated.

67

dosage is 0.15 ml/Kg, with a maximum total dosage not to exceed 6 to 8 ml. The 4 per cent paraldehyde solution should be diluted well with glucose and water and injected slowly intravenously. Although paraldehyde is sometimes effective in very difficult cases, it may cause pulmonary edema or hemorrhage and should be used only when other drugs are ineffective in controlling the status. Dosage of paraldehyde has not been satisfactorily determined, and the literature reflects a range of suggested dosages. Along with the administration of the drugs mentioned above, diphenylhydantoin sodium (Dilantin) in a dose of 5 mg/Kg per day should be given intramuscularly. Once the child is able to swallow, this long-acting drug should be given orally.

REFERENCES

1. BAILEY, D. W., AND FENICHEL, G. M.: The Treatment of Prolonged Seizure Activity with Intravenous Diazepam. J. Pediat., 73:923-927, 1968.
2. CARTER, S., AND GOLD, A.: The Critically Ill Child: Management of Status Epilepticus. Pediatrics. 44:732-733, 1969.
3. CHARLTON, M. D., AND YAHR, M. D.: Long-Term Follow-Up of Patients with Petit Mal. Arch. of Neurol. 16:595-598, 1967.
4. CHUTORIAN, A. M.: Steroid Therapy of Non-Infantile (Childhood) Myoclonic Epilepsy. Neurology 18:304-305, (March) 1968.
5. Committee on Children with Handicaps: The Epileptic Child and Competitive School Athletics. Pediatrics 42:700-702, 1968.
6. FALCONER, M. A., AND TAYLOR, D. C.: Surgical Treatment of Drug-Resistant Epilepsy Due to Mesial Temporal Sclerosis. Arch. Neurol. 19:353-361, 1968.
7. GIBBERD, F. B.: The Prognosis of Petit Mal. Brain 89:531-538, 1966.
8. KUH, H., AND McDOWELL, F.: Management of Epilepsy with Diphenylhydantoin Sodium. J.A.M.A. 203:969-972, 1968.
9. LIVINGSTON, S.: The Physicians Role in Guiding the Epileptic Child and His Parents. Amer. J. Dis. Child. 119:99-102, 1970.
10. LIVINGSTON, S., AND LIVINGSTON, H. L.: Diphenylhydantoin Gingival Hyperplasia Amer. J. Dis. Child. 117:265-270, 1969.
11. LOVELACE, R. E., AND HORWITZ, S. J.: Peripheral Neuropathy in Long-Term Diphenylhydantoin Therapy. Arch. Neurol. 18:69-77, 1968.
12. McMORRIS, SHELIA, AND McWILLIAM, P. K. A.: Status Epilepticus in Infants and Young Children Treated with Parenteral Diazepam. Arch. Dis. Child. 44:604-611, 1969.
13. MILLICHAP, J. G.: Febrile Convulsions. New York; The Macmillan Company, 1968, p. 222.
14. MILLICHAP, J. G., AND AYMAT, F.: Controlled Evaluation of Primidone and Diphenylhydantoin Sodium: Comparative Anticonvulsant Efficacy and Toxicity in Children. J.A.M.A. 204: 738-739, 1968.
15. NEEDHAM, W. E. BRAY, P. E., WISER, W. C., AND BECK, E. C.: Intelligence and EEG Studies in Families with Idiopathic Epilepsy. J.A.M.A. 207:1497-1501, 1969.

16. PATEL, H., AND CRICHTON, J. U.: The Neurologic Hazards of Diphenylhydantoin in Childhood. J. Pediat. 73:676-684, 1968.
17. PENRY, J. K., AND DREIFUSS, F. E.: Automatisms Associated with the Absence of Petit Mal Epilepsy. Arch. Neurol. 21:142-149, 1969.
18. REYNOLDS, E. H.: Mental Effects of Anticonvulsants and Folic Acid Metabolism. Brain 91:197-214, 1968.
19. SAWYER, G. T., WEBSTER, D., AND SCHUT, C.: Treatment of Uncontrolled Seizure Activity with Diazepam. J.A.M.A. 203:913-918, 1968.
20. SCHWARTZ, I. II., AND LOMBROSO, C. T.: 14&6/second Positive Spiking (ctenoids) in the Electroencephalograms of Primary School Pupils. J. Pediat. 72:678-682, 1968.
21. STEVENS, J. R.: Brief Focal Seizures vs. Petit Mal Epilepsy. J.A.M.A. 198:1203-1206, 1966.

Therapies for Autistic Children

by CHARLES WENAR, PH.D., AND BERTRAM A. RUTTENBERG, M.D.

THIS CHAPTER will review the various therapies currently employed with autistic children, with specific reference to: (1) accuracy of diagnosis, (2) description of the specific therapeutic techniques employed, (3) therapeutic goals, and (4) cost of achieving the goals in terms of time and effort.

Accuracy of diagnosis is essential to evaluating psychotherapy since the classically autistic child, as delineated by Kanner, may be the most resistant to psychotherapeutic intervention. To bypass the diagnostic problem or include a variety of disturbed children in a general category, such as childhood psychosis, confounds therapeutic efficacy with the kind and severity of disturbance. Descriptions of therapeutic techniques enable one to discern similarities and differences among therapies, and make generalizations about the current therapeutic scene. Goals and cost are interrelated. Some therapies aim to alter major personality variables, such as the ability to form a positive attachment or to tolerate frustration; others are designed to generate specific behaviors, such as verbally labeling a given number of objects or making a certain number of requests. One can rightfully expect the latter to be less costly than the former.

Unfortunately, the literature itself does not conform to these four considerations. Diagnosis is treated casually, and results and cost are described impressionistically. What therapeutic procedures were used with an autistic child, and what results were obtained at what cost? To answer the question, one must make inferences using inadequate information.

This overview will concentrate on three major therapeutic approaches. Most of them grow out of special etiological theories which, because of limitations of space, can be presented only briefly and inadequately.

EMPHASIS ON RELATIONSHIP

One group of psychotherapies regards the establishment of a positive emotional relation between child and therapist as the prime requisite for bringing about basic personality change. This concept derives from the psychoanalytic theory of early personality development. The infant has no emotional ties or no capacity for impulse control, and experiences primarily somatic sensations of distress, relief and pleasure. Through the warm, sensitive caretaking of the mother, he develops a loving, trusting relationship and object constancy which enable him to master his impulses and differentiate a self image, while facilitating perceptual and cognitive growth. The basic defect in autism is extreme emotional isolation, analogous with the lack of differentiation and unrelatedness of the infant; the basic corrective is supplying the kind of mothering experience which will enable the child to relate positively. In their goals, psychoanalytically oriented therapies emphasize broad changes in the child's emotional life, self control, motivations for mastery, and reality testing.[1,8,22,27-29,31]

Three phases of psychoanalytically oriented therapy can be distinguished. In the first phase the goal is to form a positive relationship. While there are no prescriptions for mothering, emphasis is placed on warmth, consistency, patience, understanding and meeting the child's needs. The therapist is undemanding and avoids frustrating the child, just as a mother does not demand self control of her infant nor intentionally subject him to distress. Some specific techniques for establishing contact are feeding, holding, rocking, cuddling and pleasurable visual and aural stimulation.

Once the child begins to respond positively, the therapist focuses upon helping him control primitive expression of impulses, tolerate frustration, and establish a differentiated self. This stage goes back to psychoanalytic theory that meaningful and healthy self control can be established only within the context of a positive emotional relationship, and that the infant must differentiate himself from his caretaker as the initial step in establishing his own identity. Requirements for control and restraint are made in the context of sympathetic understanding and demands are geared to the child's ability to tolerate them. Deprivations are followed by substitute gratifications when possible. Differentiation is facilitated by mirroring and reciprocal activities, such as reflecting the child's vocalizations and expressions, or playing patta-cake. Finger games help him delineate parts of his body, while peek-a-boo confirms his own continuity in the face of the alternate appearance and disappearance of the loved adult.

In the third phase treatment focuses on encouraging exploration and mastery, acquiring skills and education. At times the body is used as the starting point: the child's autoerotic activities, such as rocking, are transformed into normal motor skills; or his interest in the therapist's body and clothes is used to promote labeling, counting, and exploration of objects. Teachers, and speech, body movement and music therapists, are utilized at this stage. The general philosophy remains one of meeting the child at his own level, being non-intrusive and non-pressuring. The goal is a shift from

71

passive expectation of gratification to an active, pleasurable interest in an effort at mastery.

The above division into stages of therapy is a matter of clarity of presentation; in actuality, there is continual overlapping. There is no evidence that the first stage is easy or represents a turning point in rate of progress. Even the idea that the first phase is the critical one has been challenged by some psychoanalysts. Bettelheim[1] defines the essence of autism as the conviction that one's efforts have no influence because the world is indifferent to one's reactions. The autistic child is brought to life only as he becomes convinced that he can act meaningfully upon his interpersonal and impersonal environment.

Frostig[11] has devised a remedial program which combines psychoanalytic principles with therapeutic tutoring. Her three stages include establishing a relationship, building a body image, and stimulating perceptual, motor, cognitive and learning functions. It should be noted that an emphasis on relationship is not the exclusive property of psychoanalytically oriented therapists. Others regard it as important purely from the pragmatic point of view that it is essential to producing therapeutic changes.

The goal of psychoanalytically oriented relationship therapy is that of affecting major personality changes. The cost is high. Intensive therapy in a residential setting[27] or in a day care setting[31] and individual therapy supplemented by a special nursery school and intensive work with parents[27,29] are used. The expected length of treatment is from two to five years with case studies reported up to nine years. Clinical accounts stress the exceedingly slow, fragile and uneven progress. Bettelheim's results[1] are the most favorable reported: of 40 autistic children, 17 made a good adjustment and were functioning within normal limits, 15 made a marginal adjustment, and 8 were severely disturbed. In a study which evaluated the children's behavior objectively rather than clinically,[38] significant progress was made in relationship, psychosexual development, and, to a lesser extent, mastery, over a year's time, but no progress was made in communication and vocalization. To give a concrete idea of what "significant progress" means in the case of autism, the children changed from being resistive or attending only fleetingly to their child care worker at a distance to being able to tolerate closeness to the worker typically in the context of need gratification. The steps of progress are exceedingly slow. Another follow up study[30] presents a less favorable picture of outcome than does Bettelheim, since only 14 of 105 children were making a normal adjustment, and there was no striking difference between the treated and non-treated group. The children were "atypical", a diagnosis which includes but is broader than autistic.

Thus the issue of therapeutic efficacy is confounded with that of comparability of disturbance.

Behavior Therapy

The behavior therapist's basic thesis is that the autistic child's behavior is governed by the same principles of learning which apply to all humans and animals, particularly reward and punishment. When a response is positively reinforced (rewarded) the probability of its occurrence will increase; when it is negatively reinforced (punished) the probability of occurrence will decrease. Positive reinforcements include both positive stimuli and termination of noxious stimuli; negative reinforcements include both noxious stimuli and deprivation of positive stimuli. In the operant conditioning model, reinforcement is made contingent upon the performance of a response; only if the child does as required will he be rewarded.

Behavior therapists claim that, with the possible exception of speech, the content of the autistic child's behavior does not differ from the normal's.[9] His repertoire is impoverished, but, more important, he spends an inordinate amount of time on simple activities, such as rocking or twirling a shoestring, which have no environmental consequences. Such impoverishment may be due to parental failure to reward the child's earliest attempts to interact with them, such as vocalization. The parent may be depressed, disinterested or hostile to the child and the whole gamut of behavior which depends on social responsiveness atrophies. Of particular importance is when parental attention, praise and affection fail to acquire generalized reinforcing value. (Ironically, this etiological theory is a highly simplified version of Bettelheim's, the arch enemy of behavior therapy).

The therapeutic paradigm consists of increasing desired behaviors by positive reinforcement, and decreasing undesired ones by negative reinforcement. Positive reinforcers include food, water, social contact, fondling and music; negative reinforcers include isolation, and shock or slaps while shouting "no." In some instances, the reinforcers are decided ahead of time; in others, the therapist follows the child's lead. In certain cases, the therapist utilizes existing responses, rewarding those which successively approximate the one he wants; however, he must frequently resort to literally putting the child through the motions of a desired response.

The general therapeutic goal is for human behavior to become rewarding to the autistic child so that attention, praise and affection can exercise their enormous generative and facilitative effects on development. Expressed in a different conceptual language, this goal is compatible with the one of establishing a positive human relationship while generating, modifying or eliminating quite specific behaviors. One group of studies is concerned with

73

increasing positive and eliminating negative social responses: obeying simple commands, approaching an adult or peer, evidencing affectionate behavior, acquiring toilet training, and discontinuing temper tantrums, negativism and inattention.[2,4,6,21,23,26,39,43] Others have been concerned with speech,[13,20] imitative behavior[15,24] and reading.[14] Therapeutic results are typically reported in terms of specific behaviors, e.g., the child learned to imitate 200 body movements or learned to say 150 words.

The operant conditioning technique has been criticized as doing nothing more than training the child to make specific responses to specific stimuli. There is some truth to the criticism. Behavior therapists are concerned about the lack of generality and permanence of change in the child's inability to acquire complex behavior, and his total lack of spontaneity and initiative. At best they report that the child enjoys the sessions, responds positively to the therapist, shows an accelerated rate of learning, and generalizes to some extent beyond what he has been taught. However the change seems more a result of autism itself than a goal of operant conditioning. The pioneering study of Ferster and DeMeyer[10] showed that while autistic behavior could be modified, relatively minor changes in procedure could result in severe emotional outbursts and regression. Stimulus variability, which keeps the normal child alert, can devastate the autistic one. Subsequent therapists report they have to break down complex behavior into minute bits and proceed by exceedingly fine stages. However there is no evidence that the behavior therapist would not welcome a more rapid acquisition of molar behavior, as well as more generalization and initiative on the child's part. Specificity of change seems neither intended nor desired by them.

The cost of behavior therapy seems high. Autistic children learn slowly[4] and the processes are disrupted by inattention, negativism, tantrums and panic. The picture is also a variable one[2] with some children achieving a goal in a few trials and others taking thousands of trials over a period of a year and a half. Here as in other therapeutic approaches, the presence of speech remains the single most important prognostic sign.

There is also some evidence that behavior therapy is no more efficient than other short term therapies which set limited goals. Scanlon et al.[33] seem to have had as much success developing speech as Hewett,[13] although they did not use operant conditioning. Similarly Wolf[41] reports significant improvement on a scale going from "oblivious to sound" to "understanding words and phrases," with a week of intensive stimulation. (For review and a critical evaluation of behavior therapy, see references 12 and 18).

BODY MANIPULATION

Therapies relying on body manipulation have different theoretical rationale.

Zaslow[44] speculates that autism is due to maternal mishandling of infantile rage. The good mother not only accepts this reaction but also calms the infant by holding, rocking or talking in a soothing manner, thus insuring the transition from tension to relaxation. Certain mothers cannot tolerate rage and either withdraw from the infant or increase distress by anxious, punitive handling; Then the infant develops an extreme autonomy by which he protects himself from any psychological or physical closeness to the mother and human beings in general.

The therapeutic transaction takes place at the sensori-motor rather than at the symbolic level. The therapist induces rage by holding the child on his lap, immobilizing the child's body and arms, and physically forcing the child to look at his face. During the ensuing rage, he combines the firm but non-anxious, loving, soothing and physical control which marks the good mother's contact with her angry infant; then the child can make the essential transition from stress to relaxation.

Zaslow's "rage reduction" therapy is too new to be evaluated extensively. The cost is low compared with other techniques, and the immediate effects are dramatic. Saposnek[32] evaluated 15 autistic children for using eye contact, approaching and embracing the therapist, performing simple tasks, vocalizing normally, and relaxing muscles. After a single rage reduction session, the children shifted from the "none" or "some" categories to "moderate" or "extensive". The long range utility of the technique has not been established. Waal,[37] using a similar technique, found that he could break through the autistic withdrawal, but had to follow with more traditional play therapy.

Other therapists emphasize the role of the body in the development of the self. The earliest sense of separate and cohesive individuality is intimately connected with the emergence of the body as an entity. For the neonate, external and internal stimuli are undifferentiated. Only as he develops does he build up an image of sensations which are uniquely his: physiological distress when he is in a state of need; pleasure and excitation from being rocked, held or tickled; proprioception from the movement of his body, and visual perceptions when he recognizes himself in the mirror. The autistic child has failed to develop this basic body image; consequently he cannot develop a sense of reality because self and external world remain relatively undifferentiated. The therapist's task is to help the child establish a body identity as the basic step in evolving a differentiated self. Like Zaslow, the therapists emphasize body manipulation rather than play or verbal transactions.

Des Lauriers[7] centers his therapy around body stimulation, but both his rationale and his technique differ from Zaslow's, and in his etiological speculation he emphasizes neurophysiologic rather than psychogenic factors.

75

His aim is to overcome the affective isolation of the autistic child by means of pleasurable, or at least alluring, proprioceptive, kinesthetic and tactile stimulation. As is true of Zaslow's therapy, this stimulation can be insistent, and the child may be prevented from escaping into autistic indifference; however the approach is essentially playful instead of frustrating. Through physical contact the autistic child becomes aware not only of the existence of another human being, but also has the deeply gratifying experience that the relationship is eminently rewarding.

Schopler,[34,35] as Des Lauriers, believes autism is the result of sensory deprivation, both a constitutional deficiency and a cold mother producing a low arousal level. He especially emphasizes the infant's failure to develop from near to distance receptor usage. Sensory deprivation can be remedied by tactile stimulation, such as rocking, swinging and patting games. The stimulation must be moderately enjoyable to avoid panic. The child begins physically to feel himself as a definite entity, and bodily contact is used to develop a flexible and adaptive body schema.

Kalish[16] uses body movement to gain the child's attention, establish an emotional relation, and help him form a self-image. The therapist uses his own movements as stimuli and offers opportunities for reciprocal interaction. The child may go from the one extreme of allowing no physical contact to the other of physically trying to fuse with the therapist. The goal is for the child to achieve greater facility in expression and adaptation through greater selectivity and plasticity of movement.

Neither Schopler nor Kalish have published enough data to permit an evaluation of the relative effectiveness of their approaches. In the cases they do report, there is no evidence of the dramatic changes described by Zaslow.

MISCELLANEOUS THERAPIES

Drug Therapy.[17,19,36,40]

In general drugs are a moderately useful adjunct to therapy in diminishing hyperactivity, intensity of rage, self stimulation, or panic, and make the child more socially responsive and receptive to psychotherapeutic intervention. However results are limited and not without danger of side effects and subsequent behavioral disintegration.

Group Therapy.[3]

The meager evidence suggests that group therapy has very limited usefulness, but may be an adjunct with older children after some relationship and speech have been established.

76

Comprehensive Approaches.[25,40]

Most therapists agree that autism requires an intensive and comprehensive therapeutic approach. However, there are differences in specific strategies. Bettelheim[1] excludes the family completely from the treatment scene; others maintain contact, have the family in intensive therapy or, in the case of operant conditioning, train parents to do behavior therapy. Residential care, day care, therapeutic schools, and specialized therapies, such as speech, reading, perceptual motor coordination, music and body movement, are all part of the picture. However, there is relatively little systematic information which would enable one to evaluate their comparative efficacy.

Communication Therapy[42]

Wolf and Ruttenberg emphasize the need to motivate the child to become interested in learning to produce sounds and words, and his need for a concrete, simplified, constant physical and linguistic world. They claim that autistic children will respond to intensive communication stimulation such as is given in small doses to normal infants.

OVERALL EVALUATION

Psychotherapy with autistic children remains an extremely costly undertaking, whether one sets limited goals of affecting specific behaviors or long range goals of changing major personality variables. Many emotional roadblocks impede progress: imperviousness, inattention, negativism, temper tantrums, hyperactivity, and panic reactions. In addition the autistic child seems capable of advancing only by exceedingly slow steps. Hard earned gains are fragile and easily lost. Within this general framework, no one therapeutic approach has an established claim to advantage over another. Responsiveness to all techniques varies widely. Factors such as severity of disturbance and the presence of speech are probably more prognostic of progress rather than therapeutic approach. Only Zaslow's rage reduction therapy reports major changes in a relatively brief span of time, but more evidence is needed to establish its superiority. Until better information on comparative efficacy of all therapies is available, the experience and persuasion of the individual therapist must remain the principal guide to his strategy.

A number of controversies exist, some spurious, others genuine. The issue of relationship versus reinforcement is spurious in its polarization. Behavior therapists utilize the positive responsiveness of the child to adults, study negativism, and refer to power struggles, inattention, and temper tantrums directed at the therapist. On the other hand, relationship therapists cannot help but make use of reward and punishment as the operant conditioners define those terms. The difference is one of focus: the behavior therapists concentrate on reinforcement and let the relationship develop as it will, and the others believe the reverse. The issue of whether a relationship is an indispensable preliminary step to any therapeutic progress, however is a genuine one, yet unsettled. "Mechanical" versus "human" progress is another spurious issue. Behavior therapy tends to produce changes which are limited and situation specific, but there is no evidence that "mechanical responsiveness" is the general goal.

There are genuine differences among therapies regarding acceptance of the child, and the role of stress. At one extreme are behavior therapists and Zaslow who determine ahead of time what will be done with the child; at the other extreme are relationship therapists who follow the child's lead and try to accept, understand, and respond flexibly to him. A spurious objection is that acceptance of pathological behavior only reinforces and perpetuates it. Psychoanalytically oriented therapies are concerned with understanding causes rather than eliminating specific behaviors; their sympathetic attitude is part of a general goal of establishing a position relationship. Some behavior therapies induce stress concisely, either to punish undesirable behavior or to affect a catharsis of rage; relationship therapies are careful to keep the level of a stress within the current limits of the child's tolerance. Between the extremes are various gradations. To date there are only claims and counterclaims regarding therapeutic efficacy. Critical evidence is lacking.

REFERENCES

1. BETTELHEIM, B.: The Empty Fortress. New York, The Free Press, 1967.
2. BREGER, L.: Comments on "Building Social Behavior in Autistic Children by Use of Electric Shock." J. Exp. Res. Pers., 1:110, 1965.
3. COFFEY, H. S., AND WIENER, L. W.: Group Treatment of Autistic Children. Englewood Cliffs, N.J., Prentice-Hall, 1967.
4. COWAN, P. A., HODDINOTT, B. A., AND WRIGHT, B. A.: Compliance and Resistance in the Conditioning of Autistic Children: An Exploratory Study. Child Devel., 36:913, 1965.
5. DAVIDSON, G. C.: A Special Learning Therapy Programme with an Autistic Child. Behav. Res. Ther., 2:149, 1964.
6. DE MYER, M. K., AND FERSTER, C. B.: Teaching New Social Behavior to Schizophrenic Children. J. Amer. Acad. Child Psychiat. 1:442, 1962.
7. DES LAURIERS, A. M.: Your Child is Asleep: Early Infant Autism, Etiology, Treatment, and Parental Influences. Chicago, Dorsey Press, 1968.
8. EVELOFF, H. H.: The Autistic Child. Arch. Gen. Psychiat. 3:66, 1960.

9. FERSTER, C. B.: Reinforcement and Behavioral Defects of Autistic Children. Child Devel. 32:437, 1961.
10. FERSTER, C. B., AND DeMYER, M. K.: A Method for the Experimental Analysis of the Behavior of Autistic Children. Amer. J. Orthopsychiat., 32:89, 1962.
11. FROSTIG, M. F., AND HORNE, D.: Charting and Evaluating the Therapeutic Process with Autistic Children. Marianne Frostig Center of Educational Therapy, Los Angeles, Calif.
12. GELFAND, D. M., AND HARTMANN, B. P.: Behavior Therapy with Children: A Review and Evaluation of Research Methodology. Psychol. Bull. 69:192, 1968.
13. HEWETT, F. M.: Teaching Speech to an Autistic Child through Operant Conditioning. Amer. J. Orthopsychiat. 35:927, 1965.
14. HEWETT, F. M.: The Autistic Child Learns to Read. Slow Learning Child, 13:107, 1966.
15. HINGTGEN, J. N., COULTER, S. K., AND CHURCHILL, D. W.: Intensive Reinforcement of Imitative Behavior in Mute Autistic Children. Arch. Gen. Psychiat. 17:36, 1967.
16. KALISH, B. I.: Body Movement Therapy for Autistic Children. Paper presented at the 45th Annual Meeting of the American Orthopsychiatry Association, 1968.
17. KURTIS, L. B.: Clinical Study of the Response to Nortriptyline on Autistic Children. Int. J. Neuropsychiat. 2:298, 1966.
18. LEFF, R.: Behavior Modification and the Psychosis of Childhood: A Review. Psychol. Bull., 69:396, 1968.
19. LEHMAN, E., HABER, J., AND LESSER, S. R.: The Use of Reserpine in Autistic Children. J. Nerv. Mont. Dis., 125:351, 1957.
20. LOVAAS, O. I.: A Program for the Establishment of Speech in Psychotic Children. In: Wing, J. K. (Ed.): Early Child Autism. Oxford, Pergamon Press, 1966.
21. LOVASS, O. I., SCHAEFFER, B., AND SIMMONS, J. B.: Building Social Behavior in Autistic Children by Use of Electric Shock. J. Exp. Res. Pers. 1:99, 1965.
22. MAHLER, M. S., FURER, M., AND SETTLAGE, C. F.: Severe Emotional Disturbances in Childhood: Psychosis. In: Arieti, S. (Ed.): American Handbook of Psychiatry, Vol. I. New York, Basic Books, 1959.
23. MARSHALL, G. R.: Toilet Training of an Autistic Eight-Year Old through Conditioning Therapy. Behav. Res. Ther. 4:242, 1966.
24. METZ, J. R.: Conditioning Generalized Imitation in Autistic Children. J. Exp. Child Psychol., 4:389, 1965.
25. O'GORMAN, G.: The Nature of Childhood Autism. New York, Appleton-Century-Crofts, 1967.
26. RABB, E., AND HEWETT, F. M.: Developing Appropriate Classroom Behaviors in a Severely Disturbed Group of Institutionalized Kindergarten-primary Children Utilizing a Behavior Modification Model. Amer. J. Orthopsychiat., 37:313, 1967.
27. RANK, B.: Adaptation of the Psychoanalytic Technique for the Treatment of Young Children with Atypical Development. Amer. J. Orthopsychiat., 19:130, 1949.
28. RANK, B., AND MacNAUGHTON, D.: A Clinical Contribution to Early Ego Development. Psychoanal. St. Child. 5:53, 1950.
29. REISER, D. E.: Psychosis of Infancy and Early Childhood, as Manifested by Children with Atypical Development. New Eng. J. Med., 269:790, 1963.

30. REISER, D. E., AND BROWN, J. L.: Patterns of Later Development in Children with Infantile Psychosis. J. Amer. Acad. Child Psychiat. 4:650, 1964.

31. RUTTENBERG, B. A.: A Psychoanalytically Based Structural and Developmental Conceptualization of the Origins and Processes Involved in the Syndrome of Infantile Autism. Indiana University Colloquium on Infantile Autism, 1968.

32. SAPOSNEK, D. T.: An Experimental Study of Rage-Reduction Treatment on Autistic Children. Unpublished Master's Thesis, San Jose State College, Calif., 1967.

33. SCANLON, J. B., LEBERFELD, D. T., AND FREIBRUN, R.: Language Training in the Treatment of the Autistic Child Functioning on a Retarded Level. Ment. Retard. 1:305, 1963.

34. SCHOPLER, E.: The Development of Body Image and Symbol Formation Through Bodily Contact with an Autistic Child. J. Child Psychol. Psychiat. 3:191, 1962.

35. SCHOPLER, E.: Early Infantile Autism and Sensory Processes. Arch. Gen. Psychiat. 13:327, 1965.

36. SIMMONS, J. Q., LEIKEN, S. J., LOVAAS, O. I., SCHAEFFER, B., AND PERLOFF, B.: Modification of Autistic Behavior with LSD-25. Amer. J. Psychiat., 122:1201, 1966.

37. WAAL, N.: A Special Technique of Psychotherapy with an Autistic Child. In: Caplan, G. (Ed.): Emotional Problems of Early Childhood. New York, Basic Books, 1955.

38. WENAR, C., RUTTENBERG, B. A., DRATMAN, M. L., AND WOLF, E. G.: Changing Autistic Behavior. Arch. Gen. Psychiat. 17:26, 1967.

39. WETZEL, R. J., BAKER, J., RONEY, M., AND MARTIN, M.: Outpatient Treatment of Autistic Behavior. Behav. Res. Ther. 4:169, 1966.

40. WING, J. K.: Early Childhood Autism. Oxford, Pergamon Press, 1966.

41. WOLF, E. G.: Autistic Children: A Study of the Response to Auditory Stimuli. Unpublished Ph.D. dissertation, Boston University, School of Education, 1968.

42. WOLF, E. G., AND RUTTENBERG, B. A.: Communication Therapy for the Autistic Child. J. Speech Hearing Dis. 32:331, 1969.

43. WOLF, M. M., RISLEY, T., AND MEES, H.: Application of Operant Conditioning Procedures to the Behavior Problems of an Autistic Child. Behav. Res. Ther. 1:305, 1964.

44. ZASLOW, R. W., AND BREGER, L.: A Theory and Treatment of Autism. In: Breger, L. (Ed.): Clinical-Cognitive Psychology: Models and Integration. New Jersey; Prentice-Hall.

PART III

THE ADOLESCENT

Trends in Adolescent Psychiatry

by WILLIAM A. SCHONFELD, M.D.

A DOLESCENCE IS simultaneously a biological, psychological and social phenomenon.[17,31,75] Development at each of these levels proceeds with significant interaction and interdependence. Their integration may be appraised in the individual through an evaluation of his body or self-image.[30,69,71] Adolescence may be divided into three phases: early, mid, and late adolescence which is preceded by pre-adolescence and followed by postadolescence.[10,11,75]

The structural groundwork for adolescent development is laid by physical maturation, which is dependent on biological capacity and hereditary trends. However environmental factors, such as nutrition and general health, may delay or accelerate this process.[75,84] Biologically, adolescence begins with the acceleration of growth in height and the first signs of physical sexual maturation, and ends with the deceleration of growth, the complete development of primary and secondary sexual characteristics; although it usually encompasses the ages of 10 to 18 years in girls and 12 to 20 years in boys,[74,84] there is a wide range of normal variations with a trend for adolescence beginning at an earlier age.

Psychologically, adolescence is marked by acceleration of cognitive growth with the development of the ability to conceptualize at an abstract level.[41] This new ego capacity for abstract thinking accounts for the youth's concern with the basic meaning and values of human existence. Other psychological themes of adolescence are the search for a sense of social, sexual and personal identity,[18,30,88] and the development of what Blos characterized as the second stage of individuation.[12]

Adolescence is also a social phenomena. The primary identification of a child with his family weakens during adolescence and is replaced by a new identification with peer groups. In some cultures adolescence marks the beginning of adulthood, but in our highly technological society it has been a period of psychosocial moratorium between childhood and adulthood.[17,60] Society is progressively prolonging this period of dependency well beyond biological maturation.[46,47]

83

There have been many excellent multidisciplinary studies of the behavior and attitudes of adolescents. Some are general studies[9,43,73,79,80] while others are directed to specific problems.[8,15,24,28,68,76,77,83,85,86,87,90]

Concern in the individual centers around the evaluation of whether a youth's attitudes and behavior are a manifestation of illness, normal adolescent turmoil or merely reflect a change in mores.[50,51,52] Many in their struggle for autonomy reject adult standards of normality as a social phenomenon; others attempt to find a resolution of their internalized conflicts through aberrant behavior. We can find clues to the significance of the youth's behavior by studying his successes and failures in the maturational process, environmental influences, family stresses, self or body image, and subculture. A knowledge of the range of normality as stressed by Offer and coworkers[49,56,59] is essential for adequate diagnostic assessment of behavior.

The onset of pubescence enhances all instinctual drives, notably the aggressive and sexual ones, exacerbating all previously unresolved conflicts and initiating a variety of new conflicts. It produces in the presence of a relatively weakened ego structure, even in the normal youth, a state of great emotional upheaval, which may be called adolescent turmoil.[45,51,52] The effects range from very little in the healthy to chaotic in the seriously disturbed.[51,66] Some adolescents will not "outgrow" their maladaptations; they are apt to "grow into" them.

Masterson's five year study of 72 outpatients indicates that adolescents with psychiatric symptoms invariably suffer from psychiatric disorders and not merely adolescent turmoil.[50] The widespread practice, therefore, of calling most problems "adjustment reactions of adolescence" is misleading, and the burden of proof should be on the psychiatrist. Not all deviant behavior is sick behavior and compliance, more than revolt, may be evidence of illness. More meaningful classification is needed for the symptom complexes in this age group.[32,93,94]

TRENDS IN PSYCHOTHERAPY

Adolescents in increasing number are being referred to psychiatrists for evaluation and treatment.[3,36,65,72,74] Since they are notably difficult to reach and keep in therapy, working with them calls for special techniques. Adult-like treatment imposes responsibility and burden on adolescent egos which they often cannot carry; child-like treatment invites fixation at a children's level rather than promoting maturation.[45,74]

How intensively can one treat an adolescent? Due to the relative weakness of the youth's ego, at one time therapy was limited to conflicts that impeded growth; however improved techniques and experience have demonstrated that the adolescent should be treated as intensively as required.[10,25,29,33,51,61]

Although the youth is concerned with his roots in the past and prospects for the future, his greatest involvement is with the present. The adolescent does not usually involve himself in traditional psychoanalysis;[13,48,54] he may resent having to search for insights or even learning to cope with reality, although both are important for psychotherapy to be effective.

Individual psychotherapy should deal mainly with present relationships and concentrate on feelings as well as behavior. Therapy, if it is to succeed must make the youth stop denying reality. The adolescent must be helped to establish a realistic self image, evaluate his own behavior, accept responsibility for it, and change it if inappropriate. Some of the qualities that are especially needed in the psychotherapy of adolescents are engagement, flexibility, tolerance, partiality and willingness on part of the therapist to play a parent surrogate role as needed.[26,72,74]

Engagement means treating the adolescent as someone who is quite capable of refusing to cooperate with treatment. Many reject psychotherapy because the therapist represents the "establishment" and an attempt to make him fit into society. Yet psychoanalysts have made illuminating contributions[16,23,44,81,82] to the understanding of adolescents culminating in Peter Blos's publication of a comprehensive, integrated, pyschoanalytic theory of personality development in adolescents.[11] The task is to get the youth to see his need for treatment from his own point of view[55] and be willing to accept it.

Usually the psychiatrist has been chosen by the youth's parents, and the patient may resent having to confide in someone who he assumes to be a parental ally. This makes the first visits crucial. The therapist has to convey to the adolescent that *he* is the one the therapist is directly interested in helping, and that it is not a matter of "sickness" but of personal difficulties which can be worked out if he will think and talk about them. The patient is assured that what he says will be kept confidential and that the therapist will not conspire behind his back with his parents, school or social agencies. Therapy often requires time beyond that spent in the office, since emergencies frequently arise which require immediate attention.

The psychiatrist must be sufficiently flexible to adjust to the therapeutic needs of his adolescent patients. Some adolescents express their thoughts freely and will talk about themselves, their peers and their family. Others, particularly the younger adolescents, may need an opportunity for activity or play therapy to open the way for discussion. The relationship of therapist and patient must be active, stimulating and interesting to the youth in order for him to cooperate. Passivity of the therapist, often considered the hallmark of intensive therapy in adults, can have a disorganizing and anxiety-producing effect on the adolescent. It is also imperative for the therapist to be consistently candid in his relationship with the adolescent, and tolerant of the youth's value system even while trying to change it.

Perhaps one of the greatest problems for the therapist is assuming responsibility for curbing the youth's destructive actions. Hendrickson, Holmes and others[22,39,40] stress the need for behavior control for intensive treatment and Rinsley[63,64] regards adolescent acting-out as resistance to treatment. In so doing the therapist often serves as a parent surrogate, with the risk of bearing the brunt of the patient's negative feelings toward his parents. However it is also true that many adolescents who cannot accept limitations from a parent wish to be curbed in their behavior, and will take it from a therapist with whom the relationship is good. These adolescents want protection and fear their own impulsive behavior.

The acceptance of the psychiatrist as a parent surrogate is not always a transference response. The adolescent may be merely responding to the maturity of the therapist and seek guidance. It should be noted that many adolescents who resent the need of a parent's support accept the therapist as a surrogate parent, knowing that the relationship can always be terminated. The therapist must recognize if the emotional tie gets too strong, the restrictions too compelling or expectations too uncomfortable, the patient may run away from therapy, either in actuality or by an emotional decathexis.

One of the psychiatrist's goals in therapy should be to enhance the relationship of the adolescent and his parents. However some therapists in attempting to win the favor of the adolescent or because of over identification with him may join in condemning the parents; this may mobilize the adolescent's latent loyalty and love for his parents and turn him against the therapist.

Often the psychiatrist has to work closely with the youth's family in either concommitant or conjoint therapy. The young adolescent usually accepts this, but the older one may initially reject involving his parents, whereupon the psychiatrist must convince the adolescent that it is for his welfare. The therapist cannot meet all of the adolescent's needs. When the youth regresses to a dependent phase, he requires the kind of help from his parents that a child requires. Nor can one force independence, and insight alone will not make him so until his ego is strengthened toward emancipation. The adolescent needs to grow out of his childhood, not be freed from it.[44,74]

Even though the adolescent verbalizes problems of getting the message across still exist, and the therapist must be "tuned in on the youth's wave length." Only the psychiatrist with adequate training, interest, experience and empathy with young people can cope with this age group. The problems

86

of communication are often complicated when the psychiatrist, in an attempt to win his cooperation mimics the teenager's language and attitudes.[38]

Psychotherapeutic needs of adolescents often extend beyond individual therapy to group psychotherapy or conjoint family therapy. Group psychotherapy is an important modality of treatment adding the interaction of the adolescent with his peers.[14,21,40,64] Another approach to the therapy of adolescents has been conjoint family therapy, since so much of the adolescent's maladjustment is a result of his being the scapegoat for parents and reflects the family pyschopathology. The literature is burgeoning with descriptions of the use of conjoint family psychotherapy in the treatment of adolescents.[1,2,42,53,67,78,89]

Psychopharmacology must also be a part of the armamentarium in conjunction with psychotherapy. The objectives of psychopharmacologic agents are to control impulses, relieve anxiety, encourage patterning and render the patient amenable to significant relationships. Drugs themselves do not change established patterns of behavior, but are often able to ameliorate symptoms so as to facilitate psychotherapy, education and socialization.[19,62]

TRENDS IN TREATMENT FACILITIES

More teenagers are outpatients in psychiatric clinics than in any other decade of life. However there is a need for still more special clinics for adolescents, such as walk-in clinics and clinics stressing conjoint family therapy. The facilities for inpatient care of adolescents vary on the basis of the degree to which they depend upon education, milieu therapy, case-work, psychotropic drugs or individual, group and family therapy, as well as the professional orientation of the staff.[4,6,7]

Psychiatric services in general hospitals provide short term treatment[21,25] crisis intervention and diagnostic evaluation. However, adolescents requiring long term inpatient treatment are referred to either a psychiatric hospital[4,5,6,35] or a residential treatment center. Many would benefit if referred for part time hospitalization in day or night hospitals, half-way houses, youth hostels, youth treatment camps, treatment schools or treatment oriented residential centers. The comprehensive community mental health centers and neighborhood health centers should plan to offer many of these facilities.

There has been a great deal of discussion as to whether adolescent inpatients should be placed on an all-adolescent service or integrated with adults on a general service. Advocates of an all-adolescent unit point out the advantages of utilizing the interaction among the peers for therapeutic understanding and insight, and that group process and group pressures in the unit may exert favorable influence upon schizoid and behaviorally disturbed adolescents. The mature staff in such units, rather than the disturbed adult patients, serve as the models of behavior.[4,5,20,40,63,64,72,74,91] The advocates of housing the adolescent in an adult unit stress that those in an all-adolescent unit tend to find peers who will support sick and un-manageable behavior, whereas those on integrated services are discouraged to act out by the adults, and gain a more sympathetic understanding of the older person's problems and often a better understanding of their parents.[7,29,34] Many institutions currently combine both features having a separate facility for adolescents, while also placing certain adolescents on the adult floor.[34,37] In many hospitals, however there is either a complete disregard or merely a token concern with the education, recreational and social needs of the adolescent.

Psychiatric hospitals admitting adolescents should have a separate functioning adolescent service and program which provide an opportunity for education and remedial education, recreation, and occupational therapy and vocational planning in addition to individual, group and family psychotherapy, milieu therapy and psychopharmacology. Such service requires a well-trained multidisciplinary staff under the supervision of a psychiatrist. When adolescents have such a multidisciplinary therapeutically oriented service throughout the day, it does not make much difference where they are housed, although a separate all-adolescent unit is preferable for at least some of the patients.

Trends in Training

Training and experience in adolescent psychiatry, whether part of a residency program, a fellowship, post residency experience or junior staff position, should include all modalities of treatment in a variety of treatment settings.[27,70] Werkman[92] has described the training necessary in order to function effectively with adolescent patients. The psychiatrist must have a thorough knowledge of: (1) effective, cognitive and physical developments through all ages, and how variations effect particular adolescents; (2) dynamics of family involvements and interaction ;(3) the particular significance of peers as a transitional step toward developing autonomy; (4) the impact of school and recreational activities on character formation and emotional disturbance; (5) how to collaborate effectively as a teacher and consultant with all disciplines working with youth; (6) the total spectrum of adolescent behavior in order to understand the range of normal problems and or adolescent's emotional disorders; (7) a working knowledge of

88

psychopharmacology, group therapy, conjoint family therapy and crisis intervention techniques, and (8) the adolescent's needs help to clarify his values in relation to the current values of society. These are all secondary to and dependent upon a thorough knowledge of the dynamics and techniques of individual interviewing and psychotherapy.

Specific training programs are being developed through the National Institute of Mental Health,* but not enough in view of the great demand for psychiatrists to work with adolescents. Training of the ancillary professions to work with adolescents is also an important function of the adolescent psychiatrist.

REFERENCES

1. ACKERMAN, N.: The Psychodynamics of Family Life. New York, Basic Books, 1958.
2. ACKERMAN, N.: Adolescent Problems: A Symptom of Family Disorder. Family Process. 1:202, 1962.
3. AMERICAN PSYCHIATRIC ASSOCIATION: Position Statement on Adolescent Psychiatry. Committee on Psychiatry in Childhood and Adolescence, Amer. J. Psychiat. 123:1031, 1967.
4. BAILEY, R., BLACK, J. C., ELLIS, D. J., AND KAHN, I. R.: Mental Health Facilities for the Inpatient Adolescent, Dept. of Architecture and Psychology, Univ. of Utah, Salt Lake City, 1965.
5. BARDONA, D. T., MACKEITH, S. A., AND CAMERON, K.: Symposium on the Inpatient Treatment of Psychotic Adolescents. Brit. J. Med. Psychol. 23:107, 1950.
6. BECKETT, P. G. S.: Adolescents Out of Step: Their Treatment in a Psychiatric Hospital, Detroit, Wayne State Univ. Press, 1965.
7. BESKIN, H.: Psychiatric Inpatient Treatment of Adolescents, A Review of Clinical Experience. Compr. Psychiat., 3:354, 1962.
8. BLAINE, G. B., JR.: Youth and the Hazards of Affluence: The High School and College Years, New York, Harper & Row, 1966.
9. BLAINE, G. B., AND McARTHUR, C. C. (Eds.): Emotional Problems of the Student. New York, Appleton-Century-Crofts, 1961.
10. BLOS, P.: Intensive Psychotherapy in Relation to the Various Phases of the Adolescent Period. Amer. J. Orthopsychiat., 5:901, 1962.
11. BLOS, P.: On Adolescence: A Psychoanalytic Interpretation: New York, The Free Press of Glencoe, 1962.
12. BLOS, P.: Second Individuation Process of Adolescence. Psychoan. Study of the Child. Int. Univ. Press, 22:162, 1967.
13. BRYT, A.: Modifications of Psychoanalysis in the Treatment of Adolescents. In: Masserman, J. H. (Ed.): Adolescence, Dreams & Training, New York, Grune & Stratton, 1966, p. 80.

*National Institute Approved Training Programs in Adolescent Psychiatry are located at Children's Hospital of the District of Columbia, Neuropsychiatric Institute of the University of Michigan and McLean Hospital, Belmont, Mass.

14. CAMERON, K.: Group Approach to Inpatient Adolescents. Amer. J. Psychiat. p. 109, 1953.

15. CHWAST, J.: Depressive Reaction as a Manifestation Among Adolescent Delinquents. Amer. J. Psychoth. 31:575, 1968.

16. DEUTSCH, H.: Selected Problems of Adolescence. New York, Int. Univ. Press, 1967.

17. EISENBERG, L.: A Developmental Approach to Adolescence, Children. 12: 131, 1965.

18. ERICKSON, E. H.: Identity: Youth and Crisis. New York, W. W. Norton & Company, 1968.

19. EVELOFF, H. H.: Psychopharmacologic Agents in Child Psychiatry. Arch. Gen. Psychiat. 14:472, 1966.

20. FALSTEIN, E. I., AND OFFER, D.: Adolescent Therapy. In: Abt, L. E. and Riess, B. F. (Eds.): Progress Clinical Psychology, Vol. V. New York, Grune & Stratton, 1963, p. 62.

21. FALSTEIN, E. I., FEINSTEIN, S. C., AND COHEN, W. P.: An Integrated Adolescent Care Program in a General Psychiatric Hospital. Amer. J. Orthopsychiat. 30:276, 1960.

22. FALSTEIN, E. I., FEINSTEIN, S. C., OFFER, D., AND FINE, P.: Group Dynamics: Inpatient Adolescents Engage in an Outbreak of Vandalism. Arch. Gen. Psychiat. 9:32, 1963.

23. FREUD, A.: Adolescence. Psychoanalytic Study of the Child, New York, Int. Univ. Press, 13:255, 1958.

24. GIOVACCHINI, P. L.: Compulsory Happiness: Adolescent Despair. Arch. Gen. Psychiat. 18:650, 1968.

25. GOOLISHIAN, H. A.: A Brief Psychotherapy Program for Disturbed Adolescents. Amer. J. Orthopsychiat., 32:142, 1962.

26. GODENNE, G. D.: A Psychiatrists Techniques in Treating Adolescents. Children, 4:136, 1965.

27. GODENNE, G. D., AND KING, E. N.: An Experiment in Teaching Adolescence Psychiatry to Year V Medical Students. Adol. 2:107, 1967.

28. GOULD, R. E.: Suicidal Problems in Children and Adolescents. Amer. J. Psychoth. 19:228, 1965.

29. GRALNICK, A.: Psychoanalysis and the Treatment of Adolescents in a Private Hospital. In: Masserman, J. H. (Ed.): Adolescence, Dreams & Training, New York, Grune & Stratton, 1966. p. 102.

30. GREEN, M. R.: The Problem of Identity Crisis. In: Masserman, J. H. (Ed.): Adolescence, Dreams & Training, New York, Grune & Stratton, 1966.

31. Group for the Advancement of Psychiatry, Normal Adolescence. 6: , 1968.

32. Group for the Advancement of Psychiatry: Psychopathological Disorders in Childhood: Theoretical Considerations and a Proposed Classification. 6: , 1966.

33. HALLECK, S.: Psychiatric Treatment of the Alienated College Student. Amer. J. Psychiat., 124:642, 1967.

34. HAMILTON, D. M., McKINLEY, R. A., MOORHEAD, H. H., AND WALL, J. H.: Results of Mental Hospital Treatment of Troubled Youth. Amer. J. Psychiat. 117:811, 1961.

90

35. HARTMANN, E., GLASSER, B. A., GREENBLATT, M., SOLOMON, M. H., AND LEVINSON, D. J.: Adolescents in a Mental Hospital, New York, Grune & Stratton, 1968.
36. HENDERSON, A. S., McCULLOCH, J. W., AND PHILIP, A. E.: Survey of Mental Illness in Adolescence. Brit. Med. J., 1:83, 1967.
37. HENDRICKSON, W. J.: Gold Achievement Award, Adolescent Service, University of Michigan. Mental Hospitals, 14:525, 1963.
38. HENDRICKSON, W. J.: Treating Adolescents: Transference and Countertransference Problems. Front. Clinic. Psychiat. 4:1, 1967.
39. HENDRICKSON, W. J. AND HOLMES, D. J.: Control of Behavior as a Crucial Factor in Intensive Psychiatric Treatment in an All Adolescent Ward. Amer. J. Psychiat., 115:969, 1959.
40. HOLMES, D. J.: The Adolescent in Psychotherapy. Boston, Little, Brown, & Co., 1964.
41. INHELDER, B., AND PIAGET, J.: The Growth of Logical Thinking from Childhood to Adolescence. New York, Basic Books, 1958.
42. JACKSON, D. D., AND WEAKLAND, J. H.: Conjoint Family Therapy Psychiatry, 24:30, 1961.
43. JOHNSON, A. M.: Sanctions for Super-Ego Lacunae of Adolescents. In: Eissler, K. R. (Ed.): Searchlights in Delinquency, New York, Int. Univ. Press, 1949, p. 225.
44. JOSSELYN, I. M.: The Adolescent and His World. Family Serv. of Am., New York, 1952.
45. JOSSELYN, I. M.: The Ego in Adolescence. Amer. J. Orthopsychiat., 24:223, 1954.
46. KENISTON, K.: The Uncommitted Alienated Youth in American Society. New York, Harcourt, Brace & World, 1965.
47. KENISTON, K.: Young Radicals. New York, Harcourt, Brace & World, 1968.
48. LORAND, S., AND SCHNEER, H. I. (Eds.): Adolescents: Psychoanalytic Approach to Problems and Therapy. New York, Hoeber, 1961.
49. MARCUS, D., OFFER, D., BLATT, S., AND GRATCH, G.: A Clinical Approach to the Understanding of Normal and Pathologic Adolescence. Arch. Gen. Psychiat. 15:569, 1966.
50. MASTERSON, J. F., JR.: The Symptomatic Adolescent Five Years Later: He Didn't Grow Out Of It. Amer. J. Psychiat. 123:11, 1967.
51. MASTERSON, J. F., JR.: The Psychiatric Dilemma of Adolescence. Boston, Little, Brown & Co., 1967.
52. MASTERSON, J. F., JR., AND WASHBURNE, A.: The Symptomatic Adolescent: Psychiatric Illness or Adolescent Turmoil. Amer. J. Psychiat., 122:1240, 1966.
53. MILLER, D.: Family Interaction and Adolescent Therapy. Psychiatry, 21:277, 1958.
54. MILLER, L. C.: Short Term Therapy with Adolescents. Amer. J. Orthopsychiat., 29:772, 1959.
55. NOSHPITZ, J. D.: Opening Phase in the Psychotherapy of Adolescents with Character Disorders. Bull. Menninger Clin. 21:153, 1957.
56. OFFER, D.: Normal Adolescents. New York, Basic Books, 1969.
57. OFFER, D., AND OFFER, J. L.: Normal Adolescents Mature. In: Greenblatt, N., and Hartmann, E. (Eds.): Seminars in Psychiatry. New York, Grune & Stratton, 1969.

58. OFFER, D., AND SABSHIN, M.: The Psychiatrist and the Normal Adolescent. Arch. Gen. Psychiat. 9:427, 1963.
59. OFFER, D., SABSHIN, M., AND MARCUS, D.: Clinical Evaluations of "Normal" Adolescents. Amer. J. Psychiat., 9:864, 1965.
60. REDL, F.: When We Deal with Children. New York, Free Press, 1966.
61. RIESS, B. F.: The Treatment of Adolescents. J. Psychiat., 51:473, 1961.
62. RINSLEY, D. B.: Thiordiazine in the Treatment of Hospitalized Adolescents. Amer. J. Psychiat., 120:73, 1963.
63. RINSLEY, D. B.: Intensive Psychiatric Hospital Treatment of Adolescents: An Object-Relations View. Psychiat. Quart., 39:405, 1965.
64. RINSLEY, D. B.: Intensive Residential Treatment of the Adolescent. Psychiat. Quart. 41:134, 1967.
65. ROSEN, B. M., BAHN, A. K., SHILLOW, R., AND BOWER, E. M.: Adolescent Patients Served in Outpatient Psychiatric Clinics. Amer. J. Pub. Health, 55:1563, 1965.
66. ROTH, D., AND BLATT, S. J.: Psychopathology of Adolescence. Arch. Gen. Psychiat., 4:289, 1961.
67. SATIR, V.: Conjoint Family Therapy. Palo Alto, Science and Behavior Books, 1964.
68. SCHOFIELD, M.: The Sexual Behaviour of Young People. Boston, Little, Brown & Co., 1965.
69. SCHONFELD, W. A.: Body-Image Disturbances in Adolescents with Inappropriate Sexual Development. Amer. J. Orthopsychiat., 34:493, 1964.
70. SCHONFELD, W. A.: Psychiatric Training of Pediatric Residents and Pediatric Training of Child Psychiatry Residents. Proceedings of an Institute sponsored by the American Board of Pediatrics at Atlanta, Georgia—September 12–19, 1965. Ped., 38:740, 1966.
71. SCHONFELD, W. A.: Body Image Disturbances in Adolescents, IV Influence of Family Attitudes. Arch. Gen. Psychiat., 15:16, 1966.
72. SCHONFELD, W. A.: Adolescent Psychiatry: An Appraisal of the Adolescent's Position in Contemporary Psychiatry. Arch. Gen. Psychiat., 16:713, 1967.
73. SCHONFELD, W. A.: The Adolescent Crises Today, Socio-economic Affluence as a Factor. N.Y. State J. of Med., 67:1981, 1967.
74. SCHONFELD, W. A.: The Adolescent in Contemporary American Psychiatry. Critical evaluations by Josselyn, I., Lebovici, S., Masterson, J. Jr., Staples, H., and Boutourline Young, J. Int. J. Psychiat., 5:470, 1968.
75. SCHONFELD, W. A.: The Body and Body Image. In: Caplan, G. and Lebovici, S. (Eds.): Adolescence: Psychosocial Perspectives. New York, Basic Books, 1968.
76. SCHRUT, A.: Suicidal Adolescents and Children. J.A.M.A., 13:1103, 1964.
77. SCHRUT, A.: Some Typical Patterns in the Behavior and Background of Adolescent Girls Who Attempt Suicide. Amer. J. Psychiat., 125:69, 1968.
78. SERRANO, A. C., McDONALD, E. C., GOOLISHIAN, H. A., MAC GREGOR, R., AND RITCHIE, A.: Adolescent Maladjustment and Family Dynamics. Amer. J. Psychiat., 118:897, 1962.
79. SHAPIRO, R.: Adolescence and the Psychology of the Ego. Psychiat., 26:77, 1963.
80. SHERIF, M., AND SHERIF, C. W. (Eds.): Problems of Youth: Transition to Adulthood in a Changing World. Chicago, Aldine, 1965.
81. SPIEGEL, L. A.: Disorder and Consolidation in Adolescence. J. Amer. Psychoanal. Ass., 3:406, 1961.

82. SPIEGEL, L. A.: A Review of Contributions to a Psychoanalytic Theory of Adolescence. Psychoan. Study of the Child, New York, Int. Univ. Press, 1951, p. 375.

83. SUGAR, M.: Disguised Depressions in Adolescence. In: Usdin, G. L. (Ed.): Adolescence Care & Counseling. Philadelphia & Toronto, J. P. Lippincott Co., 1968, p. 77.

84. TANNER, J. M.: Growth At Adolescence. Springfield, Ill., Charles C. Thomas, 1962.

85. TEICHER, J., AND JACOBS, J.: Adolescents Who Attempt Suicide: Preliminary Findings. Amer. J. Psychiat., 11:1248, 1966.

86. TEICHER, J. D.: Social Isolation in Attempted Suicides in Adolescents. Int. J. Soc. Psychiat., 13:139, 1967.

87. TEICHER, J. D., AND MARGOLIN, N. L.: Thirteen Adolescent Male Suicide Attempts—Dynamic Considerations. J. Amer. Acad. Child Psychiat., 7:296, 1968.

88. TOOLAN, J. M.: Changes in Personality Structure During Adolescence. In: Masserman, J. (Ed.): Psychoanalysis and Human Values. New York, Grune & Stratton, 1960.

89. VOGEL, E. F., AND BELL, N. W.: The Emotionally Disturbed Child as the Family Scapegoat. In: Bell, N. W., and Vogel, E. F. (Eds.): The Family. Glencoe, The Free Press of Glencoe, 1960.

90. WALTERS, P. A.: Therapist Bias and Student Use of Illegal Drugs. J. Am. Coll. Health Assoc., 16:30, 1967.

91. WARREN, W.: A Study of Adolescent Psychiatric Inpatients and the Outcome Six or More Years Later. II. The Follow-Up Study. J. Child Psychol. & Psychiat., 6:141, 1965.

92. WERKMAN, S. L.: Training and Research in Adolescent Psychiatry. American Psychiatric Association Annual Meeting—Future Community Models for the Hospital Treatment of Adolescents.

93. American Psychiatric Association, Diagnostic and Statistical Manual of Mental Disorders (Second Edition), 1968.

94. Workshop Committees—American Society for Adolescent Psychiatry. Reports not published.

Therapy of the Alienated College Student

by SEYMOUR HALLECK, M.D.

A N INCREASING NUMBER of college students who consult psychiatrists
complain of vague feelings of apathy, boredom, meaninglessness,
and chronic unhappiness. Such complaints are best understood in terms of
the concept of alienation. Alienation can be defined as an estrangement
from the values of one's society and family and a similar estrangement
from that part of one's history and affective life which links him to his
society or family.

From a behavioral standpoint, the alienated student can be characterized
by the following traits:

1. *A Tendency to Live in the Present and to Avoid Commitment to People, Causes, or Ideas.* The alienated student does not look forward to assuming adult roles. He is convinced that gratification does not lie in the future
but that if good things are going to happen they must happen now. He talks
about being "washed up" at 25 years of age, and it is difficult to convince
him that people over 30 years of age are capable of enjoying sex or having
ideals.

The struggle to find commitment is perhaps characteristic of most college
students, but the alienated student is one who is on the verge of abandoning
the search for commitment. The alienated student should not be confused
with the dedicated activist. He finds it difficult to sustain interest in causes.
Nor does he find it easy to love ideals or love others. He drifts from experience to experience, either as an uninvolved observer or as a self-conscious game player who is unable to lose himself in his various social roles.

2. *An Almost Total Lack of Communication with Parents or Other
Adults.* There have always been gaps in agreement and understanding
between generations, and it is generally agreed that these gaps are becoming
wider. The alienated student is especially detached from the adult world. He

94

is not only profoundly distrustful of adults, but is convinced that closeness to adults is impossible.

3. *An Ill-defined Self-concept*. Late adolescence is a period in which young people struggle to find a solid identity. Sometimes conflicts in roles and value systems are serious enough so that the student experiences an identity crisis, a sense of profound uncertainty as to who he is, where he comes from, and where he is going. The alienated student can be described as existing in a state of chronic identity crises. His constant cries of "Who am I . . . I don't know what I believe . . . I have no self" are accompanied by anxiety that, although subdued, is nevertheless pervasive and relentless.

4. *A Tendency toward Sudden Severe Depression, Often Accompanied by Attempts at Suicide.* The alienated student is a person impervious to acknowledgement of his unconscious impulses. When exposed to situations that touch upon unconscious conflict, he has little adaptive capacity. Seemingly minor stresses produce massive affective responses, usually in the form of a depression experienced as formless, as a "cloud" coming out of nowhere. There are few affects in life as painful as depression which cannot be even partially related to ones' own existence. The student often responds with seemingly impulsive efforts at self-destruction.

5. *An Inability to Concentrate or Study.* Although alienated students are usually bright, they invariably experience blocking of their ability to perform school work.

6. *Promiscuous but Ungratifying Sexual Behavior.* Alienated students are convinced that their sexual lives can be totally open, diversified, and free of guilt. In pursuing these elusive ideals, they tend to be promiscuous. While the alienated student seems to be leading a stimulating sex life, he frequently complains that it is unsatisfying and meaningless. Intimacy, self-respect, and even orgasm are usually lacking. Female patients who are promiscuous rarely experience orgasm. Male patients increasingly complain of impotence, premature ejaculation, and inability to ejaculate.

7. *Use of Marihuana and Other Hallucinogens.* Smoking marihuana has become almost an emblem of alienation. The alienated student realizes that the use of "pot" mortifies his parents and enrages authorities. Marihuana has become a rallying cause for students, a challenge to adults, and a potent catalyst for widening the gap between generations.

The quest for exciting inner experiences through the use of psychedelic drugs represents a frustration with reality, a sense of futility with efforts to alter the external world. Many alienated students perceive the reality of their existence as so sterile and unchangeable that they expend much of their energy searching for a rapid means of changing themselves. They seek

95

a basically autoplastic adjustment in which they can create a new inner reality simply by taking a pill or smoking a marihuana cigarette.

The seven traits listed above describe the behavior of a severely alienated student. Obviously the individual student patient may be characterized by varying degrees of seriousness of each of these traits. Generally, however, these traits occur together with so much consistency that alienation can be considered as a distinct personality-pattern disturbance of young adults.

DISCUSSION

Some observers imply that alienated youth should be critically viewed as individuals who have grave psychological disturbances. Others focus upon the unusual varieties of stress currently imposed upon students and view the alienated response as an appropriate, if not admirable, adaptation to a highly troubled world. A third set of explanations are more neutral and focus upon impersonal forces that make it necessary for young people to seek new adaptational styles, one of which can be described as alienation.

Many observers view the student as an individual who has been exposed to too much permissiveness, too much affluence, and insufficient commitment to the value of personal responsibility. Much emphasis is placed upon the role of the disturbed family, especially when one or both parents have experienced some emotional disturbance, or when the mother is domineering and overprotective and the father passive and withdrawn. The sympathetic explanations view student unrest as an appropriate response to inordinate academic demands made upon young people; to the impersonality, and sometimes to the irrelevancy, of our universities; to the deterioration of the quality of life in America; to a bureaucratic and political stagnation that makes it difficult to bring about orderly change in our society; to the oppression of the American Negro; and, finally, to the war in Viet Nam.

Neutral explanations of alienation focus upon psychological changes that have taken place in man as he is forced to adapt to technological growth and a constantly accelerating rate of change in the everyday conditions of life. According to these explanations, young people distrust the past, fear the future, and are driven to live in the present. They seek immediate gratification and do not worry too much about the means by which such gratification is gained.

Other relatively impartial explanations consider the impact of media on young people. According to these hypotheses, the media first create a climate of unrest by exposing the weakness of authority and then proceed to nurture and disseminate unrest by publicizing it.

Each of the preceding theories has some validity. Alienation cannot be explained in purely psychological terms because many who are raised in permissive, affluent, or disturbed circumstances do not become alienated. Nor can it be explained exclusively in social terms because only a small number of youth adapt to our stress-laden society with an alienated response. To understand why a young person becomes alienated, it is necessary to consider all relevant stressful factors and to determine how these factors exert their influence upon a given individual.

PROBLEMS OF TREATING ALIENATION

The alienated student is not the easily treatable, late adolescent who is so often frequently described in psychiatric literature, but is actually one of the most resistant and refractory patients encountered in psychiatric practice. One of the major treatment problems is that the alienated life viewed as a social role appears to have become more acceptable to our youth. The alienated role also provides the student with considerable power.

Many students have learned to ritualize alienation so that it becomes a game which provides a highly successful weapon for hurting their parents without having to express open rage. There are few people in this world as frustrated and impotent as middle-class parents who must deal with the highly prized child who has just made a suicide attempt or who has just informed them that he is going to quit school so that he can live in Greenwich Village, find a job as a dishwasher, and write poetry. The student's artful pretense of peacefulness compounds his parents' bewilderment even further. The passive-aggressive aspects of the alienation defense are also likely to be directed against the therapist. The student's apathy, boredom, unreliability, and apparent peacefulness are often sufficiently powerful to render the psychotherapist impotent.

In treating the alienated student the following approaches, which may deviate from standard technique, are in my experience crucial.

1. The alienated student will usually project all his difficulties onto the society, and because he is partly right, the therapist can concede that the student's world is often dominated by neglect, dishonesty, or corruption. But, having ameliorated the student-therapist relationship to this extent, the therapist must then focus upon the irrational aspects of the patient's behavior. The therapist's task becomes that of helping the student to distinguish between oppressions that others impose upon him and oppressions that he imposes upon himself.

2. Some alienated students have denied their hostile feelings by adopting a pseudomature pose of having no anger but only a wistful tolerance toward parents. It may take months or even years for the student to be well enough

97

to lift the repression that contains his rage toward his parents. The therapist is faced with the task of constantly illustrating the manner in which passivity and inertia are used as aggressive weapons. Because the student eventually uses these weapons against the therapist, this issue is most often brought into clear focus through analysis of transference reactions.

3. It is important that the therapist be less of a shadowy figure or blank screen than he is in traditional psychoanalytic psychotherapy. He should at various times allow the patient to know something of his own beliefs, his values, and his motivations.

4. The therapist must pay strict attention to the misuses of the therapeutic structure. He must be even more concerned with missed hours or late arrivals of the student than he is with adult patients. Student patients often see psychotherapy as the only structure they have in their lives. Failure to impose and enforce time limits puts the therapist in the role of a nebulous figure who stands for nothing.

5. The major problems of the therapist are his impatience and his countertransference reactions. Psychotherapy for alienated students is no longer a brief matter. Favorable results are sometimes not seen for many months or years, during which the psychiatrist is likely to be ingeniously tested. The patient will miss hours, try to use his therapist for obtaining excuses, and will report activities such as stealing or cheating which may offend the therapist's sense of propriety. He will argue with the therapist and show a lack of outward respect, which contrasts sharply with the more worshipful attitude of older patients.

It is difficult at times for any therapist to avoid being jealous of, or enraged by, his alienated student patients. He is dealing with an affluent group that has few responsibilities, many of whom have experienced more sensual pleasures and enjoyed more luxuries than he will ever know. The therapist's problem is to keep countertransference reactions from hurting his patient. He is more likely to succeed in his task if he shares many of his countertransference feelings with his patient. This is an important departure from traditional psychoanalytic technique. At least some of the therapist's jealousy, some of his anger, and even some of his wish to identify with the patient must be voiced at appropriate times during the course of therapy. [*Editorial Note: According to authorities cited in previous issues of Current Psychiatric Therapies, this technique is controversial.*]

6. It is important early in therapy to interview the parents in the presence of the patient. This serves several purposes: It helps to clarify some of the intrafamilial and intrapsychic conflicts that are plaguing the patient, and provides the student with an opportunity to perceive his parents' life styles in a new light. It also reminds the student that he does have a past which con-

tinues to exert an important influence upon his present life. Finally, the family interview can be used to acquaint the parents with the nature of the problem, to set up ground rules for the extent of their communication with the therapist, and — most important — to give them some idea of their own role in the patient's illness.

7. Group therapy, can be helpfully employed as an adjunct to individual therapy. In a group setting the late adolescent has less need to justify himself or passively resist his adult therapist, and is more open to demonstrating different means of relating. Anger denied toward parents cannot be denied when it is turned against a group member. Noninvolvement is more difficult to maintain as a defensive operation. Statements such as "I just want to be left alone, I don't want to bother anybody" begin to take on a more vapid quality as group members interact with one another. After relatively few sessions the more realistic aggressive basis of their withdrawal can be safely acknowledged. Finally, the group does give young people the chance to see themselves as others see them and may provide them with a firmer sense of their own identity.

Some Troubling Questions

Would most alienated students recover from their despondent state if left alone? Are there briefer therapies? How valuable is short-term hospitalization? Are there preventive approaches that the community-oriented psychiatrist could employ?

The first three questions will be only briefly considered. We have no data as to what happens to alienated students who do not become patients. My suspicion is that most of them leave school, but what happens to them afterwards is unknown. Briefer therapy simply does not work. (See preceding editorial note.) Group therapy seems to accelerate the therapeutic process, but many alienated students are unwilling to join groups until they have first had some individual therapy. Short-term hospitalization is useful in treating acute depressions and suicide attempts, but its usefulness is quickly subverted if the patient does not continue therapy when he leaves the hospital.

The question of prevention of alienation is more complex. Preventative psychiatry based on community-oriented approaches arose primarily out of the need to provide for the mental health of the poor. Its techniques and even some of its goals may not be appropriate to treatment of an alienation engendered by affluence and privilege. Efforts to provide better educational opportunities and freedom from the shackles of poverty undoubtedly improve the mental health of the underprivileged, but there is a point at which too much freedom, too much affluence, too much leisure, and even too much psychological mindedness may be pathogenic.

99

One preventive approach, however, seems so appropriate and yet so elusive that it continually tantalizes the community-oriented student psychiatrist: This is to bring more adults into the student's life in a compassionate and realistic manner. If members of university faculties could involve themselves in the problems of students, the opportunities for identification, empathy, and intimacy that students would receive would be immensely therapeutic. But on many of our large campuses the faculty is simply not available to undergraduate students! Publication pressures, research, and commitments to granting agencies leave little time for students or leadership in a community of scholars.

Our universities have tried to fill the gap created by the professors' non-participation by hiring more counselors and more psychiatrists, with the rationale that faculty should teach and do research while professionals take care of the students' emotional needs. The student who wishes to maintain a close relationship with an adult is thereby encouraged to define his need as a psychological problem for a professional. It does not take much sophistication to appreciate that for most students a counselor or psychiatrist is a poor substitute for an interested, dedicated, and available teacher.

One difficult task for the community-oriented student health psychiatrist is constantly to urge university administrators and faculty to examine the psychological consequences that arise when faculty are estranged from students. Academicians do not see themselves as members of caretaking professions. Unlike primary and secondary school teachers and unlike case workers, they are not especially impressed with the validity of psychiatric viewpoints; even if they were impressed, it would not be easy for them to resist the pressures that keep them away from their students. Given the present structure of our large campuses, the psychiatrist who wishes to help alienated students will find his role to be that of a battle surgeon who treats the casualties but not the causes of malignant social processes.

Youthful Offenders in Psychotherapy

by HERMAN P. GLADSTONE, M.D.

OFFENDERS AS PATIENTS

THE DESIGNATION of a group of individuals as "offenders" or, more precisely, "caught offenders" does not immediately bring to mind shared psychiatric problems amenable to treatment.[1] The dispute as to whether criminal behavior can be seen as a psychiatric problem arises partly from a mistaken notion that in so doing, psychiatry identifies itself with the rules and laws of social interaction. It seems antithetic to psychiatric values and goals to "treat" an offender against society with the sole object of having him conform to the rules and laws of society.[2] Psychiatry is interested in studying society's rules, laws and values, but does not necessarily a priori identify itself with all of them. Psychiatry is interested in how individuals meet their real needs in society, what conflicts develop, and what distortions of perceptions and behavioral disorders contribute to reduction of self-fulfillment.

Certain basic principles of psychotherapy may be defined which underlie and guide any modifications of techniques with individuals or particular subgroups of our society. The nidus of this professional treatment method must be identified, learned and applied with a core group of patients before moving any distance peripherally for specialized and exceptional applications. One problem in the development of the psychotherapeutic approach has been the way in which certain laws and rules applicable to the psychoanalytic technique with specific groups of patients limited within certain diagnostic categories and social classes and settings became centrally significant. An inflexible adherence to some of these really peripheral techniques as if they represented basic principles and also the appearance of these techniques on top of a treatment prestige scale tended to delay sophisticated experimentation and widening of the psychotherapeutic approach to a greater range and variety of patients.

Psychotherapy is the planned attempt to ameliorate emotional disorder through the professional relationship. This has involved creating a kind of relationship which is honest, direct, non-manipulative, non-authori-

101

tarian, and which encourages free expression of feelings and a degree of mutual concern. The direction is toward elaborating and understanding the patient's needs, feelings and problems, while the therapist sets aside those personal concerns which originate in his own life. Goals involve reducing barriers to development and fulfillment of potentialities within realistic life conditions. Basic therapeutic values consistently upheld, implicitly or explicitly, include: (1) that it is possible to learn facts about and eventually understand human needs, motivation and behavior; (2) that these inferences may be correlated into a coherent, understandable structure; (3) that it is possible for individuals to change in their perceptions, experiences and consequent behavior, based on sufficient degree of comprehension and understanding; (4) that the alleviation of emotional disorder is a worthwhile endeavor.

Offenders have in common that they have been apprehended for violating some of the more significant rules and laws of interaction in their social world. The notable problem which may be designated as "psychiatric" in an individual who is an "offender" becomes clear-cut if the individual is seen, not as a separate isolated unit, but as part of his society. The problem may be stated as, "I do things which result in negative consequences to me (through the repercussions of others)" and furthermore "I do things which injure or threaten to destroy my relationship with others and my relationship with myself."

The common shared psychiatric problem implied in using the term "offenders" include: (1) an individual with relatively little awareness and understanding of the workings of his society's system of rules and laws; (2) a relatively less direct concern for an interest in other human beings and especially members of his society in positions of authority;[3] (3) more than usual specific immediate short-term needs and wants (such as for prestige, thrills, acceptance, material gains, rebellion) taking precedence over longer term motivating interests;[4] (4) some specific conflicts, fears, repressed feelings, organic problems or family upsets which may often and routinely be dealt with or expressed through antisocial actions; (5) a relative lack of awareness or acknowledgment of the existence of these problems; (6) an absence of interest or motivation to seek help in resolving them.

Where has psychotherapy stood in relation to each of these problems of offenders? Reviewing the items above as presented: (1) a psychotherapeutic relationship functions within the social structure and has its own system of rules and laws; (2) psychotherapy requires some interest and concern between participants; (3) psychotherapy seeks perspective in relation to short-term versus long-term motivations; (4) psychotherapy

102

takes a stand against antisocial acting out; (5) psychotherapy begins with an acknowledgment of the existence of problems; and, (6) psychotherapy requires the development of some motivation in the patients, not only to come, but to work actively.

What can be done about these initial contradictions and wide gaps to bridge? The distinctive problems manifested by offenders as differentiated from the "neurotic" or "schizophrenic" group should be kept in mind. This might suggest applicable ways of bridging the gap between the patient's attitude towards his problems and the professional's approach. Techniques with one patient group may either facilitate or present a barrier toward doing the same with another.[5] Differences in groups must also involve differences in developmental levels. For instance, in psychotherapy with adolescents, a central theme, with variations, is the degree to which any technique strengthens ego functioning and identity.[6]

CLINICAL SETTING AND PROBLEMS*

The author's major experience with therapeutic procedures with youthful offenders was through the opportunity of doing office psychotherapy with offenders on probation. This experience began with the application in toto of psychoanalytically oriented techniques to these youths and, on encountering blockage and failure, attempts at innovation and experimentation with techniques while adhering to more basic principles of psychotherapy. Eleven youths on probation were seen in psychotherapy over a period of 5 years. Forty sessions with a psychiatrist was set up as a requirement of probation. Confidentiality was maintained, and the only information shared with the court concerned progress in completing this requirement. My patients were all boys who were 16 or 17 years old, except for one who was 19. They had been involved in varieties of offenses including breaking and stealing, riding in stolen cars, threatening with a weapon, passing a fraudulent check, unlawful assembly for a gang fight, mugging, stealing from a department store and possession of a switchblade.

These patients were sent for therapy and felt little, if any, motivation of their own. They were suspicious and distrustful of law enforcement agencies and the referral for psychotherapy was one of the objects of their suspicion. Most of them were aware of the punishments possible for their offenses, and many regarded visiting the psychiatrist as the lesser of several evils, to be accepted as any other punishment might be. I began

---

*Portions of the following three sections of this chapter first appeared in my article: A Study of Techniques of Psychotherapy with Youthful Offenders, Psychiatry, 25:147-159, 1962, and are republished with the kind permission of the William Alanson White Psychiatric Foundation.

with the psychoanalytic model in working with these boys, since this represented my training and experience. I thus permitted and encouraged the patient to unfold his feelings in an accepting atmosphere with a minimum of direction, guidance or activity on my part. Some data were gathered with this approach, but little change or movement seemed to occur. In fact, a kind of deadness, repetitiveness and emptiness were noted for the most part in the patients' responses. Although psychodynamic formulations of behavior and antisocial actions could be developed, at termination the patients did not understand any more about themselves and there was no evidence that a change in delinquent behavior or in the nature of the problems had occurred. Follow-up reports after termination indicated that these initial patients were involved in essentially the same delinquent patterns as before therapy.

TECHNIQUES DEVELOPED

Innovations in technique were therefore necessary. Limits, authority and law were seen as potentially significant stimuli to growth when encountered by offenders consistently, rationally and with some sensitivity to individual development.[7,8] A conviction developed that on a deeper level the law enforcement agencies, through the psychiatrist, could in some way become stimuli for positive, rather than destructive, forces.[9] The following technical emphases were therefore developed:

(1) *Keeping the Relationship Alive*[10]

Deadness and boredom were perceived to be antitherapeutic, and holding the patient responsible for this tended to widen the gap between therapist and patient. The only alternative appeared to be for the therapist to take responsibility for this state of affairs and to counter it in various ways. One method was to include in the interaction his own personal views and reactions. Thus, freer expression of viewpoints, preferences and idiosyncrasies was made part of the therapist's communication. Also helpful here was to move with the patient into stimulating and interesting areas regardless of whether the content material appeared "therapeutic." The experience of aliveness together, if attained, would seem itself to be significantly therapeutic. The following example is illustrative:

> One youth was particularly suspicious and distrustful of the therapist from the beginning, had no interest in communicating anything, and considered coming a complete waste of time. During the first meeting he offered to make a "deal" with the therapist whereby visits would be reported to the court without their actually taking place, since both the therapist and patient could use the time to better advantage. In

subsequent sessions he would cut off inquiries about his experience and feelings, usually before he became involved, so that the relationship began to be characterized by its emptiness and formality. Thus, the patient's cynical attitude about all aspects of life seemed to him again to be justified in view of his relationship with the therapist. After several sterile sessions, the therapist learned that this boy read the newspapers each day with some interest and played out his cynical, distrustful, angry feelings in relation to the news stories. The patient was encouraged to talk about news events, and when the therapist began expressing his personal reactions to them, a distinctly alive interchange would follow which the patient did not cut off. Mutual participation increased, and free discussion of newspaper articles became a mutually rewarding experience in which real communication occurred. Not only could reactions to news events and the people involved in these events become available for therapeutic understanding, but also the type of relationship which was being established allowed for movement into areas previously avoided.

During one session, after indicating that nothing was happening in his life, the patient mentioned that he'd just read in the papers that a certain movie star was "cracking up" because he had been drinking too much. The therapist told him something he knew about alcoholism and the patient seemed interested. Then the therapist brought up the case of a baseball player who had had an emotional breakdown, about whom there had been a motion picture. The patient asked for more details about the picture and then mentioned some unusual behavior ascribed to a current baseball star, wondering if that indicated that he, also, was going to "crack up." The therapist expressed his opinion on understanding that kind of behavior, and the boy did too. This led later in the session to a discussion about what underlies various types of behavior in others and in the patient himself. It soon became evident that no matter what was discussed in this area of his apparent interest, whether competition with the Russians, political corruption, or events in the lives of famous people, his original role of objective observer would turn into that of subjective participant when the therapist actively joined in.

(2) *Stimulating the Patient's Interest in Himself, His Development and His Problems*[11]

The loosening up of communication raised the question as to what would stimulate the patient's interest to the point of seeing his relationship with the therapist as a way of discovering something useful about himself. The therapist thus began to make active attempts to bring to the fore some aspect of the patient's immediate problems or his immediate developmental level which might catch the patient's interest. If this happened, an alive interchange related to a therapeutic goal would occur. The initial interest might be called "a handle for therapeutic relatedness."

The kinds of things about which these youths could initially have some concern were immediate concrete experiences—for example, something related to the offense or possible repetition of the offense, problems with friends, difficulties with work, problems in developing a relationship with a girl friend, etc. One area which could often stimulate interest was the narrow and boring life pattern of the offender and the way in which he himself inadvertently cut off possibilities for widening his experience. It was seen that some of the antisocial acts mainly represented attempts to make life more interesting and overcome boredom. Where this kind of acting out was identified, the self-defeating and self-destructive aspects of finding excitement in this way were pointed out. At the same time the therapist expressed his feelings that there were other ways of finding such excitement without threatening the continuation of the process of development itself. An example of stimulation of a patient's interest in therapeutic investigation follows:

One youth, who was mainly answering questions but not participating, was for several sessions repeatedly posed the question, "Is there anything that others do or that you do which you don't understand?" He at first denied that there was any behavior of that sort and maintained that people have and know the reasons for everything they do. However, the repeated question seemed to "catch" his interest in a way in which other questions had not. Finally, early in one interview, he mentioned that he had been thinking of the question that the therapist had been asking. Although at that moment he couldn't recall the question, he did remember an answer he had thought of. The therapist reminded him of the question, and in an evidently pleased way the patient related that when he was playing ball with other fellows and someone missed an easy catch, some of the boys would get angry whereas others wouldn't. He wondered why they reacted differently, and he decided that it was because the ones who got angry were better players, and felt that if they could make the catch, then the other fellow should too. The therapist affirmed that this was really an example of what he was asking about, to which the patient responded with evident satisfaction. He then demonstrated that he could think of several more examples. The therapist told him at the end of this session that he certainly had the idea, then asked if he could think of something of this sort that had happened to him. Early in the next session, when things went dead, the therapist again asked this question and then the patient related an experience which had occurred when he was with a group of boys. When these boys indicated that they wanted something in a store, he stole it and gave it to them. He couldn't understand just why he had done that, since he hadn't wanted the stolen article himself. For the rest of this session and the next one, he recounted significant incidents of this sort which had occurred at various times during his life.

106

(3) *Communicating Concern about Basic Human Values*[12]

This was an area where, clearly, absence of response tended to support a pattern or problem and responding tended to interrupt it. Any contact on value issues could be an initial movement in the direction of eventual change. Thus the therapist was alert to the patient's inappropriate lack of human concern and responded with his own feelings at such moments. The therapist's expression of sensitivity toward disregard for human values was especially communicable when these patients were reacting to relationships with their peers.

Since sensitivity to human values also underlies the psychotherapeutic approach, the patient was encountering certain new dimensions necessary not only for living, but also for continuing the therapeutic relationship. This approach often had to do with recognizing what constituted the patient's concern, interest and respect for human factors in himself and in others under varying circumstances. An example will demonstrate therapeutic work in this area:

> One boy was talking with bravado about the ways in which, when he was bored, he liked to do something risky and illegal, even if he endangered himself. The therapist asked, with evident concern, whether it made any difference to him whom else he endangered. The patient said that it never made any difference. The therapist then mentioned certain people about whom this patient had begun to have feelings, and asked whether it would make any difference if their lives were in danger. After some hesitation, the patient admitted that it would. By continuing to bring such value issues to the fore, it was possible to expand this beginning concern about people for whom he cared to include people he had never met but about whom others probably cared.
>
> Another time values were communicated to this patient was when he talked in an unconcerned way of someone's dying, even though the person involved was someone for whom he might have had some positive feelings. In each such instance, the therapist expressed his sentiments about the seriousness and meaning of death, and made an effort to bring out any feelings the patient might have had for the dead or dying person. For instance, the patient showed an initial lack of concern in telling about his grandfather who was dying of cancer. The therapist's responses and questioning stimulated the patient to remember warm experiences he had shared with this man in earlier years. He subsequently began showing feelings of compassion when speaking of his grandfather.

(4) *Provoking Interest in Varieties of Consequences of Actions*[13]

The therapist attempted to focus on those kinds of reality testing which would bring actions and consequences closer together, especially self-destructive consequences of actions which a delinquent had always associated with immediate gain. Stimulation of concurrent consideration of both immediate and delayed consequences was helpful for increasing awareness of self-destructive results. For some boys the initially most striking aspect of this consideration was that preoccupation with immediate results even interfered with some of their long-term *antisocial* goals. This could then be followed by a further investigation of how their immediate and long-term needs were fulfilled by these antisocial goals. A clinical experience will illustrate this approach:

One boy seemed to be living suspended in a vacuum. He was spending most of his time lounging on certain street corners in his neighborhood. He was particularly vulnerable to becoming involved in any sort of activity which might give him a "thrill," legal or illegal, but especially illegal. After this boy felt moderately free with the therapist, he began to complain about the boredom of his everyday life and the overroutineness of what he saw as the usual activities open to him. The therapist undertook to work through with the patient in some detail the eventual consequences to himself of one or another type of risky illegal action, and, after a while, the patient experienced some discrimination in this regard. His awareness of this dimension of his behavior became sensitive enough so that soon the therapist could introduce alternative possibilities which fulfilled the boy's criteria for interests, without being illegal or having potentially serious consequences for him. At times when the therapist felt he was really engaged with and related to this patient, he felt free to make a direct value appeal to him— "what are you doing to yourself?"—as a parent might do at the right moment. That this patient was affected by these reactions of the therapist was evidenced by changes in behavior which took place soon after, such as his announcing to the therapist that he had re-entered school, this time to work seriously.

Results

Encouraging and hopeful improvements were noted in patients treated according to these transactive approaches, as compared with patients treated predominantly according to approaches following the usual psychoanalytic model. Evaluation came from follow-up reviews of probation reports as well as from observations of what was happening toward the end of therapy. Significant areas of comparison included degree of resolution of self-destructive conflicts with family and society, reduction of antisocial activity and progress in pursuit of education and life goals. An interesting finding was that for those patients with whom these dynamic techniques were used but who did not improve, the main barrier to improvement appeared to be the absence of a continuing significant outside relationship with a member of the family or parent surrogate. Improvement seemed to require such care and participation by an interested party with a longer term relationship to the patient than that of the therapist.[14,15]

REFERENCES

1. BRODY, S.: Community therapy of child delinquents. In J. H. Masserman, Ed.: Current Psychiatric Therapies, Vol. 3. New York, Grune and Stratton, 1963.
2. HALLECK, S. L.: The criminal's problem with psychiatry. Psychiatry, 23:409-412, 1960.
3. FRIGNITO, N. G., AND ORCHINIK, C. W.: The therapy of adolescent offenders. In J. H. Masserman, Ed.: Curent Psychiatric Therapies, Vol. 3. New York, Grune and Stratton, 1963.
4. PETRIE, A., McCULLOCH, R., AND KAZDIN, P.: The perceptual characteristics of juvenile delinquents. J. Nerv. & Ment. Dis., 134:415-421, 1962.
5. FRIEDLANDER, K.: The Psycho-Analytical Approach to Juvenile Delinquency. New York, Internat. Univ. Press, 1947.
6. REDL, F., AND WINEMAN, D.: Controls from Within: Techniques for the Treatment of the Aggressive Child. Glencoe, Ill., Free Press, 1952.
7. COHEN, R. E., AND GRINSPOON, L.: Limit setting as a corrective experience. Arch. Gen. Psychiat., 8:74-79, 1963.
8. LEVENTHAL, T., AND SILLS, M. R.: The issue of control in therapy with character problem adolescents. Psychiatry, 26:149-167, 1963.
9. PATTERSON, V., HARRIS, M. R., AND BEWLEY, W.: Captive outpatients: a psychotherapy program for parolees. In J. H. Masserman, Ed.: Current Psychiatric Therapies, Vol. 2. New York, Grune and Stratton, 1962.
10. EISSLER, K. R.: General problems of delinquency. In K. R. Eissler, Ed.: Searchlights on Delinquency. New York, Internat. Univ. Press, 1949.
11. OCHROCH, R.: Special difficulties in working with adolescent offenders. J. Assoc. Psychiat. Treat. Offenders, 3: Nos. 1 and 2, 1959.
12. CHWAST, J.: Value conflicts in treating delinquents. Children, 6:95-100, 1959.
13. SCHMIDEBERG, M.: Treating the unwilling patient. Brit. J. Delinquency, 9:117-122, 1959.
14. HEALY, W., AND BRONNER, A.: New Light On Delinquency and Its Treatment. New Haven, Yale Univ. Press, 1936.
15. BRUCH, H.: Activity in the psychotherapeutic process. In J. H. Masserman, Ed.: Current Psychiatric Therapies, Vol. 2. New York, Grune and Stratton, 1963.

PART IV

THERAPY
OF
ADULTS

Present Trends in Psychoanalytic Therapy

by SANDOR LORAND, M.D.

D URING THE PAST 30 years psychoanalytic rationale about therapy and the technical handling of patients has changed considerably. In 1945 I wrote, "before the 1920's analysis was more of an intellectual process and the emotional content of the transference situation was not analyzed. With preconceived ideas in mind, based on theoretical knowledge, the unconscious was investigated with a view to uncovering what the analyst presupposed to be there. The principles of technique were applied, not as the need arose, or according to the personality and flexibility of the therapist, but in accordance with a basic rule to interpret the unconscious. The technique was at times a hit and miss proposition with little or no elasticity in the application of technical rules."[39]

Freud originally defined psychoanalysis as mainly applicable to "the transference-neuroses, phobias, hysterias, obsessional neuroses, and besides these such abnormalities of character as have been developed instead of these diseases. Everything other than these, such as narcissistic and psychotic conditions is more or less unsuitable."[19] Since then, however, various reformulations and revisions have influenced the therapeutic interest, trends and clinical evaluation in analyses. Our outlook and evaluation of therapy were the direct results of a revised interest in ego psychology. Analysts with wide therapeutic experiences in somewhat different approaches tried out and added innovations, modifications to our therapeutic armamentarium in treating the borderline neuroses, cases with ego weaknesses, perversions, etc. New elaborations of the entire method were added based on clinical findings and experiences and we all make use directly or indirectly of these new technical approaches. But nearly all publications in the field maintained that the basic principles of the technique of psychoanalytic therapy, as initiated by Freud, remain valid today. Having been derived from his clinical experiences, they remain the fundamental guide in analytic therapy, although later elaborated and modified. Much attention is now given to preoedipal stages and the entire problem of early object relationships, with emphasis

113

on their relationship to the therapy of borderline neuroses, perversions, etc. These investigations made it possible to evaluate for therapeutic purposes patients who were considered not amenable for analysis.

Ego psychology also helped us gain deeper insights into the pathology of character neurosis, perversions, moral masochisms and schizophrenic regressions, and added to our better evaluation and therapeutic management of these cases. As Anna Freud wrote, . . . "the investigation of the id and its mode of operation was always only a means to an end and the end was invariably the same correction of abnormalities and the restoration of the ego with its integrity."[16] This followed Freud's earlier statement: "The quantitative factor of instinctual strength in the past opposed the efforts of the patient's ego to defend itself, and now that analysis has been called in to help, that same factor sets a limit to the efficacy of this new attempt. If the instincts are excessively strong the ego fails in its task . . . we shall achieve our therapeutic purpose only when we can give a greater measure of analytic help to the patient's ego."[17] This does not have to be taken as the ego having priority over everything else in analytic therapy, but it emphasizes the reaction of the ego to unconscious processes. All resistances, whether of the ego, superego, or id, are in the center of our therapeutic approach and have to be dealt with equally and constantly.

In the therapeutic relationships we try to strengthen the ego, but the more we can explore the earliest stages of ego development, the more fundamental factors we understand from early object relationship, the better we will be able to help the patient re-experience early frustrations and his patterns of reaction, which are then repeated in the transference relationship.

To establish a transference with patients who, as a result of early disturbances in object relationship acquired in severe neuroses with ego weakness, defects and deep regression, the analyst has to approach therapy with a special attitude. Freud referred to this when he wrote, "The ego has been weakened by the internal conflict; we must come to its aid. The position is like a civil war which can only be decided by the help of an ally from without. The analytical physician and the weakened ego of the patient, basing themselves upon the real external world, are to combine against the enemies, the instinctual demands of the id, and the moral demands of the super-ego. We form a pact with each other. The patient's sick ego promises us the most complete candor, promises, that is, to put at our disposal all of the material which his self-perception provides; we, on the other hand, assure him of the strictest discretion and put at his service our experience in interpreting material that has been influenced by the unconscious. Our knowledge shall compensate for his ignorance and shall give his ego once more mastery over the lost provinces of his mental life. This pact constitutes the analytic situation."[18]

But coming to the aid of the ego implies a number of difficulties. The patient whose object relationship in early childhood were bad, may try to maintain this bad relationship with the analyst. To prepare the groundwork for analytic therapy, the transference has first to be developed by making interpretations to the patient acceptable and well enough tolerated so as not to increase his defences.

How to reduce regression, when to stop it, when to encourage it and to what degree, is a permanent problem during the therapy. In order to undo the harm done to his ego development by his early environment, we must surmount constantly negative therapeutic reactions in the early phases of therapy. In later periods of analysis the patient's transference demands may become so violent that they demand constant attention.

The variety of opinions expressed about the theoretical as well as technical aspects of regression, give it an important place in current psychoanalytic therapy. One has to be more active in order to further the relationship with the patient and sometimes a preanalytical period is necessary to strengthen the patient's ego and help create a transference relationship.

The therapeutic management of such patients necessitates modifications and deviations of the classical psychoanalytic approach. Sometimes devices which would be called not strictly psychoanalytic are used. In furthering therapeutic success we have to change our attitudes to suit the patients' behavior. They are prone to acting out frequently in the analytical situation, which again imposes special difficulties and tolerance on the analyst. In this connection Glover stated: "Even in so-called classical analysis of the psychoneurosis, the approach of different analysts varies not only in numerous points of detail but also in many important points of policy[22] [p. 165. techniques of greater activity were adopted] due, respectively, to unsatisfactory results and to widespread feeling among analysts that analytic therapy must be speeded up."[22] (p. 166.) Glover then reminds us that long before the issue of active treatment became controversial, the technique of psychoanalysis came to include new measures of "active type." One was in the nature of a prohibition, i.e., that analysis should be carried out in a state of abstinence; the other was the positive injunction that certain cases suffering from phobias should at certain times begin to face rather than avoid situations which induce anxiety.

We accept the fact that we cannot analyze all patients the same way, and within the basic framework of established methods we have to

115

alter our therapeutic technique. It is nearly impossible for an entire analysis to be completed without the analyst at some time interfering with the patient's acting out in his social relationship and perhaps business affairs, and also in his pleasure-seeking tendencies. The therapist must manipulate the transference, dose interpretation and help the patient in an extra-analytical way. All this activity is utilized to deal with the patient's resistance and to promote analysis.[47] Again to quote Glover: "It should therefore be our object to reinforce those parts of the ego which are less affected by guilt processes and through which the patient's capacity for positive contact can be increased. The same policy should be followed when encouraging the patient to make decisions regarding his life and work which owing to a feeling of inertia he is unable to make himself."[22] (p. 241.)

Therapy, then, begins with giving some support directly to the patient to help him tolerate and cope with his daily conflicts and current difficulties. We do not attempt reconstruction or interpretation—instead we guide the patient in his everyday contacts. We then may make some inroad and modify the rigidity and resistance of the patient. Thus a transference relationship will slowly be established.

Deviation from regular procedures may be based on the personality and temperament of the analyst and yet achieve a degree of success. But deviation from classical technique should not be based on the analyst's personality and temperament alone if it is to have success in the long run. Obviously it may be connected with and have implications for the analyst's countertransference, but when it is too obviously so, results are invariably bad. What is going on in a given case must be understood apart from personal, subjective feelings on the matter. Active measures always derive out of the analyst's objectivity and understanding, and indicate empathy with his patient. Tactful application of active measures and manipulations of them will put more demands on the analyst's tolerance, elasticity and objectivity. Manipulations arising out of the analyst's countertransference imperfections, will have their effect on the therapy and its results. The post-Freudian expansion of ego psychoanalysis enriched and widened our technique of psychoanalytic therapy and placed strong emphasis not only on technical methods but also on deeper clinical investigations of technical problems in psychoanalysis.

REFERENCES

1. ALEXANDER, F.: Development of the Ego Psychology. Psychoanalysis Today, ed. Sandor Lorand. New York, International Universities Press, 1950.
2. ——: Fundamental of Psychoanalysis. London, Allen and Unwin; New York, W. W. Norton & Co., Inc., 1949.

3. ARLOW, J.: Sublimation: panel report at midwinter meeting 1954. J. Am. Psychoanal. A., 3:515, 1955.
4. BALINT, M.: The final goal of psychoanalytic therapy. Int. J. Psychoanal., 18:206, 1936.
5. ——, FAIRBAIRN, FOULKES, AND SUTHERLAND: Criticism of Fairbairn's generalisation about object relations. Brit. J. Phil. Sc., 7:——, 1957.
6. BRIERLEY, M.: Trends in Psychoanalysis. London, Hogarth Press, 1951.
7. EISSLER, E. R.: Searchlights on Delinquency. New York, Inter. Univer. Press, 1949.
8. FAIRBAIRN, W.: Endopsychic structure considered in terms of object-relationships. Psycho. Quart., 5:541, 1946.
9. ——: Obect-relationships and dynamic structure. Int. J. Psychoanal., 17:30, 1946.
10. FENICHEL, O.: Identification (1926). The Collected Papers of Otto Fenichel, First Series. New York, W, W. Norton & Co., Inc., 1953.
11. FERENCZI, S.: The Further Development of the Active Therapy in Psychoanalysis (1921). Further Contributions to Psychoanalysis. London, Hogarth Press, 1950.
12. ——: Contra-Indications to the 'Active' Psychoanalytical Technique (1926). Further Contributions to Psychoanalysis. London, Hogarth Press, 1950.
13. ——: The Elasticity of Psycho-Analytical Technique (1928). Further Contributions to Psychoanalysis. London, Hogarth Press, 1950.
14. ——: The Future Development of the Active Therapy in Psychoanalysis (1921). Further Contributions to Psychoanalysis. London, Hogarth Press, 1950.
15. —FREUD, A.: Ego and the Mechanisms of Defense. London, Hogarth Press, 1936, p. 4.
16. FREUD, S.: Analysis Terminable and Interminable. Collected Papers V, pp. 331-332.
17. ——: An Outline of Psychoanalysis. Trans. James Strachey. New York, W. W. Norton & Colk, Inc., 1949, pp. 62-63.
18. ——: New Introductory Lectures on Psychoanalysis. New York, W. W. Norton & Co., Inc., 1933, p. 212.
19. GITELSON, M.: On ego distortion. Int. J. Psychoanal. 39:245, 1958.
20. GREENACRE, P.: Problems of infantile neurosis: A discussion. Psycho. Study Child, 9:16-71, 1954.
21. ——: Trauma, Growth and Personality. New York, W. W. Norton and Co., Inc., 1952.
22. GLOVER, E.: The Technique of Psychoanalysis. New York, Inter. Univer. Press, 1955.
23. GUNTRIP, H.: Recent developments in psychoanalytical theory. Brit. J. M. Psychology, 29:82, 1956.
24. ——: Ego weakness and the hard core of the problem of psychotherapy. Brit. J. M. Psychology, 33:163, 1960.
25. HARTMANN, H.: The mutual influences in the development of ego and id. Psychoanal. Study Child, 7:9, 1952.
26. ——, AND HEINZ, AND KRIS: The genetic approach in psychoanalysis. Psychoanal. Study Child, 1:11, 1945.
27. ——, KRIS, AND LOEWENSTEIN: Comments on the formation of psychic structure. Psychoanal. Study Child, 2:11, 1946.

117

28. Hoffer, W.: Mouth, hand, and ego-integration. Psychoanal. Study Child, 3-4:49, 1949.
29. Katan, M.: Contribution to the panel on ego distortion (as-if and pseudo as-if). Int. J. Psychoanal, 39:265, 1958.
30. Khan, M. R.: Dream psychology and the evolution of the psychoanalytic situation. Int. J. Psychoanal., 63:21, 1962.
31. ———: Regression and integration in the analytic setting. Int. J. Psychoanal., 61:130, 1960.
32. Kubie, L. S.: Problems and Techniques of Psychoanalysis: Validation and Progress. Psychoanalysis as a Science, ed. E. Pumpian-Mindlin. Stanford, Calif., Stanford University Press, 1952.
33. Lorand, S.: Comments on the Correlation of Theory and Technique (1948). Clinical Studies in Psychoanalysis. New York, Inter. Univer. Press, 1950.
34. ———: On regression: technical and theoretical problems. Tokyo J. Psychoanal., 19:2, 1961.
35. ———: (Ed.): Psychoanalysis Today. London, Allen and Unwin; New York, Inter. Univer. Press, 1950.
36. ———: Psychoanalytic therapy of religious devotees. Int. J. Psychoanal., 63: P. 1, 1962.
37. ———: Technique of Psychoanalytic Therapy. New York, Inter. Univer. Press, 1946.
38. Peto, A.: Infant and mother: observations on object relations in early infancy, (1936). Int. J. Psychoanal., 30:260, 1949.
39. Spitz, R. A.: Relevancy of direct infant observation. Psychoanal. Study Child, 5:66, 1950.
40. Stone, L.: The Psychoanalytic Situation. New York, Int. Univer. Press, 1961.
41. ———: The widening scope of indications for psychoanalysis. J. Am. Psychoanal. A., 2:567, 1954.
42. Szasz, T. S.: On the theory of psychoanalytic treatment. Int. J. Psychoanal., 38: A., Parts 3-4, p. 166, 1957.
43. Winnicott, D. W.: Collected Papers: Through Paediatrics to Psychoanalysis. London, Tavistock Publications; New York, Basic Books, Inc., 1958.
44. ———: The Child and the Family. London, Tavistock Publications; New York, Basic Books, Inc., 1957.

Freedom in Analytic Therapy

by IAN ALGER, M.D.

S INCE TWO PEOPLE are involved in the analytic relationship it would seem only sensible to find out how freely each of them is able to express himself in the therapy sessions. Freedom of expression between these two participants is desirable and conducive to the growth of one or perhaps both. Traditionally there has been a difference in the role definitions. Patients have been urged and expected to express freely their thoughts and feelings. One of the justifications for the couch has been the claim that it encourages the flow of free associations, partly by allowing the patient to concentrate on inner processes without the distractions of the analyst's presence. The analyst has assumed traditionally an "objective" pose, somewhat detached, but interested, and professionally helpful. Analytic procedure in practice may be different than in theory; in actual therapy the analyst as a human often emerges.

The traditional analytic situation is basically an authoritarian one, and no matter how benign, does not encourage freedom. This authoritarian structure makes some sense when the therapeutic activity is defined as the helper giving assistance to the seeker of help. It is in the traditional medical model, and having the "patient" recline, with head lower than the doctor's is most consistent; the focus of the analytic work is on the patient's "problems". Reactions of the patient to the therapist and to the therapeutic situation are seen as important, but are explained as projections and transferences, and the distorted, aspects of the patient's reactions are emphasized. Reactions of the analyst, in turn, may be dealt with by the analyst privately as countertransference distortions or problems of his own.

Newer theories of human behavior, including contextual analysis and theories of communication field and kinesics, place greater emphasis on the importance of understanding an individual's current behavior, not just in terms of past experience, but also in terms of the present context, and the multiple levels and modes of communication. The relationship of the analyst and patient and the complex communication between them is understood as the most crucial data in the therapy, and only in understanding the context in which other material about a person's life is presented can that other material be validly comprehended.

If the analyst is going to work in this newer framework he will include his own behavior and personal reactions in the exchange he has with his patient, and the degree to which he can be direct and open in communicating this information will determine the freedom of his expression in the therapy. The corollary of this is that the patient will include his feelings and reactions in the same way, and indeed will be encouraged to be more free in this way himself by the example of the analyst. Both participants must take more risk as persons because they are revealing and acknowledging intimate human reactions. This relationship requires not only trust in the other, but more importantly trust in oneself, and recognition of one's human frailties, and reactions. This human approach of one person to another overrides the standard role assignments. Even though the analyst has certain skills which still give him insight, the patient has unique capacities to include personal material to which only he has access. Certainly the consideration of the realities of the patient's past and present life, and dreams and hopes for the future is pertinent, but therapy is basically an encounter between two very human beings.

Communication can be classed in three categories: (1) objective data, at varying levels of abstraction, often using language, but not exclusively; (2) meta-communication or communication which is about or modifies other communication, such as instructions to the receiver which help him understand the significance of messages; and (3) para-communication which designates messages which define the sender, such as indications of background, status, or current mood. All are used by participants in a relationship continually to define and redefine its current nature. With these methods communications are more free, direct, and open, there is less contradiction and double-binding. Thus the traditional authoritarian model of therapy will shift to a more equalitarian encounter.

Much of therapy is not verbal, but communicated by the setting, (including furniture and lighting) by the dress and address of the therapist, and by the rules set forth in regard to time and money. The therapist becomes as bound by the standard and accepted practices as the patients, but when the therapist changes traditions, both participants can experience new freedom of expression. Because of the usual hierarchical authoritarian structure, any changes will most likely be in the direction of a peer relationship.

I no longer ask patients to use the couch. A bolster pillow used as a backrest can be moved for a pillow if someone does want to lie down. I have one chair in the office which is larger than any of the others (traditional analyst-authority chair), but also I have two other chairs in the office and at times sit in one of those. When I moved to my present office several years ago I brought a Lawson couch which had been in my former waiting-room. It wouldn't fit into the new waiting-room, so I put it in my office. Now I have two couches and three chairs.

Shortly after I moved, a woman who was sitting on the Lawson couch began to cry. On similar occasions in the past I had wanted to move towards someone who was crying, but the usual furniture arrangement did not allow much freedom. When a patient is reclining on the couch it is awkward to sit beside him (and with such a situation the medical doctor might revert to an impulse to take the patient's pulse). With the new arrangement I found it easy and comfortable to move over and sit beside the woman on the couch. This position of side-by-side seating also reflects more the collaborative, peer quality of relationship, than the across-the-desk or behind-the-couch authority positions.

This expanded seating arrangement has also led to more movement. I sit in different places with different patients or with the same patient at different times, and the patients also change the places they sit. There is more sprawling at times, and there is much more change of position during hours. Patients and I feel freer to stand or move about. At times one or both of us has felt free to sit on the floor. A new patient talked in the first session about her feelings of constriction during some previous therapy, and her fear of her former analyst. I suggested she might like to sit on the floor with me while we talked about it. She immediately did. She kept looking down, and I asked her how it felt to look directly at me. She said that she felt uncomfortable when we both seemed so much at the same level. She moved back a little until she found a comfortable space between us, and then did look at me. Later she reported that from that time she was more able to look at people in other situations, and also found that she was able to change her position in situations where she previously had felt frozen.

The freedom of movement has led some patients to suggest that we go for a walk during some hours, and we have. Occasionally a patient and I have spent the hour in a nearby coffee-shop. Both the patients and I feel much less formal and constricted, and the definition of our relationship as persons has shifted markedly.

When I first mentioned the setting as defining the relationship, I also noted that rules about time and money play an equally significant part. These rules too need not be inflexible. On occasion when a patient is intensively involved at the end of his hour, I have gone to the waiting-room and asked the next patient if he would be willing to postpone his appointment so I could continue with the person I was with. Often there is agreement, and indeed patients have told me that it made them feel good that they could give something to the other person, and also they felt that if

121

they sometime felt the need, the same possibility would be open for them. In one instance the woman who was waiting said that she had something very important to deal with, and she herself suggested that she go out for a cup of coffee for half her time and then return. I believe that my willingness to break the time stricture encouraged her willingness to break the rigidity of her self-centeredness which was a more usual kind of reaction on her part.

Surprisingly money rules can on occasion be bent as well. During the course of one session I reacted to a rather covertly blaming statement from one man by becoming depressed. I stopped participating actively and grew increasingly sulky for about 20 minutes. I realized finally how I was behaving and began to tell the man about my depressed and angry feelings. He at first responded angrily, and then we came to understand more and more about our reciprocal effect on each other. When the hour ended I felt embarrassed, and told him that I thought we should schedule another time because I didn't want to charge him for that hour. He asked why, and I replied that I felt I was the one who had gained from the session. In a kind way he explained to me that this was what therapy was all about; we both gained from the experience, and of course he expected to pay me for the time.

One of the strongest of the unwritten analytic rules does not have to do with the matters of setting, time or money, but rather with the prohibition against the analyst openly sharing his personal emotional reactions with the patient. The non-professional and the non-therapeutic effects of such openness is often cited as reason for suppressing such "acting-out", and it is recommended that these "counter-transference" reactions be worked through. In such reasoning the importance of the patient's becoming aware of the actual human qualities of the analyst as another person, with failings and conflicts as well as strengths and successes, is missed. In an opening session a woman finally looked up at me in an apparent mixture of anguished, embarrassment and apology, and turning over her hands confessed, "My palms are sweating." I turned over my hands, and said to her, "Mine are too". She let out a sigh and said, "I feel so much better. Then you're human too! I thought analysts didn't have feelings, that they were all analyzed." From that time I felt we had made contact as two people. We were able to begin to understand better the way we had been operating before; she had seen me as a frightening figure, and I had thought of her as having some power to judge me by virtue of her responses in therapy.

Another example of openness in revealing reactions had to do with my lateness for an appointment. The patient was a young man in his twenties who was scheduled for the final hour in the afternoon. All day I had been running about ten minutes late, but before his session I took another phone call, spoke to my secretary and went into the kitchen for a Coke. The result was a twenty-five minute delay in starting the session. He was furious at me, and told me directly that he was angry and if he had any self-esteem he would have walked out 15 minutes ago. He then spoke to me more quietly, and said that he really thought that I was not taking him into consideration, thinking of the pains he had taken to come on time, or realizing that he might have other appointments later. At first I felt quite stiff and defensive, especially since I recognized the justification in his complaint and indictment. I told him I felt he was very justified in his feeling and that I could understand his anger. He only seemed more enraged and frustrated. I then said that I felt uneasy, anxious, and cornered; I had felt increasingly tired during the afternoon and dreaded the last hour. I had wished that I didn't have to work more that day, but had felt an obligation to complete the schedule and to see him since he had come all the way to see me. Instead of being in touch with those feelings at the time and telling him directly about my dilemma, I had communicated it to him indirectly. I finished by telling him I felt sorry now for his discomfort and inconvenience. He reacted by saying that he had missed considering how I might be feeling. He realized he had been hurt and furious when he had yelled at me. Further, if I wasn't there next week right on time, he was warning me that he was walking out! I told him that if I was late he had the alternative of walking out. This did not give him full relief because, although he would be showing me he could take independent action, he also would be losing the time together, which was important to him. He said that he knew he had trouble seeing me as human, and seeing that I could do inconsiderate things; he saw now that I had hang-ups too. As he left he turned and smiled, "If you're late next week, I'll wait a while".

The use of videotape playback in therapy sessions has been of value in helping me become more aware of my personal reactions, and more directly to confirm their presence to the patient. A recording of one session was being played back to a patient. It showed the two of us sitting beside each other. He was talking, and I looked distracted and apathetic. He asked that the videotape be stopped, and said "You look as if you were bored and far away." I had been surprised myself to see how bored I appeared, because at the time I had been unaware of it. Now as I watched the picture I became aware of the very dull, apathetic feeling I had experienced as he had been talking in a monotonous tone. At the time of the actual incident, I had not found a way to interrupt and had avoided a direct challenge to him, although I had earlier been unaware of this avoidance. I now turned to the patient saying that I knew I had been bored, and acted aloof and detached. He looked somewhat taken aback and tears came to his eyes. In a few moments he said, " You know, I'm really touched. I just don't expect anyone to affirm something like that, and I've gotten used to sealing over the feeling of hurt I get."

A psychiatrist asked recently, "You have been talking about openness of expression. Suppose you have an attractive woman patient who tells you she is sexually attracted to you, and wants to know if you feel that way about her. And you do. What do you tell her?"

In answer I said, "I'd tell her that she was a very attractive gal, she was sexy, and I really went for her." I went on to say that she already would know of your attraction whether you told her or not, so it was very important to acknowledge your feelings in order to maintain an open relationship. When the feelings are acknowledged it then is easier to look together at the way sex has been used possibly in a flirtatious and competitive way, and how it may have been used to avoid the development of a human relationship with close personal involvement.

Direct Psychoanalysis

by JOHN N. ROSEN, M.D.

D IRECT PSYCHOANALYSIS is a method of psychotherapy based upon
the discoveries of Freud. Although it was originally developed for
the treatment of psychotic individuals, it has also been used successfully
with individuals who were neurotic rather than psychotic.

Essentially, direct psychoanalysis is a psychiatric recreation and revision
of the individual's relationship with his early maternal environment. We
regard this environment as being pre-eminently influential in the psychosexual development of every individual. For some, it is a beneficent
"mother" which can be incorporated and assimilated comfortably; for
others, it is a malevolent "mother" which may never be "digestible" in
the psychological sense. According to our theory, psychosis is a regression
to pregenital, neoinfantile experience, in which the individual seeks hallucinatory or symbolic representations of the indispensable but deadly
"mother he knew." Neurosis is a less drastic, less regressive attempt to find
substitutes for the original "mother" and early maternal environment.
Both the psychotic and the neurotic individual tend to project the original
"maternal" qualities upon current environmental objects, either animate
or inanimate. This tendency is related to the phenomena of transference
and repetition-compulsion which Freud observed.[1]

Unlike a conventional psychoanalyst, the direct psychoanalyst accepts
the parental role which is thrust upon him, in treatment, by the psychotic
or neurotic individual. The direct psychoanalyst serves as a kind of psychiatric "foster-parent," in the sense that "foster" as defined in Webster's
Dictionary means one who feeds or nourishes; he "nourishes" the psyche
of the individual whom he is treating. This therapeutic responsibility has
been formulated as the "governing principle" of direct psychoanalysis:
the psychiatrist must be a loving, omnipotent protector and provider for

the patient. With a psychotic, he must act like an idealized parent who now has the responsibility of bringing up this neoinfantile individual all over again.[2] With a neurotic, or with an individual who has recovered from psychosis but is still "neoneurotic," the direct psychoanalyst must function parentally to guide the individual towards maturity and independence. Although there is no "governing principle" of conventional psychoanalysis, for purposes of comparison Freud and his associates specified that the psychoanalyst conventionally functions as a "mirror,"[3] or as "a blank page on which the patient can inscribe his transference-fantasies."[4] This emphasis upon impersonality and non-involvement suggests a fundamental difference between conventional psychoanalysis and direct psychoanalysis. Conventional psychoanalysis is a method of *research,* while direct psychoanalysis is a method of *treatment.* As Franz Alexander pointed out in a recent paper, "Freud never changed his view that remembering of repressed traumatic situations is the ultimate goal."[5] In direct psychoanalysis, we find that we cannot support this view. For therapeutic success in the treatment of a psychotic or neurotic individual, insight and abreaction are not enough. The specific therapeutic agent seems to be the complex, emotionally-charged parent-child kind of relationship between the psychiatrist and the individual whom he is treating.

During the two decades of its development, much has been written about the "techniques" of direct psychoanalysis. Some commentators, with or without the benefit of first-hand observation and experience, have said that direct psychoanalysis is largely a matter of a single technique: the "direct" interpretation. Others have said that direct psychoanalysis is largely a matter of the personality or attitude of the psychiatrist who is using it. Logically, these two are not the only possibilities; and in fact, neither of these opinions would seem to be correct.

Since 1956 we have been engaged in an extensive study of the procedures used in direct psychoanalysis. In that year the Institute for Direct Analysis was established at Temple University Medical Center, with the help of generous grants from the Rockefeller Brothers Fund, the Doris Duke Foundation, and other benefactors. To study the techniques of direct psychoanalysis, many psychiatrists and other specialists observed me treating a series of 12 psychotic individuals. There were hundreds of hours of such observed treatment, with additional hours of seminars and discussions. Also, there was an extensive analysis of tape-recordings and motion-pictures made during treatment sessions.

Several publications have emanated from this research program. Besides a number of papers in professional journals, there have been three books published: *Observations on "Direct Analysis",* by Dr. Morris W. Brody;[6]

126

A Psychotherapy of Schizophrenia, by Dr. Albert E. Scheflen;[7] and *Direct Analysis and Schizophrenia,* by Dr. O. Spurgeon English and his associates, Drs. Bacon, Hampe, and Settlage.[8]

While these publications disagree on many specific points of procedure or of theory—thus reflecting the independent and objective attitudes of their authors—they all seem to agree that the interaction between the direct psychoanalyst and the psychotic individual is a complicated one. None of them maintains that direct psychoanalysis is a matter of one or a few techniques such as the "direct" interpretation, and none of them insists that direct psychoanalysis is largely a matter of the psychiatrist's personality or attitude. Instead, these publications propose that direct psychoanalytic treatment consists of a wide variety of procedures. Dr. Scheflen's book is the most specific and the most comprehensive in this regard; for instance, it enumerates 16 "techniques of forceful persuasion," and gives examples of each of them from the verbatim recordings of treatment sessions. The book by Dr. English and his associates is similarly documented with specific examples of various procedures which the authors have observed in direct psychoanalytic treatment; for instance, Dr. English describes a number of "tactics" ranging from "Attacking Parental Image in Super Ego" to "Calling Attention to Patient's Potentialities."

Most of the observers at the Institute for Direct Analysis have attempted to construct their own theoretical explanations of the therapeutic process; for example, Dr. Bacon discusses direct psychoanalysis "from the viewpoint of identity," while Dr. Settlage discusses a relationship in which "the therapist establishes himself as being clearly dominant and the patient's ego becomes submissive to the ego of the therapist." In these and other discussions, the various authors make use of many different Freudian or non-Freudian concepts to account for or characterize different aspects of direct psychoanalysis. As I consider them, some of these choices are particularly apt and illuminating, but others seem to be improvised, unsuitable, or perhaps misleading.[9]

Many of the procedures which a direct psychoanalyst may use in a particular situation of treatment, either with a psychotic individual or with a neurotic, are not "techniques" in any strict sense of the word. For instance, during the treatment of a psychotic individual, the direct psychoanalyst might eat a meal with him and the assistant therapists in the treatment unit. Or the direct psychoanalyst might take him to the barbershop for a haircut. Or the direct psychoanalyst might grip his hand tightly while discussing a feeling that his hand was "limp and weak, like a woman's," as one individual complained. Such procedures are not rigidly

127

formulated "techniques," nor are they random gestures which have no therapeutic purpose. Instead, they are comparable to the procedures which a parent ordinarily and naturally uses in relating to a child. As such, they may be affectionate or stern, approbative or critical, spontaneous or deliberate, according to the demands of the particular situation which arises. The direct psychoanalyst makes use of many different "parental" procedures in his role of the "good parent" to the psychotic individual.

At the same time, unlike most parents, the direct psychoanalyst is also mindful of the psychological aspects of his relationship with the neo-infantile psychotic. For therapeutic results, it would not be sufficient to act like a "good parent" only at the conscious level; good intentions and kindly behavior would not be sufficient to meet the psychotic's unconscious needs. He is not, after all, an infant in fact. He is a person who has grown up physically without growing up psychically.

The needs of the psychotic individual are numerous, and many of them are subtle. To begin with, he needs to be informed of the fact that he is psychotic. It may be obvious to those around him, even to the casual layman, without being obvious to him. At the outset of treatment, the direct psychoanalyst gently but firmly tells the individual: "You are suffering from insanity. That is why you have been brought here to this psychiatric hospital. I am going to take care of you." It is not uncommon for the individual to react with surprise and relief, and to exclaim, "So that's what it is that's been bothering me."

Secondly, the psychotic individual needs to feel that he is understood, beyond the mere fact that he is psychotic. He needs to feel that someone is paying attention to his verbal or non-verbal "cries for help," his desperate efforts to conjure up "the mother he knew" through hallucinations, delusions, symbolism and other devices of the unconscious portion of the ego. To meet this need, the direct psychoanalyst pays close attention to the individual's behavior, attempts to understand it psychoanalytically, and attempts to convey his understanding in terms which the psychotic individual is likely to accept. For instance, if a psychotic is insisting that people are trying to kill him by poisoning his food, the direct psychoanalyst does not classify and pigeon-hole this as a colorful example of a "delusion of persecution." Instead, he discusses this specific complaint with the individual; drawing upon his prior knowledge of the sense in which "poisoned food" may be a concretistic reference to the inadequacies of the early maternal environment, he tries to lead the individual towards conscious understanding of this unconscious meaning. The direct psychoanalyst may convey this meaning immediately to the psychotic individual, by means of one or more interpretations; or he may lead the individual to it by asking a series of questions about food, eating, and the mother's

128

role as feeder of the infant. Or the direct psychoanalyst may also deal with the individual's fear by demonstrating that the food is not really poisoned, that it can be eaten safely; and then he may begin to pursue the symbolic meanings of "food-poisoning."

In each instance where he has acquired a psychoanalytic understanding of the psychotic's manifest behavior, the direct psychoanalyst proceeds as in the instance just described. It is through these proofs of his interest and comprehension that the direct psychoanalyst gradually makes the psychotic individual come to feel understood.

However, the cry of an infant is intended not only to be comprehended by his environment but also to be acted upon appropriately; and similarly, the "cry" of the psychotic individual must be acted upon by the psychiatrist. What is the psychotic seeking? In essence, he is seeking "mother." The individual is seeking the original qualities of his early maternal environment, which he perceived as being indispensable but deadly to him. Or speaking in terms of psychodynamics, we would say that the ego is seeking somehow to become fused, integrated, with the superego— which we regard as the psychical representation of the early maternal environment.

The direct psychoanalyst deliberately assumes the role of a "good parent" towards the psychotic individual whom he is treating. At the same time, he deliberately strives to weaken the individual's libidinal attachment to the "bad parent," the "bad mother," represented by the malevolent superego. As a "good parent," the direct psychoanalyst provides the individual with understanding, control, protection, physical comfort, and other evidences of his benevolent attitude. He calls the individual's attention to these benefits; and he refers to them explicitly in connection with his "love" of the individual. Often he may say to the individual, in so many words, "I love you. I am going to take care of you. You are just like a son (or daughter) to me."

As an attacker of the "bad parent," which is represented by the individual's malevolent superego, the direct psychoanalyst often refers explicitly to the hostility or indifference of "mother." He may cite actual instances which are recorded in the individual's history; for instance, "Didn't your mother abandon you, and leave you with your aunt, when you were just a baby?" Or, the direct psychoanalyst may refer to more recent happenings as if they signified a maternal deficiency; for example, he might ask: "If your mother really loves you, then why hasn't she called you up or tried to visit you here?" In reality, the direct psychoanalyst himself may have prohibited such visits by the mother or other members of the family.

This aggressive aspect of direct psychoanalysis has been confusing to

129

some observers, partly because its theoretical basis has not been appreciated fully. Direct psychoanalytic theory takes into account the psychotic individual's tendency to concretize as "mother" his impressions of his superego, his actual mother, his early maternal environment in general, and his various maternal surrogates. For the psychotic individual, "mother" is a conglomeration of all these elements. Accordingly, when the direct psychoanalyst wishes to discuss one or more of these elements with the individual, he must do so in the concretistic terms to which the psychotic is accustomed. Instead of referring to abstractions such as "superego" or "early maternal environment," he must refer specifically to "mother." This recognition of the psychotic's tendency to concretize his experience is essential to the direct psychoanalytic approach. It is valuable not only in the general understanding of the psychotic individual's dilemma, but also in the immediate understanding of specific happenings as treatment progresses; for instance, in understanding the psychological implications of "food-poisoning" which was mentioned earlier.

The direct psychoanalyst continues to function in the role of a "good parent" as the psychotic individual gradually moves towards maturity. Between psychosis and the level of mature adulthood, we find an intermediate level of immaturity which we refer to as the "neoneurosis." A "neoneurotic" individual requires close attention and psychiatric treatment especially designed to meet his psychical needs. While he has ascended from the neo-infantile level of psychosis, this individual is still in need of "parental" care and guidance from the psychiatrist. Like a neurotic individual who has never been psychotic, he is located psychosexually at the oedipal level of development, and he cannot progress further towards full maturity until his oedipal problems have been resolved. Unlike the ordinary neurotic, however, this individual has undergone a considerable revision of his psyche—through the experience of being psychotic, and through the experience of being treated by direct psychoanalysis. Consequently, he has acquired a familiarity with his own psyche which the usual neurotic individual might acquire only after extensive treatment by conventional psychoanalytic means. In addition, the neoneurotic individual has acquired new superego-components from the direct psychoanalyst: elements of benevolence and judiciousness in the place of, or in compensation for, his superego's original malevolence. Direct psychoanalytic treatment for the neoneurotic individual includes the further revision and improvement of the ego-superego relationship, as well as guidance and education to assist him in coping with realistic problems of the environment to which he has returned.

At the present time, we are giving special attention to the possibility

130

of using direct psychoanalytic procedures in the treatment of neurotic individuals who have not been psychotic. It appears to us that with these individuals as well as with psychotics, the psychiatrist can properly and effectively accept those parental responsibilities which the individual is eager to thrust upon him.

REFERENCES

1. ROSEN, J. N.: Transference: a concept of its origin, its purpose, and its fate. Int. J. Psychotherapy, Psychosomatics, Special Education. 2:300, 1954.
2. ———: Direct Analysis: Selected Papers. New York, Grune and Stratton, 1953.
3. FREUD, S.: Recommendations for physicians on the psychoanalytic method of treatment. In: Collected Papers, Vol. II. New York, Basic Books, 1959.
4. FREUD, A.: The Ego and the Mechanisms of Defense. New York, International Universities Press, 1946.
5. ALEXANDER, F.: Current problems in dynamic psychotherapy in its relation to psychoanalysis. Am. J. Psychiat. 116:322, 1959.
6. BRODY, M. W.: Observations on "Direct Analysis." New York, Vantage, 1959.
7. SCHEFLEN, A. E.: A Psychotherapy of Schizophrenia. Springfield, Illinois, Charles C Thomas, 1961.
8. ENGLISH, O. S., HAMPE, W. W., BACON, C. L., AND SETTLAGE, C. F.: Direct Analysis and Schizophrenia. New York, Grune and Stratton, 1961.
9. ROSEN, J. N.: Direct Psychoanalytic Psychiatry. New York, Grune and Stratton, 1962.

Existential Theory and Therapy

by ROLLO MAY, PH.D.

AND

ADRIAN VAN KAAM, PH.D.

WILLIAM JAMES once said that every new theory goes through three stages. First, it "is attacked as absurd; then it is admitted to be true, but obvious and insignificant; finally it is seen to be so important that its adversaries claim that they themselves discovered it."[1]

Existential psychotherapy certainly went through plenty of the first stage, lasting until about two years ago. It also has survived the second stage. The most recent period seemed marked by the third stage; everyone claimed his school invented it. There were voices which said that existential psychology is Adlerian, others that it was all in Jung, others that it was encompassed in Freud, still others that it was identical with Zen Buddism and anti-intellectual trends on one hand; or with a super-intellectual philosophy composed of untranslatable German terms on the other. It was said to be therapy which everyone does when he is doing good therapy, and also to be—especially in its classical phenomenological wing—a philosophical analysis which has nothing to do with the practice of therapy as such. These spokesmen seemed blithely unaware of their patent contradictions: if existential psychotherapy is one of these things, it cannot be the others.

But more and more the attitude of psychiatrists and psychologists in America seems to have become a serious and questioning interest in the existential approach; and it is therefore finding its constructive way into our thinking. Increasingly the books coming off the press as outlines or surveys of psychology and psychiatry have their chapter on this approach. The difficulty, of course, experienced by the authors of most of these books lies in the fact that this psychology does not fit our usual categories. In America we try to test our psychologies behavioristically, but the existential viewpoint denies that this is possible: its concept of "being-in the

---

[1] W. JAMES,: Pragmatism: A New Name for Some Old Ways of Thinking. New York, Longmans, Green, and Co., 1949, p. 198.

world" implies that no item of behavior can be understood apart from its subjective meaning to the person involved, just as there is no subjective meaning which does not have its objective pole. Also in books on psychotherapy we tend to categorize therapies in terms of techniques: but although existential psychology has made and will make significant and in some ways radical contributions to many therapists' manner of treatment, it is not essentially a technique, and therapists of many different technical schools may rightly be called existential.

A number of psychiatrists and psychologists who have been important for the development of psychotherapy in this country have held viewpoints to a greater of lesser degree existential long before that term was heard in America. William James, Adolph Meyer, Harry Stack Sullivan, Gordon Allport, Carl Rogers, Henry Murray, Abraham Maslow are examples. But what has been lacking (with the possible exception of William James) has been a consistent underlying structure which would give unity to the work of these psychiatrists and psychologists who are concerned with man in his immediate existence. This underlying structure must necessarily be both on the philosophical and psychological levels. We propose here that the existential approach, re-cast and re-born into our American language and thought forms, can and will give this underlying structure.

By good fortune several of the classical works in existential psychiatry and psychology have just been translated and are in process of being published in English. One of these is Erwin Straus' The Primary World,[1] a basic treatment of sense experience in psychiatry and psychology. Another is a collection of Straus' papers, including such works as the widely quoted "Upright Posture."[2] Medard Boss' Psychoanalysis and Daseinsanalysis will also be available in 1963.[3] Prof. Herbert Spiegelberg's two-volume work on phenomenology makes that field at last accessible to us in English.[4] A number of other basic works are appearing, and thus the serious student will be able to study original works and come to his own judgments.

PRINCIPLES UNDERLYING THEORY

Since any adequate psychotherapy rests upon a theory of personality, we shall present here several principles indicating how a comprehensive theory can be and is being developed in the existential approach.

---

[1] To be published in 1963 by Free Press, Glencoe, Illinois.
[2] To be published by Basic Books, New York.
[3] To be published by Basic Books, New York.
[4] The Phenomenological Movement, A Historical Introduction, Martinus Nijhoff, The Hague, Holland, 1960.

A comprehensive theory of psychotherapy presupposes the integration not only of findings in various schools of psychology and psychiatry but also of their interrelationships with one another and with human nature as such. Such an over-all integration is feasible only on the basis of a synthesizing idea or theoretical construct concerning man's nature which is comprehensive enough to connect all those findings without distorting their original contribution. First, *phenomenological descriptions* are necessary in order to uncover the original phenomena on which the interpretations of the various schools are based. Second, in order to find what binds those phenomena with one another and with the nature of man, we need the method of *existential* phenomenology, which tries to describe man's nature as such, that is, its essential characteristics.

The construct of "existence" is one of those comprehensive concepts and thus refers to the fact that it is man's essence to find himself bodily together with others in the world. This concept unites the subjective, physiological, objective and social aspects of the reality of man. The student of psychology has to split up this reality of man into many aspects in order to study them in isolation. As a result we are confronted with a variety of psychologies, such as social, behavioristic, physiological, introspectional, psychoanalytic and so on. In contrast, the existential approach seeks to *reintegrate* the phenomena which are discovered when man has been studied from those various, isolated viewpoints. But this reintegration presupposes a return to the original experience of man in his unity before he was split up into a variety of profiles by the various methodologies. It is for this reason that the construct of man's existence is used in psychology and psychotherapy as an integrational construct. In this context we define an integrational construct as: *a concept that refers to observed phenomena and that can be used for the integration of the greatest number and variety of phenomena and relationships observed by the different schools of psychology and psychiatry.*

Although "existence" or "existential" is the fundamental construct used in this comprehensive theory of personality, many more constructs are needed to develop a full theory. We shall here call them subordinated constructs, such as "mode of existence," "existential world," "existential transference," "the centered self," "ontological security and insecurity," and so on. They have the function of connecting the phenomena uncovered by the various schools of psychotherapy with the fundamental construct of existence.

The existential psychotherapist profits from the work of various existential philosophers without aligning himself with any particular school or system of philosophy. He borrows some of their existential concepts which prove useful for his integrating task. The status of the concepts, however, in a scientific psychological theory differs essentially from their previous position in philosophy. First, the existential psychologist neither affirms nor denies their ontological validity. For this would imply a philosophical statement which the psychologist and psychiatrist with only empirical methods at his disposal cannot make. Second, he changes them into hypothetical constructs from which he derives postulates which can be put to the empirical test. Third, he allows the original meaning of these constructs to change while being attuned to the phenomena uncovered in the various areas of psychology and psychiatry.*

The Existential Approach to Therapy

We may now consider the application of the existential constructs to the practice of psychotherapy in one area, namely, *will* and *decision*. The capacity for self-conscious will and decision (we shall define these terms later) is taken as one of the essential, distinguishing characteristics of the being called man.†

The existential approach in psychology and psychotherapy holds that we cannot leave will and decision to chance. We cannot work on the assumption that ultimately the patient "somehow happens" to make a decision, or slides into a decision by ennui, default, or mutual fatigue with the therapist, or acts from sensing that the therapist (now the benevolent parent) will approve of him if he does take such and such steps. The existential approach puts decision and will back into the center of the picture—"The very stone which the builders rejected has become the head of the corner." Not in the sense of "free will against determinism"; this issue is dead and buried. Nor in the sense of denying what Freud describes as unconscious experience; these deterministic "unconscious" factors certainly operate, and the existentialists, who make much of "finiteness" and man's limitations, obviously know this. We hold, however, that in the revealing and exploring of these deterministic

---

*An example in theoretical physics of the change of the meaning of such a construct during the dialogue between philosophical concepts and observed data is the hypothetical construct "atom" that was first formulated by Democritus.

†It is well known that the existential thinkers such as Kierkegaard, Nietzsche, Sartre, Paul Ricoeur and Tillich have dealt centrally with the problem of will and decision. "Man becomes truly human only in moments of decision," stated Tillich in his demonstration that "will" is one of the essential characteristics of man as man. Probably the most accessible and readable book in this whole area is *The Courage to Be* by Paul Tillich (Yale: 1952). The endeavor has also been made to formulate psychologically the problem of will and decision; see Rollo May, "Existential Bases of Psychotherapy," *American Journal of Orthopsychiatry,* October, 1960, Vol. 30, No. 4.

forces in his life, the patient is orienting himself in some particular way to the data and thus is engaged in some choice, no matter how seemingly insignificant; is experiencing some freedom, no matter how subtle.

But the existential attitude in psychotherapy does not at all "push" the patient into decisions. Indeed, we are convinced that it is only by this clarification of the patient's own powers of will and decision that the therapist can avoid inadvertently and subtly pushing the patient in one direction or another. The existentialist point is that self-consciousness itself—the person's potential awareness that the vast, complex, protean flow of experience is *his* experience—brings in inseparably the element of decision at every moment. This conative element is present to some degree in experiences as simple and non-world shaking as any new idea one finds oneself entertaining, or any new memory that pops up in a seemingly random chain of free association. It is these and similar considerations which have led the existential psychotherapists to be concerned with the problems of will and decision as central to the process of therapy.

But when we turn to the endeavor to understand will and decision themselves, we find our task is not at all easy. Our problem hinges upon the terms "will" and "wish" and the interrelation between the two. The word "will," associated as it is with "will power," is at best dubious, and perhaps no longer helpful or even available. But the reality it has historically described must be retained. 'Will power" expressed the arrogant effort of Victorian man to manipulate nature and to rule nature with an iron hand (*vide* industrialism and capitalism) and to manipulate himself, rule his own life in the same way as an object (shown particularly in Protestantism but present in other modern ethical and religious systems as well). Thus "will" was set over against "wish" and used as a faculty by which "wish" could be denied. We have observed in patients that the emphasis on "will power" is often a reaction formation to their own repressed passive desires, a way of fighting off their wishes to be taken care of; and the likelihood is that this mechanism had much to do with the form "will power" took in Victorianism. Victorian man sought, as Schachtel has put it, to deny that he ever had been a child, to repress his irrational tendencies and so-called infantile wishes as unacceptable to his concept of himself as a grown-up and responsible man. Will power was then a way of avoiding awareness of bodily and of sexual urges or hostile impulses that did not fit the picture of the controlled, well-managed self. The process of using will to deny wish results in a greater and greater emotional void, a progressive emptying of inner contents which must ultimately impoverish intellectual experience as well.

136

In attacking these morbid psychological processes, Freud produced his far-reaching emphasis on the *wish*. In view of the fact that in our post-Victorian day we still tend to impoverish the word by making it a concession to our immaturity or "needs," let us hasten to say that the term "wish" may be seen as related to processes much more extensive than the residue of childhood. Its correlates can be found in all phenomena in nature down to the most minute pattern of atomic re-, action; for example, in the context of what Whitehead and Tillich describe as negative-positive movements in all nature. Tropism is one form in its etymological sense of the innate tendency in biological organisms to "turn toward." However, if we stop with "wish" as this more or less blind and involuntary movement of one particle toward another or one organism toward another, we are inexorably pushed to Freud's pessimistic conclusion of the "death instinct," the inevitable tendency of organisms to move back toward the inorganic. Therefore, in human beings "wish" can never be seen without relation to "will."

Our problem now becomes the inter-relation of "wish" and "will." We shall offer some suggestions which, although not intended to make a neat definition, show us some of the aspects of the problem that must be taken into consideration. "Wish" gives the warmth, the content, the child's play, the freshness and richness to "will." "Will" gives the self-direction, the freedom, the maturity to "wish." If you have only will and no wish, you have the dried up Victorian, post-Puritan man. If you have only wish and no will, you have the driven, unfree infantile human being who as an adult may become the robot man.

We propose the term "decision" to stand for the human act which brings both will and wish together. Decision in this sense does not deny or exclude wish but incorporates it and transcends it. Decision in an individual takes into the picture the experiencing of all wishes, but it forms these into a way of acting which is consciously chosen.

THERAPEUTIC DIMENSIONS

The process of therapy with individual patients involves bringing together these three dimensions of wish, will and decision. As the patient moves from one dimension to the next in his integration, the previous level is incorporated and remains present in the next.

In practical therapy, the first dimension, wish, occurs on the level of *awareness,* the dimension which the human organism shares with all nature. The experiencing of infantile wishes, bodily needs and desires, sexuality and hunger and all the infinite and inexhaustible gamut of wishes which occur in any individual, seems to be a central part of prac-

137

tically all therapy. Experiencing these wishes may involve dramatic and sometimes traumatic anxiety and upheaval as the repressions which led to the blocking off of the awareness in the first place are brought out into the open. On the significance and necessity of unmasking repression—the dynamic aspects of which are beyond the scope of our present discussion—various kinds of therapy differ radically; but we cannot conceive of any form of *psycho*therapy which does not accord the process of awareness itself a central place. The experiencing of these wishes may come out in the simplest forms in the desire to fondle or be fondled, the wishes associated originally with nursing and closeness to mother and family members in early experience, the touch of the hand of a friend or loved one in adult experience, the simple pleasure of wind and water against one's skin; and it goes all the way up to the sophisticated experiences which may come, for example, in a dazzling instant when one is standing near a clump of blooming forsythia and is suddenly struck by how much more brilliantly blue the sky looks when seen beyond the sea of yellow flowers. The immediate awareness of the world continues throughout life, hopefully at an accelerating degree, and is infinitely more varied and rich than one would gather from most psychological discussion.

From the existential viewpoint, this growing awareness of one's body, wishes and desires—processes which are obviously related to the experiencing of identity—normally also brings heightened appreciation of one's self as *a* being and a heightened reverence for Being itself. Here the eastern philosophies like Zen Buddhism have much to teach us.

The second level in the relating of *wish* to *will* in therapy is the transmitting of awareness into self-consciousness. This level is correlated with the distinctive form of awareness in human beings, consciousness. (The term *consciousness,* coming etymologically from *con* plus *sciere,* "knowing with," is used here as synonymous with self-consciousness.)* On this level the patient experiences I-am-the-one-who-has-these-wishes. This is the level of accepting one's self as having a world. If I experience the fact that my wishes are not simply blind pushes toward someone or something, that I am the one who stands in this world where touch, nourishment, sexual pleasure and relatedness may be possible between me and other persons, I can begin to see how I may do something about these wishes. This gives me the possibility of *in-sight,* of "inward sight," of seeing the world and other people in relation to myself. Thus the previous alternatives of repressing wishes because one cannot stand

---

*The relationships of awareness to self-consciousness have been developed elsewhere, (May, op. cit.). Strictly speaking, "self-consciousness" is redundant: consciousness already implies relation to the self.

138

the lack of their gratification on one hand, or being compulsively pushed to the blind gratification of the wishes and desires on the other, are replaced by the experience of the fact that I myself am involved in these relationships of pleasure, love, beauty, trust and I hopefully then have the possibility of changing my own behavior to make these more possible.

On this level *will* enters the picture, not as a denial of wish but as an incorporation of wish on the higher level of consciousness. To refer to our example above: the experiencing of the blue of the sky behind forsythia blossoms on the simple level of awareness and wish may bring delight and the desire to continue or renew the experience; but the realization that I am the person who lives in a world in which flowers are yellow and the sky so brilliant, and that I can even increase my pleasure by sharing this experience with a friend, has profound implications for life, love, death, and the other ultimate problems of human existence. As Tennyson remarked when he looked at the flower in the crannied wall, ". . . I could understand what God and man are."

The third level in the process of therapy is that of *decision* and *responsibility*. We use these two terms together to indicate that decision is not simply synonymous with will. Responsibility involves being responsive, *responding*. As consciousness is the distinctively human form of awareness, so decision and responsibility are the distinctive forms of consciousness in the human being who is moving toward self-realization, integration, maturity. Again, this dimension is not achieved by denying wishes and self-assertive will, but incorporates and keeps present the previous two levels. *Decision* in our sense forms the two previous levels into a pattern of acting and living which is not only empowered and enriched by wishes and asserted by will but is responsive to and responsible for the significant other persons who are important to one's self in the realizing of the long-term goals. This sounds like an ethical statement, and *is* in the sense that ethics have their psychological base in these capacities of the human being to transcend the concrete situation of immediate self-oriented desire and to live in the dimensions of past and future and in terms of the welfare of the persons and groups upon which one's own fulfillment intimately depends. The point, however, cannot be dismissed as "just" ethical. If it is not self-evident it could be demonstrated along the lines of Sullivan's interpersonal theory of psychiatry, Buber's philosophy and other viewpoints, that *wish, will* and *decision* occur within a nexus of relationships upon which the individual himself depends not only for his fulfillment but for his very existence.

139

Reality Therapy

by WILLIAM GLASSER, M.D. AND LEONARD M. ZUNIN, M.D.

Reality therapy is based upon the premise that all people in all cultures possess from birth to death a need for an identity; that no other person thinks, looks, acts, and talks exactly as each individual does. Reality therapy differs from psychoanalysis, from operant conditioning, or from some of the newer therapeutic ideas in that it is applied not only to the problems of irresponsibility and incompetence, but also to the modes of daily living.

Formation of a success or failure identity becomes most obvious at age 6, when the child enters the first grade and is first challenged to develop intellectual, verbal, and social skills which determine if he will be a successful or unsuccessful person and associate with others accordingly. Individuals who identify with failure either *deny* reality or *ignore* it. What is traditionally called mental illness are the various methods by which an individual avoids reality.

The Basic Principles of Reality Therapy

Basic to reality therapy is the concept of involvement, which is necessary to motivate a person toward success. The following are ways in which the therapist becomes responsibly involved with the person he is trying to help and guides him toward working for a success identity.

Principle I: Personal

The therapist must communicate that he cares, that he is warm and friendly. Aloofness and cool detachment are not therapeutic. Understanding and realistic concern are the cornerstones of effective treatment. The use of personal pronouns by both the therapist and the patient such as *I* and *me* and *you,* rather than *it* or *one does* or *out there* or *they,* facilitates involvement.

Being personal also means that the therapist is willing, if indicated and appropriate, to discuss his own experiences and to have his values challenged and discussed. He demonstrates that he acts in a responsible manner and admits that he is far from being perfect or free of concerns. The therapist conveys to the individual, usually nonverbally, his sincere belief that the patient has the ability to be happier and do better, and that he is capable of functioning in a more responsible, effective, and self-fulfilling manner. In fact, if the therapist does not believe this about the patient, he is doing the patient a disservice by continuing to engage him in a treatment situation.

It is not possible for a therapist who leads a responsible life of his own to become deeply involved in friendships with everyone who comes to him for help except within the context of the office. The therapist has to be honest about this and explain it to the patient, rather than imply promises which he cannot fulfill. The warmth, the concern, the involvement in the therapeutic relationship, is what is essential, rather than the content of the verbal exchange. This means that anything is open for discussion; if the individual is talking about subjects other than his own misery or problems, this is not seen as resistance but rather as something worthwhile and of interest to both the therapist and the patient.

Principle II: Focus on Behavior Rather Than Feelings

There is a basic fallacy in the notion "When I feel better, I will do more;" when people do more, they feel better. It is far easier to enter this cycle at the "doing" rather than the "feeling" point.

For example, if an individual comes to the office and states, "I feel miserable and depressed," rather than one of the traditional answers such as silence or "Tell me more about it," or "Have you had any suicidal thoughts? " or "Have you ever felt this depressed at any other time in your life? " the reality therapist might respond by saying, "Is it possible that what you are doing is depressing you? " When patients begin to outline what they are doing and what they have done over the last few days, it often becomes apparent that any normal, average human being would also be depressed with similar conduct. The therapist might then ask the patient why he was not more depressed—a provocative question for most individuals seeking help. When they begin, with the help of the therapist, to outline the various modes of conduct that support them emotionally and prevent their becoming ever further depressed, we assist them in becoming aware of their own inner strengths, potentials, and attributes.

This second principle is poignantly illustrated in intimate love relationships. Unless two individuals enjoy each other as human beings, the feelings of love and warmth and closeness begin to fade. Only by sharing behavior, whether sexually or in constructive and creative enjoyment, can the relationship be sustained and grow.

Principle III: Focus on the Present

Reality therapy is based upon a conviction that whatever we are today is the sum total of everything that has happened in our lives; however, all that can be changed is the immediate present and the future. When the past is discussed, incidents are never left as entities in and of themselves but are always related to current behavior. For example, if a person described a crisis experience that

141

occurred several years ago, the therapist will ask him what he learned from it, and how it is related to his present behavior and attempts to succeed in life. In contrast to traditional psychotherapeutic approaches, which emphasize past traumatic encounters, failures, and difficulties, (1) we discuss strengthening and character-building experiences that occurred in the individual's past and relate them to current attempts to succeed, (2) we explore constructive alternatives that the individual might have taken at the time, and (3) we discuss especially what he did do that assisted him in avoiding greater difficulty.

Contrary to this principle, case histories in the traditional format, whether by probation officers, psychiatrists, psychologists, or social workers, sometimes concentrate on failures, shortcoming, traumas, and problems with which the person has had to cope, whereas a person's successes and hidden potentials are sadly neglected.

Principle IV: Value Judgments

Every patient must make a value judgment as to what he is doing to contribute to his own failure before he can be helped to change. Part of emotional health is a willingness to work within the framework of society. However, the therapist should not impose his own social judgments on the patient, since this would relieve the patient of the responsibility for his own behavior.

Principle V: Planning and Commitment

One of the continual problems in therapy, as well as in all aspects of life, is that, once a good plan is made, we must develop the strength and the responsibility to carry it through. A significant portion of therapy involves making plans that are realistic. It is far better to err on the side of programs that are simple and easily implemented, than those that are complex and stand a greater risk of failure. Patients gain a success identity only through successes and not through failures.

An important advantage is to put the plan in writing, particularly in the form of a contract betwee n patient and therapist. The differential weight that is attached to the written versus the spoken word was long ago utilized by the legal profession, and the reality therapist may find this an exceedingly useful device.

Principle VI: Evasions

Plans may fail, but it is the obligation of the reality therapist to make clear to the patient that no excuses are acceptable. Far more therapeutic benefit is gained from working with the patient on redeveloping the plan than in discussing the reasons for the plan's failure. The therapist should not deprecate the patient for failing, but the joint task is to make a new plan or to modify the old one.

142

Principle VII: Eliminate Punishment

Punishment works most poorly on individuals with a failure identity. Therefore, we avoid ridicule, sarcasm, or hostile statements such as "You just don't have what it takes."

Punishment is different from the natural consequences of failure. To the extent that the reality therapist is able to eliminate punishment and not accept excuses for failure, to help the patient substitute constructive value judgments and make plans accordingly, and then help him to make a commitment to follow through, the therapist is assisting his patient to achieve success.

Transference, as described in other therapeutic approaches, occurs not only in the therapeutic experience but in the experiences of everyday life. Rather than attempt to enhance this phenomenon and then "analyze" it, the reality therapist attempts to decrease attendant distortions. If the patient relates to the reality therapist by saying, "You remind me of my father," the reality therapist may say, "I am not your father, but I would be interested in knowing what you see in us as similar." The therapist thus attempts in every way possible to present himself as a genuine, concerned person, helping the patient to understand and deal with reality.

Behavior Therapy

by EDWARD DENGROVE, M.D.

Behavior therapy consists of a number of treatment methods derived from the application of learning principles, both classical and operant. These techniques constitute a break with traditional insight therapy, emphasizing symptoms rather than personality review and change. They do not handle unconscious dynamic factors; the symptoms, or behavior as a whole, are considered the disease, but cognizance is taken of the person behind the symptom, and consideration is given to values, attitudes, and beliefs. Neurosis is defined[29] as learned behavior that is persistent and unadaptive, and which is acquired in anxiety-generating situations. Historically, symptoms arise by training or trauma, by purpose or accident, during the life span of the individual who is more or less predisposed toward them.

Reciprocal inhibition[32] is a process of relearning whereby, in the presence of an anxiety-evoking stimulus, a nonanxiety-producing response is continually repeated until it extinguishes the old, undesirable response. Various treatment methods are based upon this principle and include systematic desensitization; active, graded therapy; assertive techniques; sexual responses; and numerous others. These approaches require four essentials:

1. Contact with the feared object, situation, or feeling.
2. A graduated approach to this contact.
3. Motivation of the patient to make this contact on a regular basis.
4. Fear reduction—induced by reassurance, relaxation training, medication, distraction, hypnosis, or other technical means.

Additionally, these four essentials are preceded by a proper behavioral diagnosis in order to "target in" upon the symptom.

Systematic desensitization is done through visual imagery in the doctor's office; in this process the patient lives through his fears and anxieties while in a relaxed state. Active, graded therapy requires contact with the feared object, situation, or feeling in a realistic manner.

History taking is essential to a behavioral diagnosis. The patient's complaints are sought and found in the manner usually accomplished by a competent psychotherapist, and his past and personal history are recorded so that a better idea of the patient may be formed. A list of fears is then requested. Some behavior therapists utilize a Fear Survey[31] or other questionnaire. I also ask for an autobiography of undetermined length, to help fill in the gaps.

An executive who stuttered excessively while dictating to his stenographer changed his stenographer, but to no avail. When asked to close his eyes and reconstruct the scene, he concluded that it was not the stenographer who caused him to become tense, but the fact that what he was saying was being made a matter of public record and he would be held accountable for it. Desensitization was directed thereafter to his concern for his stated words.

A useful technique for identifying source and reinforcement of a symptom or behavior is letter association.[3]

The patient is asked to sit back in the chair and relax, to close his eyes and think of a particular symptom, to relate it to the last setting or event (or the first, or any) in which it was felt, and to attempt to relive or reconstruct—to whatever extent is possible—the feeling tone of the complaint. He is then asked to give the very first letter that comes to mind, then the next one. When five letters are noted—the number is arbitrary—they are listed vertically in order. At this point the patient is allowed to open his eyes if he wishes; he is requested to give the first word—again only the first one—that comes to mind and which begins with each of the letters previously chosen. He is to make up sentences using each word or freely to associate the words. In the majority of instances one is able to pinpoint the immediate cause of the symptom or to trace it back to its source.

A complete list of fears is secured from the patient and anxiety hierarchies are set up for each one. A hierarchy is a list of stimuli to which the patient reacts with anxiety, from the least disturbing to the most frightening.

For instance, to the woman who is afraid to leave the house, the least disturbing stimulus would be just looking out of the window or opening the door and putting out one foot. The most frightening would be walking about town freely. Relaxational methods are then taught, using a modified Jacobson technique[29-31] of differential relaxation of various muscle groups, or hypnosis, or medication. Only when she is completely at ease will treatment be effective. As she lies on the couch or sits in the chair with her eyes closed and at peace with herself, the least anxiety-provoking stimulus from the hierarchy is presented to her visual imagination. For instance, she is asked to visualize herself looking out the window of her home. If she retains her composure and continues at ease while viewing the scene, she informs us by a signal that it is not disturbing to her. She may have been asked to raise her hand slightly or to move her head a bit, up and down for yes, side to side for no; not enough to disturb her equanimity. The next stimulus on the list is then presented. She is asked to view herself putting a foot out of the door; then to walking a few steps; to view herself walking to the street in front of her house; to walking on the street as far as the house next door; and so on. If there is anxiety at any one presentation, she is asked to view the preceding scene, which she can do again with greater ease. At this point the session is terminated, although a number of fears may be so handled in the one session. At the next session, the desensitization process starts with the last item that did not evoke anxiety at the previous meeting, and treatment moves ahead from there. In the interim, the general level of anxiety has apparently diminished so that she can cope with further elements in the hierarchy. Transfer of the relief from anxiety in these fixed situations to real life situations occurs.

Psychological desensitization is much like chemical desensitization for an allergic disorder, wherein the patient is injected with minute quantities of the allergen and gradually exposed to larger and larger doses until he or she is able to cope with the natural environment. As a rule, there is an acceleration of progress as one moves along.

In active, graded therapy, real-life approaches are made to the feared feeling, object, or situation.

Consider the child who is afraid of dogs. The child is held by a trusted person who allows him to suck on a lollipop (food is used as a counter to anxiety also) and points to a dog on a leash in the distance. A little later, the child, still held, is encouraged to view a dog through a pet-shop window. Still later, he is brought closer to a dog; and later, closer still. With the pleasure of the food and the security of being held by a trusted person, the child gradually experiences a reduction of his fear. One may use pictures of dogs or toy dogs at first, gradually progressing to small, friendly dogs and then to medium-sized dogs. In the end, the child is able to reach out and touch a dog.

One must do the very things that one fears. A fear cannot be overcome by avoiding it, nor by trying to drown it out with continued medication. Medicine, while useful, is to be reduced gradually and finally discarded. Avoiding the phobic situation or object only perpetuates the fear by reinforcement of the escape response. So, while giving the patient the tranquilizer or sedative, insist that he or she make attempts toward overcoming the fears, in a graduated fashion and with reassurance, persuasion, or the security of your presence.

The patient is not expected to attempt any activity that produces overwhelming anxiety. But he is encouraged to try tasks that are mildly upsetting, at the same time attempting to quiet himself. If the anxiety persists, he is to stop what he is doing, for this will only set him back. Instead, he is to return to doing those things that he can do without getting upset. The patient is

146

exposed at first only to those fears he can cope with, gradually increasing contact with those productive of more and more anxiety. One can get accustomed to almost any new situation that is approached gradually.

Interestingly, as the milder fears are overcome, the more disturbing ones concurrently lose their intensity. However, the patient must proceed at his own pace; he is assured that there is no reason to feel guilt or shame if progress is slow. At times, under pressure of need or anger, large strides are made, but this is the exception. Sometimes it is only after the patient has completed an activity that he realizes what he has accomplished without apprehension or anxiety.

Assertive Responses

Some patients fear to raise their voices to the therapist, or to swear even mildly, or to express anger in any form. Such patients are encouraged to shout or scream; to swear, first without looking at the therapist and then looking at him; to smash his fist into the couch or on the arm of the chair. In effect, the patient is taught to express his anger toward the authoritative figure of the therapist. Of course there are limits to how much can be expressed outwardly, but at least the patient can allow himself to feel the anger and not repress or suppress it. The learned freedom is carried over to real life. The patient is made happier and more capable by this character change.

Wolpe and Lazarus[31] emphasize that although the most common class of assertive responses involved in therapeutic action is the expression of anger and resentment, the term "assertive behavior" is used broadly to cover all socially acceptable expression of personal rights and feelings. A polite refusal to accede to an unreasonable request; a genuine expression of praise, endearment, appreciation, or respect; an exclamation of joy, irritation, adulation, or disgust—all may be considered examples of assertive behavior. Diminishing the object of fear by poking fun at it also makes it easier to overcome. Making fun of one's emotional responses will do the same. The "paradoxical intention" of Frankl[5] is based upon this type of approach.

Sexual Responses

Learning to relax during coitus is another shortcut to overcoming impotence and, often, frigidity. Wolpe's method[29], which has been particularly effective in many cases of impotence, consists of teaching the patient to relax in the act and not become anxious over inability to produce an erection. The wife is told not to expect performance on her husband's part for a while; partners are just to caress and enjoy each other, whatever the outcome. When the man no longer feels that he is obliged to perform, he discovers that he is able to do so once again. No effort is made to work through long periods of life history. Of course there are some situations in which impotence is due to lack of love and the

147

absence of real interest in the spouse, but in the absence of this, many patients will respond successfully to this simple Wolpeian approach within two to six sessions.

Symptom Substitution

It has been my experience in the years during which I have used these techniques that symptom substitution or replacement does not occur if the underlying base for the symptom is no longer operative.

Clinical Problems

No therapeutic approach is without difficulties that challenge the alert and inventive therapist. The following problems are illustrative.

Improper Behavioral Diagnosis

Stevenson and Hain[25] insist that one does not consider merely a specific phobia; for example, fear of barber shop. There may be a dread of scrutiny by others, a rebelliousness against social customs, impatience with delays, aversion to confinement, fear of mutilation, anxiety-arousing experiences with chairs resembling barber chairs; sexual arousal; issues of seniority; and other explanations for the phobia—a multiplicity of stimuli that touch off the central response.

The presence of historically earlier sources of anxiety, according to Meyer and Crisp,[20] may complicate recovery until ferreted out. Clarke[4] has shown that relearning, too, will fade if it is not reinforced. Lazarus and Serber[17] concede that maladaptive behavior may not be due to anxiety, but to naiveté or poor verbal skills; therapy therefore aims not at desensitization but at re-education, modeling, and practice. Other instances they cite include complaints secondary to psychotic processes that respond to antipsychotic medication and phobic disorders in patients suffering with depression. These patients are better treated with antidepressant medication or by advice to secure employment, invitation to join a supportive therapeutic group, and training to develop assertive response.

Difficulties in Relaxation

Relaxation is indispensable to success in most cases using reciprocal inhibition, but the method used to relax the patient is not so important as the depth of relaxation it produces. There appears to be only one criterion of adequacy of depth: the patient's subjective estimation. The patient must feel not partially or nearly relaxed, but completely so. Wolpe[28] asks a patient to imagine a situation in which he has felt panic and to label this "100." Then he is asked to imagine a situation in which he has felt most calm and at ease, and to label this

"0." The percentage of relaxation must be over 85 per cent to be effective for desensitization.

It is my custom to ask a patient to nod his head up and down or side to side in answer to the question, "Do you feel relaxed. Are you at ease?" Often, if I am not sure of the answer, I will add, "Are you completely relaxed, completely at ease?" Interestingly, these may differ, the patient nodding yes to the former and no to the latter. I have found, too, that when a patient indicates that he is still not at ease, it is most helpful to ask him to put himself at ease, without further suggestions from myself, over the next few minutes. Often this is effective.

Sometimes progress is slowed because the patient indicates that he is relaxed when he is really only resting, i.e., merely lying still but with continuing muscular tension. A greater difficulty lies with patients whose bodies are relaxed but who remain obsessed with trying to retain control.

Difficulties in Desensitization to the Hierarchies

Lazarus[18] comments: "The patient may not be picturing the scenes described; he may fail to signal anxiety only because the time interval is too short to permit vivid imagery; he may introduce extraneous variables without the therapist's knowledge; he may experience immediate associations of which the therapist ought to be aware; and so forth. . . ."

I have found an occasional patient whose facile mind races ahead, and although he is not anxious about the scene being presented, he is disturbed by the scene he is associating on his own; he anticipates me. A minority of patients do not experience anxiety at all when they imagine situations that in reality are disturbing.[29,30] In some of these patients, anxiety can be evoked when they are asked to describe the scene they imagine.[11] Others may have to resort to active, graded desensitization.

Differences in Individual Conditionability

Phobic conditions are seen in three separate groups of patients: obsessive-compulsives, schizoid, and post-traumatic. The obsessive-compulsive perfectionistic pattern is the most common and the most intensively affected. These people are neat, systematic, conscientious, orderly, concerned that everything should be in its right place and that there is a right place for everything. They want to please everyone excepting their spouse. Feelings of inadequacy are always present. Assertive techniques and role playing are utilized in order to develop an increased self-confidence, less perfectionism, ability to cope with dominant people, and an "I don't really care" attitude.

The schizoid personality develops phobic complaints within a pansymptomatic picture, the central issue being an inner helplessness and difficulty in coping with hostile feelings. Desensitization to both are necessary, assisted by therapeutic group techniques.

Other Means of Reciprocal Inhibition

When a patient cannot be sufficiently relaxed for reciprocal inhibition to take place, other means of countering the phobic anxiety must be employed. Sexual and assertive feelings are often used together with a variety of techniques limited only by the ingenuity of the therapist.

> Lazarus[13,14] used anger as a counterdevice in systematic desensitization. In place of relaxation, his patients overcame each item in the hierarchy by an angry response. He also reported the use of directed muscular activity, such as pounding one's hands against a padded stool. With children, he and Abramovitz[12] employed a process of visual imagery, with the child incorporating his phobic symptoms into a fantasy situation, using the hero to overcome the feared object. Similar techniques[18], using emotive or assertive imagery and cognitive variables, have been employed with adults. I have found it of value, where relaxation is not sufficient, to ask the patient to signal me when he is taking his fearful situation "in stride," rather than being completely without anxiety; or to visualize himself helping others in similar situations and being constructively useful. Some situations (*e.g.*, sexual ones) do not call for relaxed responses, but for pleasurable ones.

The literature of behavior therapy is filled with the inventiveness of therapists who have devised ways to get around the relaxational barrier. Whatever method is used, however, must reduce fear from one session to the next one.

Faith, Trust, and Expectation: The Placebo Effect

The patient comes to the therapist expecting help and motivated toward getting better. Beecher[2] has pointed out that 35.2(±2.2) per cent of patients are placebo reactors and that placebo reactivity is directly related to experienced distress or suffering. Wolf[27] considers this the effect of meaningful situations, whereas Gantt and Stephens[7] credit a positive expectancy reaction. Truax[26] points out that therapists who are low in communicated empathy, nonpossessive warmth, and genuineness are ineffective.

Anticipation or the Fear-of-Fear Itself Phenomenon

There is a difference between fear of an object or situation and fearful anticipation of them. It is the difference between the armed bandit's actually pointing the gun at you, and your expectation that you might be held up. In the former, one is actually faced with the threat; in the latter, it may never happen.

Often a patient will say that it is not the actual happening of an event that bothers her but the worry about it ahead of time. As one woman related, "I worried and worried about it, but when I finally forced myself to go there, it wasn't at all what I thought. I got along fine." Many of us have undergone similar experiences when taking examinations; yet once we were engaged in writing the examination, we quieted down. We had somewhere to go with our aroused state, and provided we had done our work beforehand, we could concentrate on the task at hand with a certain amount of equanimity. Frequently the task is to convince the patient to make the try.

Physiologic Components

MacLean[19] relates expectation to the brain's electrical activity. A slow, negative shift in potential builds up in the frontal cortex and does not collapse until the subject has made a decision. Goldstein[10] characterizes individuals by their mode of response, some responding chiefly by means of the autonomic nervous system, some by muscle tension, and others with overt muscle activity. Autonomic components are often the only discernible symptoms in neurotics.

One needs to desensitize not only to the act, but to anticipation of the act, as a separate hierarchy. I attempt to decondition the patient to anxiety by having him feel fright: open his eyes widely, suck in air, and hold his breath in an inspiratory position, urging him to re-experience the feeling of dread as much as possible. Imitation of anxiety responses must be actually felt. Additionally, the patient is made aware of the heart beat, and assisted in becoming used to the visceral sensations, to accept the inevitable and say "to Hell with it!" Operant techniques[8] may be used to reinforce autonomic responses. Sometimes the anticipation takes on an obsessive quality, at which time we must revert to thought-blocking procedures[31] or aversion relief methods.[23]

Delay or Inability to Transfer Improvement from Office to Real Life

The difficulty carrying over "improvement to everyday real life results from problems involving behavioral diagnosis and motivation.

A 20-year-old woman was doing well in the office with systematic desensitization to her fears of walking and driving from her home, whereas elsewhere she had made no progress at all. Asking her to make attempts in real life produced only excuse after excuse during each session as to why it had been impossible for her to do anything that week. She had an anticipatory fear response, of such degree that she would not make the slightest attempt, even with help. Further diagnostic exploration revealed her fear that if she were free to come and go as she pleased, she would simply go and not return. She had no respect for her immature husband, yet feared to give up her kind of life.

151

There are cases in which there is no solution to a conflict of conscience, in which secondary gain outweighs the pain of the neurotic solution and inhibits the danger of psychotic breakdown. When patients are making out reasonably well with monies received from insurance schemes, treatment may become well nigh impossible. The passive-dependent personality is only too happy to retire from the stresses and strains of competition and responsibility. When pressed, even lightly, the symptoms simply return or are aggravated.

Stevenson[24] instructs a patient not to come for her next appointment unless she drives alone, or insists that a timid woman not call for her next appointment until she has discussed a feared operation with a surgeon, or offers a fee reduction to another patient if she will discuss her annoyance directly with her mother-in-law. He, himself, began riding elevators with a woman who feared doing so. The latter active, graded therapy, or *in vivo* training, is an important addition to systematic desensitization, and often the patient can be led to make attempts outside the office in a gradual manner.

Avoidance of Setbacks during Treatment

Relapses occur when the patient is pushed too fast, the phobic situation is reinforced, or a general overall increase in anxiety occurs. In a study of speed of generalization in systematic desensitization, Rachman[21] showed that reductions in fear from imaginal to real-life situations occur almost immediately. Relapses, however, occurred in slightly less than 50 per cent of the occasions tested during the succeeding hours and days. Though his experiments were conducted under limited test conditions, the need for reinforcement was indicated.

Gelder and Marks[9] note that single panic attack, whatever the reason, may undo the effects of weeks of treatment, and if less severe attacks of anxiety are repeated, the fear may also be relearned. Much of the skill of behavior therapy, they add, lies in tracing environmental causes for these unexplained attacks of panic.

A male patient had a recurrence of fear in church. After four Sundays without difficulty, he again began to sweat and shake. It was quite hot in church, and he had started to sweat, which temporarily reinstituted his phobia.

According to Franks[6], there are two ways to cope with relapses: either develop new counter conditioning techniques that minimize regression or provide "booster" follow-up conditioning sessions.

152

Recurrence of Symptoms after a Lapse of Time

One of the first patients whom I treated with systematic desensitization was a woman in her early forties. She had suffered a phobic state for about 12 years. When treated with systematic desensitization, she progressed to a point where she could travel, not only from her home, but also to great distances. After a lapse of several years, she phoned for an appointment. She was frightened; her symptoms had returned. Examination, however, proved her alarm to be unfounded. She was suffering from some of the symptoms of menopause, had mistaken them for the return of her previous illness, and had panicked. Reassurance and estrogens limited her visits to one. She phoned to say that she was her renewed self again.

The Importance of Concurrent Physical and Interpersonal Problems

Any circumstances that increase the general level of anxiety may delay progress.[22] Concern over physical disorders, justified or not, inhibits systematic desensitization. A doctor does not wish to overlook an undiagnosed physical disorder because of a mistaken notion that the basic trouble is a psychological disease.

When a patient complains of attacks of panic, with feelings of faintness, numbness, dread, perhaps chest and head tightness, and the like, one must give immediate thought to the hyperventilation syndrome. Having the patient breathe rapidly, with forceful expiration for 1 min. in the office quickly reproduces the same effects and reassures the patient. She is advised that all she needs to do to control these symptoms is to slow down her breathing, breathe into a paper bag, or take a sedative. Many symptoms of gas (eructations, borborygmi, abdominal pains, and spasms) are explained on the basis of throat tension, muscle spasm, or air swallowing.

As to interpersonal obstacles in treatment, I advise patients that an understanding and cooperative spouse is not only helpful but also an essential part of treatment. Marital problems tend to retard progress and should be resolved.

Lazarus[14] emphasizes the part played by others in the persistence of a symptom. In one instance he had to call in the patient's husband and mother and inform them that they were reinforcing the patient's dependency by displaying concern and expressing reassurance whenever she complained of minor somatic discomfort. They were requested not to pay attention to these negative statements, but to reward by attention, encouragement, and approval all positive self-reference and independent responses. He states that it is presumably impossible to become an agoraphobic without the aid of others who will submit to the inevitable demands imposed upon them by the patient. They play a vital role thereby in sustaining and maintaining the agoraphobic behavior, and make lasting therapeutic change unlikely unless they are treated concurrently.

153

None of the present-day sedatives and tranquilizers quiet the patient without also producing a certain amount of drowsiness. This is a hindrance or danger to the patient who must work, think, drive, or use machinery. Many therapists do not prescribe medication, but treatment is made much easier and carried out more effectively in a shorter period of time when the patient has the reassurance that the pill in her hand will effectively terminate her anxious spell. Placebos have no place here, for even those responding to placebos will not do so on every occasion; once a patient is fooled, it becomes a difficult matter to get him to try to face the feared object, situation, or feeling once again. I have found it most useful to diminish the anxiety, on occasion, with medication. As the patient continues to expose herself to the noxious stimulus, I gradually cut down the dosage so that he or she is exposed to smaller amounts of anxiety and thereby to effective desensitization. This approach is helpful when a patient must work in the presence of the phobic stimulus.

One further problem with medication is the development of dependency upon the drug. A few patients use the pill as a crutch, taking it in anticipation of an attack, rather than during one. These, too, must gradually be weaned from medication.

Although some therapists use behavior therapy techniques exclusively,[33] it seems best to employ them as an added tool in a broad armamentarium of therapeutic modalities.[1,15] In doing so, however, it is important to keep in mind that the behavioral approaches are quite different from those of insight therapy, and one must adopt this different orientation in order to utilize these techniques successfully.

REFERENCES

1. Abramovitz, C. M.: Personalistic Psychotherapy and the Role of Technical Eclecticism. Psychol. Rep. 26:255, 1970.
2. Beecher, H. K.: Measurement of Subjective Responses. New York, Oxford University Press, Inc., 1959.
3. Dengrove, E.: A New Letter-association Technique. Dis. Nerv. Syst. 23:25, 1962.
4. Clarke, A. D. B.: Learning and Human Development. Brit. J. Psychiat. 114:1061, 1968.
5. Frankl, V. E.: Paradoxical Intention. A Logotherapeutic Technique. Amer. J. Psychother. 14:520, 1960.
6. Franks, C. M.: Clinical Application of Conditioning and Other Behavioral Techniques. Cond. Reflex 1:36, 1966.
7. Gantt, W. H., et al: Effect of Person. Cond. Reflex 1:18, 1966.
8. Gavalas, R. J.: Operant Reinforcement of an Autonomic Response: Two Studies. J. Exp. Anal. Behav. 10:119, 1967.
9. Gelder, M. G., and Marks, I. M.: Severe Agoraphobia: A Controlled Prospective Trial of Behavior Therapy. Brit. J. Psychiat. 112:209, 1966.

10. Goldstein, I. B.: Study in Psychophysiology of Muscular Tension. I. Response Specificity. Arch. Gen. Psychiat. 11:322, 1964.
11. Jaspers, K.: General Psychopathology. Chicago, University of Chicago Press, 1963.
12. Lazarus, A. A., and Abramovitz, A.: The Use of "Emotive Imagery" in the Treatment of Children's Phobias. J. Ment. Sci. 108:191, 1962.
13. Lazarus, A. A.: A Preliminary Report on the Use of Directed Muscular Activity in Counter-conditioning. Behav. Res. Ther. 2:301, 1965.
14. Lazarus, A. A.: Broad Spectrum Behavior Therapy and the Treatment of Agoraphobia. Behav. Res. Ther. 4:95, 1966.
15. Lazarus, A. A.: In Support of Technical Eclecticism. Psychol. Rep. 21:415, 1967.
16. Lazarus, A. A.: Learning Theory and the Treatment of Depression. Behav. Res. Ther. 8:83, 1968.
17. Lazarus, A. A., and Serber, M.: Is Systematic Desensitization Being Misapplied? Psychol. Rep. 23:215, 1968.
18. Lazarus, A. A.: Variations in Desensitization Therapy. Psychotherapy: Theory, Research and Practice. 5:50, 1968.
19. MacLean, P. D.: The Brain in Relation to Empathy and Medical Education. J. Nerv. Ment. Dis. 155:355, 1967.
20. Meyer, V., and Crisp, A. H.: Some Problems in Behavior Therapy. Brit. J. Psychiat. 112:367, 1966.
21. Rachman, S.: Studies in Desensitization, III: Speed of Generalization. Behav. Res. Ther. 4:7, 1966.
22. Rachman, S.: Phobias: Their Nature and Control. Springfield, Ill., Charles C Thomas, Publisher, 1968.
23. Solyom, L., et. al.: Evaluation of a New Treatment Paradigm for Phobias. Canad. Psychiat. Assoc. J. 14:3, 1969.
24. Stevenson, I.: The Use of Rewards and Punishments in Psychotherapy. Comp. Psychiat. 3:20, 1962.
25. Stevenson, I., and Hain, J. B.: On the Different Meanings of Apparently Similar Symptoms, Illustrated by Varieties of Barber Shop Phobia. Amer. J. Psychiat. 124:3, 1967.
26. Truax, C. B.: Some Implications of Behavior Therapy for Psychotherapy. J. Consult. Psychol. 13:160, 1966.
27. Wolf, S.: Placebos: Problems and Pitfalls. Clin. Pharmacol. Ther. 3:254, 1962.
28. Wolpe, J.: Personal Communication.
29. Wolpe, J.: Psychotherapy by Reciprocal Inhibition. Stanford, Stanford University Press, 1958.
30. Wolpe, J.: The Systematic Desensitization Treatment of Neuroses. J. Nerv. Ment. Dis. 132:189, 1961.
31. Wolpe, J., and Lazarus, A. A.: Behavior Therapy. New York, Pergamon Press, Inc., 1966.
32. Wolpe, J.: Psychotherapy by Reciprocal Inhibition. Cond. Reflex. 3:234, 1968.
33. Wolpe, J.: Editorial. IN: Newsletter, Assoc. Adv. Behav. Ther. 3:1, 1968.

Art Therapy

by Mardi J. Horowitz, M.D.

Art therapy, along with various nonverbal therapies, is enjoying a renaissance of interest among mental health workers. When therapists change from talking with patients to encouraging some form of graphic communication, it is usually because they want to obtain more information, or to establish more closeness or rapport with the patient, or to evoke emotional expressions and work through feeling states, or to transform the patient's mood or attitude.

Some types of information may be communicated in images rather than verbal thoughts or statements. The emotional and conceptual differences between modes of representation, and the special properties of image formation, have been discussed in detail elsewhere.[1] To summarize somewhat oversimply, many repressed memories and fantasies are accessible to consciousness in image representation, but are unexpressed or untransformable into word meanings. Often such memories or fantasies emerge in a series of drawings or paintings without awareness on the part of the patient as to what is communicated. For example, the nature of patients' self-representations and object relationships can sometimes be quite obscure in their verbal statements, especially if patients are inarticulate. However, a therapist may be able to infer a great deal from their drawings of themselves, their family, and their peer groups.

Sometimes a therapist talks with a patient for many interviews and yet cannot establish an internal representation of that patient's existential world. Every therapist, of course, has his own style of relating to different types of patients. However, many develop a kind of image-model based on the patient's reports: They have some idea of what his parents were like, what his dreams and fantasies are like, and how he sees himself and the world. When verbal communication does not lead to that type of rapport, some therapists shift the mode of communication to pictorial form, hoping that the patient's images will be more readily grasped at the feeling, intuitive, or "gut" level.

The case is much clearer in patients who are mute, severely withdrawn, or who simply mistrust any talking relationship. While some therapists remain physically present but silent with such patients until they are willing or able to talk, other therapists believe they can reach a patient by a nonlexical approach such as attempting to draw with them.

156

Expression and Working-through of Emotions and Memories

Some patients use intellectualization, isolation, splitting off, and suppression to such an extent that their verbal cognitions and communications are virtually devoid of feeling. For example, a patient may have a blocked grief reaction after the loss of an important person. He may not avoid verbal description of the loss, the memories relevant to the relationship, or the consequences of the separation. Therefore, each repetition is neutral, without the feelings that the therapist infers "ought" to be present if the mourning process is to be carried to completion. In such circumstances, some therapists may ask the patient to evoke an image or draw the person who has been lost, or some variant on this theme. In some patients this process of shifting the mode of representation from lexical to image is accompanied by a marked shift in the subjective experience of affect. The image may evoke the feelings not experienced when descriptive words were used, leading to subsequent translation of the feelings and the images into lexical representation for more secure and complete cognitive processing.

One important aspect of working-through involves modification of the defenses that before treatment were used to ward off the conflicted affects and associated ideas. The motives for defense often include a wish to avoid guilt, shame, fear, or anger. In many patients there is also anxiety over their inability to control affective states. The shift to graphic media may allow patients with relatively weak defenses to externalize the control process: Because they control the drawing or painting production, they may feel more in control over the formation of their internal cognitive and affective states. With some expression of affect and with a sense of greater capacity for volitional control, such patients may shift impulse-defense configurations and thus reduce symptom formation.

Transformation of Emotion or Attitude

Because image formation is closely linked with emotion, images can be used to change mood or attitude. This process is complex in actual practice and not without hazards, but a simple illustration is that of a depressed person who is asked to draw a happy scene. If he cooperates, his mood may lift (temporarily) and the experience may indicate to him that it is possible to feel better, thus supplying hope. In an opposite manner, a patient troubled with great rage may be encouraged to express some of this affect, within controlled limits, in painting. Some affect is discharged and there is some sense of being in control of what was once feared as out of control.

More complex routes to a change in attitude involve using the image production and the images produced as a mode of externalized thinking and trial action. The picture remains after the mental image has failed; additional responses and various possibilities can then be investigated. Through such experimental versions of action plans, he may discover routes out of a

157

predicament which were not so anxiety provoking as he feared. The therapist may in some instances "show the way." Thus, the patient, through trial actions and changes, may gain courage to try real actions and changes.

In a similar manner, because of the durability of the graphic product over time, a patient can review what he has done. Some cognitive operations that have escaped his conscious reflection may become apparent to him or be shown to him. Through such clarification and awareness it is sometimes possible to motivate change in cognitive operations. For example, a patient may always use "undoing" as an unconscious defensive operation. In a series of paintings he may always paint and then paint over in form, that is, cancel out any aggressive statement. By witnessing this pattern, he may become aware of the anxieties that he has avoided by continually undoing. He may then attempt to transform his defensive attitudes into conscious controls.

Disadvantages

While the foregoing purposes express some of the advantages of image formation and graphic communication in psychotherapy, a therapist should also recognize the disadvantages. Lexical representation is the most secure form of representation because the meanings of words are relatively stable and are generalized across persons. The meanings of images, anchored in early memories, tend to be more idiosyncratic, symbolic, and overdetermined. These factors may lead therapists to misinterpret the graphic products of patients; equally important, it may lead patients to misinterpret the graphic symbols of art therapists.

The second disadvantage is closely related to the first. It is easy to blur or change the attributed meaning of an image, since images lend themselves to multiple signification. If left at the image level of representation, an idea or emotion can be split off, re-repressed, or otherwise avoided. For full integration into the personality, ideas and feelings expressed as images should be translated into lexical representation (and perhaps vice versa). In fact, one usually resorts to art therapy when dealing with persons who have inhibited cross translation of modes and so have avoided converting images into word meanings.

The third disadvantage concerns the filters placed by transformational processes between image representation in subjective experience and concrete or graphic representations. As Gombrich[2] notes, drawing skills require not only accurate perception but also acquisition of graphic conventions or abbreviations. A person learns schemata for use in drawing. Also, eye-hand coordination must be finely tuned in order to produce a desired image. For such reasons, persons of differing skill, capacity, and experience vary in their ability to produce an external replica of an internal image. A poor drawer, or a person with a tremor, could be humiliated by the experience unless carefully supported.

A fourth disadvantage relates to the aesthetic property of graphic products. Either patients or therapist may become caught up in producing an artistically pleasing work. While in some instances this may allow a desirable sense of mastery or self-esteem, it can also be a preoccupation that occurs at the expense of therapeutic work. I believe it is seldom wise, for example, to use the products of art therapy in any kind of exhibition unless it is for scientific or educational purposes or unless the art therapy is strictly a form of occupational therapy.

The final disadvantage of art therapy relates to one of its strengths—it deals closely with fantasy life. Some patients may lose their distress in thinking the fantasy and find it relatively free of anxiety because nothing in it is real. They may enthusiastically pour out a rich fantasy life in graphic products, but use this entire activity to avoid dealing in reality with real problems. I believe that this danger is great enough that art therapy should not be the sole technique of any therapist; rather, it should be in contact with lexical forms of therapy. Sometimes patients have two therapists, one for each form. If so, the closest cooperation is necessary to avoid a split between the ego functions of reality and fantasy cognitions and communications (as well as to manage splitting in transference responses).

Styles of Art Therapy

Since image formation and graphic communication comprise a system of representation, they resemble lexical thinking and verbal communication in that the system of representation can be put to a variety of uses. Thus, any school or theory of therapy could use images and graphic media. Whatever the theoretical persuasion of the therapist, the interpersonal structure of the art therapy situation can be grouped as individual production, group production, or graphic interaction.

Individual art therapy was pioneered in this country by Margaret Naumberg.[3] Classically, the patient produces a series of drawings and paintings and may provide verbal associations to the contents. The therapist, in this tradition, uses verbal rather than graphic communication to offer interpretations, ask questions, give suggestions, or encourage further production. The agents of therapeutic change are usually regarded as establishing a trustful relationship with the therapist, interpretation of meaningful symbols, and expressing and working through conflicted emotions and ideas.[4-5] Some therapists emphasize synthesis and growth rather than analysis and insight, and use art productions to provide a sense of mastery and control, identity, self-esteem, clarity, and creativity.[7-9]

Art therapy techniques can also be used in group settings. The most common use is with psychiatric inpatients with whom the graphic production can be used to foster social communication among patients who become too tense with the verbal interchanges of conventional group psychotherapy. The therapist can, for

159

example, suggest a common topic. Patients can work together, focusing both on their own work and the presence of each other. They may work with separate media or together (as on a mural). Periodically, the work can be discussed verbally, with return to the graphic production when anxiety or resistance levels rise above a useful threshold.

The group setting can also be used to study the role structures of small organizations such as the family. When assigned a common graphic task, they may reveal in a verbal family interview[10] the interactional dynamics and feelings that are unavailable or concealed.

An additional ingredient can be added to situations of individual or group art therapy if the therapist uses the image mode of communication rather than the verbal one. I have found this manner of approach to be especially useful in reaching withdrawn schizophrenic patients.[11] The patient and I usually sit side by side and use the same media. I try to keep conversation to a minimum and to respond to the patient by graphic production. In this technique, content may be objective (for example, stick figures), but quite often it is abstract. A great deal is learned, however, from the patient's pattern of response, use of tools, selection of shape and color, and his use of territory on the surface used. Almost always the first phase is a testing phase, to see what the boundaries, permissions, and prohibitions of the therapist will be. An expressive phase, in which the patient reveals some of his current concerns, usually does not emerge until the seventh to tenth session—provided the therapist successfully manuevers through the testing phase. These phases of testing and expression probably occur in many other therapeutic situations. Once in the expressive phase of therapy, the therapist may take different approaches to the images produced.

The Therapist's Response to the Patient's Images

The degree of structure or intervention imposed by the therapist varies in art therapy just as it does in verbal therapy. The mildest intervention is inquiry; the most directive is telling the patient what to express or doing it for him.

In inquiry the therapist simply asks the patient to communicate more; for instance, to talk about a picture he has made, or to make a picture of some memory, fantasy, dream, or hallucination he has experienced mentally. Inquiry may extend to suggestions to the patients of modes or directions of expression. For example, the patient may be asked to do a picture of how he feels when angry, or to depict his bodily feeling in a graphic way, or to show members of his family. Or, the therapist may suggest a shift in media; for example, he may suggest large brushes or fingerpaint for a patient who is overcontrolled and rigid. Also, the therapist may suggest image formation, as in guided daydreaming, and then ask the patient to draw or paint his subjective images.[12-14]

Such directive daydreaming techniques have some hazards if improperly or unskillfully used. The patient often has relatively less regulatory control over image formation than over word representation, and can sometimes have emergent memories or affect states that are too powerful to be integrated with other cognitive structures.

Directive techniques are, of course, not always oriented toward remembering or expressing. The therapist may deliberately direct a patient to draw recurrent intrusive images repeatedly, on the grounds that through such repetition the patient may learn control of the image, complete cognitive processing of the relevant ideational and affective associations, and so master a previously overwhelming experience or fantasy. A similar technique could be supported, theoretically, on the basis of learning theory and the concept of desensitization in behavior therapy.

The therapist may intervene graphically or verbally in other ways either to increase or decrease the level of the patient's defensive and controlling functions. As an example of increasing controlling functions, consider a patient who has just depicted an extremely threatening situation where a symbol, representative of himself, is in danger or endangers another symbol (a common theme in the expressive phase of interaction painting or drawing). The therapist can reduce the threat by drawing interactions demonstrative of how conflict can be acceptably reduced without the annihilation of either "symbol." If the patient has drawn a situation where "he" is impossibly menaced by a monster, the therapist can draw in weapons, candy to appease the monster, or a friendly monster. Naturally, such techniques would be used only if a patient is relatively out of control and anxious over his impulse; they would not be used when his expression has been within tolerable limits.

In less disturbed patients, the therapist may make interventions that reduce or counteract avoidance of expressing areas of conflict. For example, a patient afraid of relating to women may avoid depiction of women in his drawings. Once he is sheltered by sufficient relationship with the therapist, the latter may introduce or suggest depiction of female figures. Or, if aggression is a behavioral problem, but is avoided in verbal communications, the therapist can introduce the theme symbolically. Currently, art therapists use techniques along the spectrum from simple encouragement to draw or paint, to specific and focused interventions. The more specific and directive the intervention, the greater the training, experience, and skill needed on the part of the therapist.

Summary

Art therapy uses images as a mode for representation of ideas and feelings. As is true of representation in words, the resultant communication can be utilized for any kind of therapeutic purpose. Art therapy techniques range from individual to group role structures. The therapist has available either a verbal or graphic influence on the patient. These influences can range from support to uncovering to manipulation of the patient's cognitive processes. It is to be hoped that the increased prevalence of graphic communication will not be a fad or be claimed as property by any school of therapy, but will lead instead to a deeper understanding of the cognitive processes involved in image formation, symptom formation, and conflict reduction.

REFERENCES

1. Horowitz, M.: Image Formation and Cognition. New York, Appleton-Century-Crofts, Publisher, 1970.
2. Gombrich, E.: Art and Illusion: A Study in the Psychology of Pictorial Representation. New York, Pantheon Books, Inc., 1969.
3. Naumberg, M.: Psychoneurotic Art: Its Function in Psychotherapy. New York, Grune & Stratton, Inc., 1953.
4. Naumberg, M.: Dynamically Oriented Art Therapy: Its Principle and Practice. New York, Grune & Stratton, Inc., 1966.
5. Stern, M.: Free Painting as an Auxiliary Technique in Psychoanalysis. In Bychowski, G., and Despert, J. L. (eds.): Specialized Techniques in Psychotherapy. New York, Basic Books, Inc., Publishers, 1952.
6. Pickford, R.: Studies in Psychiatric Art. Springfield, Ill., Charles C Thomas, Publisher, 1967.
7. Ulman, E.: Art Therapy in an Outpatient Clinic. Psychiatry 16:55-64, 1953.
8. Kramer, E.: Art Therapy and the Severely Disturbed Gifted Child. Bull. Art Ther. 10:3-20, 1965.
9. Kellog, R.: Understanding Children's Art. Psychol. Today 5:16-25, 1967.
10. Kwiatkowska, N.: The Use of Families' Art Productions for Psychiatric Evaluation. Bull. Art Ther. 1:52-69, 1967.
11. Horowitz, M.: Graphic Communication: A Study of Interaction Painting with Schizophrenics. Amer. J. Psychother. 17:320-327, 1963.
12. Kubie, L.: The Use of Induced Hypnagogic Reveries in the Recovery of Repressed Amnesic Data. Bull. Menninger Clin. 7:172-182, 1943.
13. Reyher, J.: Free Imagery: An Uncovering Procedure. J. Clin. Psychol. 19:454-459, 1963.
14. Leuner, H.: Guided Affective Imagery (GAI). A Method of Intensive Psychotherapy. Amer. J. Psychother. 23:4-22, 1969.

Contributions of Hypnosis
to Psychotherapy

by Lewis R. Wolberg, M.D.

Most practitioners who experiment with hypnosis, and seriously attempt to blend it with their habitual techniques, find that it can be productive under certain conditions, even turning the tide from a threatened failure to a therapeutic success.

I wish I could say that hypnosis has been triumphant in all my cases. It has not. I have had my share of disappointments. But the more I have utilized hypnosis over the years, the more respect I have gained for its potentialities. Indeed for me it has continued to be the most important of all the instrumentalities that I have employed in concert with my general therapeutic techniques. Obviously hypnosis must be blended with basic psychotherapeutic procedures because employed in isolation it has limited value (Conn[1]).

How hypnosis works is still a matter of conjecture. In assaying its impact we are confronted with the same confounding variables that envelop all of the psychotherapy. We are slowly beginning to understand some of these variables, but we have not yet been able to expose them completely to the searchlight of scientific exploration (Frank[4]). In psychotherapy we are still balanced precariously on the peak of mounting ambiguities. We do not even yet possess a conceptually valid paradigm around which we can organize our ideas of interpersonal processes. The complexities of chemical, neurophysiological, intrapsychic, spiritual, and social interactions defy description, let alone analysis. We are reduced to accepting the pragmatic proposition that if a method works we should utilize it (Orne[8]). After all we still do not know how electricity operates, but we are constantly employing and enjoying its miracles.

A convenient way of looking at hypnosis is to regard it as a form of communication which expedites a number of healing processes common to all forms of psychotherapy. One of the most important is that hypnosis enhances the multiple roles the therapist must willy-nilly play with his patients as he leads them through the emotional labyrinths of their illness.

Let us outline a few of these roles. A good deal of relief from tension and restoration of homeostasis is generally scored in psychotherapy as a consequence of the placebo influence. Here the therapist, without design or intent, is regarded as the miraculous healer, a *magician*. In the mind of the patient he possesses the means and the wizardry to bring a halt to his suffering and illness. Faith in the therapist's tactics is an important element in all healing processes. It is especially enhanced by the maneuvers of trance induction and utilization (Shapiro[11]).

A second role the psychotherapist assumes is that of *confessor*. Unlocking the door to one's inner burdens unleashes feelings and fears habitually guarded as too reprehensible to reveal. In addition to the immediate and temporary release from tension, there is in such emotional catharsis the added dividend of exposing onself without disguise to an empathic authority. When the expected conventional shock reactions are not forthcoming, the patient usually responds with greater self-tolerance and self-acceptance, and this may register a permanent imprint on his superego. Hypnosis quickly opens up founts of bottled-up emotion owing to its effect on repression. It thus enhances the confessor roles of the therapist.

Suggestion enters into every authority-subject, professional-client relationship (Weitzenhoffer and Sjoberg[13]). As an expert the professional functions wittingly or unwittingly in the role of *demigod* whose pronouncements are subtly absorbed, often without challenge. In hypnosis, suggestibility, as is well known, is greatly enhanced and hence this therapeutic dimension is accordingly magnified.

Perhaps the word *philanthropist* denegrates the fourth role the therapist plays with his patients by virtue of their relationship. The patient projects his hopes for an encounter with an idealized parental figure who will supply him with the understanding and bounties he feels he failed to receive from his own parents. Obviously this unrealistic camouflage is sooner or later swept away when the therapist fails to come up to expectations, but while it lasts the idealization promotes the acceptance of the therapist's theories and practices which will hopefully continue to exert a therapeutic impact when the therapist eventually becomes a mere flesh-and-blood figure. Hypnosis has a remarkable effect on the relationship and even during the first trance session may cut through resistances that would ordinarily delay the essential establishing of rapport. This is especially important in detached and fearful individuals who put up barriers to any kind of closeness and hence obstruct the evolvement of a working alliance.

The fifth role assumed by a productive therapist is that of an *identification model*. Often without awareness the patient's values are recast in the mold of the therapeutic relationship. The patient quickly senses the kind of human being with whom he is dealing from a variety of verbal and nonverbal cues. An amalgamation of the therapist's with his own values occurs gradually, sometimes stirring up conflict. Signs of conflict may not appear in direct form. Value change occurs when the patient works through his need for spurious gratifications inherent in the retention of his neurotic way of life. We assume, of course, that the therapist's values are more realistic and constructive than those of the

164

patient. Hypnosis often elevates the image of the therapist as an idealized authority and expedites his role as an identification model (Dreikurs[3]).

The sixth role of *benefactor* is one that the therapist usually does not deliberately assume, but which may be bestowed on him by a hopeful recipient eager to incorporate palliative subsidies. Even though the patient's incentives may be spurious, the end result can be an incorporation of reinforcements that can shape behavior toward a more healthful adaptation (Dorcus[2]). Once a new behavioral response has been established, or neurotic sequences controlled, certain favorable consequences may occrue to the benefit of the individual, and these positive reinforcers help to maintain accelerated change. There is little question in studying the dreams and associations of subjects in and following a trance that they are inclined to augment the powers of the hypnotist as a potential benefactor.

As a transferential object in the form of a *parental surrogate,* the therapist plays his seventh role in the therapeutic drama. Once the idealization of the therapist crumbles to the dust of disappointment, the frustrations and furies of childhood, compounded out of significant early conditionings, may contaminate the relationship with the therapist (Gill and Brenman[6]). The distortion of the image of the therapist is often concealed by pleasantries, defenses, and facades; but dreams, fantasies, and associations may expose the undercurrent interpersonal climate. Unless the therapist is trained to detect and to deal with transferential symbols, resistance may soon block therapeutic progress. Hypnosis can expedite the release of transference in a remarkable way and lay open insidious roadblocks to memory recovery.

The eighth common role of the therapist is that of *educator.* Patients will obviously look up to the therapist for constructive guidance. They will seek counsel and direction to usher them out of the middle of their neurotic plight. But unfortunately they will block their own path with resistances—resistances to the development of a proper working relationship, to the understanding of the nature and source of their problems, to the use of the therapist's techniques, to the employment of reparative and restorative patterns, to the control of their own destiny. Dealing with these resistances is perhaps the most important task in moving a patient from dead center. Hypnosis not only serves an important function in detecting and exposing the myriad resistances to change, but it helps the patient to challenge and work them through.

When we consider the multiple roles that the therapist must play in psychotherapy, we come to the conclusion that the quality of his personality which will enable him to assume the varied roles demanded of him will be as important as his expertise. Hypnosis will not overcome deficiencies in the therapist that interfere with capacities to function in various therapeutic roles. The therapist will respond to the patient, not only as one who needs his help, but also as an individual onto whom he can project certain of his own needs and

165

problems. These may run counter to the essential roles he must assume. We may anticipate varied strivings in the therapist, his reactions being influenced by the sex, status, age, attitudes, symptoms, and personality characteristics of the patient. Thus the same therapist may react sadistically toward a strong male patient, with pathological tenderness toward a weak passive male, with seductive feelings toward an attractive female, with violent disgust toward a drug addict, and with hopelessness toward a schizophrenic. The presence in the therapist of therapeutically destructive attitudes can be antagonistic to improvement with any kind of psychotherapy. The mere fact that he employs hypnosis will not make up for bankruptcy in any of his personality assets.

The basic requirements for good hypnotic therapy are no different from those for any kind of brief psychotherapy. The therapist must be able to perceive rapidly the underlying dynamics and immediate emotional needs, and to recognize what constructive defenses and other assets exist that will aid him in helping his patients respond positively to him and to his techniques.

The value of hypnosis is thus no greater than the proficiency of the practitioner who employs it. There are many professionals who do well with other techniques, but who refuse to use hypnosis because they are not able to employ it competently. Actually not all doctors make good surgeons, and not all therapists can become competent hypnotherapists. Some fail miserably when they attempt to practice the hypnotic method. Skill is an ingredient in any technique and hypnosis is no exception. What is important for each therapist to establish is the utility for him of hypnosis in his work. Does he feel comfortable in utilizing hypnosis? Does inducing a trance make him feel powerful, sadistic, or anxious? Does he sense a change in his feelings toward his hypnotized subject which differ from how he feels when the patient is in the waking state? Is he able to remain objective about the material produced by the patient? Can he apply the same dynamic criteria to the behavior responses of the patient in hypnosis, and to the patient's reactions to the trance experience posthypnotically, as he would to any other of the patient's reactions? Does hypnosis have a personal meaning for the therapist that makes him overvalue its effects? These questions can be answered only when the therapist applies his hypnotic technique to a variety of patients and carefully observes his own responses as well as those of his subjects. Where untoward feelings are mobilized in him, he may ask himself whether he can control these feelings in order to operate as objectively as possible. If he cannot, hypnosis is not a technique that is suitable for him.

One common defect is excessive passivity in the therapist. There is a tradition in training that dictates that one must be as inactive and noninterfering as possible. The presumption is that the patient must dictate the terms of his own destiny, as well as the pace he pursues in approaching a cure. The therapist must do nothing to interpose his own values on the patient since the patient must work these out for himself. Theoretically this sounds fine. The only problem is that the methods that derive from these precepts help very few patients. In most cases a structured and rational kind of activity guarantees the best results. A good therapist does not impose his standards on his patient; however, he has a responsibility to interfere with ideas and attitudes that are part of cherished value systems which the patient insists on retaining even though they are to his continued disadvantage.

What is vital also is that the therapist feel free to interrupt neurotic symptoms if necessary without worrying too much about whether or not he is doing something antitherapeutic. An unwholesome shibboleth in psychiatry is the belief that although symptoms may be temporarily ameliorated by suggestion, a cure cannot be achieved until the motive for recovery overwhelms the ends achieved by the illness, or until the dynamic psychological processes which mediate the disease are thoroughly understood by the patient himself. Remove a symptom and its return in the same or substitutive form will hang over the patient like the sword of Damocles. An illustrative but apocryphal story is that of a hiccuping applicant at an airline office who requested a ticket from an unusually attractive clerk. "Here you are," remarked the girl, "and you owe us an additional $150." "What!" exclaimed the man indignantly. "I paid for my ticket completely." He continued excitedly, "I don't owe you a cent more." "I know," smiled the clerk flirtatiously, "but you see, I cured your hiccups." Looking surprised the man replied, "You are absolutely right. Now what can you do for high blood pressure?"

There is still, in spite of overwhelming clinical evidence of its safety, controversy about symptom removal. In a few experimental situations that have been reported by several investigators, symptoms removed by direct command without any suggestion as to replacement have produced some substitute symptoms (Seitz[9,10]); however, the same kind of experiments done by other observers have not shown this result. In either case, the attitude and expectations of the operator may be somehow communicated to the patient, perhaps nonverbally. I have personally tried to bring on vicarious symptoms by forceful suggestions. At least with my techniques I have either successfully removed or ameliorated the symptoms without ill effect, or else the patient has refused to abandon them in spite of my best efforts. In the latter instance I presume the patients needed their symptoms to preserve their psychological balance. The goal of symptom relief is a legitimate one, for any disturbing symptomatology results in a pyramiding of tension which may cue off a variety of physical and emotional ailments not directly related to the original complaint. It follows that removal of an offensive symptom can restore the individual's sense of mastery rather than vitiate it, and restoration of emotional homeostasis may then result.

There is considerable evidence that supportive and palliative techniques may

167

sometimes result not only in lasting relief from complaints, but also, in some cases, even in reconstructive character change (Wolberg[14]). These developments are not fortuitous. They follow the working through of conflict initiated by a constructive use of the therapeutic interpersonal relationship. What happens, it may be asked, if a patient insists upon retaining a certain symptom though he realizes it is neurotic and even self-damaging? I believe that it is within a patient's rights to retain a symptom if he really desires to do so. But when a patient comes to me with a crippling symptom, and tells me that he does not want to give his symptom up, I feel it to be an obligation to help him to reposition his sights. Many patients forced to see me by their physicians because of excess tension or improper life habits would like to get well without altering in the least the destructive patterns responsible for their troubles. Sometimes they will want me to force them to want to get well. Obviously this is impossible with hypnosis or with any other technique; however, I will try to educate them into recognizing for themselves their improper thinking processes that make them adhere to values and patterns that are hurtful to them. But in the long run they are the arbiters of their own destiny and eventually must make the choice between retaining strivings that make for illness and those that will promote health.

Another common question is why if a patient really wants to get well, he is sometimes unable, even when his motivation for recovery is strong, to overcome his neurosis in spite of our best skills as hypnotherapists. One deterrent to our therapeutic designs is the emergence of outmoded coping mechanisms that survive in almost pristine form, even though the paths toward which they are pressed serve destructive ends. Much as cultures retain folkways of primitive lineage that have no functional utility, so the human being repetitively and compulsively is committed to anachronistic means of attack, retreat, entrenchment, and other defenses. These we employed in defiance of reason as preferred modes of interpersonal operation. Flexibility to shifts in the environment is the keynote of adaptation; inflexibility cannot help but interfere with mental health.

What actually accounts for the peculiarly tenacious persistence of mal-adaptive and functionally useless patterns is difficult to say. Neither psycho-analytic theory nor learning theory nor any other theory has adequately explained them. One would expect that the absence of positive reinforcements would eventually extinguish certain traits particularly where they have created problems for the individual. But even though no rewards are apparent, some neurotic patterns persist to the mutual dismay of the victim and the professional person who proposes to help him.

It is in the therapy of such apparently nonresponsive patients that a dynamic approach can prove valuable above and beyond the benefits of symptom removal. One cannot discount the effectiveness of nondynamic behavioral

168

approaches in the average individual. These often depreciate the delving into unconscious material and the disgorging of repressed and repudiated aspects of the psyche. But in many recalcitrant patients we find that a mere search for immediate environmental reinforcements of maladaptive behavior, and efforts to remove these or to substitute for them unpleasant consequences yields little for our efforts. Moreover, where the behavioral repertoire needs broadening and attempts are made to remove behavioral deficits by techniques which reward for proper responses, we are disappointed in the hoped-for shaping of healthy conduct.

Where a therapist has had some psychoanalytic training he may be able to expand his effectiveness by probing into the sources of conflict in his nonresponsive patients. It is not always essential to burrow into the depths of the unconscious with all the techniques that Freud has given us. The patient will usually reveal basic problems to us without effort by his defiant responses to our methods and to our personalities as we induce hypnosis and utilize the trance to pursue our therapeutic objectives. Resistance to hypnotherapy will reflect fundamental characterologic distortions and surviving childish needs and defenses which act as initiating foci for neurotic illness. In bringing the patient to an awareness of his resistances and manipulations, we are often enabled to break through the impediments that without challenge will surely cripple our best therapeutic tactics. The hypnotic experience becomes a biopsy of the existing pathology and ultimately a means to its resolution.

What may happen then is an insightful working through of neurotic patterns. Theoretically repressions are restored to keep certain pathogenic conflicts from awareness. A more harmonious balance occurs among the various components of the psychic apparatus. A sense of mastery permits the discarding of regressive defenses. Positive reinforcements are then imparted for productive behavior while neurotic behavior receives negative reinforcement.

Where resistances to verbalization, free association, and the remembering of dreams and early memories exist, hypnosis may lift these obstructions (Wolberg[15]). Hypnosis may light up archaic interfering transference and bring fundamental problems to the surface. It may also aid in the working-through process, particularly the conversion of insight into action by dealing directly with resistances to change.

It is difficult to see how the dimensions of transference and resistance which occur in one form or another in many patients even in the briefest hypnotic therapy can be managed without some knowledge of, and capacity to work within, a dynamically oriented framework. Furthermore, countertransference is so often mobilized in active approaches such as hypnosis that its understanding and control are mandatory to effective operation. Actually the understanding of psychoanalytic principles may enable us to follow more accurately a patient's progress and to detect resistance even where our goal is mere symptom relief. Such understanding may spell the difference between success and failure.

The notion that in the trance state we bypass resistances to deal exclusively with the unconscious (Freud[5]), only to have the conscious barriers restored with awakening, is another of the persistent misconceptions about hypnosis. Any experienced analyst is aware of the need to work with resistances rather than with the repudiated drives and conflicts that evade the resistances. The uncovering of repressed material may come about with the hypnotic induction or the use of certain hypnoanalytic techniques. This is insufficient in itself. What is required is that the patient be challenged to understand why it is difficult for him to countenance or to acknowledge this material to the waking state. Pointed questions and injunctions to work on his resistances, and to accept, reject, or modify the material that has been revealed while pondering its implications, may register their effects on the patient's ego. The changes wrought will be manifest in the patient's dreams—for instance, in less distorted symbolism and conscious associations. "Spontaneous" insights may then emerge.

We must overemphasize the need for insight in all cases. In my experience, and that of many of my colleagues, the overcoming of an established neurotic pattern can occur without the subjective appearance of insight. What often happens is that insight *follows* upon the resolution of a problem, rather than precedes it. For example, a frigid woman who experiences her first orgasm may be rewarded with a flood of insights into why she feared yielding control, which will help her to face intercourse with expectations of enjoyment rather than frustration.

This is not to minimize the impact of true understanding of the repetitive and compulsive nature of contemporary neurotic behavior, and its origins in early life experience with significant authority figures. This type of insight may act as a liberating force from the primary and secondary gains of the neurosis. It upsets the balance between the repressed and repressing elements. It fosters a desire to test the reality of one's attitudes and values. It gives the person an opportunity to challenge the very philosophies that govern his life. But insight alone is not enough to arrest the neurotic process and to promote new and constructive ways of handling reality. Instead, insight may produce not change but an accentuation of anxiety, since it defies the individual to approach life on different terms. He is perhaps for the first time outraged at his customary defensive tactics. He may then throw up a smoke screen of resistance and retreat into old defensive patterns. Therapy may grind to a halt induced by intolerable fantasies associated with action.

It is at this point that the dynamic therapist can utilize the precepts of those who are dedicated to symptom-oriented therapy, as are the behavior theorists. He can encourage his patients, once they have acquired "insight," to expose themselves actively to situations which will ablate unhealthful and reinforce constructive behavior. Hypnosis can be singularly effective in promoting such an exposure (Spiegel,[12] Moss[7]). There is much in the methods of both behavior therapists and those who are psychoanalytically oriented for mutual study and blending if they retain experimental open-mindness and discard their distrust of each other.

We may challenge another questionable traditional precept: the idea that hypnosis is unsuited for certain vulnerable patients: for instance, borderline cases who are notoriously unstable and who are likely to shift over into a psychotic phase at the least sign of stress. In my experience I have found hypnosis particularly suited to the treatment of many borderline patients. By promoting relaxation, it can have a calming effect on the individual. I believe that it may, in the existing protective atmosphere of a relationship with a projected idealized supportive, nonpunitive authority figure, be singularly reassuring. The interested, nonthreatening encouraging manner of the operator, with absence of hostile and seductive maneuvers, may be most supportively rewarding. This is not to say that the patient will not respond with misinterpretation and unstable behavior irrespective of how gently he is appraoched. But a proper bearing on the part of the operator reduces such incidents and may be therapeutically rewarding.

Obviously one must expect in some borderline patients during hypnosis a greater degree of emotionally disturbed reactions than in more stable patients. These reactions may spontaneously erupt irrespective of the approach or behavior of the operator. They are easily provoked by overt aggressive activities, or probing. They are most frequently mobilized by psychotherapeutic techniques that challenge defenses and resistances, or that deal with preconscious or unconscious trends and impulses. They are less frequently present when during hypnosis suggestions are confined to tension alleviation or pain reduction. They are reduced by a reassuring and supportive attitude on the part of the operator.

There is, therefore, no reason why hypnosis should not be used in borderline and even psychotic patients. But where an operator finds that he is excessively upset by occasional disturbed reactions, or is unable to control them, or observes that he stimulates more than occasional explosiveness in such patients, he may prudently avoid hypnosis. This is not to say that in the waking state he may not be confronted with similar upsetting reactions in his sicker cases, particularly where his techniques or the relationship is interpreted as threatening. However, it may be that his own unconscious manipulations and aggressive or seductive tendencies may not reveal themselves so easily in his tactics without hypnosis.

There is no way of predicting in advance the exact influence that hypnosis may have on any patient or his problems, since each individual will respond uniquely to the techniques in line with the special meanings they have for him. The mental set with which he approaches hypnosis, his motivations to be helped, the depth and quality of his resistances, his conception of the therapist and the image he conjures up of him, the skill of the therapist, the kinds of interventions administered, the management of the patient's doubts and oppositional tendencies, and the nature of the patient's transference and therapist's countertransference will all enter into the responsive Gestalt.

Potentially hypnosis may catalyze every aspect of the therapeutic process. Whether or not the therapist will want to employ it will depend largely on how much confidence he has in hypnosis and how well he works with hypnotic techniques. I believe that every therapist owes it to himself to experiment with hypnosis as an adjunct to his customary psychotherapeutic methods, for if he gives himself the proper opportunity, he may as a consequence be able greatly to enhance his effectiveness as a psychotherapist. The least that can happen is that he will learn a great deal more about the workings of the human mind than he knew before in his prehypnotic days. And this in itself can be a cherished blessing.

REFERENCES

1. Conn, J. H.: The Psychodynamics of Recovery Under Hypnosis. Int. J. Clin. Exp. Hypn. 8:3-15, 1960.
2. Dorcus, R. M.: The Influence of Hypnosis on Learning and Habit Modifying. In: Dorcus, R. M. (Ed.), Hypnosis and Its Therapeutic Applications. New York, McGraw-Hill Book Co., Inc., 1956.
3. Dreikurs, R.: The Interpersonal Relationship in Hypnosis. Psychiatry 25:219-226, 1962.
4. Frank, J.: Persuasion and Healing: A Comparative Study of Psychotherapy. Baltimore, Johns Hopkins Press, 1961.
5. Freud, A.: The Ego and the Mechanisms of Defense. New York, International Universities Press, 1946.
6. Gill, M. M., and Brenman, M.: The Metapsychology of Regression and Hypnosis. In: Gordon, J. E. (Ed.), Handbook of Clinical and Experimental Hypnosis. New York, The Macmillan Company, 1967, pp. 281-318.
7. Moss, C. S.: Brief Crisis-Oriented Hypnotherapy. In: Gordon, J. E. (Ed.), Handbook of Clinical and Experimental Hypnosis. New York, The Macmillan Company, 1967.
8. Orne, M. T.: Implications for Psychotherapy Derived from Current Research on the Nature of Hypnosis. Amer. J. Psychiat. 118:1097-1103, 1962.
9. Seitz, P. F.: Symbolism and Organ Choice in Conversion Reactions: An Experimental Approach. Psychosom. Med. 13:255-259, 1951.
10. Seitz, P. F.: Experiments in the Substitution of Symptoms by Hypnosis. II. Psychosom. Med. 14:405-424, 1953.
11. Shapiro, A. K.: Attitudes Toward the Use of Placebos in Treatment. J. Nerv. Ment. Dis. 130:200-211, 1960.
12. Spiegel, H.: Hypnotic Intervention as an Adjunct for Rapid Clinical Relief. Int. J. Clin. Exp. Hypn. 10:23-29, 1963.
13. Weitzenhoffer, A. M., and Sjoberg, B. M.: Suggestibility with and Without "Induction of Hypnosis." J. Nerv. Ment. Dis. 132:204-220, 1961.
14. Wolberg, L. R.: The Technic of Short-Term Psychotherapy. In: Wolberg, L. R. (Ed.), Short-Term Psychotherapy. New York, Grune & Stratton, Inc., 1965, pp. 127-200.
15. Wolberg, L. R.: Hypnoanalysis. In: Wolman, B. B. (Ed.), Psychoanalytic Techniques. New York, Basic Books, Inc., 1967, pp. 533-559.

Practical Pastoral Counseling*

by CALVERT STEIN, M.D.

The Pastoral Mystique

Pastors outnumber psychiatrists by about 35 to 1, and psychologists by about 15 to 1. Although no longer the awesome witch doctor and traditional medicine man of his tribe, the pastor is frequently the first port of call in times of trouble. Pastors often make heroic efforts to bridge the generation gap and to facilitate expression of contemporary concern in the search for a meaning to life.

Traditional tools of the pastoral calling still include an ecclesiastic mantle, brief prayer, appropriate scriptural quotation or incantation representing a higher authority, and an attentive ear. These procedures promote a natural hypnotic receptivity per se, even without the bowed head and priestly touch. They are also inherent in the spiritual aura which the pastor carries with him to homes, meetings, and hospitals.

Regardless of setting, however, the daily observance of simple ritual, religious symbols, and sacred music serve as excellent tranquilizers for the anxious and troubled believer, but agnostics and atheists are not entirely immune.

As with ancient high priests the clerical garb may be scant defense against staunch defenders of tradition. Consequently the modern pastor risks much when he attempts radical departures from prescribed ritual by bringing into a previously conservative house of worship such changes as vernacular prayer books, rock and roll, folk masses, "sensitivity" groups, and other "heretical" abominations. Emotional turmoil can be minimized when changes are made gradually.

When to Consult or Refer

Self-Referral. Like miracle workers of old the pastor usually recognizes the intimate relations between mind and body—the psychosomatic pain, the flush, flutter, tremor, dry mouth, and other tensions (cf. *pulpit jitters;* Job 17:1, 19:14). He also respects the efficacy of adjunctive faith healing as well as the restraining potency of an implied "hex" via spiritual disapproval. Nevertheless,

---

*Some of the material in this chapter appeared in somewhat different form in *Practical Pastoral Counseling,* by Calvert Stein, Springfield, Ill., Charles C Thomas, 1970. Courtesy of the publisher.

he too must learn to deal with personal pressures including temptation, seduction, betrayal, disillusionment, guilt, and self-reproach from his own mistakes—especially failure to deal with transference and countertransference.[6] He must also "play it cool" with competitive colleagues and obstreperous lay associates who frequently reject what they actually need.

Recognition of Emotional Depression. The patient or client with morbid and sometimes unrecognized emotional depression often has physical complaints which are resistive to all therapy except temporarily to euphoric drugs or alcohol. He makes many promises but few friends and cannot keep them because he is usually dull company except when he can have "just one or two" drinks. As Al-Anon repeatedly reminds the spouses, alcoholics are experts at the confidence game, but physical as well as moral degradation are close behind, and the treatment is neither short nor simple.[1,2] Families, employers, or "friends" who cover up for addicts are doing them no favors. The addiction not only serves as a camouflage for self-destruction—it also offers a quasi alibi for involving and endangering others.

Taking unnecessary risks, ignoring customary safety precautions, habitual overwork, habitual clowning, and giving away valuable personal belongings may be the first clues to underlying depression. Too many emergency wards still fail to insist on psychiatric care.

Another risk is the borderline would-be suicide who will not give his name or extracts a promise not to tell anyone or appeals to the counselor's vanity: "You're the only one I can trust." Such a precarious client needs strength, not honor or sentiment. Calling the police may be distasteful and embarrassing yet easier to face than guilty negligence and irreversible death.

Sharing Responsibility. In general, what is true for the alcoholic, drug user, and suicidal client also applies to the homosexual, habitual gambler, criminal, shoplifter, and recidivist juvenile delinquent. Their misconduct represents both rebellion and a thinly veiled cry for help.

Parents who physically abuse their children need sterner correction than a pastor can usually supervise, but the field is still wide open for his constructive influence. Too much negligence, indulgence, and leniency not only on the part of parents but also by judges and society is largely responsible for each community's having the kind of morality and safety which it deserves.

Miscellaneous Challengers. The isolate or loner is an expert at avoiding commitments. The harder one tries to help him, the more he resists.

The chronic disrespecter of other people's rights or privacy appeals to sympathy, expects extra privileges, and pays little attention to what others say or think. Giving him "enough rope" may hang the project as well as himself. This is especially true of the "eager beaver" helper who wants to be in on

174

everything, tries to hog the credit, but lets others carry the ball and do the work.*

Sociopathic dropouts make their own rules yet follow them only when convenient. For these misanthropes argument and reason are usually futile. In a captive audience, as in an institutional setting, they have been known to respond to group confrontation by their peers as well as renewed religious pressure. However, hard-core homosexuals, alcoholics, and drug addicts are usually the result of long-standing emotional deprivation and warping. Consequently, preventive treatment requires early detection, complete abstinence, and intensive long-term reconstruction by devoted experts.

Common Denominators in Counseling and Psychotherapy

Pastoral counseling arose from the universal demand for protection from the great unknown, for an explanation of the mysteries of birth, puberty, sickness, death, floods, and other disasters, and for control of the unseen spirits that affected man's destiny. ". . . for with authority commandeth he even the unclean spirits, and they do obey him" (Mark 1:27).

Faith healing is based on the universal power of positive suggestion in a group of two or more—patient, clergyman, and God. Suggestibility and receptivity are enhanced by the priestly touch, concentrated attention, exclusion of extraneous stimuli, heightened expectation of gratifying results, and the willingness to make some personal sacrifice. These are also the phenomena of the hypnotherapeutic trance state. Assuredly no psychedelic drug could be expected to accomplish more.

Major procedures in counseling, faith healing, and psychotherapy are also universal, regardless of varying "new" doctrines and tongue-twisting terminology. They can be recognized as familiar principles of worship: meditation, ventilation of grievances, emotional release or abreaction of tension from anxiety, cleansing via confession and ritual, atonement via sacrifice, payment, or penance, and reformation of behavior.

These psychotherapeutic procedures serve the faithful followers by affording favorable opportunities to "cool it" and to learn how to "hang loose" when they are "uptight." They can be as productive over the telephone or at the bedside as in the sanctuary—especially with the additional bonus of the benediction.

The benediction or summing up should also review such issues as: What has been accomplished thus far? What are the long-range objectives? What must be tackled immediately? What liabilities must be overcome? And what strengthening assets make the task less difficult than it had appeared at first? For the

---

*A second reading of the parable of the prodigal son may help to refocus attention on the underlying injustice of an overindulgent father toward a conscientious and hard-working brother (Luke 15:11-32).

175

self-styled atheist one may suggest approval from some appropriate VIP whether living or dead as a substitute for divine approval. In everyone's life some mortal had to care.

Productive Techniques in Personal Counseling

Initial Contact. When on call the pastoral counselor should be available at all times yet avoid making commitments he cannot keep. In the initial summons he should note omissions, repetitions, contradictions, gross errors, and freudian slips; he should make a house visit if indicated or suggest another telephone or office conference soon, and perhaps a letter meanwhile. The caller may be completely in the wrong, yet the pastor usually does better with a soft answer. He can always be sorry for something; e.g., "I'm sorry you feel this way" or "I'm sorry so few people agree with you, but I'm glad you're thinking the problem through" or "I appreciate your calling to express your views."

Like the country doctor of old the pastor is always on call. Nevertheless, to protect his health and privacy, he must also learn how to say "no" diplomatically; e.g., "I have an emergency call at the hospital but I can make time for you later in the day" or "Drop in for a chat right after the next service" or "Please write me a letter and I'll certainly make the time to read it. Meanwhile, shall we pray together. . . ? " or "Let's bring it up at tomorrow's open conference" or "Several others have had a similar problem and are eager for a group discussion. We meet right after vespers; and you don't have to talk about yourself if you don't want to. . . . I'm sure you'll feel lots better. . . . I'll be looking for you; and thank you very much for calling."

When brief services are held regularly several times each day, they operate as a continuing therapeutic group experience. A familiar example of this among orthodox and conservative Jews is the breakfast minyan at which 10 or more bereaved mourners gather for daily kaddish memorial prayers followed by fellowship and food which they prepare themselves.

Useful relaxing procedures while talking in the pastor's study include such "busy work" as knitting, doodling, finger painting, and clay modeling. They serve as constructive nonverbal outlets like caressing a rosary. They displace conscious attention and also afford some feelings of accomplishment as well as security.

Maintaining a strong image by the counselor requires cultivation of appropriate diction and meticulous attention to personal cleanliness—especially shoes, nails, and breath. Levity, off-color stories, inappropriate diction, and personal anecdotes are inappropriate. The counselor should not confide similar mistakes or doubts of his own. When a personal anecdote seems indicated, it can be told in the third person as though it had happened to a friend or acquaintance.

Clay Modeling. From an assortment of small plastic jars of modeling clay on

176

the counselor's desk, the client is invited to select a sample. His choice of color usually harmonizes with tie, shirt, blouse, or dress and usually reflects the mood of the day. "While we are talking just let your hands do whatever they feel like doing with the clay." A perfectionist frequently models a sphere or "perfect world." A hostile client may refuse yet make a crude baseball which he would obviously like to throw at someone. The counselor may then invite him to punch a pillow held by the counselor, or bang down on a chair or sofa, or play a game of darts on the board on which any VIP or s.o.b. may be projected. When a client models a flower (the sex organ of plants), he may be preoccupied with spiritual love for a departed soul; however, when a hangman's noose or a lethal weapon is fashioned, confrontation and consultation are usually in order. Clients will often hastily destroy their creations if the models are too obviously associated with an embarrassing conflict. Nests, eggs, and fruit bowls suggest home and family. Vague or impressionistic creations usually conceal the sculptor's hidden message. Snapshots can be taken of the production and the subject reviewed at a later conference.

Role playing is a simple adaptation of an old counseling procedure: "Well, what would you do in my place? " It is an effective game of make-believe. The counselor says, "All right. Now you know this person who's been upsetting you. Let's pretend you are that person. You try to mimic him so I'll have a fairly clear idea of what he's like. I know you, and I'll try to think, talk, and act as you might do."

When the client is unable to assume another's role or to remain in that role, a personal hang-up is obviously indicated. The counselor then relieves the tension or embarrassment by changing the subject or reversing roles or even playing both roles. Role playing stops when it has accomplished its objective or is no longer productive. Frequently no words are needed at all. A spontaneous gesture, whether hostile, friendly, or indifferent, may convey one's feelings more eloquently.

Roles are reversed whenever clarification is needed. After a few starts the client may exclaim, "Oh, but she wouldn't *say* that" or "It wouldn't happen that way." The counselor then invites role reversal so the client can show just what "she" would have said or done. Insights usually develops rapidly but the experienced counselor does not have to confront the client or spell it out every time. It is usually enough to say, "How do you feel now? "

When role playing and role reversal are used in groups, others are invited to express how they feel. Common denominators are usually reported in the form of childhood frustrations, injustices, unexpressed grievances, and inability to deal with people who habitually impose. Presently, additional psychodramas with rehearsal for dreaded future interviews are enacted among smaller subgroups in various parts of the room. The leader merely invites the members to "rap" or chat with anyone they like while he either leaves the room or makes

177

the rounds and visits with each group as auditor or participant after asking the group's permission.

Additional Rewarding Group Procedures

Warm-up techniques include music, songs, hymns, a processional march, dancing, games, projects, busy work, and other community center routines. Natural dominance will emerge from leaderless groups left to themselves, but the dominance is not necessarily constructive—even well-meaning catalyzers often need controls.

The simulated hot line introduces hypothetical situations for "safe" confrontation. Several volunteers man a simulated 24-hour telephone answering service for "troubled callers." The pastor may act as observer or director. The "caller" may refuse to reveal his name or telephone number but the "panelist" may also fail to make adequate contact and consequently loses his chance to help. Statements such as the following can be productive: "Thank you very much for calling. You may call me John, and I'd like you to choose some name by which I can call you. It doesn't have to be your real name. I also want you to know that I will not hang up on you but you do know that telephone disconnections sometimes happen; so if you'll let me have the number I could call you right back. You'd rather not? Okay. I just wanted you to know. Now, how can I help you? "

A "caller" may choose to report some crisis such as a "trip" with LSD or may threaten suicide or may describe some domestic scene. Personal identifications and analysis should be avoided. "How do the rest of you feel? " is a safe yet provocative question which offers the leader an opportunity to suggest, "Well then, suppose you reverse roles and let's see how it might go. Pretend that you (on the panel) really have this problem. Now change places with the 'caller' and show us what you would want someone to do about it? "

Management of Aggression

Verbal. A tense person is invited to think of a poem, song, or story, or to select someone from the group to take the role of an annoying person in his life (teacher, employer, member of family, a former buddy, or even the pastor himself) and to tell him or her off as a blankety-blank so-and-so, using whatever language he deems proper. Groups do not shock easily, and verbal retaliation with choice diction often releases unsuspected hostility or provokes unexpected laughter. Insight into identity of the real culprit often develops quickly.

A simple verbal warm-up procedure for any size group is to pair off the participants, who then choose a family or members of a team or make up a skit. One may say to the other, "There's something about you that I don't understand," or "Sometimes I think you don't like me," or "You bug me the

178

wrong way," or some such remark. In short order each partner recognizes the need for further communication, and since it's a make-believe structured situation, they are usually able to accept and deal with the confrontation without too many defensive reactions.

Nonverbal. Members of the group pair off and choose a cast for a pantomime or charade. Or, facing each other, they lock hands and take turns trying to push each other around the room. Hand or "Indian" wrestling serves a similar purpose. A time limit of 5 to 10 seconds serves as a safety precaution. Or someone who feels left out can try to break into a circle of people who lock arms and try to exclude him. Similarly a timid person may be placed within a circle of his peers from which he is invited to try to break out. The rules should be clear: trickery or feints may be in, but foul play is out. When a member of a minority group succeeds on his own initiative, group approval usually appears spontaneously—even when someone in the circle lends a little help.

An excellent boost for morale results when eight volunteers (three on each side and one at head and feet) gently lift and then rock a prone isolate who has had a rough time and needs a little TLC: tender, loving care. Just sitting or reclining on a carpeted floor usually facilitates relaxation and simplifies the warm-up.[3]

Projective techniques are "make-believe" games in which everyone is invited to participate. As with a parable from scripture each auditor can identify as much as he chooses. A suggested verbalization using soothing tones follows: "Fix your gaze on some spot on the ceiling or wall. Keep watching it until your eyes get too heavy to stay open. Meanwhile let your breathing slow down, relax your body, make yourself very comfortable, and pretend to go sound asleep. Now the moment your eyes close I'd like you to imagine yourselves at a very special party. You've just won a door prize—something special and wonderful. You do not have to reveal the nature of your prize. However, when the party's over, just come back here, alert yourselves, and feel free to share with us as much as you are willing for us to know." [8]

For marriage counseling, any of the above procedures may prove effective. In addition, a study of the client's scrapbook, graduation and wedding pictures, reports on courtship, in-laws, honeymoon, work, eating, and other personal habits usually reveals the real culprit in the form of uncut apron strings and futile attempts to please or rebel against too many former competitors or VIPs. Be sure to ask who was *not* at the graduation, wedding, or other special event, and *why*.

Finally, the pastoral counselor is a patient teacher and a neutral referee—not a judge, jury, or partisan. The responsibility for accepting counseling and initiating change belongs with the individual client, who should be required to make his own appointments and commitments. You yourself are a VIP. Your own reputation for wisdom and firmness with finesse is being tested repeatedly; so do not hesitate to seek expert counseling when indicated. The world's best specialists for any problem are no further away than your own telephone.

For the dying patient one should provide truthful but compassionate reassurance, encouragement to sound off, and periodic suggestions to remember happier times. A gentle reminder of some of the wonderful "mystery trips" one used to take with a trusted adult serves as a positive influence to neutralize pessimism concerning the "last mile."

REFERENCES

1. Masserman, J. H.: Neurosis and Alcohol. In: Principles of Dynamic Psychiatry. Philadelphia, W. B. Saunders Company, 1946, pp. 210-215.
2. Masserman, J. H.: Causes and Dynamics of Alcoholism (#114). Pfizer Medical Film Library, New York, N.Y.
3. Schutz, E. C.: Joy. New York, Grove Press, Inc., 1969.
4. Stein, C.: Practical Psychotherapy in Nonpsychiatric Specialties. Springfield, Ill., Charles C Thomas, Publisher, 1969.
5. Stein, C.: Practical Family and Marriage Counseling. Springfield, Ill., Charles C Thomas, Publisher, 1970.
6. Stein, C.: Trance, Transference and Countertransference in the Resistive Patient. Amer. J. Clin. Hypn. 12:213-221 (April), 1970.
7. Stein, C.: Practical Pastoral Counseling. Springfield, Ill., Charles C Thomas, Publisher, 1970.
8. Stein, C.: Hypnotic Projection in Brief Psychotherapy. Amer. J. Clin. Hypn. pp. 143-155, 1970.
9. Stein, C.: Sex in the Bible. Unpublished data.

PART V

SEXUAL DEVIATIONS

Aversion Therapy of Homosexuality

by N. McConaghy, D.P.M.

In evaluating the efficacy of the various treatments of homosexuality the same questions require answering as with the investigation of any psychiatric therapy. These are: What are the aims of treatment? Can the achievement of these aims be attributed to the specific effects of the treatment? How can the achievement of different aims by various treatments be compared?

In studies utilizing either relationship psychotherapy or aversion therapy for homosexual patients, a common aim has been that the subjects adopt heterosexual patterns of behavior. Other aims have varied, e.g., to what extent should the patients cease homosexual behaviour, and should they obtain "insight" into the postulated origins of their homosexuality? As regards the achievement of the common aim, psychotherapy and aversion therapy have not been shown to differ significantly. Woodward[16] reported that 36 percent and Bieber[2] that 27 percent of their homosexual patients became exclusively heterosexual following psychotherapy; MacCulloch and Feldman[8] reported a similar response in 33 percent of their subjects following aversion therapy. The last authors also stated that 58 percent became heterosexual as judged by the Kinsey scale.[7] Mayerson and Lief,[9] using a similarly less rigorous definition of heterosexuality, concluded that 50 percent of their group achieved this state following psychotherapy. Freund[6] considered that 18 percent of the patients he treated showed a satisfactory response in that they had heterosexual intercourse regularly for several years following aversion therapy. He was the only one of these workers to follow up his subjects for such a long period of time, and the only one to report that some of his patients at later interviews admitted they had lied about their degree of response earlier.

Conclusions concerning the efficacy of the two forms of therapy have varied considerably. Coates[4] considered that psychotherapy was superior, whereas MacCulloch and Feldman[8] claimed the advantage for their form of behavior therapy. Freund[6] and Bieber[3] decided the results of both were similar, in respect to changing sexual behavior. As none of the groups treated can be accepted as comparable, in the absence of data from controlled trials evaluating the two forms of therapy, such conclusions are likely to continue to vary.

Regarding the degree to which the results reported above can be attributed to the specific effects of the treatment, uncertainty must again prevail. Most psychiatrists have had the experience of seeing patients or other acquaintances

183

cease homosexual or other deviant forms of behavior under the influence of religious beliefs or guilt-provoking pressures and at times become unaware of the existence of the feelings that led to the deviant behavior. To the extent the above therapies produce changes in patients' conscious feelings and sexual activity, these therapies could be operating in similar ways, without producing any actual change in the strength of the patients' homosexual or heterosexual drives.

In an attempt to overcome this problem a series of studies were carried out to determine whether an objective technique could be developed which measured the strength of such sexual drives, and if so, whether such a technique could be used to demonstrate changes due to treatment. Facilities were not available for the psychotherapeutic treatment of a large series of homosexual patients, and aversion therapy alone was studied. It was additionally decided to investigate the mode of action of this therapy—in particular to determine if it acted by setting up conditioned reflexes, as has been generally accepted.[5]

Measuring Sexual Orientation

The objective measure investigated was the recording of changes in the subject's penile volume while he watched a travelogue-type moving film. At approximately 1-minute intervals there were inserted into the film 10 segments of 10-second shots of an orange circle followed by 10-second shots of nude young women, alternating with 10 10-second shots of a blue triangle followed by 10-second shots of nude young men. The sexual orientation of the subject was determined by measuring the 10 penile volume changes to the shots of women and the 10 to shots of men and testing the significance of the difference between the two groups of 10 scores using the Mann-Whitney U test.[10]

As a control group 11 medical students who were confident of their heterosexual orientation volunteered to undergo this film assessment. All showed greater penile volume increase to the pictures of women, 10 to a statistically significant extent. An unexpected finding was that these subjects commonly showed a penile volume decrease to pictures of the males. Penile volume increases to the orange circles preceding the female nudes and decreases to the blue triangles preceding the male nudes occurred as conditioned responses.[13] Similar results were obtained in a larger study investigating 60 psychology student volunteers.[1]

Comparison of Apomorphine Aversion and Aversion-Relief Therapy

The initial aversion treatment study investigated the response of 40 homosexual patients. As expected, in the film assessment they tended to show penile volume increases to the pictures of the males, decreases to those of the females, and appropriate conditioned responses to the preceding circles and triangles. The conditioned responses were used to provide a measure of each of the homosexual subje.ts' ability to set up conditioned responses—his so-called conditionability.

The primary aim of the first treatment study was to compare the efficacy of two forms of aversion treatment, using as measures of response both the patients' subjective reports of change in sexual feelings and behavior and the changes in penile volume reactions to the shots of male and female nudes. As stated earlier, the aversion therapies are widely considered to act by setting up conditioned responses. A secondary aim was to obtain evidence for or against this theory by examining the relationship between each subject's ability to respond to aversion therapy and his ability to set up conditioned responses in the sexual orientation film assessment. In the first study the two treatments compared were apomorphine aversion and aversion relief. Both methods have been claimed to be effective in treating homosexuality.[6,15]

With apomorphine aversion, the subject was initially given a subcutaneous injection of 1.5 mg. of apomorphine. After a variable interval, usually about 8 minutes, he commenced to feel nauseated. Severe nausea lasting 10 minutes without vomiting was aimed for and the dose constantly adjusted throughout treatment to maintain this response. The patient timed the onset of the nausea and one minute prior to its expected onset switched on a slide projector and viewed a slide of a nude or seminude male which he found sexually exciting. Prior to the nausea reaching its maximum he turned off the projector. Twenty-eight such treatment sessions were administered at two-hourly periods over five days, each patient being admitted to the hospital for the five days.

With aversion-relief therapy, for each patient 14 slides were made of words and phrases considered by the patient to be evocative of aspects of homosexuality which he found exciting. These slides were projected at 10-second intervals. The patient read each one aloud. Immediately after he finished reading he received a painful electric shock through electrodes attached to the fingertips. Following the 14 slides, one was projected which related to aspects of normal sexuality. This was left on for 40 seconds and not accompanied by a shock. The appearance of this slide produced a sense of relief as the patient learned it would not be accompanied by a shock. In one treatment session this procedure was carried out five times, with intervals of 2½ minutes intervening. Three treatment sessions were given daily for 5 consecutive days during which the patients were hospitalized. Hence each patient received a total of 1050 shocks during treatment.

Subjects. Forty persons conscious of homosexual feeling who wished to have this reduced and who were not overtly psychotic were accepted for treatment. Eighteen had been arrested for homosexual behavior, eight on more than one occasion. Legal action had led to 6 of the 18 coming for treatment, the other 12 no longer being under any form of constraint. Ten patients were married and 20

185

considered they were sexually aroused by women or had been in the past, four stating that their heterosexual interest was greater than their homosexual interest. These four had all been arrested for homosexual behavior—one on three occasions. Thirty-eight had had homosexual relations with a number of partners. Two had had no overt homosexual experience since adolescence; one of these was distressed by his strong feelings of attraction to other men, the other by homosexual sadistic fantasies.

Method. The 40 patients were randomly allocated to two groups of 20, one group to receive immediate treatment, one delayed treatment. Each group of 20 was further randomly allocated to two groups of 10, one group to receive apomorphine, the other aversion-relief therapy. The immediate treatment group viewed the sexual orientation assessment film immediately prior to treatment and again 3 weeks later. The delayed-treatment group viewed the film 3 weeks prior to treatment as well as on these two occasions. This enabled any changes occurring in the immediately treated group after treatment to be compared with changes occurring over the same period of time, without treatment, in the delayed-treatment group. At three weeks following treatment the patients were also interviewed about change in sexual feelings and behavior.

Results. In the delayed-treatment group there was no significant change in penile volume responses in the film assessment without treatment intervening. Following treatment, the immediate treatment group showed significantly less penile volume increase to the pictures of nude men, compared to their response prior to treatment. As regards the penile volume response to the pictures of women, those patients who showed penile volume decrease to these pictures before treatment showed significantly less decrease following treatment. There was no change in the responses of those patients who before treatment showed no change or penile volume increase to these pictures. The changes in penile volume to pictures of men and women were still present without any weakening at follow-up a year later.

The patients also reported reduction in their homosexual and increase in their heterosexual feelings and behavior. The reported reduction in homosexuality was greater at 2 weeks than at 1 year following treatment; the reverse was true in respect to heterosexuality. These reported changes in sexual feelings correlated significantly with the changes to the sexual orientation film at 1-year follow-up, but not at 2 weeks following treatment. It was concluded that the reported changes at 1 year were more reliable than those at 2 weeks, the longer time allowing the patients to assess their feelings more accurately.

At 1 year following treatment, approximately half the patients reported reduction in homosexual feelings and a half—not necessarily the same patients—an increase in heterosexual feelings. A quarter reported they had ceased homosexual behaviour and a quarter—not necessarily the same—that they had commenced or increased the frequency of heterosexual intercourse. However, all

186

patients were still aware of some degree of homosexual feelings. There were no significant differences in the results of the two treatments, either in changes to the film assessment or in reported sexual feelings and behavior. There was no consistent relationship between each subject's outcome with treatment and his conditionability as measured by the amplitude of his conditioned responses in the film assessment. This study has been reported in greater detail elsewhere.[11,12]

Comparison of Apomorphine Aversion and Avoidance Conditioning

MacCulloch and Feldman[8] reported a much better outcome, at least in terms of complete loss of homosexual feeling, in patients treated with an aversive technique using avoidance learning. With this technique, the patient viewed the slide of a male and was instructed to leave it on as long as he found it attractive. After 8 seconds he commenced to receive an electric shock if he had not removed the slide by means of a hand switch with which he was provided. The shock continued until he removed the slide. Once he avoided the shock three times in succession, by switching the male slide off before 8 seconds had elapsed, he was placed on a schedule of reinforcement. On one-third of the trials he could still switch the slide off whenever he wished; on another third he could switch off the slide after a variable delay; and on the final third he could not switch the slide off until after he received a shock. On some occasions following the removal of the male slide and cessation of the shock, the slide of a woman was shown—with the expectation that this might increase heterosexual feeling.

This aversive technique was compared with apomorphine aversion in a further study, similar in design to the initial one, comparing apomorphine aversion with aversion-relief. The subjects were approximately comparable to those of the first study. Avoidance conditioning was given in 14 sessions of treatment over 5 days. During each session the male slide was shown 30 times. The apomorphine treatment procedure was basically unchanged.[14] The aims were to attempt to replicate the findings of MacCulloch and Feldman as to the greater efficacy of avoidance learning and to replicate the findings of the first study as to the changes following apomorphine aversion.

Only the second aim was realized. There was no significant difference in outcome with the two treatments. Both treatments produced a similar degree of reduction in homosexuality as indicated by the patients' subjective reports and by the changes in their response to the sexual assessment film. There was again a significant correlation between these two measures of outcome. No weakening in the change in response to the sexual assessment film occurred at follow-up 6 months later. There was no consistent relationship between response to treatment and the subjects as measured in the film assessment.

Most subjects are unaware of the changes in penile volume measured in the

187

sexual assessment. It would seem unlikely that these changes could be under conscious control. Hence their modification with treatment and the correlated reduction in reported homosexual feeling would appear to be valid indicators that the treatment is at least to some extent effective. The disconcerting finding of the two studies is that three widely different aversive techniques have produced essentially the same results. Feldman and MacCulloch stated they designed the elaborate technique of avoidance learning to fully exploit the many thousands of experiments on animal and human learning with the expectation that it would prove a much more effective therapy. If the aversion therapies act by setting up conditioned responses, this application of learning principles to obtain better conditioning must result in a more effective therapy. That it did not suggests strongly that these therapies do not act in this way. This is further suggested by the fact that there was no consistent relationship between a patient's ability to set up conditioned responses in the assessment film and his degree of response to aversion therapy.

Comparison of Classical, Avoidance, and Backward Conditioning

To investigate this further, a third study was carried out. A similar design was followed to the previous ones, except that three aversive techniques were compared—avoidance learning, classical conditioning, and backward conditioning. With classical conditioning, 10 to 15 slides of nude or seminude males to which the patient showed and felt a significant sexual response were selected. Three of these slides were shown to the patient for 10 seconds in each treatment session. Overlapping and continuing beyond the last second of exposure of each slide, a shock of 2 seconds' duration was administered, of an intensity as high as the patient could tolerate. The three slides were shown at intervals of approximately 4 minutes. The patient received 14 such sessions of treatment over 5 days.

With the backward conditioning procedure the patient received a 1-second shock of the same order of unpleasantness as that used in the avoidance learning procedure. A half second after the shock terminated he was shown for 4 seconds the slide of a male to which he was sexually responsive. Two seconds later either he was shown a slide of a nude or seminude girl or the screen was left blank for 16 seconds. After a further half second he again received the shock which preceded the male slide. This sequence was followed 30 times in each treatment session. The patient received 14 such sessions of treatment over 5 days. The procedure was designed to expose the patient to slides of men and women and to a series of shocks for approximately the same duration as with the avoidance procedure. The major variable altered was the relationship of the stimuli. With the backward procedure the unconditioned stimulus—the shock—preceded rather than followed the conditioned stimulus—the slide of the male. Backward conditioning has been widely found to produce minimal if any stable conditioned responses. Hence, if aversion therapy acts by setting up such responses, it would be expected that this form of treatment would be significantly less effective than avoidance or classical conditioning.

Another variable investigated was the effect of booster treatment. Each patient returned for follow-up film and clinical assessment 3 weeks after termination of treatment. Following these, he was given a session of treatment similar to that he had received previously. He continued to return monthly for such booster treatments for 6 months. He then had a film assessment and received the final booster. After a further 6 months he was interviewed to obtain his reported response at that time. In the first two studies no evidence of weakening in response to aversion treatment occurred over the follow-up period, as measured by the changes in penile volume to pictures of men and women. If aversion therapy acts by setting up conditioned responses, such weakening should occur by the process of extinction, and booster treatment should prevent this weakening, at least in part.

Again all three treatment procedures produced changes in the patients' reported feelings and behavior and in their penile volume responses to the movie shots of men and women comparable to the changes in the first two studies. There were no significant differences in the efficacy of the three treatments, nor did this efficacy appear to be increased by the monthly booster treatments.

Clinical Relevance

The studies carried out indicate that 6 to 12 months following aversion treatment about half the patients report an increase in heterosexual feeling and a decrease in homosexual feeling. A quarter have ceased homosexual activity and a quarter have commenced or increased the frequency of heterosexual intercourse. These changes are paralleled by a decrease in the patients' penile volume response to movie films of nude males, a change which does not appear to be under conscious control. Furthermore, those patients who show penile volume decreases to pictures of women have these significantly reduced following treatment. As all patients were unaware that they showed these penile volume decreases, it seems unlikely that their reduction can be due to the suggestion effects of aversion therapy and argues that a change in the strength of sexual feelings is produced by this treatment. However, techniques of aversion therapy which should maximize conditioning are no more effective than those which should minimize it. It would seem that aversion therapy does not act by producing conditioned responses.

The immediate relevance of these studies to the clinician who wishes to use aversion therapy in the treatment of homosexuality is that it appears unnecessary to use elaborate equipment or treatment procedures. A form of

189

classical conditioning similar to that used in the third study would seem easiest to use. Though, in the studies reported, treatments involving showing pictures of girls did not result in more heterosexual behavior by the patients, there was a trend for more heterosexual feelings to be reported, at least in the first weeks following treatment. It would seem worthwhile to incorporate pictures of girls also.

These studies provide no data on the ideal frequency of treatment, though they indicate that booster treatments are unnecessary if a series of treatments are given intensively over 5 days. However other clinicians using aversion therapy with homosexual patients in office practice have informed the author that they have obtained results which appeared comparable to those obtained in these studies, with treatments given in weekly sessions over a few months. This would not seem surprising in view of the present finding that the efficacy of treatment remained unaffected by grossly manipulating variables which theoretically should be much more important. Until further data become available the clinician can plan the course of aversion treatment with the primary determinants being his and his patient's convenience.

A reasonable procedure would be for the patient to select about 10 slides each of nude adolescent and young men and women to which he felt a sexual response. In each session of treatment three male slides would be shown for 10 seconds, the patient receiving a 2-second shock commencing during the last second of exposure of the male slide. The level of shock should be as unpleasant as the patient will tolerate. Following the shock a slide of a woman would be shown for 20 seconds. Variable intervals of 3 to 5 minutes would be left between showing the three sets of male and female slides. Such sessions of treatment would be given three or more times in the first week and gradually reduced in frequency over the following few months.

Treatment additional to aversion therapy was avoided in the above studies. Of course, a supportive psychotherapeutic attitude is necessary, if not purely on humanitarian grounds, then at least so that the relationship with the therapist is such that it will encourage the patient to continue treatment. Patients who are anxious about sexual involvements with women could be expected to benefit from desensitization therapy in addition. However, the author has not had significant success when he has used this in patients who wished to continue treatment after final follow-up. Systematic study of this treatment both in comparison with and in addition to aversion therapy is indicated.

Adverse psychiatric reactions occurred in less than 10 percent of patients following aversion therapy, when they took the form of depressive or, more rarely, anxiety symptoms. Similar symptoms had occurred in the patients prior to treatment and the author did not consider they were "symptom substitutions." In fact, they were more likely to occur in patients who had failed to respond to treatment.

190

As to the selection of patients, obviously psychopathic patients do not persist with treatment, nor do many patients who come in a crisis situation. It is best to delay treatment in the latter group until they have a better understanding of their feelings. This of course also applies to patients who are depressed, when their wish for treatment may be motivated by the associated guilt. The author did not treat patients who were overtly psychotic. It has been reported[8] that patients over 30 years old do not respond as well to aversion therapy. In the author's experience they are less likely to completely cease homosexual activity and to initiate heterosexual intercourse. However, they report reduction in their homosexual feelings and behavior as commonly as do younger subjects. This older group of patients are more likely to indulge in illegal activities, such as making sexual contacts in public lavatories, often in an apparently compulsive manner. Reduction in homosexual drive appears to give them more control so they are able to continue their homosexual behavior without being subject to arrest. Many of these older and some of the younger patients state they appreciate the freedom from the continual preoccupation with homosexual thoughts which was present prior to aversion therapy. It would seem to the author that reduction of homosexual feelings without increased heterosexual feelings and behavior, though not an ideal treatment response, may still be a worthwhile one. In *The Republic* Plato said: "Old age has a great sense of calm and relaxation. When the passions have relaxed their hold you have escaped, not from one master, but from many."

Probably few heterosexuals would welcome the sense of calm and relaxation which was won by a loss of sexual passion, but this may not be so for many people whose deviant drives force them to behave in ways which are likely to result in severe social and legal sanctions.

Acknowledgments

The National Health and Medical Research Council of Australia is thanked for providing a grant enabling these studies to be carried out.

REFERENCES

1. Barr, R. F., and McConaghy, N.: Penile Volume Responses to Appetitive and Aversive Stimuli in Relation to Sexual Orientation and Conditioning Performance. Brit. J. Psychiat. 119:377-383, 1971.
2. Bieber, I.: Homosexuality. New York, Basic Books, Inc., 1962.
3. Bieber, I.: Aversion Therapy of Homosexuals. Brit. Med. J. 2:372, 1967.
4. Coates, S.: Clinical Psychology in Sexual Deviation. In: Rosen, I. (Ed.), The Pathology and Treatment of Sexual Deviation. New York, Oxford University Press, 1964.
5. Feldman, M. P., and MacCulloch, M. J.: The Application of Anticipatory Avoidance Learning to the Treatment of Homosexuality. I. Theory, Technique and Preliminary Results. Behav. Res. Ther. 2:165-183, 1965.

6. Freund, K.: Some Problems in the Treatment of Homosexuality. In: Eysenck, H. J. (Ed.), Behaviour Therapy and the Neuroses. London, Pergamon Press, 1960.
7. Kinsey, A. C., Pomeroy, W. B., and Martin, C. E.: Sexual Behavior in the Human Male. Philadelphia, W. B. Saunders Company, 1948.
8. MacCulloch, H. J., and Feldman, M. P.: Aversion Therapy in Management of 43 Homosexuals. Brit. Med. J. 1:594-597, 1967.
9. Mayerson, P., and Lief, H. I.: Psychotherapy of Homoxexuals: A Follow-up Study of Nineteen Cases. In: Marmor, J. (Ed.), Sexual Inversion. New York, Basic Books, Inc., 1965.
10. McConaghy, N.: Penile Volume Change to Moving Pictures of Male and Female Nudes in Heterosexual and Homosexual Males. Behav. Res. Ther. 5:43-48, 1967.
11. McConaghy, N.: Subjective and Penile Plethysmograph Responses Following Aversion-Relief and Apomorphine Aversion Therapy for Homosexual Impulses. Brit. J. Psychiat. 115:723-730, 1969.
12. McConaghy, N.: Subjective and Penile Plethysmograph Responses at Two Weeks and One Year Following Aversion-Relief and Apomorphine Aversion Therapy for Homosexual Impulses. Brit. J. Psychiat. 117:555-561, 1970.
13. McConaghy, N.: Penile Response Conditioning and Its Relationship to Aversion Therapy in Homosexuals. Behav. Ther. 1:213-221, 1970.
14. McConaghy, N., Proctor, D., and Barr, R.: Subjective and Penile Plethysmography Responses to Aversion Therapy for Homosexuality: A Partial Replication (to be published), Arch. Sex. Behav.
15. Thorpe, J. G., Schmidt, E., Brown, P. T., and Castell, D.: Aversion-Relief Therapy: A New Method for General Application. Behav. Res. Ther. 2:71-82, 1964.
16. Woodward, M.: The Diagnosis and Treatment of Homosexual Offenders. Brit. J. Delinq. 9:44-59, 1956.

Group Psychotherapy of Male Homosexuals

by SAMUEL B. HADDEN, M.D.

T HE PROBLEM OF HOMOSEXUALITY is deserving of more considerate psychiatric attention than it has received. Only in recent years have reports of the successful treatment of homosexuality by psychotherapy begun to appear in psychiatric literature. Previously, pessimism not only prevailed in published works, but it also dominated psychiatric thinking and teaching. This negative attitude has no doubt contributed to the poor results obtained because a therapist schooled to believe that treatment will not be helpful will unconsciously communicate this attitude to the patient and will therefore accomplish very little. Some therapists still inform the homosexual that a change in his sexual pattern cannot be expected and that treatment may accomplish little more than to help him to live more comfortably with his affliction. However, Bergler,[1,2] Bieber,[3] Munzer,[4] and I[5,6] have recently reported favorable results, and I firmly believe that when therapists endeavor to dismiss the prejudicial pessimism which now exists and commit themselves to a more hopeful approach, they will find their results will improve.

One significant factor which contributes to the perpetuation of this defeatist attitude may be the frequent quotation of Freud's statement: "The removal of genital inversion or homosexuality is, in my experience, never an easy matter. On the contrary, I have found success possible only under special favorable circumstances, and even then the success essentially consisted in being able to open to those who are restricted homo-sexually the way to the opposite sex which has been until then barred, thus restoring to them full-bisexual function. . . . To undertake to convert a fully developed homo-sexual into a heterosexual is not more promising than to do the reverse, only for good practical reasons the latter is never attempted."[7]

There are many groups, made up primarily of homosexuals, that announce their dedication to "the improvement of the legal and social status of the homosexual." These organizations consistently quote these negative views and thereby discourage the afflicted from seeking help. Some publications of such organizations express resentment that homosexuality is regarded by physicians as an illness and maintain that it is no more an abnormality than left-handedness.

A few of these associations are promoting a praiseworthy effort to educate the public to the fact that homosexuals can be constructive and useful citizens and that not all of them are obvious and objectionable. Such efforts deserve psychiatric support. These organized groups should not continue their hostility to the efforts of psychiatrists to have the disorder regarded as a symptom of a neurosis or character aberration which is a treatable condition. Until such antagonistic efforts are changed, many homosexuals who could be helped will continue in their disturbed state of maladaptation. I personally feel that homosexuality is a most unfortunate condition but that society has just as much right to expect those affected to seek treatment and join in efforts to stamp out the disorder as we have to expect the cooperation of the tuberculous patient and his family in eradicating this disease.

My interest in this problem was greatly advanced when a colleague, in referring a patient to me for treatment, used every conceivable derogatory epithet in making the referring appointment by phone in the presence of the patient. I sympathized with the young man who turned to a fellow physician for help and received humiliating abuse instead. Too often the psychiatrist regards the homosexual as a socially undesirable individual and communicates this feeling to him. Many homosexuals have been harshly rejected and treated so contemptuously that their hostile attitude toward medicine and psychiatry is easily understood. It is time for us to try to comprehend the condition better, to enlighten the community, to aim to devise more effective measures for its treatment and guides for its prevention.

As my interest increased in the problem of the homosexual, treatment results began to improve. Since I was using a group approach to the treatment of many neurotics at the time, I felt that their integration into these groups of neurotic patients might be helpful. However, when these homosexual patients revealed their problem to the group, they felt rejected in spite of my efforts to protect them and they withdrew. Because of this experience, I felt that it would be desirable to treat them in exclusively homosexual groups. I now realize that those patients revealed their homosexuality—possibly as an unconscious desire to be rejected— too early, before they had found acceptance or before the group was sufficiently mature to accept their deviant behavior. I now know that a

194

relatively mature group can accept homosexuals and that they can do well in mixed groups, but I still feel I have obtained better results with exclusively homosexual groups.

Practically all of the homosexuals I have treated in groups have been cases in which the prognosis was somewhat favorable.[1] They were all patients seen and treated in private practice and were diagnosed as neurotic or character disorder. All were referred by other psychiatrists or physicians, and while the initial treatment contact was forced upon some through arrest or family pressure, others sought treatment because of depression, fear of discovery, or mounting anxiety. Some were well motivated while others were pressured or forced to continue in treatment by legal edicts or family insistence.

When a patient who resents being forced into treatment enters, he is prone to announce that he has no intention of changing his homosexual pattern and maintains that he finds homosexuality a most desirable way of life and is quite happy with it. Invariably this statement is challenged by a member of the group, and the newcomer is asked to describe those things about homosexuality which make it so desirable. Soon he realizes that he is in a group of homosexuals who know the problems and heartaches of the afflicted. They accept his statement as a necessary rationalization, but they soon convince him that at one time all of them had expressed similar views themselves. It is surprising how effective the group is in breaking down this rationalization, but having done so they ease the resultant anxiety by reassurance that the patient can be helped to a way of life for which he will not have to be apologetic.

This breaking down of the rationalizations is something which the group quickly accomplishes that is difficult to achieve otherwise.

At the beginning of a new group, assurance that benefit can be derived must come largely from the therapist. However, in a going group, a new member can be reassured by the older members as they discuss changes which they have experienced themselves and have observed in others. This reassurance that others have undergone change and even reversal of their sexual pattern has a gratifying effect in that it encourages members to stay in treatment.

The group sessions are conducted along psychoanalytically oriented lines. Each member gives a meaningful account of his life and in so doing activates memories in other members so that the cathartic phase is accelerated and deepened. Fantasies activated by experiences are shared and discussed. Strong lines of identification are established and vicarious catharsis and abreaction becomes apparent. The therapist endeavors to do little more than direct the group so that each member becomes in-

195

volved and benefits. Interpretation of dreams and other material is left to the group with the therapist playing a catalytic role.

Before patients are brought into the group, they are seen in several individual sessions in order that we may have some knowledge of their ego strength and other traits. We gain basic information about the constellation into which they were born, knowledge of their relationships with the various members of the family, and all other information that might give clues to the important factors in the development of their homosexuality. I also evaluate each individual as to how he will fit into the group, for we endeavor to maintain our groups with persons of approximately the same intelligence level and to avoid too wide a spread in age. When I feel that he will be a suitable member for an existing group, I present to him the desirability of entering it, emphasizing the fact that I am placing him there because my experience has shown that the greatest likelihood of successful treatment lies in the group approach. Of this I am firmly convinced, and I feel that it is most important that whenever a patient is moved from individual therapy into group psychotherapy, regardless of what his condition might be, it is necessary that the therapist really believe that it is the best approach to his problem. If he does not believe this and arranges the admission of a patient to the group only as an expedient measure, this lack of conviction is quickly communicated to the patient.

In my discussion with the patient before referring him to a group, I make it clear that I regard homosexuality as but one symptom of a pattern of maladjustment and seek to bring other symptoms to the fore. I also present to him the belief that homosexuality is an experientially determined state and that it does not develop as a result of any glandular imbalance or anything that was inherent in him at the time of birth. I impress upon him that experiences in early life contributed to his inability to make an effective attachment in his peer groups, and assure him that in the group others who have had the same problem will help him as they explore the experiences, the fantasies and fears which have arrested their psychosexual development at their present level.

As each member attends his first session, we review these beliefs which we hold about homosexuality, and quite often there is a spontaneous affirmation of their validity from members who have recognized their truth as they progress in treatment. We impose upon each a gentleman's agreement to attend at least six sessions before he withdraws, and then ask that no matter when he may wish to withdraw from the group, he will agree to present his reasons for withdrawing during one of the sessions. We also impress upon the newcomer that he will be expected to reveal truthfully feelings that may be activated in the group and that eventually he will bring to it meaningful autobiographical material and discussion of his own fantasies, dreams, and other material which will help him to understand the development of his maladjusted state. Each individual is known only by his first name, and in the group at all times his anonymity is protected. We impose no restrictions on patients' relationship with each other outside the group except to suggest that should any pertinent material develop through discussions or activities outside, it is to be brought into the group in order that all may benefit. We make it clear that our objective is the complete reversal of the sexual pattern, and we express our belief that this can be accomplished. Each patient is asked to present to the group some sketch of his homosexual problems, including the time his activity began, the circumstances under which it began, the attitudes he may have toward his homosexuality, and those circumstances which led up to his seeking treatment. We have found this procedure helpful because it gives the therapist the opportunity of repeating at the time of introduction of each new member certain material such as the concepts we hold of the nature of homosexuality, the fact that it is a treatable condition and that it grows out of experience in early life.

As can well be imagined, each patient at the time of introduction into a going group reveals a good bit of anxiety. However, it is quite common for a new member, before the end of the session, to report that he actually feels better now that he has made a start in treatment, and many will state that it is comforting to be with people who are trying to do something about a common problem rather than reassure each other that nothing can be done. This we have observed even in patients who were figuratively forced into treatment by a demand that the law or their families has placed upon them.

If a new member is already anxious about his homosexuality on coming into a group and hopes to undergo change, he very frequently expresses concern about the possibility of being pressured into giving up homosexuality when he is not ready for a heterosexual pattern of existence. The group quickly assures him that no demand will be made upon him to terminate his homosexuality until he knows he is ready and able to do so. Many participants, during their first session with the group, ask for some reassurance about changes that can be achieved, and the older members are likely to encourage them by speaking of progress which they have made; in so doing, they usually refer to improvement in symptoms and behavior other than their homosexual practices. They speak of other neurotic traits or character deficiencies which have im-

197

proved and invariably allude to changes in their feelings about homosexuality since coming into treatment. Some report actual changes in their sexual attitude. Most members are able to report some changes and encourage the anxious member to persist in treatment.

In our conduct of the group, we never question the extent of any member's homosexual activity, and any diminution in this activity or alteration of sexual outlook is made known to the group only when a new member inquires about improvement which others have experienced. The only time the group shows any intolerance toward a member is when they believe the individual is not participating effectively and obviously is not trying to contribute to his own improvement or that of others.

Each member quickly realizes that he is accepted by the others in the group, and many comment that it is very comforting to be accepted for what you are and to find yourself among fellows who understand and are motivated toward change. Those who have been integrated exclusively in gay circles find this experience unique and comment that they feel liberated from the pressures of the gay groups which constantly aim to reassure each other that the homosexual way of life is wonderful. The true interest of the group members in each other's progress is reassuring. As a result of this experience, they gain confidence in venturing into more heterosexually oriented groups—e.g., the young man who remains aloof from the other people with whom he works for fear of discovery may soon venture joining with a group of fellow workers for lunch, and because of the confidence gained in this experience, his way back to an integration with straight groups begins.

Some homosexuals who have been ridiculed for swish propensities are often quite hostile to the whole group, but this is quickly interpreted and the group assures him that he doesn't have to defend his swish appearance or mannerisms. He will soon find that they will not gain him any status in the therapy group, and on some occasions when he flaunts his obvious homosexuality in the group, he has been requested not to join them on leaving the sessions. Although this might be considered a traumatic experience, it is usually done with such sincerity that the individual who has insisted on being obvious soon undergoes change in dress and mannerisms. He knows they are seriously trying to change, and soon he, too, comes to grips with his problem. The group presents a constant reality demand on its members.

The group, having accepted the fact that their homosexuality is an outgrowth of difficulty in making normal adaptations, begins to review early patterns of behavior and experiences, and the members readily recognize that with few exceptions they have never been able to make

198

effective relationships with their peers at any period of their lives. Inevitably, discussion of the parental relationship and those relationships within the home that prepare them for their entrance into the world outside occur. Practically every homosexual I have studied has come to recognize evidence of maladjustment at the time he first entered school, and this fact naturally focuses attention sharply on the experiences in the home in relationship to the parents.

We feel that while no two homosexuals have had identical histories, there are traumatic experiences in their parental relationships which contribute to their initial maladjustment and eventual homosexuality. Maternal dominance is an important factor. With some, the mother is a hostile rejecting figure, who becomes a consistent threat to the child. As a protective device, he may establish a negative identification with the mother, deny his aggressiveness and become figuratively castrated in order to avoid the hostility of the mother figure. In some situations, the mother is sweetly seductive, dominates the life of the child by cajolery, and prevents him from making masculine identifications or developing normal aggressiveness. The father also plays a very important role; the hostile, rejecting father may cause the son to deny aggression, become passive, and turn away from a masculine pattern of sexual behavior. In other instances, the absent or weak, passive father does not provide an effective pattern of identification; does not encourage the boy in his masculine identifications. With this lack of guidance and direction, the child accepts a passive life role. Various combinations of these parental traits may be found in the family of the homosexual. The relationship with brothers and sisters is also an important factor in some instances. An older harsh, domineering sister may be a more threatening figure than the mother. The rejecting, ridiculing older male sibling may cause the initial withdrawal of the young brother. It is, indeed, unusual to find a homosexual in whose home there was no conflict or complete dominance of the constellation by one parent. There is usually conflict between the parents which revolves around a struggle for dominance between them.

As parental and family relationships are discussed by one member of the group, there is bound to be release of feelings activated in others in the group. This emotional reliving of traumatic experiences with others lends an impact to the reliving that seldom occurs in the one-to-one relationship. I have seen a patient in a group reveal for the first time an awareness that the mother he adored never let him do anything he wanted to do but always assured him that he would be more pleased doing as she wanted him to do. He at first may say this never made him angry, because his mother was such a lovely person. This will bring into the discussion a patient who had a somewhat similar experience, and

199

since he may reveal that he did resent this, there may then be released real angry feelings that had to be suppressed. Those angry feelings are then related to the fact that this led to an over-all denial of aggressive impulses, and very often in a number of successive sessions, members of the group will bring forth one experience after another with which every member will to some degree identify and report having had similar experience. This mutual reliving is a most important dynamic factor in the group therapy of the homosexual.

In the review of early life experiences, overly protective attitudes of one or both parents are frequently revealed, and the fact that parents kept them out of the rough-and-tumble play of their peers in the preschool period is frequently brought to the fore. I feel that it is in this period, before any semblance of organized play is initiated, that the child by going through the wrestling, pulling, tugging, and scrambling phase has the experience of close physical contact with his peers and gets the feel of belonging. Naturally there is risk of injury, but this is usually minor and I think there is no more important period in child development than this scrambling preschool period. Those who have not had it are timid as they approach the active play in the schoolyard, and their withdrawal has already been established. The absence of close intimate contact in early child life often leaves a void which is filled in adult life by a quest for male peer contact in the sexual embrace.

A very significant experience provided by the group is the discussion of the meaning of and the feelings and fantasies associated with the homosexual act. Feelings of loneliness and aloofness are revealed to be impelling factors in intiating cruising for an outlet. The need to be wanted becomes so intense at times that they may enter an act without appreciable sexual excitement, even erection, to gratify the need to be meaningful to another person. Wanting to be wanted and accepted—even as a sexual object—is often a most important compelling factor to some homosexuals. There are times when one may react to some rebuff with intense anger, and on such occasions one who is usually quite passive may become aggressive and seek a passive partner on whom he acts out his hostility and hate. In such discussions, members become aware of the significance of their drives and interpret their own and the others' behavior as a distorted effort to become a meaningful part of the lives of others and of a society to which they recognize they are maladjusted. More than once patients have said in such a discussion that to be acceptable only by the unacceptable is no longer gratifying. They seek more satisfying acceptance and move more willingly toward change.

Once the members of a homosexual group have accepted themselves as

200

abnormally oriented, their progress toward health is like that of any person with a neurosis or character disorder. They are treated as other maladjusted patients and their conflict approached and resolved by the psychotherapeutic measures of the group therapist. At times many sessions may pass without any mention of homosexuality.

When a member begins to reorient and reintegrate with heterosexual groups, anxiety again mounts. Fear of exposure is quite disturbing, and at this time the group is very effective in supporting the member as he commits himself to a new way of life. Frequently, he announces that he cannot give up his homosexual friends; the group usually reassures him that he need not do so but can retain them as he acquires others. We have seldom had reports that homosexual friends object, and they are more likely to encourage than to object. Eventually the patient reaches a point where he can reject the behavior of homosexual friends while still maintaining contact with them. However, as he finally commits himself to a heterosexual life, his homosexual friends diminish in importance to him and are often dropped.

Those who go on to a reversal of sexual pattern may begin by dating girls, often considerably older or younger than themselves. Their early dates are often quite casual and are for dinner, theatre, or movies. As acquaintances broaden, double dates and party dates become common and are often commented upon enthusiastically. Acceptance in other groups has ego-strengthening significance and is often followed by more courageous dating. As a member finds a girl he loves and is thinking of becoming married or engaged, the feelings involved are freely discussed in the group. The comforting warmth and the feelings of greater significance as they face the responsibility of marriage are emphasized. Where marriage has occurred, the group is interested in knowing only that the new way of life is pleasing and gratifying.

The members anticipate well in advance the departure of a patient from a group. The member decreases his verbal participation but makes very pertinent comments on the material under discussion, relating his experience to those whose productions are being considered. His role is not that of the patient who moves into a cotherapist role, but rather that of a reassuring, confident comrade. He is seemingly employing the knowledge and insights he has acquired to reassure himself and encourage the others. Eventually he announces his intention of leaving the group, and at this time they question him about his attitude toward his experiences, toward others, and toward himself. He is in effect called upon to review his progress and describe the changes that have occurred. This examination of the results obtained is reassuring to those who remain and usually

201

initiates in subsequent sessions a discussion of how those who remain are progressing. The experience is reassuring to the group and contributes to the strengthening of the purpose of its members.

No patients have been considered as having been treated who attended less than 20 sessions (approximately 30 clock hours). Those who have been successfully treated have attended, as a rule, 100 or more sessions and have ranged in age from 23 to 35 at time of initiation of treatment. I cannot report any success with anyone over 40, but I believe more intensive work with this group by combining individual and group psychotherapy should offer considerable hope of reversal.

The evaluation of the results of treatment of the homosexual is no easier than an assay of the results of psychotherapy in any condition. As group psychotherapists generally recognize, the group can rather realistically appraise the progress of the various members, and in the final assessment this is given consideration. The views of the family are considered, and the progress on their jobs or at school is evaluated. The overall appearance of the individual undergoes change. In addition to considering the fact that the patient feels that he has changed, he often presents evidence that others consider advancement. With all of these considerations and the report of the patient, we feel justified in stating that about one-third of the patients we have treated have experienced a reversal of their homosexual pattern.

The utilization of a group approach offers promise, and we sincerely hope that as more attention is focused upon his problem, there will not only be an increase in beneficial results obtained but additional information will be gained about experiences leading to the development of homosexuality so that means of its prevention can be recognized.

REFERENCES

1. BERGLER, E.: What every physician should know about homosexuality. Internat. Rec. Med. #171:685, 1958.
2. BERGLER, E.: Homosexuality—Disease or Way of Life. New York, Hill and Wang, Inc., 1957.
3. BIEBER, I.: Homosexuality—A Psychoanalytic Study. New York, Basic Books, Inc., 1962.
4. MUNZER, J.: Treatment of the homosexual in group psychotherapy. In Topical Problems of Psychotherapy. Vol. 5. Basel, Switzerland, Karger.
5. HADDEN, S.: Attitudes towards and approaches to the problem of homosexuality. Penn. Med. J. 60:1195, 1957.
6. HADDEN, S.: The treatment of homosexuality by individual and group psychotherapy. Amer. J. Psychiat. 114(9):810, 1958.
7. FREUD, S.: The Psychogenesis of Homosexuality in a Woman. Internat. Psycho-Analyt. Library Collected Papers Sigmund Freud. Vol. 2. London, The Hogarth Press, 1948, p. 206.

The Treatment of Transvestism and Transsexualism

by ROBERT J. STOLLER, M.D.

THERE IS NO ADEQUATE TREATMENT for either transvestism or transsexualism; what follows will only emphasize this opinion.

Our discussion will be confused unless transvestism and transsexualism are defined. Not all conditions in which there is dressing up in the clothes of the opposite sex—cross dressing—are transvestism. Momentary transvestic tendencies are seen in many children; some homosexuals cross-dress on occasion; and if one judges by the frequency of transvestic references nowadays, in books, plays, movies, and jokes, many adults who do not need to cross-dress are nonetheless interested in its manifestations. However, transvestism is different from the above. The transvestite wishes to be accepted in society as a woman at the same time as he wishes to remain a male.* He starts (except in children, who will be discussed later) as a fetishist, with a single garment producing excitement, gradually progressing until an equally impelling need develops —the desire to appear, when dressed, so much like a woman that he can pass undetected for one. That part of transvestism which is fetishistic serves, as do all perversions, as a preserver of sexual gratification, (potency), without which, either in practice or when used in fantasy, the man's sexual capacities are severely crippled. The fact that the transvestite's sexual response is so restricted by this unusual practice contributes to the fierceness of the need and the intensity of the pleasure, making treatment—since it aims at removing this pleasure—so difficult. However, in addition to the fetishism, with its sexual excitement, is the nonsexually exciting need to take on the role, especially the femininity, of a woman. This is a matter of having identified with women (not merely imitating them) and can lead the transvestite to run the great

---

*The word "woman" will be used to imply an identity, a gender, and a role—psychological qualities; "female" implies only biological attributes of sex; likewise for "man" and "male."

risks of social humiliation or arrest if he is caught trying to pass as a woman. In addition to passing, almost every transvestite also lives part of each day undisguisedly as a man. There is great satisfaction for him in telling himself he is able to be *both* a man and a woman. Crucial is his constant awareness, whether sexually excited or not, that he has a penis and thus is a "woman with a penis."

The above description excludes all other types of people who cross-dress, even the transsexual. The transsexual is different in that he does not wish to alternate between being a man and woman but rather wants to be changed by any devices known to medicine to be both a woman and a female.* He gets no sexual excitement from clothes and will gladly sacrifice his genitals to live a woman's role.

THERAPY

In the first place, the transvestite does not wish to stop being a trans-vestite. He would like society to change so that he would be safe; this not having happened, he will occasionally seek out a psychiatrist to learn how to avoid the fear, shame, and guilt produced by society's attitudes. Although he may ask the psychiatrist to cure him of the transvestism, what he is really asking is to be cured of his pain. He generally does not consider his transvestism to be painful. Quite the opposite, it is most enjoyable; what it stirs up in others is what leads to the pain.† So when the transvestite discovers that the doctor's goal is the removal of the syndrome, the patient leaves.

There are variations in the above discussion of ego syntonicity. In adolescence the transvestite will feel evil and a freak, but the pleasure is too intense to be stopped. Later on, the man may have fits of remorse and disgust after orgasm, throw away the clothes and, if he has been caught at it, come to the psychiatrist filled with strong motivation to change. This almost always passes off after one or two visits. Rarely, a patient will continue in treatment for months or years, but the reports in the literature of extended treatment end with such a statement as: "The patient was improved but moved before treatment ended."

I would consider a transvestite to be cured of transvestism if, without

---

*Note that the transvestite wants to be a male and a woman but not, as the transsexual wishes, a female and a woman.

†I have been unable to determine, either from the literature or from patients evaluated or seen in research-treatment, to what extent their guilt is an inherent part of the complex psychodynamics at the heart of the condition and to what extent it is the effect of society's fear of and indignation at cross-gender impulses. Practically speaking, the amount of guilt felt by the transvestite is insufficient to galvanize the treatment, once he learns how to deal with society.

the need for conscious control—inhibition, suppression, denial, avoidance, or courage—he no longer cared to cross-dress, had not substituted barely disguised but similar forms of sexual or gender role behavior, and was now potently and pleasurably using a woman with whom he had an affectionate relationship for his sexual gratification. (This would be asking a lot of most men, not just transvestites.) In other words, his character structure would have so changed that he now wished to maintain the differences between men and women, no longer needing to merge with women now that his excessive identification with them had withered.

Certainly such changes do not seem impossible. To a lesser degree they may occur in the normal development of children and adolescents and in the treatment of some effeminate men, whether practicing homosexuals or not. Oddly enough, there is no case reported in which one can feel this has occurred with a transvestite.* The few psychoanalytic wrtings on the subject reveal that the treatment has illuminated the psychodynamics, but in no case in which the descriptive material is that of a real transvestite is it clear that the patient lost his perversion—either the sexual (fetishist) aspect or the gender (the desire to pass as a woman).[2-9] This holds true for the rest of the psychiatric literature except for a very few recent papers to be discussed.†

The only recently reported treatment for which more than one author shows enthusiasm is that called aversion therapy, conditioning, negative conditioning, or behavior therapy. These reports show a resurgence of interest in the use of repeated applications of pain or vomiting that were in vogue 50 years ago and sporadically since (e.g., in the treatment of alcoholics). While the theory has become more sophisticated, the techniques have retained their simplicity: painful electric shock to the edge of agony or monumental bouts of vomiting, these administered while the patient dresses in his favorite garments, looks at photographs, or listens to tapes of himself describing himself as a transvestite, etc.[16-29]

I am prejudiced against these techniques‡ and worried that learning

---

*Although one report, suggesting personality change, is optimistic, the follow-up is superficial.[1]

†Because this is a biased statement, I should note there are sporadic reports[5,6,10-15] of patients who are described as better, relieved, improved, etc., but it is not really clear what was done in treatment, why the patient changed and what were the manifestations of the change or in some cases even if the patients were transvestites or more simply fetishists.

‡So are others.[30-34] ". . . I submit that electric shocks [faradic aversion treatment] are in the same category as the flogging, ducking, and cannon-firing of the past, and that good intentions do not justify the means employed."[34]

205

theory is being prostituted into a device for flailing at psychoanalytic theory and data, and fearful that such forms of treatment might become facile techniques for cruelty in unscrupulous hands. Still one must be cautious about claiming the only true faith. There are many treatments in medicine which may be brutal for patients but when properly used are the best that we as yet have to offer (e.g., EST in the psychotic depressions). If the goal of the treatment of the transvestite is set as being the removal of cross-dressing, if nothing else has been of use, and if aversion treatment removes the activity, then it should be used—if. The next series of "if's" takes us into an even soggier swamp, the whole issue of who defines what is antisocial behavior and the extent to which this behavior endangers society or its individuals. How much pain should be inflicted on a patient to make him conform? For the homicidal individual, a great deal. How much for the transvestite? To what extent does society's lenient attitude cause deviant behavior to increase? Does deviant sexual and gender behavior weaken a society? What does "weaken a society" mean? How do we discuss transvestism and its treatment if we haven't the answers to these kinds of questions?

The recent optimistic reports of the aversionists leave a therapist hungry with hope and a skeptic skeptical. If the treatment works and there are patients who want it, the misery should be worth suffering; we must not discard a treatment that is of use simply because it is not the kind we prefer for theoretical, moral, or idiosyncratic personal reasons. Thus far, however, the number of successes is very small, the follow-ups too short, and the method of checking if the treatment has worked either skimpily reported or skimpily applied. ("Are you better?" "Yes." Good—the patient is better.)

Let me report briefly a "cure" that I observed but played no significant part in, and as one picks holes in the argument he can experience the kind of skepticism some of us feel regarding any cures of transvestism ascribed to *any* method of treatment.

I had been seeing this man, a typical transvestite, for about a year. He would not consider himself a patient but rather a research subject, though I was aware that his occasional visits were motivated by more than his willingness to assist in the research. As distinct from most transvestites, he had a clear though mild paranoid quality, which put him into closer contact with some of his psychodynamics than the typical transvestite. Sometime before his first visit, he had gotten from some reading the idea that transvestism and homosexuality were connected. To determine if this were true for himself, over a period of several months he talked with homosexuals, visited "gay" bars, and read increasingly about homosexuality. (I take this to be evidence of homosexual desires, still forbidden, nonetheless moving toward conscious gratification.) Along with this interest, he coerced his wife into sexual games in which homosexual qualities were increasingly manifest. This was accompanied by a crescendo of anxiety, irritability, suspiciousness, depressive fits, and hyperactivity, culminating in a paranoid psychosis precipitated by his having his wife, dressed like a prostitute, attach to herself an artificial penis he had made, with which she then performed anal intercourse upon him. Following this finally quite conscious gratification of his homosexual desires, he became suicidal and homicidal. As we talked throughout the several hours of this emergency, he vividly expressed his opinion, derived possibly in part from his readings but mainly from his own psychotic thoughts, that his transvestism had been an attempt to keep himself from sensing his homosexual desires. As he absorbed what he was saying, he became calmer. He also stopped his transvestism. Since that moment, a year ago, he has not practiced it again.

A psychodynamic remission. He now has insight, the product of his psychosis and the cause of his remission. Where formerly a potential psychosis was held in check by the complex character structure we have called transvestism, the psychosis is now contained by insight. But is that the answer? Is there proof this is so? Would a recurrence of the psychosis prove the thesis wrong?

The patient now says that he no longer has any desire to dress. He has given away the clothes, makeup, wigs, transvestite magazines and books, and the clothes catalogs. When he sees a woman wearing articles of clothes the sight of which would formerly excite him, he feels no lust (nor disgust either). His wife corroborates all this, although, since she cannot climb into his mind and know all he thinks, she still fears it might start up again. (To what extent do her fears that he might indulge press him toward doing just that?)

Yet it is with as inadequate data as the above that we must judge the results of treatment reported in the literature. In this case, the time of remission has been too short to say that his "self-cure" has worked. Many transvestites are known to have periods of disgust or fear in which they swear off their perversion and get rid of their paraphernalia. Under sufficient provocation—and a terrifying psychosis may be as effective as a course of apomorphine, electric shock, or a jail sentence—transvestites can refrain from months to years.

The point is this: It is too early to be enthusiastic about results of aversion treatment. If it turns out that its users can effect long remissions in many cases, without a high price in substitute symptom formation or

207

overlying crippling inhibitions, then this painful therapy will be valuable. Until then it cannot be reported that it is the proper treatment for transvestism.*

Another form of treatment that might be considered is castration. Legislation permitting this under certain circumstances for managing "sexual psychopaths" has been enacted in California and Scandinavia. The loss of testosterone would undoubtedly drastically reduce the number of orgasms the transvestite enjoys from the fetishistic aspect of his perversion; it probably would not effect his desire to pass as a woman. Transvestites who have lived into their 60's and 70's note a decrease in sexual desire but none in the desire to cross-dress.

Since transvestites do not endanger other people, there is no rationale for forcing them to be castrated.

For the sake of completeness, we can note reports on two other types of treatment. The first[35,36] is that of a borderline patient who was a transvestite and gave up his transvestism under nialamid, meprobamate, and chlorpromazine; after maintenance dosage for four years he is reported in "good mental health." It is not clear how extensive the follow-up evaluation has been. At any rate, this method has not yet produced a wave of former transvestites successfully treated with phrenotropic drugs.

The second report is that EST made two transvestites feel better.[37]

So far, this discussion has concerned only men. What about women? While women cross-dress, they do not fulfill the other criteria for a diagnosis of transvestism. Our society permits normal women to wear mannish clothes or even men's clothes. In addition, cross-dressing is seen in some homosexual women. However, this is not fetishistic, and they are not trying to pass as men. On the contrary, it is a preoccupation with them to let the world know that they scorn men and feel them unnecessary.

There are, however, a very small number of women who wish they were men and who pass as men. They are not transvestites but transsexuals and do whatever they can to obtain sex transformation operations.

In other words, although there are many *transvestic* women, I doubt if there are any *transvestite* women.[38]

TRANSSEXUALISM

It is impossible to discuss the treatment of transsexuals without becoming involved in moral issues. The transsexual, unlike the transvestite, does not wish to remain a male† but wishes to have his body changed so that

---

*See also Coates[31] for a reasoned display of skepticism.

†For simplicity I shall discuss this primarily in terms of males.

208

he becomes as completely female as medical techniques can contrive. In addition possibly to threatening the masculinity of the physicians to whom the transsexual makes his request, the patient treads on ancient feelings in society regarding the preservation of fertility. Then too, of a more practical nature, the surgery is extensive and not without danger; being of a completely elective nature—the indications are purely psychological—one hesitates to embark on cosmetic procedures that are so much more intricate and hazardous than fixing a nose.

The most troubling aspect is that the easier it is to have such procedures done, the more patients request them. As the word gets around, as it has in the last decade or so, more and more effeminate men request to be changed. Lumping them all together in one category leads to the implication that anyone making such a request is a transsexual.[39,40] If it is a surgeon who oversimplifies these differences in gender identity, and there is no one to stay his hand, there will be tragic consequences. For the effeminate homosexual who prizes the pleasures his penis brings him with other men or for the transvestite who so enjoys his fetishism and the sense of being a woman with a phallus, the realities of having been castrated can be disastrous. For the patient, this may mean a severe depression or paranoid psychosis, and for the physician the treacherous uncertainties of the medical-legal issues which have still not been clarified by the courts.

The general rule that applies to the treatment of the transsexual is that no matter what one does—including nothing—it will be wrong.

First, what happens if the procedures are completed? It is a fact that can be proved only by having seen transsexuals (not pseudotranssexuals) in intensive follow-up from months to years after they have completed their "sex transformation" procedures that many are better adjusted (we won't pause to document that vague term) postoperatively than they were before. Their anguish before the procedures is intense and genuine (one of the many points distinguishing their reactions from pseudotranssexuals). Nonetheless, they are left more or less dissatisfied, feeling that although the procedures have feminized some of their appearance and functions, the results are far from complete. The transsexual will wish not only breasts, vagina, and femalelike external genitalia, absent facial and body hair (all of which can be supplied) but also ovaries, uterus, and fertility. So if the surgeon complies with the patient's request, he is likely still to be harassed by the patient, who wants more. Some are sexually promiscuous and some become entertainers who capitalize on their notoriety. In addition, these patients are exhibitionistic and unreliable as manifested in the office by a high rate of missed appointments, lateness, and peculiar distortions of their history even in areas outside of the development of gender. These qualities make working with such patients distasteful for some physicians.* (It adds nothing to our knowledge to apply the coup de grace by dismissing them with the statement, "They're all psychopaths.") Pauly, in his excellent review of 100 cases of transsexualism, concludes that, "Follow-up studies at the present time indicate some apparent success, but these results must be interpreted with caution."[41]

On the other hand, if one does not assist them they are deeply unhappy. The argument against treating this unhappiness by surgery or hormones is exemplified by the following: ". . . if . . . the demand for a change of sex operation is based upon a delusion [sic] conviction, then only the treatment of the underlying psychoses or personality disorder is in my view admissable or correct.

"Sometimes such patients are suffering from schizophrenia and are overtly psychotic; sometimes it is hard to see where, apart from their singular and absolute rejection of their own sexuality, their judgment is in other ways abnormal. In either case only such treatment as will enable them to come to terms with the reality of their condition is open to the psychiatrist to offer or endorse."[42]

One would not give a throne to a psychotic who delusionally felt he was a king; is it not as irrational to grant the transsexual his request just because he is unhappy? The cases are not parallel, however. Psychotics who want thrones do not become less disturbed even when they become kings, but most transsexuals are less depressed and anxious, more sociable and affectionate, etc. after "the change." Also, very few transsexuals are clinically psychotic. (While I have heard of such, in my limited experience, I happen not to have seen one who was, although one or two were a bit frayed at the edges.) Their "delusion," coming from sources we have not yet found, is placed in a setting of intact reality testing. Almost all of these patients know their request is strange; they do not question that society considers them bizarre; there is nothing grandiose or persecutory in their thinking; they are not trying to change the world or to construct a philosophic system to impose on others, etc. I go into this detail only so that we can avoid the simple answers that come by using simple words like "psychotic" and "delusion" rather than describing the data as we observe them.

---

*These qualities have not been present in the few transsexual females with whom I have worked. Such patients have been dependable, quietly determined, and without flamboyance. As a result they became quite successful in living their inconspicuous lives as men.

210

However, for all this, if there were any psychiatric treatment that were even partly useful, it would probably be better than this disquieting "psychosurgery." It has been suggested[43] that "no psychotherapeutic procedure less than intensive, prolonged, classic psychoanalysis would have any effect. If properly done, it could probably reduce the patient's agitation and the level of his unhappiness. It is not impossible that his major symptoms may decrease in frequency and urgency." This statement has the vigorous ring of sober caution; it also must have been written by someone who has never tried to get such a patient into analysis. Unfortunately, no one has ever reported such success by any psychotherapeutic technique. We must search for such techniques, but in the meanwhile it seems haughty to say that "only such treatment as will enable them to come to terms with the reality of their condition is open to the psychiatrist to offer or endorse." Since we have nothing to offer or endorse that can give these patients any relief, to make this a rule to put into practice when sitting in one's office with the patient who asks your help means to do nothing. The problem for the psychiatrist then is only should he do this nothing gracefully or horsewhip the bloody beggar off the compound.

Benjamin, who has treated more patients requesting sex transformation procedures than anyone else, has a method of evaluation and treatment on which he has reported favorably.[44,45] After weeding out those patients who are psychologically obviously unsuited, he suggests to his candidates that they actually pass as women for many months. He has found that for some, while the fantasies of being a woman are very rich, the rigors of living as a woman are either too frightening or the person is too masculine to be able to keep it up. During this time, Benjamin prescribes estrogens, feeling that they not only give the patient an inner sense of femaleness and an observable change in body contours, but that the estrogens in themselves have a tranquilizing effect on males. If after this trial, it is Benjamin's opinion that the patient is still highly motivated and sufficiently feminine, he then refers the patient for surgical procedures. When these have been performed, he continues to follow up these patients indefinitely. He has reported on 40 patients followed postoperatively; 34 were "satisfactory" (on a three point scale of satisfactory, doubtful, or unsatisfactory).

At this point it is worth mentioning a practical difficulty that arises should the psychiatrist choose to recommend a patient for such surgery. Practically no such procedures have been performed in the last few years in major American medical centers (with the exception of patients who had already gotten parts of the operation done somewhere else or where

211

the patients had already mutilated themselves). There is a lot of secrecy involved in finding a surgeon who will cooperate, and even then the patient must have thousands of dollars. These operations are not being done in medical centers with facilities for nonpaying patients except in the rarest of instances. Although there are clinics in foreign countries where "sex transformation" surgery is performed, it is alleged that not all routinely adhere to the rigid standards of asepsis familiar in American operating rooms.

It is unsettling to realize that transsexualism was scarcely an issue for physicians until a few years ago. This knowledge may annoy physicians who are aware that had the techniques not been applied to transsexuals and then publicized, such people would have contained themselves, as hopeless people certainly can do. Considering the nature of this subject, it may be unwise to say that Pandora's box has been opened, but it is true that we have to come to terms with the problem. We cannot legislate it away, probably, and we do not know how to treat it psychiatrically.

I would suggest, because these procedures may be disastrous if used with the wrong patient, that they not be used except as research techniques. This would mean that they should not be done simply because the patient has the money to afford bootlegging. They should not be used unless the patient has been studied in depth and for at least six months by a team of psychiatrists, psychologists, endocrinologists, and urologists. For those who do go to surgery, the follow-up should be intensively pursued for at least a year and then at least several times a year for years, with the patient actually being talked to by members of the team. Participating physicians should be legally protected from suits. In the course of such a program, we shall not only learn about the treatment of transsexualism, hopefully so much that one will not need to continue using these procedures, but, more important, about the sources and manifestations of gender identity.

CHILDREN WITH GENDER PERVERSIONS

This chapter can be closed with some comments, partly chilling and partly hopeful, about children with gender perversions. It is becoming apparent from reports in the literature,[46,47] which are confirmed by my own experience and that reported informally by colleagues in this country and in Europe, that childhood transvestism is much more common than we had imagined and that it may start very early, sometimes before age 1.[48] I do not mean the unremarkable manifestations of occasional, low intensity transvestic behavior, but rather the overpowering, flagrant, habitual urge to cross-dress. There are no reports of any child with this true transvestism being followed into adulthood, but considering the hold with which this passion seizes the child, it is most likely that its natural history leads to adult cross-dressing. (I would guess that it is from these children that the transsexuals come, both male and female).

What is hopeful is that we have a few clues that the process might be modified. There are a couple of reports of transvestite boys[49,50] who, with their mothers being simultaneously analyzed, gave up their cross-dressing and other feminine interests, this accompanied by changes in character structure beyond those naturally occurring with growing up. However, there are as yet no adequate follow-ups.

At this time then, it seems that prevention by education of parents or treatment of the few who can be given such treatment are the best hopes in childhood transvestism. Unfortunately, the former requires a revolution in the attitudes of many parents and of our society (which is moving all too rapidly toward massive blurring of gender differences), while the latter is still terribly time consuming and experimental.

REFERENCES

1. McKenzie, R. E., and Schultz, I. M.: Study of a transvestite. Evaluation and treatment. Amer. J. Psychother. 15:267-280, 1961.
2. Fenichel, O. (1930): The Psychology of Transvestism. Collected Papers I. New York, Norton, 1953, pp. 167-180.
3. Freud, S. (1927): Fetishism. Standard edition. 21:149-157, London, Hogarth Press, 1961.
4. —— (1938): Splitting of the Ego in the Defensive Process. Collected Papers 5. London, Hogarth Press, 1950, pp. 372-375.
5. Gutheil, E. A.: The psychologic background of transsexualism and transvestism. Amer. J. Psychother. 8:231-239, 1954.
6. Harnik, E. J.: Pleasure in disguise—The need for decoration and the sense of beauty. Psychoanal. Quat. 1:216-264, 1932.
7. Lewis, M. D.: A case of transvestism with multiple body-phallus identification. Int. J. Psychonal. 44:346-351, 1963.
8. Segal, M. M.: Transvestitism as an impulse and as a defense. Int. J. Psychoanal. 46:209-217, 1965.
9. Stoller, R. J.: Transvestism and transsexualism. Presented at Symposium on Sex Disorders in Clinical Practice, San Francisco, March 1965.
10. Deutsch, D.: A case of transvestism, Amer. J. Psychother. 8:239-242, 1954.
11. Edelstein, E. L.: Psychodynamics of a transvestite. Amer. J. Psychother. 14:121-131, 1960.
12. Grant, V. W.: The cross-dresser: A case study. J. Nerv. Ment. Dis. 131:149-159, 1960.
13. Lukianowicz, N.: A rudimentary form of transvestism. Amer. J. Psychother. 16:665-675, 1962.
14. ——: The cases of transvestism. Psychiat. Quart. 34:517-537, 1960.
15. Philippopoulos, G. S.: A case of transvestism in a 17-year-old girl. Acta Psychother. 12:29-37, 1964.

16. ALLEN, C. E.: Electrical aversion therapy. Brit. Med. J. i:437, 1964.
17. BARKER, J. C., THORPE, J. G., BLAKEMORE, C. B., LAVIN, N. I., AND CONWAY, C. G.: Behavior therapy in a case of transvestism. Lancet i:510, 1961.
18. BARKER, J. C.: Aversion therapy on sexual perversions (correspondence). Brit. J. Psychiat. 109:696, 1963.
19. BARKER, J. C.: Electrical aversion therapy. Brit. Med. J. i:436, 1964.
20. BARKER, J. C.: Behavior therapy for transvestism. Brit. J. Psychiat. 111:268-276, 1965.
21. BLAKEMORE, C. B., THORPE, J. G. BARKER, J. C., CONWAY, C. G., AND LAVIN, N. I.: The application of faradic aversion conditioning in a case of transvestism. Behav. Res. Ther. 1:29-34, 1963.
22. ——, ——, ——, ——, ——: Followup note to: the application of faradic aversion conditioning in a case of transvestism. Behav. Res. Ther. 1:191, 1963.
23. CLARK, D. F.: Fetishism treated by negative conditioning. Brit. J. Psychiat. 109:404-407, 1963.
24. COOPER, A. J.: A case of fetishism and impotence treated by behavior therapy. Brit. J. Psychiat. 109:649-652, 1963.
25. GLYNN, J. D. AND HARPER, P.: Behavior therapy in a case of transvestism. Lancet i:619-620, 1961.
26. LAVIN, N. I., THORPE, J. G., BARKER, J. C., BLAKEMORE, C. B., AND CONWAY, C. G.: Behavior therapy in a case of transvestism. J. Nerv. Ment. Dis. 133:346-353, 1961.
27. McGUIRE, R. J., AND VALLANCE, M.: Aversion therapy by electric shock: A simple technique. Brit. Med. J. i:151-153, 1964.
28. RAYMOND, M. J.: Case of fetishism treated by aversion therapy. Brit. Med. J. ii:854-856, 1956.
29. ——: Behavior therapy (correspondence). Brit. J. Psychiat. 110:108-109, 1964.
30. ALLCHIN, W. H.: Behavior therapy (correspondence). Brit. J. Psychiat. 110:108, 1964.
31. COATES, S.: Clinical psychology in sexual deviation. In The Pathology and Treatment of Sexual Deviation. I. Rosen, Ed. London, Oxford University Press, 1964.
32. MacDONALD, I. J.: Behavior therapy in a case of transvestism. Lancet i: 889-890, 1961.
33. MATTHEWS, P. C.: Behavior therapy (correspondence). Brit. J. Psychiat. 110:108, 1964.
34. WHITLOCK, F. A.: (correspondence). Brit. Med. J. i:436, 1964.
35. PENNINGTON, V. M.: Phrenotropic medication in transvestitism. J. Neuropsychiat. 2:35-40, 1960.
36. ——: Treatment in transvestism. Amer. J. Psychiat. 117:250-251, 1960.
37. EYRES, A. E.: Transvestism: Employment of somatic therapy with subsequent improvement. Dis. Nerv. Syst. 21:52-53, Jan. 1960.
38. STOLLER, R. J.: Female (versus male) transvestism. Read at the American Psychoanalytic Association Annual Meeting, New York, May 1965.
39. HAMBURGER, C., STÜRRUP, G., AND DAHL-IVERSON, E.: Transvestism. J. Amer. Med. Ass. 152:391-396, 1953.

214

40. HAMBURGER, C.: Desire for change of sex as shown by personal letters from 465 men and women. Acta Endocr. 14:361-375, 1953.
41. PAULY, I.: Male psychosexual inversion: transsexualism. Arch. Gen. Psychiat. 13:172-181, 1965.
42. STAFFORD-CLARK, D.: Essentials of the clinical approach. In The Pathology and Treatment of Sexual Deviation. I. Rosen, Ed. London, Oxford University Press, 1964.
43. OSTOW, M.: Transvestism (correspondence). J. Amer. Med. Ass. 152:1553, 1953.
44. BENJAMIN, H.: Nature and management of transsexualism with report of 31 operated cases. West. J. Surg. 72:105-111, 1964.
45. ——: Clinical aspects of transsexualism in the male and female. Amer. J. Psychother. 18:458-469, 1964.
46. GREEN, R., AND MONEY, J.: Incongruous gender role: nongenital manifestations in prepubertal boys. J. Nerv. Ment. Dis. 131:160-168, 1960.
47. ——: Effeminacy in prepubertal boys. Pediatrics 27:286-291, 1961.
48. STOLLER, R. J.: The mother's contribution to infantile transvestism. Presented at 24th Internat. Psychoanalytical Congr., Amsterdam. The Netherlands, July, 1965.
49. SPERLING, M.: The analysis of a boy with transvestic tendencies. Psychoanal. Stud. Child, 19:470-493, 1964.
50. GREENSON, R. R.: Discussion of Stoller's presentation. 24th Internat. Psychoanalytic Cong., Amsterdam, The Netherlands, 1965.

Psychiatric Treatment of the Sex Offender

by Asher R. Pacht, Ph.D.; Seymour L. Halleck, M.D.; and John C. Ehrmann, Ph.D.

D URING THE LAST DECADE, increasing public attention has been focused on the sexual criminal. In an effort to cope with this perplexing problem, many states have developed special legislation for dealing with this group. For the most part, this legislation has been wholly inadequate. Public concern tends to emphasize the responsibility of psychiatry for developing effective treatment programs. To date, the psychiatric treatment of these offenders has been considered unrewarding and only a limited body of knowledge has come from the profession. This paper offers information in this area by detailing some of the unique experiences involved in the effective treatment of a large group of sex offenders.

Based on nine years experience with an operative Sex Crimes Law, the authors have developed a cautiously optimistic outlook toward the psychiatric treatment of this disorder. Favorable therapeutic results are, however, dependent upon the incorporation of specific factors in the program. Briefly stated, these are:

A. The necessary administrative machinery for differential handling which stresses indeterminate sentencing for those who need psychological treatment.

B. Over-all support from progressive judicial and correctional administrators as well as appropriate institution facilities and adequate staff.

C. A diagnostic appraisal which insures intensive study of the psychodynamics of the individual offender.

D. A flexible program which includes all modalities of psychiatric treatment.

While the emphasis in this paper is directed toward treatment, brief attention must be given to the first three factors which are considered necessary prerequisites.

The administrative and legal structure of our program is based on the Wisconsin Sex Crimes Law which was instituted in July, 1951. This law specifically recognizes the psychological nature of many sex offenses and establishes the machinery both to identify and provide specialized treatment for the "deviated" sex offender. Under this program any person convicted of rape, attempted rape or indecent sexual behavior with a child, *must* be committed to the State Department of Public Welfare for a pre-sentence social, physical and mental examination. Any other offense prompted by a desire for sexual gratification may be examined at the discretion of the Department. During a sixty day examination period, the Department attempts to determine if the individual is in need of specialized treatment for "mental or physical aberrations." If the individual is found in need of such treatment, the court *must* either recommit him indeterminately to the Sex Deviate Facility at the State Prison, or place him on probation with mandatory outpatient psychotherapy. Unlike most sex crimes laws, this program fulfills two needs. It provides treatment for those who can benefit from it and maximum custody for life, if necessary, for those who cannot utilize treatment and who remain a danger to society.

No law, regardless of how well it has been written, can be effective unless it has the wholehearted support of all those concerned with its operation. The Wisconsin Sex Crimes Law was developed by a large committee which included judges, lawyers, correctional administrators, mental health personnel, and representatives of civic and religious groups. These groups have maintained an active interest in the operation of the program and continue to lend their support. Equally vital has been the cooperation received from all levels of personnel at the State Prison where the program is conducted. Despite the limits imposed by a maximum security setting, modalities of rehabilitation comparable to adjunctive therapies in mental hospitals are available. Where specific treatment needs cannot be met at the Prison, the facilities of mental hospitals and other correctional institutions can be used. In addition, after-care services are provided by a large, well trained state parole service. Most important, it has been possible to maintain (although with considerable difficulty) an adequate staff of qualified psychotherapists and consultants.

Adequate diagnostic facilities are available during the pre-sentence observation period. Social history material is obtained from two sources. Trained social workers in the field submit a report based on direct contacts with the individual's family, acquaintances, and appropriate agencies. In addition, an intensive psychiatric social history is obtained from the individual at the prison. Each offender receives a battery of psychological tests and has a series of interviews with a psychiatrist. When the different disciplines have completed their examinations, the offender is discussed at a staff conference and a group decision is made with respect to his diagnosis and his proper committability under the Sex Crimes Law. A report of the staff decision is then submitted to the Department of Public Welfare and from there to the committing court.

The law is worded in a manner that makes it unnecessary to conform to a rigid rule of responsibility or committability in recommending a person for treatment. The staff is free to develop their own criteria for selecting the most suitable candidates for recommitment into the treatment program. In practice, we recommend commitment under the Sex Crimes Law for those people who present two basic qualities in their personality and behavior. First, we look for an immaturity in the development of sexual functions, which also encompasses other areas of the individual's personality and social behavior. Second, we look for a deviation of the individual's normal sexual aim or object which he has little ability to control by conscious rational thought. We then speak of this individual as having a compulsive need to live out his sexual immaturities.

Although our population presents a wide variety of social backgrounds, intellectual abilities, and previous levels of achievement, it is rare that we see an offender with a relatively intact personality. The majority of our patients demonstrate few ego strengths and few conflict-free areas in their lives. Histories of severe trauma and emotional deprivation during early childhood are commonplace. Approximately 40 per cent of our population has had previous correctional experience and many others have been wards of the State. Our experience indicates that sex deviates as a group function in the world as inadequate individuals.

Sexual behavior, for most of our patients, is associated with tremendous needs to satisfy passive wishes, bolster self esteem, find identity and, in a figurative sense, be fed. Many of these individuals would fall into the category of ambulatory schizophrenic or borderline states.

The treatment begins when the individual has been recommitted to the prison under the law. At this institution, he immediately becomes involved in a program which includes orientation, classification and job assignment. The scope as well as limitations of our treatment may be clarified by examining the personality patterns of our offenders, particularly as related to the impact of the prison milieu. Given the inadequate ego skills and passivity of our patients, we are faced with problems created by placing these individuals in a prison environment. Their overwhelming passivity is accentuated by arrest and commitment. The impact of arrest on a sex offender leads to feelings of shame and humiliation. When the passive, inadequate individual encounters these emotions, he becomes

218

even more helpless. He seeks easily grasped concepts or structures that will afford him an explanation for his behavior. Many sex offenders dismiss their behavior as being entirely the product of overindulgence in alcohol. Sometimes the offense is denied in its entirety both to the authorities and to themselves. More often attempts are made to rationalize deviant behavior by claims that the patient was seduced by sexually aggressive, precocious young boys or girls. Given the personality limitations of our patients and the impact of the prison milieu, there is a need for immediately creating a climate of acceptance which at the same time discourages rationalization, denial, and projection.

Each new inmate is placed in an orientation group led by two members of the psychiatric staff. These groups contain between ten and twenty patients and meet for a total of ten sessions. Basic principles of mental health as well as the mechanics of normal sexual behavior are explained and discussed. Wherever possible, relevant films are used and free discussion is encouraged. These meetings attempt to create a climate devoid of blame or punitiveness toward the sex offender. The orientation group also serves the purpose of giving our staff a second chance for evaluating the patient's potential for psychotherapy, and it is not until the end of this period that a specific treatment program is outlined.

A majority of offenders are offered psychotherapy. We currently provide both individual and group psychotherapies ranging from insight therapies to supportive and even didactic approaches. For those individuals who we feel are able to make personality changes, the major goal of treatment is to provide a degree of self understanding sufficient to help them resolve their impulsive sexual motivations. For those who do not demonstrate a potential for personality change, treatment may consist of strengthening useful defenses, education, and emotional support.

Based on their needs, many individuals are recommended for expressive individual or group psychotherapy. While all members of our staff accept the role of unconscious processes in determining behavior, the backgrounds and training of different individuals leads to a variety of approaches. Thus, free association is frequently supplemented by a variety of techniques based on client-centered and learning theory. Success in therapy seems to depend more upon the offender's motivation and the therapist's skill than on specific theoretical investment. In general, therapists tend to use techniques directed at uncovering unconscious material when working with patients who are appropriately motivated and can tolerate anxiety. Group therapy was originally inaugurated to provide for a maximum number of contacts with a limited professional staff. It has, however, proved so markedly effective in helping establish positive self-identification quickly, and in bringing about the development of social and interpersonal insights that we now regard it as a treatment of choice for many.

Psychotherapy is less frequent than we feel to be optimal, and runs the gamut from a few who receive therapy twice a week to a greater number who are seen weekly or biweekly. The average length of treatment time for both group and individual therapy is approximately fourteen months.

The process of our reeducative therapy with sex offenders may be broken down into three phases. The initial phase is devoted to creating a climate which allows the establishment of a therapeutic relationship. This period may encompass several months to a year. Only after the development of such a relationship can the individual begin to examine his behavior without resorting to defensiveness or intra-punitive mechanisms. The second phase is the period of working through nuclear conflicts. During this period, therapy focuses upon those factors in the background of the individual that have contributed to the development of deviant trends. Considerable attention is also directed toward the day to day interactions in the prison setting emphasizing those vignettes of behavior that are similar to self destructive actions that have led to incarceration. The last phase of therapy is devoted to problems of separation and planning for the future. This is often a very complicated process. Returning to the free world from a closed institution presents an additional burden to the stresses of community attitude, vocational problems, family attitudes, and separation from the therapist.

Termination of therapy does not necessarily mean automatic release from the institution. The final responsibility for release rests with a Special Review Board which is independent of the treatment service and consists of a social worker, a lawyer, and a psychiatrist. The majority of offenders released are assigned to an after-care program which includes supervision and counselling by trained social workers.

The combination of a correctional setting, an indeterminate sentence, and the inadequate personality structure of the sexual deviate tends to produce specific problems in psychotherapy which may not be encountered elsewhere, The most outstanding of these is the type of resistance in which the patient eagerly grasps onto a psychological or moralistic formula which provides him a rationalization for his behavior. This serves as a superficial explanation for his difficulties which may also lead him to the conviction that he will not repeat the offense. If he merely promises to stop his aberrant behavior, and holds to his belief on the basis of an alleged change in his morals or an alleged understanding of his difficulties, he sets up a tremendous road-block to treatment. The patient who clings to such a position effectively removes the need for a therapist or any further therapeutic change. The most satisfactory way to avoid this resistance is for the therapist to be constantly aware of any tendencies in himself toward adopting a psychiatric "partyline" which the inmate can learn and parrot back to him. The inmate must be constantly questioned as to what he actually does understand about himself and both he and the therapist must realize that the areas involved are so complex that they can never be treated with certainty.

It is essential that the offender take responsibility for his actions. Rationalizing behavior through invoking alcoholism, unfortunate circumstances, or even psychoanalytic formulations, does not lead to therapeutic progress. The offender must recognize that it is he who has committed the crime. It is neither the alcohol, nor the environment, nor the neuroses. Optimally therapy should be conducted in a situation where the offender is moderately anxious and both uncertain and concerned about his propensity to repeat the offense. The inmate who leaves the institution with doubt and apprehension is perhaps a better risk than the one who leaves with an ultimate assurance of being cured.

A sizeable number of offenders are not selected for expressive therapy primarily because they either show little motivation or do not have sufficient ego strength to cooperate in this type of treatment. For this group we have been experimenting with a wide variety of other techniques including supportive educational sessions, environmental manipulations, and even exhortative approaches. Many of these offenders have been unable to tolerate close contact with another person without feeling aroused by all sorts of infantile sexual and aggressive feelings. Few are able to appreciate that a close benevolent relationship with another individual is a possibility. These men are provided therapeutic contacts ranging from "friendly chats" to specific didactic sessions on sexual problems. Through such techniques many offenders are able to discover a new type of interpersonal relationship and to markedly strengthen their internal controls. Adjunctive services such as religious, occupational, and educational counseling are used.

There are a few offenders who are neither interested in nor able to cooperate in any type of psychotherapeutic venture, but who will respond to the basic correctional program of the institution. For those who do not, our program functions primarily to protect society. Some of these individuals will be committed far longer than they would have been under ordinary sentencing. We feel that the failure of ordinary psychological treatment techniques with this group represents an inadequacy of psychiatric knowledge, and that until techniques are more refined, treatment must consist of indeterminate custodial care. This is analogous to the case of the chronically psychotic patient in the mental hospital who often

221

must be institutionalized even though there is little definitive treatment available.

All in all, our experience in working therapeutically with this group has taught us to be flexible in our thinking, daring in our experimentation with new techniques, and realistic with respect to the establishment of meaningful goals. Only by modifying orthodox concepts have we been able to produce positive results.

The parole experience and discharge record of individuals who have received treatment under the law is encouraging. Only a few of the more relevant statistical results will be presented. Of 1,605 male offenders examined under this law over a nine year period, only 783 were found to be in need of specialized treatment. Parole experience with this group has been excellent. Of the 475 individuals granted parole through May 31, 1960, only 81 have violated that parole—a rate (17 per cent) considerably lower than that found with parole granted to the general prison population. It is particularly noteworthy that only 43, or 9 per cent of the total paroled, violated their parole by commission of a further sex offense. For individuals who have been discharged following a period of institutional treatment and parole supervision, the results are even more outstanding. Through May 31, 1960, 414 individuals were discharged from Departmental control; only 29, or 7 per cent of this group, committed a new offense following discharge. We feel that this law has been most effective, not only in providing protection to the public, but also in demonstrating that most sex offenders are capable of responding to treatment.

PART VI

PSYCHOPATHY AND PSYCHOSES

The Treatment of Psychopaths

by MELITTA SCHMIEDEBERG, M.D.

PSYCHOPATHY and criminality overlap, but are not synonomous. Some ordinary persons break the law under pressure or temptation; habitual criminals however are abnormal or abnormalised and usually psychopathic. On the other hand, many well-to-do psychopaths manage to remain within the law. Psychopathy is not an entity, nor a rarity. With three million serious felony offenders in the USA the number of psychopaths must run into millions, yet they have hardly been studied, even diagnostically. They range from the borderline psychotics, such as those committing horrible types of murder or bizarre acts, to the borderline neurotics, who often still have some social or family ties, suffer from depressions if they fail, and may commit suicide if the game is up. Even the ordinary person may, under the pressure of certain situations, as in wartime, develop psychopathic reactions and even become psychopathic. The neurotic, again, does not always correspond to the textbook version of overconscientiousness, and even obsessionals may show psychopathic reactions and act antisocially. This is still more true of borderline psychotics, schizoid and paranoid personalities. Some psychiatrists tend to minimize antisocial traits in their patients and call them "character cases" or "passive aggressive dependents." The line between the "bad boy" in adolescence and the psychopath is not easily drawn, and it is hard to distinguish the product of the slums, devoid of moral and other training, from the "true" psychopath. Many alcoholics and other "acting out" patients are actually psychopathic; most drug addicts many of whom are former gang boys.

The psychopath behaves antisocially and has antisocial ideals and fantasies; he both "wants to be a villain" and is forced to be one, since he is unable to succeed socially. Often there is deep underlying hopelessness. Psychopaths are not altogether devoid of anxiety and guilt, but they manage effectively to cut off these levers of socialisation, the temporary awareness of which frightens them excessively. While anxiety and guilt

225

help to make the neurotic and normal person more social, they incite the psychopath to antisocial acts in his attempts to prove himself master of these emotions which he fears and despises.

A patient felt guilty towards his wife whom he mistreated; to punish her for having made him feel bad, he beat her and when she cried he beat her harder.

The cliché that psychopaths "fail to learn from experience" is only partially true. Time teaches them to become a more skillful criminal, but not to socialize, though some give up their fight against society as they get older. Their failure to learn from social experience is based on their ability to take their behavior out of its social context, to break the continuity of cause and effect and the continuity of time. Punishment to them is not consequence, but merely ill luck or injustice. They continue to believe that they will go scot-free, irrespective of how often they have been caught, and are almost delusionally convinced of their superior intelligence. Their excessive narcissism makes them immune to social pressures and rational thinking. The problem for therapy is that they want no treatment, because they have no wish to change and find no fault with themselves, but only blame others and society. Their denial mechanisms and narcissism make them, as a rule, immune both to severity and kindness. The only time they are somewhat amenable to influence is when their narcissistic bubble of grandeur has been burst, when they have been caught and await trial. Incidentally, the anxiety they then experience and the desperate efforts they make to avoid punishment is proof that they desire punishment neither consciously nor unconsciously. Although I have examined thousands, I have not yet seen a single serious offender who was motivated by an unconscious wish for punishment. The fact that antisocial personalities and psychopaths have been mistaken for "neurotic offenders" and been treated as such has had disastrous consequences, likely to bring psychiatry into disrepute in legal circles.

Probation which developed empirically, has hit intuitively on the one avenue by which many offenders can be influenced, namely a combination and delicate balance of fear and kindness, by approaching the offender when the apprehension of punishment and the experiences of trial have stirred him and he is relieved because he has not been sent to prison.

Though the patient usually can be reached when the harsh reality has pierced his narcissistic defences, such influence is as a rule only short-lived, owing to the psychopath's remarkable ability to reestablish his antisocial mental balance with the help of his ideas of grandeur and denial. Hence we need a situation of continuing pressure. The attempt of some psychiatrist to win an antisocial patient over by siding with him

226

against authority and removing external pressure, usually results in the patient feeling relieved and staying away. The patient comes for treatment unwillingly, and his good resolutions are attempts to manipulate the therapist. He must be allowed such hope for manipulating or he would not try, but the therapist must be careful how far he allows himself to be manipulated; rather, he must manipulate the patient to socialize him. The enforced attendance must be used to establish a more genuine relation; this can only be done by showing understanding and by giving help in teaching the patient to solve his problems and to gain satisfaction in a social manner. We must constantly fight the patient's tendency to denial and to insensitizing himself by evoking two opposite emotions almost simultaneously, i.e., giving him sympathy for having been wronged, yet highlighting the wrong he has done and warning him of the consequences of his behavior, thus evoking guilt and building on whatever rudiments of social feelings he possesses. This must be done so that he feels the doctor is on his side, e.g., would regret it if he went to prison. Unbearable anxiety or guilt stimulate his antisocial mechanisms, yet no influence is gained unless sufficiently strong emotions are evoked.

These patients have tremendous energy, probably because so little of it is inhibited and sublimated and are able to wear out their environment and the therapist. Effective therapy should turn the tables on the patient and wear him out: create situations for him to which he must conform rather than allow him to control the situations. The more persons are involved in the treatment situation, provided they are well co-ordinated, the better. In the Association for the Psychiatric Treatment of Offenders in New York City we utilize many persons, each playing his own role. The clinical director sees the patient on intake, trying to motivate him, thus making the task of the therapist easier. She remains a figure of authority to whom the therapist can refer. The probation officer, with the judge behind him, plays his legal role and represents final authority. The therapist is more on the patient's side. Then there may be a reading instructor, medical doctor, members of family or friends, with all of whom the therapist seeks contact and whom he tries to co-ordinate.

I had, as Clinical Director of APTO, succeeded in getting a young recidivist out of detention, after he had been arrested for new offenses during treatment. He needed a letter from APTO for the court hearing and I insisted that he see me. When he phoned for an appointment I discovered that he had no job. "Look here Billy, what can I write in this letter? The judge knows that you have been in trouble before, that you stole cars again while on probation. If I write that you have no job, what will he think? I give you a piece of advice. Do not see me till you have a job." But there were only three days left to the hearing. Next day Billy had a job, the first one in his life.

227

Treatment of the psychopath, then, is the opposite of the passive, detached, nonjudgmental therapy currently used for neurotics, since this type of patient contrasts in all essentials with the neurotic. The latter is too inhibited, overconscientious, worries too much, acts too little and too slowly, is afraid of change; the former is consumed by restlessness, is in constant motion, acts on the spur of the moment, is underconscientious, and asocial. The task of therapy is to build inhibitions, social feeling and conscience, to teach him to delay action, to think within the context of reality, to establish a sense of continuity, to solve his problems and gain satisfaction in a social manner. To do this we must be active and alert, manipulate him and his environment; not only be judgmental, but teach the patient values and judgment.

Cooperation with the courts is essential. For this it is necessary to know and respect the prerogative of the courts, have some knowledge of law, institutions, criminal mentality, know what, can and, cannot be condoned, what recommendations to make to the Court and how reports should be written, what information should be given or withheld, etc.

Since this highly specialised knowledge and approach is essential for the treatment of offenders, and even for evaluating them diagnostically, criminal psychiatry should be developed and taught as a specialty. Psychiatrists lacking such experience should not advise courts, educators, parents, etc. on the handling of delinquents as analogies drawn from private practice with neurotics are misleading.

Treatment of Depression

by PAUL HUSTON, M.D.

Introduction

Many qualifying terms are attached to the word depression. Some of these describe characteristics such as agitated or anxious, psychotic, or suicidal; others refer to probable etiologic factors as drug depression, reactive, involutional, neurotic, or postpartum. Official American Psychiatric Association diagnostic nomenclature lists four categories: manic-depressive, involutional, psychotic depressive reaction, and neurotic depression. The existence of so many types of depression may perplex the therapist who wishes to apply specific treatment. However, for practical purposes, general guidelines exist which broadly determine the therapy employed. These depend upon the clinical picture, available treatment techniques, and practical problems of management.

Clinical

We shall first present a picture of depression that responds to antidepressant drugs and electrotherapy and which is also managed by supportive psychotherapy. The patient complains of low spirits, sadness, despondency, lack of enjoyment of life, and gloomy outlook. He looks downcast, smiles little or half-heartedly, and has a slumped posture and a listless gait. Many patients respond and move slowly; their thoughts flow sluggishly and they cannot concentrate or make decisions. Some patients, instead of retardation, exhibit restlessness, anxiety, or even marked agitation. Simple daily tasks seem mountainous; and poor appetite causes weight loss. Sleep disturbance appears as awakening in the early hours of the morning. In mild and moderate stages of depression, some patients feel more depressed, anxious, and retarded in the morning hours, but by evening complete or partial relief occurs.

Depressed patients may experience a wide variety of somatic sensations and physical complaints for which they seek medical relief. These include headache, usually of occipital location, dull feelings in the head, blurred vision, paresthesias, tightness in the chest, urinary frequency, diminution in libido, reduction or cessation in the menstrual flow, muscle tremors, soreness and pain, fatigue and weakness.

A depressed patient may have delusions of unworthiness, sin, guilt, and hopelessness, with the conclusion that only suicide will bring relief. He may reveal his suicidal intent by allusion, speaking of getting his affairs in order, making a will, where he wishes burial, of being tired of living, and by giving away personal effects. Other patients speak directly of suicidal thoughts or plans. A few depressed patients suffer from paranoid delusions, falsely believing others intend to harm him or refer to him in derogatory terms. Whatever the mental content of the depression, it has as essential features retardation (or marked agitation), diurnal rhythm, poor appetite, and early morning awakening. This type of depression, sometimes referred as endogenous, on the average, runs a course of 8 to 12 months, and in about 50 per cent of cases recurs again during the life of the patient. Changes in the external environment and attempts to cheer and reassure the patient meet with only quite temporary effects lasting a few hours or a day or two. Many episodes of depressive feelings do not meet these general criteria. Their characteristics and treatment will be discussed later.

Indications for Hospital Care

Two important questions arise immediately in the treatment of depression. One concerns the presence of suicidal ideas; the other, a decision whether to hospitalize the patient.

Suicidal ideas in a patient always concern the physician. Such ideas are likely to be found more often in lonely patients, in depressed alcoholics, and in those with a family history of suicide. Suitable questions to elicit suicidal ruminations are: Did you ever wish you could go to sleep and never wake up? Have you ever hoped you would never awaken after taking your sleeping medicine, or have you felt so badly you have thought of doing something to yourself? Airing suicidal thoughts frequently relieves the patient, who then feels the physician knows and understands the worst about him. The physician discusses all the reasons the patient has for suicide. In this he holds out hope for recovery. The patient is told that no matter how black the future seems, patients with depression recover. Strong or impulsive suicidal ideas require immediate steps to protect the patient by hospitalization or by arranging capable 24-hr. attendants.

Besides suicidal danger, indications for hospitalization include severe depressions not responding to treatment, inability of relatives to give care, or complicating physical problems that require further diagnostic study or treatment. Outpatient electrotherapy needs relatives able to provide special care.

Psychotherapy of Depression

The psychotherapy of the endogenous depressed patient is primarily supportive. Probing into unconscious factors or emotional conflicts possibly

230

related to the depression may make the patient more introspective, anxious, depressed, and more suicidal.

If the patient has thoughts of hostility and guilt, the physician minimizes them. Attempts are made to build up the patient's self-esteem by recounting his laudable qualities and accomplishments. Sometimes the patient will accept his depressive symptoms better if they are interpreted as a temporary malfunction of his nervous system. He should be reminded of the nervousness that appears in hyperthyroidism, of premenstrual tension and blues, of unaccounted-for mood swings in his past experience. Usually these efforts to minimize depressive ideas are transitory, but they provide partial relief until more definitive treatment with antidepressive drugs or electrotherapy can be applied.

The patient should be encouraged to continue daily activities within the limits of his available energy. Activity draws attention away from his depressive preoccupations and keeps the routine of customary living. But the patient should not be pushed beyond his energy reserve, for then he will feel more depleted and discouraged. Nor should the physician push the patient into human contacts if he believes others can detect his depression, for this may give rise to feelings of estrangement and guilt. To assess how much work the patient can do, the physician should learn the routine of the patient's typical work day and week. This information serves as a base for prescribing activities and helps the therapist to judge the response to treatment. The practical questions involve the time of arising and retiring, the constancy of sleep, the hours of work, the social and recreational contacts.

The patient should be advised to maintain his nutritional status by adequate food intake. If he has great concern about insomnia, meprobamate or chloral hydrate may be prescribed. Do not continue hypnotics for long, since sleep improvement is one of the best indicators of response to definitive treatment.

Persons entrusted with the general supervision of the patient, whether in the hospital or out, should convey a supportive and optimistic attitude of wanting to help. Relatives should avoid discussion of interpersonal conflicts that may arouse animosity and guilt. The physician should instruct them on what to observe so that they can report the progress of treatment when the patient returns for outpatient or office visits.[1,3,4,5]

Drug Therapy

For mild endogenous depressions with diurnal rhythm where the patient feels normal or nearly so in the late afternoon or evening, the use of amobarbital sodium (1.5 to 3 gr.) and amphetamine sulphate (5 to 15 mg.) at breakfast and lunch may largely relieve the patient of his symptoms. The fixed ratio of these drugs in Dexamyl tablets is appropriate for the average case. If the patient has tension, amobarbital sodium alone is often better; for patients without tension,

231

amphetamine alone may be more effective.* A disadvantage of amobarbital and amphetamine in combination or singly is that after six to eight weeks, the medication loses its effectiveness and the dosage needs to be increased. Continuation of this process reaches toxic levels. However, stopping the drugs for 10 to 14 days renews their effectivenss when readministered.[5]

The best antidepressant drugs are the tricyclic compounds, and widely used are imipramine (Tofranil) and amitriptyline (Elavil).[2] For both, the dose is commonly begun at 75 mg., daily divided into three equal parts and given with meals. The dosage level can increase over a two- to three-week period up to a level of 250 mg., per day, occasionally to 300 mg., per day. An average daily level is 150 to 200 mg., in three or four equal doses. Amitriptyline possesses the advantage of a slight sedative effect, which calms tension and promotes sleep. With use of these drugs, improvement begins to appear in one to two weeks after initiating treatment. The maintenance level is the minimal daily dose that produces maximal response. Other tricyclic compounds in use are despramine, doxepin, nortriptyline, and protriptyline. Side effects are usually not serious and include dry mouth, sweating, blurring of vision, fine tremor, and postural hypotension. The patient may adjust to the last effect by arising from a recumbent position slowly. Most of these side effects disappear after the first few weeks of treatment. Others, rarely seen, are urinary retention, aggravation of glaucoma, skin rash, jaundice, and agranulocytosis.

Another class of antidepressants, the monoamine oxidase inhibitors (MAO), are generally less effective than the tricyclic compounds, and are used only if the tricyclic drugs have failed or if the patient has a history of responding to a MAO inhibitor in a previous depression. The MAO inhibitors are phenelzine, isocarboxazid, nialamide, and tranylcypramine. Trycyclopramine is the most effective, but the most toxic; phenylzine is the best for general use. The daily dosage range for these drugs differs from that for the tricyclics; for example, for phenylzine it is 30 to 60 mg. Serious hyperpyrexial coma may develop with the MAO inhibitor when administered with other drugs such as insulin, barbiturates, meperidine, amphetamines, ephedrine, phenylaphrine, and tricyclic antidepressants. Because of this, when shifting from a tricyclic drug to a MAO inhibitor, a drug-free period of seven to ten days should intervene. Patients on MAO inhibitors should not drink alcohol or eat foods (such as ripened cheeses, pickled herrings, chicken liver, yeast extracts, chocolate, and broad beans) that may cause a hypertensive crisis.

How long should a patient be kept on a drug? The vast majority of depressed patients recover after a variable length of time without definitive treatment. The

---

*EDITOR'S NOTE. The deleterious effects of the barbiturates on driving and other essential skills must be seriously considered, as must psychologic addiction to amphetamine compounds.

range is from a week or two up to several years, with an average period of eight to ten months. So far as known, drug treatments do not shorten the duration. After the patient has been on a maintenance dose for six to eight weeks, the daily dose is reduced to 50 mg., in the case of imipramine or amitriptyline, for a two-week period. If no sign of relapse appears, the dose is lowered another 50 mg., per day, for an additional two- to four-week period. But if, following reduction, depressive symptoms appear or worsen, increase the dosage level to the previous level for another four- to six-week period, after which repeat the reduction process.

In following the course of a patient on drug therapy, the use of a check list of depressive symptoms helps judge progress considerably. The literature contains several lists such as those by Zung[8] and Hamilton.[4] Since patients may have idiosyncratic symptoms, the writer prefers to construct a list for each patient. In it are included also the common depressive symptoms. Each symptom is rated from 0 to 3: 0 indicates absence of the symptom; 1, present in mild degree; 2, moderate; and 3, severe. On return visits, usually at weekly intervals at the beginning of treatment and every two to three weeks after reaching the maintenance dose level, the symptoms are graded. The list becomes a record of the course, proving of particular value in establishing the maintenance level and in the process of drug reduction.

If a patient fails to respond to a drug in four to eight weeks, he may be considered a candidate for electrotherapy.

Electrotherapy

Electrotherapy, a time-tested treatment for depression, produces recovery in two to three weeks in 85 per cent of cases.[6] For severe depressions, usually six to eight treatments at the rate of three per week suffice; cases of moderate or mild severity need fewer treatments. Few contraindications or complications to electrotherapy exist. The contraindications are a coronary attack within the preceding four months, esophageal varices that might hemorrhage (as in liver cirrhosis with portal hypertension), bleeding peptic ulcer, acute infections, or aortic aneurysm. Complications in the early days of electrotherapy were mild compression fractures of the anterior lips of the vertebral column, usually in the region of dorsal 4, 5, and 6, and dislocation of the jaw or shoulder. Muscle relaxants now prevent these.

Techniques of Electrotherapy

The skin over the temples is rubbed with gauze soaked in alcohol, after which succinylcholine chloride (Anectine), 10 to 15 mg. is injected rapidly intravenously to produce muscle relaxation. For the alternating-current stimulus, electrodes are placed tightly against the temples to conduct a current of sufficient voltage and duration (10 to 15 sec. after the intravenous injection of anectine) to cause a petit mal response (Medcraft apparatus, voltage 100, current time 0.1 sec.). The petit mal response abolishes memory for respiratory distress due to the succinylcholine. At the time of maximal relaxation, which comes 30 to 40 sec. after the injection, a second electrical stimulus of sufficient voltage and time to produce a grand mal type of reaction is administered. This voltage falls between 120 and 140, and the duration of current is 0.3 to 0.5 sec. The patient is aerated with 100 per cent oxygen through a face mask during the major reaction and until normal respiration returns.

Patients usually show some memory loss for recent events after four to five treatments. The patient and his relatives are told about this and also informed that normal memory will return in two to three weeks after the last treatment. Most patients show complete recovery after five to seven treatments. An additional treatment helps prevent immediate relapse. Electrotherapy relieves a current attack, but does not prevent subsequent depressions.

Electrotherapy is sometimes used prophylactically to prevent relapse. An occasional patient will again show signs of returning depression four to eight weeks after a successful course of therapy. Giving such a patient one or two treatments will abort the full-blown depressive syndrome. Antidepressant drugs may prevent relapse.

Other Types of Depression

Depressive Symptoms Associated with Other Illnesses

Depressive symptoms may appear with diseases such as general paresis, multiple sclerosis, viral infections, or the ingestion of certain drugs, such as rauwolfia compounds. If the depression should persist, after treatment of the primary condition, antidepressant drugs or electrotherapy may be indicated.

Depressive Symptoms Following Losses

Most significant loss is the death of a spouse or other close relative. The ensuing grief lasts four to eight weeks, and the bereaved may show a variety of manifestations: preoccupation with the image of the deceased; self-accusations of negligence in relation to the deceased; hostility toward doctors and nurses, alleging inadequate care of the deceased; and an aversion to normal activities. The griever feels sad, his sleep is fitful, his appetite poor, his mental concentration difficult, and he complains of a variety of physical troubles. The visits of widows and widowers to general practitioners increase twofold in the first six months after the death of the spouse. Ordinarily, temporary grief requires only symptomatic relief such as hypnotics for sleep or a mild tranquilizer for general tension. Occasionally the grief passes over into a depressive state for which antidepressant drugs or electrotherapy are necessary.

The elderly and physically ill also may experience depressivelike feelings. Prominent symptoms include poor energy, easy fatigability, anorexia, constipation, insomnia, hypochondriasis, loss of interest, fault finding, irritability, excessive demands on others, sadness, or apathy. To understand such reactions, we need to consider the meaning of aging or of a physical illness to the individual. If being old lowers the patient's status, he may suffer a deflation of self-esteem. If the patient has an illness with a poor prognosis or a permanent disability, adjustments are necessary to preserve ego stability. All these may affect the patient's family relationships, his occupation, and his economic and social position. Some persons can accept aging or illness with a minimum of difficulty; others overcompensate with hitherto dormant resources, or by excessive attempts to control their milieu. Still others retreat into helplessness, show hostility or dependency, and refuse to accept their disability. Mutilating surgery poses the problem of the loss of a valued portion of anatomy; for example, the amputation of an extremity or a breast. Depressive reactions may occur in anticipation of, as well as after, the surgery. All these situations must be handled on an individual basis; if they can be solved, the depressive symptoms lift. If the symptoms become more pervasive and serious, antidepressant drugs or electrotherapy should be considered.

Neurotic Depressive Reaction

Neurotic depressive reaction,[7] is a diagnostic entity with vague conceptual boundaries and is treated almost exclusively with insight psychotherapy, frequently over a prolonged period. The neurotic depression most commonly occurs in persons who have a life-long history of neurotic traits in response to a personal loss. Generally, the depression fluctuates in severity and rarely reaches profound degrees. It responds temporarily at least to strong reassurance and especially to a satisfying dependent emotional relationship with another person. Mental and physical retardation is not present, and appetite and food intake, as a rule, are not diminished; occasionally these patients eat more and gain weight. These patients characteristically feel worse in the evening, and their sleep is apt to be broken, although some sleep profoundly. Anxiety, trouble in concentration, irritability, easy fatigability, and a wide variety of somatic complaints plague the patient. The mood in neurotic depression seems closely tied to the patient's relationship to other persons. The patient displays a clinging need for sympathy and attention or, failing to secure this, reacts in a critical, demanding, or even hostile way, which in turn alienates his relatives and friends. This makes the patient feel more rejected. Suicidal gestures may occur as acts of spite against a person from whom the patient had sought more emotional support.

Psychotherapy begins by combating ideas of lowered self-esteem, after which attention is directed toward clarifying the precipitating circumstances of the current depression as well as any previous ones. The aim in this inquiry is to discover those of the patient's reactions to other people that led to depressive feelings, and to make the patient gradually aware of them. The patient's frustrations, ineffective defensive maneuvers, anxieties, guilt, and anger become more conscious. His immature way of giving and receiving affection often emerges as a central fault. Continued analysis of the problem may trace the origin of the defect to early childhood. In the process of uncovering past feelings and developing insight, the patient may act toward the physician as he did toward other people in his life. These occasions present opportunities to help develop insight into the basic defect. The goal of treatment is to help the patient learn more mature techniques of developing interpersonal relationships.

In the treatment, mild tranquilizers such as meprobamate or mood elevators such as amphetamines may be employed to help the patient through difficult periods of depression.

The therapist must remember that some cases of retarded or endogenous depression begin with a clinical picture more nearly resembling a neurotic depression. Gradually, over weeks or a month or two, the symptoms change and a clinical picture indistinguishable from endogenous depression becomes apparent. Treatment of this condition then follows the outline previously presented for the use of antidepressant drugs or electrotherapy.

REFERENCES

1. Cohen, R. A.: Manic-Depressive Reactions. In: Freeman, A. M., and Kaplan, H. I. (Eds.), Comprehensive Textbook of Psychiatry. Baltimore, The Williams & Wilkins Co., 1967.
2. Cole, J., and Davis, J. M.: Antidepressant Drugs, *ibid.*
3. Ford, H.: Involutional Psychotic Reaction, *ibid.*
4. Hamilton, M.: A Rating Scale for Depression. J. Neurol. Neurosurg. Psychiat., 23:56, 1960.
5. Huston, P. E.: Psychotic Depressive Reaction. In: Freeman, A. M. and Kaplan, H. I. (Eds.), Comprehensive Textbook of Psychiatry. Baltimore, The Williams & Wilkins Co., 1967.
6. Kalinowsky, L. B.: The Convulsive Therapies, *ibid.*
7. Mendelson, M.: Neurotic Depressive Reaction, *ibid.*
8. Zung, W. W. K.: A Self-Rating Depression Scale. Arch. Gen. Psychiat. 12:63, 1965.

Outpatient Therapy of Chronic Schizophrenia

by WERNER M. MENDEL, M.D.

A MAJOR TASK FACING PSYCHIATRY TODAY is the development of techniques and treatment personnel for the large patient population requiring prolonged care and management. Included in this population primarily are the chronic schizophrenic patients, as well as some patients with borderline states. Unfortunately, the specific etiology of those disorders generally grouped under the heading of chronic schizophrenia remains obscure. At present, we can do no more than to view this group of illnesses as complex psychobiological reactions to a multitude of somatic, psychological, genetic, environmental, and social forces. In this chapter we propose to describe the theory, technique, and results of an outpatient treatment program for chronic schizophrenia in which 166 patients and 18 therapists participated for four and one-half years. The specific therapeutic skills utilized in this program can be taught easily to non-professional personnel and can be effectively carried out by them with psychiatric supervision.

The phenomenological approach to illness concerns itself with a detailed study of the disordered existence. Analyses of disorganized schizophrenic existences have repeatedly demonstrated that schizophrenia can be understood in terms of disorganization of the world of the patient and that this is primarily a perceptual disorganization.[8] The individual is what his world is.[4] This world which the individual has created and in which he takes a stand is, in fact, the individual. This world can be studied in terms of time, space, and causality. Such an approach to understanding schizophrenic illness leads to the type of therapeutic intervention which views the treatment task in terms of the reorganization of perceptual processes. The perceptual disorganization must be treated by a therapeutic intervention which fosters reorganization of the world design of the patient.

Within the framework of the transaction between the therapist and the patient, three simple reorganizational tasks can be structured. These are directed to the facilitation of the reorganization of the perception of the internal world, the reorganization of the perception of the external world, and a reorganization of the perception of the future.

The correction of the disorganized perception of the internal world can be carried out by a selected listening for, and emphasis on the action of the patient. This results in a concomitant de-emphasis of wishes, fantasies, thoughts and dreams which are listened to but are not placed in the position of primary importance as they are in more "psychoanalytically-oriented" treatment.

In essence, the attitude is conveyed to the patient that the therapist is primarily interested in action. This emphasis enforces a realignment and reorganization of the perception of the internal world so that patients can function (act) more effectively in the external world.

Therapeutic measures directed to the correction of the perceptual distortion of the external world consist of helping the patient to recognize the possibility of interpreting the same events in a number of alternative ways. Even if the patient can not accept the possibility of a different world construction, the therapeutic transaction fosters at least a suspicion that there are other possibilities.

It has been demonstrated in a number of existential studies that for the schizophrenic patient, the future is closed.[2,6] The forceful reopening of the future is evolved out of the therapeutic transaction. Once the future reopens, it is held open both in the therapeutic transaction and in the world of the patient. In the therapeutic transaction, the non-ending quality of the relationship, the definite appointment in the future, the reliability and availability of the therapist keep the future open. In the transaction of the patient with his world, the future is kept open by preventing the patient from placing himself in situations which will lead to failure. For with each failure there is a progressive closing of the future as the existence moves from, "it will be, it may be, it might be, it might have been," to "it will never be."[6]

DESCRIPTION OF THE TREATMENT TEAM AND PATIENT POPULATION

This program of outpatient treatment[7] utilized both professional and non-professional personnel as psychotherapists. The professional individuals were psychiatrists, clinical psychologists, and psychiatric social workers. The non-professional personnel were a group of carefully selected and experienced psychiatric aides,* all of whom had demon-

---

*In the California State Hospital system these aides are called Psychiatric Technicians. They have no formal psychiatric training prior to employment. However, they do have on-the-job training during the first several weeks of employment.

strated their ability to deal with chronic, emotionally disturbed patients in the hospital setting.

The patient population treated in this program consisted of 166 chronic schizophrenic female patients, ranging from 20 to 66 years of age with an average of 32. The duration of hospitalization prior to entering the treatment program ranged from one month to eighteen years with an average of 2.6 years. Many of the patients had histories of previous long hospitalizations with an average of three prior hospitalizations per patient. All patients were seen individually on a once a month basis* for a 20 to 30 minute interview. Fifty-seven per cent of the patients were given tranquilizers in conjunction with their psychotherapy.† All medications were prescribed and supervised by the psychiatric physician, who also provided supervision for the psychologists and social workers participating in the treatment program. The supervising psychiatrist met with all the aide therapists in group supervision once a week, at which time the aides discussed each of their patient contacts with the psychiatrist.

Specific Description of Treatment Technique

Reorganization of the Perception of the Internal World

In the interview, the focus is always on action. The patient is encouraged to talk about activities. More specifically, it is constantly emphasized that what is important to the therapist and to other significant people is what the patient did, rather than wishes, fantasies, thoughts, or hallucinations. No interpretations are offered, no dynamic speculations made. The emphasis is on the here and now and the you and I.

Reorganization of the Perception of the External World

A persistent attempt is made to get the patient to report perception of the external world in specific and concrete action terms. The therapist questions perceptions which appear distorted and disorganized, and reinforces a more accurate and conventional view of the world. This provides the patient with some degree of validation and assistance in organizing perception of the external world. Such an approach to reality makes it necessary for the patient to entertain a continuing suspicion that the construction of the world is not entirely as he sees it, but rather that alternate world perceptions and constructions are possible.

---

*On occasion, a few patients were seen once every two weeks or once a week for brief periods of time. The frequency of visits was increased when the patient demonstrated increasing disorganization.

†Patients who had been receiving medication in the hospital continued on medication after leaving.

The chronic schizophrenic patient has a tendency to see the future as closed. The treatment transaction reopens the future. The pre-existing relationship to the helping situation is utilized whenever possible by assigning the patient to the therapist with whom he has developed a relationship while still in the hospital. The therapist attempts to provide the patient with the assurance of an indefinite or permanent therapeutic relationship by communicating the attitude that it will continue as needed. Each therapeutic interview ends with the emphatic statement, "I will see you next month" and the patient is given a specific appointment slip with time and date. Even though at times it becomes necessary for the therapist to be replaced by another, a continuing relationship is guaranteed to the patient. Patients are able to handle changes in therapists without apparent disruption of their level of adjustment.

At all times, the therapist assists the patient to avoid situations which would lead to failure. Patients are always reassured that they would not be rejected by the therapist if they could not function in certain areas. The therapist acts as a buffer between the sick patient and the unrealistic demands and expectations of others by helping the patient to evaluate his limitations in terms of the disordered existence. This protects the patient from placing himself in situations which are doomed to failure by his incapacities. Such failure would lead to a closing of the future.

Specific Instructions to the Treatment Team

The psychiatrist in charge of the program emphasized the following points to the treatment personnel:

I. The patients selected for this outpatient treatment program are those who have lived a constricted, isolated and alienated existence for years. In all probability for most of these patients, the monthly or bimonthly contact with the therapist is one of the high points of their existence. It serves the purpose of reassuring them of the reality of the helping situation which is represented by the hospital, the doctors, and all the adjunctive personnel.

II. It is important for the patient that each therapist comply with the basic structure of the interview. It should begin on time and should end on time. If possible, it should be conducted in the same room and the patient should sit in the same chair each month. Each time the patient should be given an appointment slip before leaving; if appropriate, he should be given a prescription. Everything should be as much the same from appointment to appointment as possible. All of this serves to reassure the patient that the therapeutic situation is structured, that we know what we are doing, and that he can count on being treated consistently by us. This structured 20 minute interview may be the only encounter he can predict during the entire month.

III. The general attitude during the therapeutic encounter is essentially non-judgmental and non-demanding. However, we explore with him the consequences of his past and contemplated future actions, and we may lead him to the recognition that specific consequences are indeed undesirable for him. We are non-demanding of the patient in terms of his need for success. The only demand we make of the patient is that he come for his appointments, come on time, and talk with us. Demands for success and function are made by society, by family, and by the patient's own needs. Our job is to soften these demands for the patient, particularly if we feel he can not meet them.

IV. We get the patient out of impossible situations whenever necessary. Patients very much want to please their therapist. They frequently respond to our therapeutic zeal and need for observing improvement by attempting to engage in complex interpersonal relationships or work tasks for which they are not ready. The result will be failure, exacerbation of symptoms, and inability to continue the treatment encounter. Whenever a patient tells us that he is going to take a job, that he is going to get involved in a new complex relationship, or that he is going to change his life situation, we must respond with much caution. After careful exploration of all aspects of the reality of the situation and the possible consequences of the contemplated action, we must judge whether the patient can handle it.

V. During each interview, we listen to the patients' verbalizations and respond selectively, but focus attention on action and reality. This serves the purpose of helping to demonstrate to the patient what is real as contrasted to fantasy. It demonstrates to him that his actions count and that he is held responsible for them, while his fantasies, dreams, delusions, and hallucinations are his own private domain. For example, if a patient comes in stating, "This morning when I came to the appointment the bus passed me by. I know that the driver was told by the Communists not to pick me up," one of two responses may be made. First, one might focus on activity and state to the patient, "How did you get here, finally, after missing the bus?" One emphasizing the importance of his action in contrast to his fantasies and delusions, thus, might also show him that he could possibly re-interpret the event in a more realistic way by saying, "Is there any other reason you can think of why the bus passed you by?" Even if the patient can not accept any other reason and states, "You probably think it passed me by because it was full, but that wasn't the reason", he at least maintains some level of recognition that the events can be quite differently perceived.

241

VI. Built into the transaction between the doctor and the patient is hope and the possibility of change. The very fact that the patient comes to the doctor (or doctor symbol) implies that he has hope that things might be better. Even if the patient does not have hope but only the suspicion that things can be different, this keeps the future open. The therapist in the encounter demonstrates interest, effort, and concern, and thus he, too, assumes an open future. We further reinforce this open future by the clear statement of the next specific appointment time.

RESULTS

Thirty per cent of the total 166 chronic, schizophrenic patients demonstrated such disorganization of behavior that they needed to be returned to the hospital during the fifty-one months treatment and observation period which this study reports. A total of fifty patients returned to the hospital. Thirty-six of these, or 72 per cent of all returnees, came back into the hospital within the first year. One hundred and sixteen patients (70 per cent) remained functional outside of the hospital for the entire 51 months' period while receiving the outpatient treatment described in this chapter.

The treatment results obtained by the psychiatrists were the same as those obtained by the psychiatric aides. Exactly the same techniques have been employed with chronic schizophrenic patients who have not been previously hospitalized. There patients were not treated by technicians but by minimally experienced medical students. The results of such an approach to outpatient treatment were comparable to those reported for aftercare patients.

REFERENCES

1. ARIETI, S.: Psychotherapy of schizophrenia. Arch. Gen. Psychiat., 7:112, 1962.
2. BINSWANGER, L.: The Case of Ellen West, In Existence. New York, Basic Books, 1958, pp. 237-363.
3. FROMM-REICHMANN, F.: Psychotherapy of schizophrenia. Am. J. Psychiat., 111:410, 1954.
4. HEGEL, G. W.: The Phenomenology of the Mind, II Ed. New York, Mac-Millan, 1931, pp. 335-336.
5. MAZZANTI, V., AND BESSELL, H.: Communication through latent language. Amer. J. Psychother., 10:250, 1956.
6. MENDEL, W.: The future in the model of psychopathology. J. Exist. Psychiat., 2:363, 1962.
7. ——, AND RAPPORT, S.: Outpatient treatment for chronic schizophrenic patients. Arch. Gen. Psychiat., 8:100, 1963.
8. ——: Hospital treatment for chronic schizophrenics. J. Exist. Psychiat., 4:49, 1963.

Comprehensive Therapy of Schizophrenia

by ELVIN V. SEMRAD, M.D.

A COMPREHENSIVE clinical approach[8,9] to assist the schizophrenic person in his improvement, rehabilitation, and possible recovery has as a general objective—the development of his capacity to love, live, and work in a reasonable degree of subjective comfort.[4] The approach is primarily psychotherapeutic. Medications are adjunctive and used when recovery cannot be initiated or maintained on a relationship basis. The responsible physician serves as a resource, a support, and a gratification to all personnel involved as they take the initiative and responsibility to relate to the patient psychotherapeutically.

The symptoms, as elicited by stressful life events, are respected as real, with minimum concern with unconscious fantasies. Rapport relationships imply experiences or series of experiences with objects that are sustaining, supportive, gratifying, rewarding, and growth stimulating. Always clinically relevant is "who is doing what to whom, when, why, and apropos to what life issues?" The patient learns from his experience with his therapist and the care-taking associates who furnish new relationships and experiences and introduce a necessary and permanent factor into the patient's mental economy.[6]

Therapy is usually conducted face to face in an atmosphere of mutual understanding and rapport, and depends on what type of help the patient needs, and is willing to receive, as well as on what assistance the physician is able and willing to give. Long-term therapy of schizophrenic persons becomes essentially a character analysis, comprising an educative process and a corrective ego experience in acknowledging and keeping in perspective life experiences, be they painful or pleasurable.

The processes of comprehensive therapy may be discussed as follows:

a. The personal diagnostic processes
b. Prescription and use of impersonal processes
c. The ego compensation processes
d. The ego maintenance processes
e. The analysis of the psychosis-vulnerable ego
   (intensive-dynamic psychotherapy)

PERSONAL DIAGNOSTIC PROCESSES

A personal diagnostic summary is designed primarily to guide the therapy by the negotiations of the patient with the therapist. Before one decides to explore his mental life or to establish a deep rapport, the clinical questions must be answered—i.e., "What does he need help in doing that he cannot do for himself?"

Identification of the life impasse which occasioned the ego decompensation is primary.[14] If acute and overwhelming, it requires therapeutic activity to enable the patient to integrate the overwhelming traumatic experience, usually a loss. If it is debilitating and occasions a chronic step-by-step regression, it requires replacement or substitution. If realistic acceptance of frustrations is not possible, reintegrative mourning activity becomes necessary. Patients who manifest denial patterns of "not minding" (catatonic features) call forth demonstration in that they matter to the therapist. Projection patterns (usually in paranoid patients) call for responsibility sharing on the part of the therapist by his awareness of painful ideas and affects that the patient cannot bear by himself. The more the patient progresses out of his narcissistic regressed position, the more he functions as a depressed patient. Part of the diagnostic processes is the careful consideration of activity programs,[7] and the worker's skill therein, that will have a specific place in total treatment planning.

PRESCRIPTION OF IMPERSONAL PROCESSES

Chlorpromazine (thorazine) is particularly useful[12] when there is overwhelming, intolerable psychic pain which has to be mitigated.[1,5] In the therapeutic relationship intolerable affects in states of excitement, turmoil, or regression occur most frequently under two conditions: (1) where there has been disturbance in the equilibrium between the therapist and the patient; (2) when the patient is in a state of transition from one level of ego functioning to another, whether regressive or progressive. "Energizers," and "antidepressants" have less value. Often overt demands for drug treatment are made by the patient and sometimes by the staff. Although the patient's demand may be legitimate and appropriate, often it represents a specific therapeutic issue—e.g., it may be symbolic of the patient's demanding, and feeling entitled to, something other than medication, from someone other than the doctor. Those demands can be extremely difficult to meet, since the patient, when frustrated, may become accusatory and difficult and may act in destructive ways. The staff may also demand medication for patients when the therapeutic milieu is unable to contain the patient's demands. Electroconvulsive therapy is limited to patients who do not react to the ataractic drugs and are out of control. Insulin coma therapy and psychosurgery are most rarely recommended.

The compensation process, that is, a return from regression to optimum ego functioning, begins with the initial step of supplying the patient's emotional needs. Object-providing procedures, such as occupational therapy, nursing, etc., become an integral part of the team-planning activities. The therapist himself, as a resource, serves the patient as an object for ego identification. He encourages the patient to internalize the therapist's ways of dealing with experience. Through candid, respectful interaction, a corrective ego experience is structured. Mourning is a necessary part of treatment, and termination begins with the original working arrangement from the very first clarification or interpretation. The therapist helps the patient learn that to forget is not the way to get relief from intolerable life pain and that mastery, remembering, reliving, acknowledging, bearing, and putting in perspective go hand in hand; security is gained when the patient acquires the capacity to think, tolerate loneliness, and deal with life experiences as they are rather than as one would like them to be.

This type of support[9] requires that the patient likes, trusts, wants to understand, and is dependent upon the therapist. The patient desires expression of endearment and affection and reports things about himself as worse than they are to prove to himself that the therapist could still appreciate and understand him even if these reports were true. Allowing the patient to reach this state of dependent attachment should be done cautiously. The depth of the patient's confidence should always depend upon the depth of rapport established. The ideal way is to make him wish to talk about serious and unpleasant topics, not to force him to do so against his will. Regression indicates that the patient feels he is not accepted as a person in his own right and requires re-evaluation of the therapist's role.

The tendency of the patient to magnify difficulties that would excuse failure may be due to the therapist's expecting reward for his efforts by improvement on the part of the patient. It often begins when the patient is symptom free but is reluctant to leave the hospital, in a neurasthenic-like state.[10] It is imperative for the maintenance-supportive contact to continue in some form until the patient no longer needs it. The clinician's problem at this point is to diagnose and re-evaluate dynamically the patient's need for ego maintenance, intensive psychotherapy, or analysis of the psychosis-vulnerable ego.

THE EGO MAINTENANCE PROCESSES

After recompensation, there follows a period of 9 to 12 months during which the patient works to re-establish his relationships with his own objects, aided by the patterns of his experience with his therapist. He is helped to recognize his own contributions to his maladjustments by analysis of his ego functioning in relation to vital life issues. This is often referred to as the long-haul period, the 9 to 12 months after the initial 3 or 4 month's regression. Longer periods of regression require a modification of the time table. In the hospital with the personnel and the therapist as "trustful objects" the patient tries through trial and error to negotiate his interpersonal relationships more realistically and satisfactorily, primarily by thinking instead of acting, stopping, looking, listening and taking in data, especially cues from other people, as well as from within himself. Now, in essence, he tries to apply this lesson to unsolved relationships with the "particular people" in his life to achieve skill in social adaptation and success in self-expression and in great measure to "mend" violated relationships occasioned by his assault on them through regressive behavior. Aids to psychotherapy at this time come primarily from rehabilitation procedures, day or night programs, and the objects therein who serve as resources. Group psychotherapy and family therapy may be helpful. The patient tries to find conventional manners of living that are preferable to his psychotic value system.

By mutual agreement, therapist and patient often agree to terminate official visits at this point. Availability for maintenance support must remain a possibility[3,6,8] no matter at what distance in fact or time; even a reply to a Christmas card may be a maintenance contact.

REFERENCES

1. COLE, J. ET AL.: Progress in Neurology and Psychiatry, Vol. 16. New York, Grune & Stratton, 1961, pp. 539-574.
2. EWALT, J. R., AND FARNSWORTH, D. L.: Textbook of Psychiatry. New York, Blakiston Division, McGraw-Hill Book Co., 1963.
3. EWALT, J. R.: Psychotherapy of schizophrenic reactions. In: Current Psychiatric Therapies, Vol. III. New York, Grune & Stratton, 1963.
4. FREUD, A.: A. Aichhorn, an obituary. Int. J. Psychoanal. 32:51-56.
5. HAVENS, L.: Problems with the use of drugs in psychotherapy of psychiatric patients. J. Psychiat. 26 (3):289-296, 1963.
6. MANN, J., AND SEMRAD, E. V.: Conversion as process and conversion as symptom in psychosis. In: On the Mysterious Leap from the Mind to the Body. Felix Deutsch, Ed. New York, Int. Univ. Press, 1959, pp. 11-26.
7. SEMRAD, E. V., AND DAY, M.: Technique and procedure used in the treatment and activity program for psychiatric patients. In: Changing Concepts and Procedures in Psychiatric Occupational Therapy, published by the American Occupational Therapy Association. Dubuque, Iowa, William T. Brown Company, 1959.
8. SEMRAD, E. V.: Long-term therapy of schizophrenia (formulation of the clinical approach). Paper read as part of Symposium "Psychiatry in the Mid-Sixties," presented by the Division of Psychiatry and Neurology, Touro Infirmary,

Nov. 19, 1964, New Orleans, La. Philadelphia, J. B. Lippincott Company. In press.

9. SEMRAD, E. V., BINSTOCK, W. A., AND WHITE, B.: Brief Psychotherapy. Presented as the Maudsley Bequest Lecture on Short-Term Psychotherapy at the Royal Society of Medicine, London, May 13, 1965. In press.

10. SEMRAD, E. V.: Discussion of Part I, Mental Patients in Transition. Greenblatt, M., et al. Springfield, Ill., Charles C Thomas, 1961, p. 46.

11. SEMRAD, E. V.: A discussion of Dr. Arnold H. Modell's paper, "Primitive Object Relations and the Predisposition to Schizophrenia," read before the Massachusetts Mental Health Center Semicentenary, Oct. 12, 1962. In press.

12. SEMRAD., E. V., AND KLERMAN, G: Discussion of M. Ostow's paper "The Complementary Roles of Psychoanalysis and Drug Therapy." Read before the American Psychiatric Association Research Conferences on Psychiatric Drugs. Boston State Hospital, Boston, Mass., April 3, 1965.

13. SEMRAD, E. V.: Discussion of Dr. Herbert Rosenfeld's paper on Object Relations of the Schizophrenic in the Transference Situation, Psychiatric Research Report, #19, American Psychiatric Association. Titled Recent Research in Schizophrenia. Edited by Philip Solomon, M.D., and Bernard Glueck, Jr., M.D.

14. ZASLOW, S. L., AND SEMRAD, E. V.: Assisting psychotic patients to recompensate. Ment. Hosp. 15:361-366, 1964.

15. STANDISH, C. T., AND SEMRAD, E. V.: Group psychotherapy with psychotics. J. Psychiat. Soc. Work, 20; 143-150, 1951.

247

PART VII

DRUGS
AND
ADDICTIONS

Pharmacotherapy of Tension and Anxiety

by Heinz E. Lehmann, M.D. and Thomas A. Ban, M.D.

Definition of Minor Tranquilizers

The word tranquilizer first appeared in the literature around 1822, used by DeQuincey, the author of *Confessions of an Opium Eater*. Thomas Hardy also used the term in the 1890s but after that the word practically disappeared from the language.[1] In the early 1950s it made a spectacular comeback, when the first effective drugs in the treatment of psychotic symptoms were discovered, i.e., chlorpromazine and reserpine.[2-4] It also happened that both these first two antipsychotic drugs produced drowsiness. They were therefore, somewhat hastily, labeled tranquilizers in order to distinguish them from other sedative and hypnotic drugs which produced drowsiness but which were ineffective against psychotic symptoms and which did not produce extrapyramidal manifestations. Within a short time a great number of drugs effective against psychosis and capable of inducing extrapyramidal signs were developed.[5] These also were called tranquilizers, along with new drugs which otherwise might or might not have fallen into the older classification of sedatives. So, in an attempt to prevent utter confusion, a distinction was made between "major" and "minor" tranquilizers—the major tranquilizers referring to the antipsychotics or neuroleptics and the *minor tranquilizers* referring to the antianxiety drugs which do not have any antipsychotic or neuroleptic effects.[6]

More recently the term anxiolytic sedatives has been proposed by the World Health Organization Committee[7] to cover any drugs which previously had been referred to as *minor tranquilizers*. The WHO defined anxiolytic sedatives as substances which reduce pathological anxiety, tension, and agitation without therapeutic effects on cognitive or perceptual processes. The qualification

251

"anxiolytic" was added to the old term sedative in order to indicate clearly that the focus of the classification was on the anxiety-reducing properties of these drugs. Hypnotics, sedatives, and minor tranquilizers were all grouped together as anxiolytic sedatives because the Committee agreed that there was insufficient evidence of a true pharmacological difference between them. All hypnotics—primarily sleep-inducing drugs—can be used effectively as anxiety-reducing sedatives when given in small enough doses, and all the drugs which are primarily and traditionally used for the treatment of anxiety and tension states—minor tranquilizers—induce drowsiness and sleep when given in sufficiently high doses.

Pharmacological Control of Anxiety

The history of the pharmacological control of anxiety, psychomotor restlessness, and insomnia can be separated into three periods: the first from the introduction of general anesthesia, which came into general use around 1850 (and subsequently of old-time sedatives), until the development of the first clinically used barbiturate in 1903; the second from the discovery of the barbiturates to the discovery of minor tranquilizers in the 1950s; and the third from that time until today's anxiolytic sedatives.

Minor Tranquilizers

There are three major groups of minor tranquilizers: propanediols, diphenyl-methanes, and benzodiazepines.

Propanediols. In the course of studies with phenylglycerol ethers in the 1940s—to develop compounds with antibacterial effects—Berger[8] found that some of the drugs produced flaccid paralysis of the voluntary skeletal muscles. Furthermore the phenylglycerol ether mephenesin exerted a quieting effect which was described as tranquilization in the first publication reporting on its pharmacological action.[9] It was of particular interest when it was shown that mephenesin could allay anxiety without clouding consciousness.[10,11] The rapid oxidation of mephenesin, however, seemed to be a clinical handicap, and attempts were made to produce a compound with longer duration of action. Various substitutions and esterifications of mephenesin finally resulted in meprobamate, a compound with a longer duration of action and a wider margin of safety. Among the propanediol derivatives which have found clinical application are ethinamate, primarily prescribed as a sleep-inducing agent, phenaglycodol, a daytime sedative, emylcamate, a substance with muscle-relaxing and tension-relieving properties, and tybamate, which has recently been introduced as an antianxiety drug.[12]

Both meprobamate and tybamate—the two most extensively employed propanediol preparations in the treatment of anxiety—are readily absorbed from the gastrointestinal tract. Meprobamate reaches its peak plasma levels 2 hours

252

after ingestion and tybamate in less than 2 hours. This is followed by a steady decline in blood concentration. The half-life of meprobamate in the organism is 11 hours, whereas the half-life of tybamate is only 3 hours. Interestingly, physical dependence on tybamate has not been reported. Shelton and Hollister[13] attribute the absence of dependence and withdrawal reactions to the unusually short half-life of tybamate, which is only a third or a fourth of that of meprobamate.

Diphenylmethanes. Of the four minor tranquilizers in this category—benactyzine, captodiamine, hydroxyzine, and phenyltoloxamine—only one, hydroxyzine, is widely used in the treatment of anxiety. According to Lehmann,[14] an ideal anxiolytic should produce enough side effects to keep it from becoming habit forming ("to keep it a treatment rather than a treat"), but not so many as to reduce the patient's willingness to take it as prescribed. A recent study conducted by Silver et al.[15] suggests that hydroxyzine may approach these criteria.

Benzodiazepines. The benzodiazepines were derived from compounds known in the literature as 3,1,4-benzoxadiazepines. Since the discovery of chlordiazepoxide a large number of 1,4-benzodiazepines have been synthesized, studied pharmacologically, and investigated clinically. Among the benzodiazepine derivatives which have found clinical application are nitrazepam and flurazepam, primarily prescribed as sleep-inducing agents, and diazepam, oxazepam, medazepam, chlorazepate, and prazepam—all antianxiety drugs.

Other Anxiolytic Sedatives

There are several other relatively new groups of anxiolytic sedative drugs, e.g., carbinols, piperidinediones, quinazolones. Most recently doxepin, a dibenzoxepin derivative, was shown to have antianxiety effects. In a number of clinical studies doxepin was found to be at least as effective as an anxiolytic as some of the frequently employed minor tranquilizers, e.g., chlordiazepoxide, meprobamate, hydroxyzine, and phenobarbital. No case of dependency on doxepin has been reported to date.[16,17]

Are Minor Tranquilizers Effective?

In contrast to neuroleptics, the demonstration that minor tranquilizers have a therapeutic action encountered considerable difficulties. In two consecutive United States Veterans Administration (VA) studies, for example, no evidence could be found that the addition of an active drug has a superior therapeutic effect to an inactive placebo in the treatment of anxious patients.[18-20] On the other hand, the Philadelphia group, Rickels and his collaborators,[21] were able to demonstrate the superiority of minor tranquilizers—barbiturates, meprobamate, chlordiazepoxide, diazepam, oxazepam, and tybamate—over an inactive placebo.

In the case of meprobamate, for example, Rickels and Snow[22] found that it was definitely more effective in the treatment of the moderately to mildly anxious neurotic patients than placebo (or even phenobarbital). Yet in a further analysis of this study Shader[23] noted that when the psychiatric and medical patients were kept separate the use of meprobamate was not significantly better than placebo at the 5 percent level in the psychiatric patients on physicians' ratings of anxiety, depression, irritability, or headache. Only for insomnia relief was meprobamate superior ($p < 0.02$) to placebo.

Klein and Davis[24] provided definitive evidence that at least the most frequently employed minor tranquilizers do have a therapeutic effect. They presented "box scores" based on the comparative effectiveness of six minor tranquilizers with placebo in 97 double-blind controlled studies. They found that in most studies barbiturates or meprobamate were more effective than placebo (11 out of 17 and 16 out of 25 studies, respectively). Furthermore, out of 13 studies, diazepam was found to be statistically better than placebo in 11, and out of nine studies, oxazepam was found to be significantly superior than an inactive preparation in eight. In all of 22 studies reviewed chlordiazepoxide was significantly better than placebo. The same applies to the 11 studies reviewed on tybamate.

For some time it has been seriously considered that differences among the clinically used minor tranquilizers are slight or absent, at least insofar as overall therapeutic efficacy is concerned. More recently, however, there are indications that there are some differences among the overall therapeutic efficacies of at least some of the minor tranquilizers. For instance, it has been shown in double-blind controlled studies that most minor tranquilizers are more effective (seven studies) than or equal to (18 studies) barbiturates. Out of six studies, diazepam was found to be statistically significantly better than barbiturates in three; out of seven studies, chlordiazepoxide was significantly better in three, and out of 12 studies, meprobamate produced significantly more improvement in one.[24] Furthermore, Rickels[25] asserts that, in most controlled studies which report no statistically significant differences between minor tranquilizers and barbiturates, simple inspection of data gives the following rank order of drug efficacy: (1) minor tranquilizers, (2) phenobarbital sodium or amobarbital sodium, and (3) placebo.

Do Anxiolytic Sedatives Differ in Their Action?

The slight improvement in overall therapeutic efficacy with the new drugs does not justify the rather large number of clinically available minor tranquilizers. Nevertheless, if the new minor tranquilizers would qualitatively differ in their therapeutic action from the older ones, this alone would justify their existence.

It was considered that acute patients—independent of diagnosis and nature of anxiety—responded best to barbiturate treatment whereas chronic patients did not respond to it. Supporting data for this contention were obtained in a study by Rickels et al.,[26] who found that patients with acute symptoms (6 months or less) responded comparatively best to phenobarbital (and also to placebo), but that meprobamate and chlordiazepoxide seemed to be superior to phenobarbital (and also to placebo) in patients with chronic symptoms. Similar findings were reported by Jenner et al.[27,28] and Wheatley.[29]

Rickels in 1967 presented a comprehensive review of the pharmacotherapy of anxiety and tension.[25] He pointed out important relationships between psychopathological symptom profiles and responsiveness to specific pharmaco-therapeutic agents. At first, Overall et al.[30] demonstrated that depressed patients could be subdivided into three symptom profiles: anxious-depressed, hostile-depressed, and retarded-depressed; and they observed that a large number of depressed patients, namely, anxious-depressed and hostile-depressed patients, did better with the neuroleptic thioridazine than with the tricyclic antidepressant imipramine, whereas imipramine was most affective in the nonanxious, retarded-depressed patients. More recently Hollister et al.[31] reported similar differential results for perphenazine, a neuroleptic phenothiazine, and amitriptyline, a tricyclic antidepressant.

Whereas Overall et al.[30] found neuroleptics (major tranquilizers) therapeutically effective in anxious-depressed patients, Rickels et al.[32] found minor tranquilizers useful for the same group. In their study, meprobamate produced as much symptomatic improvement in depressed neurotic outpatients as did protriptyline, a tricyclic antidepressant with no antianxiety properties. In fact, during the first 2-week study period, meprobamate caused significantly more symptom reduction than protriptyline. By dividing depressed neurotic patients into high and low anxious groups, in further analysis they found that low anxious-depressed patients improved most and high-anxious depressed patients least with protriptyline, and the latter patients improved most with meprobamate or a combination of meprobamate and protriptyline.

Rickels et al.[33] found another symptom dimension of prognostic value: the dimension of emotional (psychological) versus somatic symptom focus. Applying this dimension in the analysis of data they were able to demonstrate that deprol, a combination of meprobamate and benactyzine, was more effective in somatizing, anxious-depressed patients than imipramine, whereas imipramine was more effective in less anxious, less somatizing depressed patients. In the same frame of reference fluphenazine, in anxious as well as depressed patients, produced significantly poorer results in somatizing medical clinical than in less somatizing, more emotionally focused general practice patients.[21,34] It was also demonstrated that meprobamate alone and chlordiazepoxide alone were about

255

equally effective in both somatic and emotional neurotic symptoms.[33,35,36] Tybamate was most effective in patients with a somatic symptom focus. Diazepam and phenobarbital, on the other hand, seemed to be slightly more effective in patients displaying emotional symptom focus.[25]

Using an entirely different framework, Feldman[37] was able to show differences among the three most frequently employed benzodiazepine preparations. Anxiety reduction was approximately the same with the three compounds, but when hostility was considered, chlordiazepoxide produced a 7 percent improvement, diazepam produced no improvement, and oxazepam was associated with a 50-percent improvement rate. If hypoactivity was considered, chlordiazepoxide, diazepam, and oxazepam produced improvement rates of 0 percent, 36 percent, and 12 percent, respectively, and if hyperactivity was considered, the rates were 46 percent, 0 percent, and 39 percent, respectively. These findings were supported by Shader,[23] who found that the use of chlordiazepoxide and diazepam was associated with increased hostility levels in normal male volunteer subjects whereas the use of oxazepam did not produce such hostility increments. On the basis of these data, Shader[23] suggests that for the inhibited, motor-retarded, but anxious patient, diazepam may be the ideal drug; for the overactive anxious patient, chlordiazepoxide may be preferable; and for the anxious patient with a history of hostile outbursts or temper tantrums, oxazepam may be the drug of choice.

Practical Considerations

Suicide

The rate of suicidal attempts made with any drug prescribed for neurotic or depressed patients increases with the number of years the drug has been on the market; it may be only a question of time when suicidal attempts will be made as frequently with other drugs as they are made now with barbiturates. In the meantime, the fact that barbiturates are among the most toxic of all psychotherapeutic drugs should be fully realized. Some drugs, e.g., chlordiazepoxide (CDZ) or the benzodiazepines in general, seem to be almost suicide proof to the extent that suicidal attempts with as high a dosage as 2250 mg. of CDZ remained unsuccessful. Other minor tranquilizers like the propanediols in general, or meprobamate in particular, can produce fatal poisoning, but are, nevertheless, safer than the barbiturates. Still less toxic are the neuroleptics. Therefore, in consideration of the danger of possible suicide, a physician might sometimes prescribe neuroleptics rather than minor tranquilizers, in spite of the fact that neuroleptics are less effective in reducing anxiety than minor tranquilizers.

256

Driving

In spite of considerable investigative effort devoted to the question of the interaction of minor tranquilizers with driving skill and performance, the evidence reported in different studies is still conflicting. There is general agreement, however, that the combination of even moderate doses of alcohol with minor tranquilizers produces significant impairment of the judgment and skills necessary to drive a car. Kielholz et al.[38] showed in a carefully designed and conducted study that single therapeutic doses of minor tranquilizers did not significantly impair driving performance unless the drugs were combined with alcohol. However, in the same experiment, alcohol alone impaired driving performance as much as it did in combination with drugs.

Theoretical Considerations

Pharmacotherapy of anxiety may be rendered somewhat less complex if anxiety is viewed in terms of three essential components.

The first component, arousal, is a diffuse and fundamental property of all behavior and it is mainly responsible for the intensity of anxiety. Physiologically it is a function of the reticular ascending system (RAS). The second factor, affect, refers to the specific qualities of feeling, behavior, and somatic response which characterize anxiety. It is now generally accepted that affects are elaborated in the limbic system, which is responsible for the interpretation of all personal experience in subjective terms of feeling. The third component is apperception, i.e., articulate awareness and cognitive evaluation of any affective experience, a function of the neocortex.

All three components—RAS, limbic lobe, and neocortex—are involved in the subjective experience of anxiety, forming a mutual feedback network. Barbiturates inhibit this entire feedback network in a nonselective, global manner.[39] The newer minor tranquilizers have less inhibitory effect on the RAS and on the neocortex. They exert most of their inhibitory action on the limbic system.[40,41] The neuroleptics sometimes, but not always, inhibit the RAS and have even less inhibitory effect on the neocortex than the newer minor tranquilizers. Neuroleptics also effect the limbic system in a way which differs from the minor tranquilizers; the neuroleptics tend to increase the activity of some limbic structures, e.g., the hippocampus. Increased limbic system activity, induced by neuroleptics, is associated with a slowing of the cortical EEG; on the other hand, decreased limbic system activity, induced by minor tranquilizers, is associated with a faster EEG, which is also characterized by a lower energy content.[42,43]

On the biochemical level there is increasing evidence that plasma and urinary catecholamine levels are elevated in anxious patients[44,45] with a subsequent rise in nonesterified fatty acid concentration in the blood and with an increase in the

257

urinary output of hippuric acid.[46] Because of this it is important that most minor tranquilizers decrease catecholamines or antagonize their effects.

An entirely new concept in the treatment of anxiety was presented by the introduction of propranolol,[47] a beta-receptor blocking agent[48] which was shown to be useful in the treatment of neurotic patients with manifest anxiety and cardiac symptoms, e.g., tachycardia.[49,50] Whether the anxiolytic effects[51,52] of propranolol are due to its peripheral action, i.e., interference with physical abnormalities which result in anxiety,[53] or to direct central effects, as has been suggested by Leszkovsky and Tardos,[54] still remains to be seen.

Heuristically most important, however, is that anxiety can be artificially induced by a variety of drugs with well-defined chemical structures and pharmacological actions. Under the influence of these substances the common and the differential characteristics of anxiety can be studied and the treatment of anxiety can be systematically investigated. A number of drugs have been reported to induce anxiety and/or tension, among them autonomic-sympathomimetics (ephedrine, epinephrine, or amphetamines) and various psychotomimetic substances, among which yohimbine, lysergic acid diethylamide, psilocybin, and mescaline are the most important. Parallel with the increase in anxiety and/or tension, under the influence of these drugs, there is also an increase in nonesterfied free fatty acid concentrations in the blood.[55] There are indications that the high free fatty acid levels can be prevented or counteracted by both somnolent insulin or high doses (3000 mg. per day) of nicotinic acid. Nicotinic acid can also prevent stress-induced mobilization of free fatty acids.

Artificially induced anxiety is perhaps one of the best available methods for the intensive study of specific anxiety and also for the systematic exploration of its specific prevention and/or treatment. But artificially, drug-induced anxieties also present themselves today as clinical conditions with increasing frequency. To understand this developing area of psychiatry and to define its scope and treatments are beyond the topic of minor tranquilizers and are among the great new challenges psychiatry and clinical psychopharmacology will have to meet.

REFERENCES

1. Oxford Dictionary. London, Oxford University Press, 1961.
2. Delay, J., and Deniker, P.: 38 cas de psychoses traités par la cure prolongée et continué de 4568 RP. Ann Medicopsychol. (Paris) 110:364, 1952.
3. Lehmann, H. E., and Hanrahan, G. E.: Chlorpromazine: New Inhibiting Agent for Psychomotor Excitement and Manic States. Arch. Neurol. Psychiat. 71:227, 1954.
4. Kline, N. S.: Use of Rauwolfia Serpentina Benth in Neuropsychiatric Conditions. Ann. N.Y. Acad. Sci. 59:107, 1954.
5. Ban, T. A.: Psychopharmacology. Baltimore, The Williams and Wilkins Company, 1969.
6. Lehmann, H. E., and Ban, T. A.: Pharmacotherapy of Tension and Anxiety. Springfield, Ill., Charles C Thomas, Publisher, 1970.

7. WHO: Report of a Scientific Group on Research in Psychopharmacology. Technical Report Series No. 371, Geneva, 1967.
8. Berger, F. M.: Anxiety and the discovery of the Tranquilizers. In: Ayd, F. J., and Blackwell, B. (Eds.), Discoveries in Biological Psychiatry. Philadelphia, J. B. Lippincott Co., 1970.
9. Berger, F. M., and Bradley, W.: The Pharmacological Properties of a β-Dihydroxy-(2-methylphenoxy)-propane (Myanesin). Brit. J. Pharmacol. 1:265, 1946.
10. Gammon, G. D., and Churchill, J. A.: Effects of Myanesin upon the Central Nervous System. Amer. J. Med. Sci. 217:143, 1949.
11. Schlan, L. S., and Unna, K. R.: Some Effects of Myanesin in Psychiatric Patients. J.A.M.A. 140:672, 1949.
12. Splitter, S. R.: A New Psychotropic Drug: Evaluation of Tybamate in the Treatment of Anxiety and Tension States. Psychosomatics 5:292, 1964.
13. Shelton, J., and Hollister, L. E.: Simulated Abuse of Tybamate in Man. J.A.M.A. 199:338, 1967.
14. Lehmann, J. E.: Tranquilizers, Clinical Insufficiencies and Needs. In: Cerletti, A., and Bové, F. J. (Eds.), The Present Status of Psychotropic Drugs. Amsterdam, Excerpta Medica Foundation, 1968.
15. Silver, D., Beaubien, J., Ban, T. A., Saxena, B. M., and Bennett, Jean: Hydroxyzine, Amitriptyline and Their Combination in the Treatment of Psychoneurotic Patients. Curr. Ther. Res. 11:663, 1969.
16. Beaubien, J., Ban, T. A., Lehmann, H. E., and Jarrold, Louise: Doxepin in the Treatment of Psychoneurotic Patients. Curr. Ther. Res. 12(4):192, 1970.
17. Sterlin, C., Ban, T. A., Lehmann, H. E., and Jarrold, Louise: A Comparative Evaluation of Doxepin and Chlordiazepoxide in the Treatment of Psychoneurotic Outpatients. Curr. Ther. Res. 12(4):195, 1970.
18. Lorr, M., McNair, D. M., Weinstein, G. J., Michaux, W. W., and Raskin, A.: Meprobamate and Chlorpromazine in Psychotherapy. Some Effects on Anxiety and Hostility of Outpatients. Arch. Gen. Psychiat. (Chicago) 4:381, 1961.
19. Lorr, M., McNair, D. M., and Weinstein, J.: Early Effects of Chlordiazepoxide (Librium) Used with Psychotherapy. J. Psychiat. Res. 1:257, 1963.
20. Caffey, E. M., Hollister, L., Klett, C. J., and Kaim, S. C.: Veterans Administration (VA) Cooperative Studies in Psychiatry. In: Clark, W. G., and del Giudice, J. (Eds.), Principles of Psychopharmacology. New York, Academic Press, Inc., 1970.
21. Rickels, K., Raab, E., Gordon, P. E., Laquer, K. G., DeSilverio, R. V., and Hesbacher, P.: Differential Effects of Chlordiazepoxide and Fluphenazine in Two Anxious Patient Populations. Psychopharmacologia (Berlin) 12:181, 1968.
22. Rickels, K., and Snow, L.: Meprobamate and Phenobarbital Sodium in Anxious Neurotic Psychiatric and Medical Clinical Outpatients. A Controlled Study. Psychopharmacologia (Berlin) 5:339, 1964.
23. Shader, R. I.: Antianxiety Agents: A Clinical Perspective: In: Dimascio, A., and Shader, R. I. (Eds.), Clinical Handbook of Psychopharmacology. New York, Science House, 1970.
24. Klein, D. F., and Davis, J. M.: Diagnosis and Drug Treatment of Psychiatric Disorders. Baltimore, The Williams and Wilkins Co., 1969.
25. Rickels, K.: Antineurotic Agents: Specific and Non-specific Effects. In: Efron, D. H. (Ed.), Psychopharmacology: A Review of Progress. Washington, Public Health Service Publication No. 1836, 1968.
26. Rickels, K., Clark, T. W., Ewing, J. H., Klingensmith, W. C., Morris, H. M., and Smock, C. D.: Evaluation of Tranquilizing Drugs in Medical Outpatients. Meprobamate, Prochlorperazine, Amobarbital Sodium and Placebo. J.A.M.A. 171:1649, 1959.

259

27. Jenner, F. A., Kerry, R. J., and Parkin, D.: A Controlled Trial of Methaminodiazepoxide (Chlordiazepoxide, "Librium") in the Treatment of Anxiety in Neurotic Patients. J. Ment. Sci. 107:575, 1961.

28. Jenner, F. A., Kerry, R. J., and Parkin, D.: A Controlled Comparison of Methaminodiazepoxide (Chlordiazepoxide, "Librium") and Amylobarbitone in the Treatment of Anxiety in Neurotic Patients. J. Ment. Sci. 107:583, 1961.

29. Wheatley, D.: Chlordiazepoxide in the Treatment of the Domiciliary Case of Anxiety Neurosis. In: Proceedings of the Fourth World Congress of Psychiatry. Amsterdam, Excerpta Medica Foundation, 1968.

30. Overall, J. E., Hollister, L. E., Meyer, F., Kimbell, I., and Shelton, J.: Imipramine and Thioridazine in Depressed and Schizophrenic Patients. J.A.M.A. 189:605, 1964.

31. Hollister, L. E., Overall, J. E., Shelton, J., Pennington, V., Kimbell, I., and Johnson, M.: Drug Therapy of Depression. Arch. Gen. Psychiat. (Chicago) 17:486, 1967.

32. Rickels, K., Raab, E., DeSilverio, R. V., and Etemad, B.: Drug Treatment in Depression: Antidepressant or Tranquilizer? J.A.M.A. 201:675, 1967.

33. Rickels, K., Ward, C. H., and Schut, L.: Different Populations, Different Drug Responses. Amer. J. Med. Sci. 247:328, 1964.

34. Rickels, K., Snow, L., Uhlenhuth, E. H., Lipman, R. S., Park, L. C., and Fisher, S.: Side Reactions of Meprobamate and Placebo. Dis. Nerv. Syst. 28:39, 1967.

35. Rickels, K., Baumm, C., Raab, E., Taylor, W., and Moore, E.: A Psychopharmacological Evaluation of Chlordiazepoxide, LA-1 and Placebo, Carried out with Anxious Neurotic Medical Clinic Patients. Med. Times 93:238, 1965.

36. Rickels, K., Downing, R. W., and Downing, M. H.: Personality Differences Between Somatically and Psychologically Oriented Neurotic Patients. J. Nerv. Ment. Dis. 142:10, 1966.

37. Feldman, P. E.: Current Views on Antianxiety Agents. Pamphlet from Scientific Exhibit presented at the Annual Meeting of the American Medical Association, Houston, Texas, 1967.

38. Kielholz, P., Goldberg, L., Obersteg, J., Poeldinger, W., Ramsay, A., and Schmid, P.: Circulation routière, tranquillisants et alcohol. Hyg. Ment. 2:39, 1967.

39. Aston, R., and Domino, E. F.: Differential Effects of Phenobarbital, Pentobarbital and Diphenylhydantoin on Motor Cortical and Reticular Thresholds in the Rhesus Monkey. Psychopharmacologia (Berlin) 2:304, 1961.

40. Kletzkin, M., and Berger, F. M.: Effect of Certain Tranquilizers in the Reticular Endothetical System. Proc. Soc. Exp. Biol. Med. 102:88, 1959.

41. Schallek, W., Zabransky, F., and Kuehn, A.: Effects of Benzodiazepines on the Central Nervous System of the Cat. Arch. Int. Pharmacodyn. 149:467, 1964.

42. Itil, T. M.: Electroencephalography and Pharmacopsychiatry. In: Freyhan, F. A., Petrilowitsch, N., and Pichot, P. (Eds.), Clinical Psychopharmacology. Basel, Karger, 1968.

43. Pfeiffer, C. C., Goldstein, L., Murphee, H. B., and Jenney, E. M.: Electroencephalographic Assay of Anti-anxiety Drugs. Arch. Gen. Psychiat. 10:446, 1964.

44. Woolfson, G.: Recent Advances in the Anxiety States. In: Coppen, A., and Walk, A. (Eds.), Recent Developments in Affective Disorders. Ashford, Headley Brothers Ltd., 1968.

45. Levi, L.: Neuro-endocrinology of Anxiety. In: Lader, M. H. (Ed.), Studies of Anxiety. Ashford, Headley Brothers Ltd., 1969.

46. Sourkes, T. L.: Biochemical Changes in the Expression of Emotion. Canad. Psychiat. Ass. J. 7:529, 1962.

47. Turner, P. G., Grossman, K. L., and Smart, J. V.: Effect of Adrenergic Receptor

Blockade on the Tachycardia of Thyrotoxicosis and Anxiety States. Lancet 2:1316, 1965.

48. Ahlquist, R. P.: Study of Adrenotropic Receptors. Amer. J. Physiol. 153:586, 1948.

49. Besterman, E. M. M., and Friedlander, D. H.: Clinical Experiences with Propranolol. Postgrad. Med. 41:426, 1965.

50. Nordenfeldt, O.: Orthostatic ECG Changes and the Adrenergic Beta Receptor Blocking Agent Propranolol (Inderal). Acta Med. Scand. 178:393, 1965.

51. Grossman, G. K. L., and Turner, F.: The Effect of Propranolol in Anxiety. Lancet 1:788, 1966.

52. Wheatley, D.: Comparative Effects of Propranolol and Chlordiazepoxide in Anxiety. Brit. J. Psychiat. 115:1411, 1969.

53. Frohlich, E. D., Dustan, H. P., and Page, I. H.: Hyperdynamic Adrenergic Circulatory State. Arch. Int. Med. 117:614, 1966.

54. Leszkovsky, G., and Tardos, L.: Some Effects of Propranolol on the Central Nervous System. J. Pharm. Pharmacol. 17:518, 1965.

55. Hollister, L. E.: Drug-Induced Psychoses and Schizophrenic Reactions: A Critical Comparison. Ann. N.Y. Acad. Sci. 96:80, 1962.

Therapy of Non-Narcotic Psychoactive Drug Dependence

by William E. Bakewell, Jr., M.D., C.M.
and John A. Ewing, M.D., D.P.M.

Although toxic reactions may occur in response to administration of many psychoactive drugs (amphetamines, bromides, LSD, cannabis, phenothiazines, etc.) there is a specific clinical syndrome associated with dependence upon drugs associated with depressed nervous system activity. The Diagnostic and Statistical Manual of the American Psychiatric Association (DSM II) classifies this syndrome as *304.2 Drug dependence, barbiturate* and *304.3 Drug dependence, other hypnotics and sedatives or "tranquilizers"*.

The eventual recognition of the dangers of barbiturate dependence motivated search for central nervous system depressant drugs free of this liability. Since the early 1950's a number of "non-barbiturate" CNS depressant drugs have been introduced. Clinical experience with these newer agents has shown that abuse of some of them can result in intoxication, tolerance and dependence, and an abstinence syndrome almost identical to that caused by barbiturates. Thus barbiturates can be considered the prototype, and much of the information on them can be applied to the other central nervous system depressant drugs such as: chloral hydrate (Noctec, Somnos, etc.), chlordiazepoxide (Librium), diazepam (Valium), ethchlorvynol (Placidyl), ethinamate (Valmid), glutethimide (Doriden), meprobamate (Equanil, Miltown), methaqualone (Revonal), methyprylon (Noludar), oxazepam (Serax), and paraldehyde (Paral).

Intoxication, Tolerance, Dependence, and Abstinence

Barbiturate intoxication is marked by confusion, intellectual impairment, personality change, emotional lability, motor incoordination, staggering gait, slurred speech and nystagmus. Tolerance refers to the need for increased amounts of the drug to produce effects formerly produced by smaller doses. This physiological adaptation is not of much moment with ordinary clinical use of the drug, but becomes crucial when a person taking the drug in an

262

uncontrolled fashion has an urge to seek more and more drug effect. As the dose is progressively increased physical dependence may develop, after which abruptly stopping the drug results in the intense disturbances of abstinence. The barbiturate abstinence syndrome can be a serious, even life-threatening state, which may include delirium and grand mal convulsions. The physical and psychic responses of the abstinence syndrome seem to represent an over-swing or rebound CNS hyperexcitability following removal of the drug's depressant action. The effects of abstinence can be relieved by giving the drug itself or by another drug of similar pharmacologic activity. Considerable cross-tolerance or cross-dependence seems to exist among these CNS depressant drugs. However drug dependent states are not to be seen solely as "chemical diseases"; they all involve a complex interaction of social and psychological, as well as physiological and pharmacological, factors. The potential for drug dependence of the barbiturate type is greatest in patients with a history of dependence upon other substances, including alcohol. Special caution must therefore be used in prescribing CNS depressant drugs for the management of alcoholic patients. Experience suggests that serious drug dependence probably occurs in the maladjusted who seek relief from feelings which are to them unbearable. The drug offers an escape route which they find preferable to more personal and direct forms of coping. Typical sources of mental anguish are intrapsychic conflicts over aggressive, sexual and dependent wishes; feelings of inadequacy and being overwhelmed; or the symptoms of specific psychiatric syndromes. Dependence upon barbiturates, although a fairly specific entity, is to be found superimposed upon all types of psychiatric disorganization.

A common sequence is for the patient to begin using barbiturates for relief of anxiety or insomnia, and to increase dosage gradually, usually without the knowledge of his physician. Tolerance is only partial in that a slight increase in dosage can produce definite signs of intoxication. Sometimes patients try to balance the sedative drug against stimulants, such as amphetamines. Once the average adult is taking more than seven or eight 100 mg. barbiturate capsules daily, he cannot suddenly discontinue the drug without discomfort and the possible dangerous complications of abstinence. Isbell[6] found that subjects taking 800 mg. or more daily of a short-acting barbiturate developed weakness, tremors and anxiety upon withdrawal. Seventy-five per cent of these patients had convulsions and 60 per cent showed a picture similar to delirium tremens. Subjects taking 600 mg. daily developed anxiety, tremors and weakness; those taking less than 400 mg. daily had only minor symptoms of abstinence. Thus physical dependence occurs in cases of abuse and not within normal dose ranges of the drugs.

Complete information about the occurrence, distribution and patterns of abuse of the non-narcotic CNS depressant drugs is not available, but some indication of the size of the problem is gained from surveys of the incidence of drug dependence among patients admitted to hospital. Hamburger[5] reported that about 23 per cent of patients admitted to the Public Health Service Hospital in Lexington, Ky., were dependent upon barbiturates as well as narcotics. Bakewell and Wikler[1] reported a 6.8 per cent incidence of physical dependence on non-narcotic CNS depressant drugs among patients admitted to a university hospital psychiatric ward. Ewing and Bakewell[4] found a 7.6 per cent incidence of drug dependence in 1,686 patients admitted to another university hospital psychiatry service. Clinical experience teaches that drug dependent patients are by no means found exclusively on psychiatric wards. Experience also indicates a trend towards the simultaneous abuse of several depressant drugs, often in combination with alcohol. Chelton and Whisnant[3] found from thin layer chromatography tests of blood and urine of 100 consecutive alcoholic patients admitted to an Atlanta hospital that 38 had taken a depressant drug in addition to the alcohol. Some patients take relatively minor overdoses of several different depressant drugs. The actions seem to be additive and the effect is similar to gross over-dosage of only one drug, but the history may be more confusing and the diagnosis more difficult.

DIAGNOSIS OF DRUG DEPENDENCE

The first essential to establishing the diagnosis of drug abuse is, of course, a detailed history which includes questions concerning the use of sleeping pills, sedatives, tranquilizers and "nerve pills". Drug dependent patients typically are reluctant to reveal the full details of their drug abuse, and a "negative history" given by the patient does not necessarily exclude the possibility of the drug dependent state. People who have ready access to such medications should be considered especially liable to develop this syndrome. This includes a variety of workers in the health professions and even their relatives. Certainly we have been impressed by the number of physician's wives whose undiagnosed illness eventually led to their psychiatric referral and the discovery of drug dependence.

Past or current alcoholism, previous abuse of drugs, more than average familiarity with the names and doses of sedative drugs and the possession of prescriptions from several physicians should increase the examiner's suspicion. Relatives may be able to supply corroborative information, and it is often useful to have them bring in for identification all of the medicines used by the patient. Usually the patient should be hospitalized for withdrawal from the medication, and an attempt must be made to explain to him the importance of candor and cooperation. Nonetheless a careful search of his personal belongings for a cache of drugs is indicated at the time of admission. Laboratory studies can assist in the appraisal of such patients. The presence of barbiturates in the blood can confirm the suspicion of drug dependence, but the absence of detectable barbiturates in body fluids does not exclude the diagnosis. Abnormal EEG tracings tend to occur with intoxication. Mixed rhythmic fast and slow waves, mainly in frontal and parietal tracings are seen. Wulff[10] described the common EEG as being "spiky" with an abnormal amount of fast activity. However 39 per cent of his patients addicted to short acting barbiturates had a normal EEG at rest. In the general hospital some cases of drug dependence are revealed by the onset of the abstinence syndrome which can first be suspected from the occurrence of insomnia, anorexia, weakness, restlessness, sweating and shakiness. The patient may complain of feeling anxious, suffer nausea and vomiting, and display irritability. Examination usually reveals postural hypotension along with muscular twitching. This is followed by psychotic signs with hallucinations, usually visual and tactile. The peak incidence of convulsions occurs between 24 and 48 hours after the last dose, but some seizures may occur as late as the fourth or fifth day. Especially on a busy general hospital ward where the patient may not be carefully re-examined after the initial workup, it is not unusual for an epileptiform seizure to be the first sign noticed by the staff. A neurological survey is often sought for such cases and consideration of the drug dependency syndrome is delayed. Psychotic symptoms typically appear later than convulsions, from the third to the seventh day. The abstinence syndrome, if untreated, may last up to a week and involves much delirium. The hyperactivity, insomnia, confusion, tremors, hallucinations and delusions are very much like the delirium tremens of the alcohol abstinence syndrome. Hyperpyrexia is a grave sign. Clinical improvement is rarely seen until a prolonged sleep has occurred.

TEST DOSE METHOD

Whenever CNS depressant drug abuse seems a possibility, a "test dose" of pentobarbital (Nembutal) is indicated. This test, designed to demonstrate drug tolerance (and hence drug abuse), is conducted when the patient is sober, has an empty stomach and is in bed. For the average adult 200 mg. of pentobarbital by mouth is used as the test dose; half this amount may be used in testing an elderly or debilitated patient and occasionally a 300 mg. dose is selected to test a patient in whom extremely high levels of drug intake are suspected from the history. The patient is examined for drug effects one hour after swallowing the test dose. The majority of non-drug-tolerant patients will be heavily sedated by 200 mg. of pentobarbital and usually show nystagmus, slurred speech and incoordination.

In a recent experiment 10 normal volunteers were given 200 mg. of pentobarbital or placebo in a double-blind fashion.[8] One hour after receiving pentobarbital 7 of the 10 subjects were found to be asleep and the 8th was heavily sedated. The two remaining subjects were relatively alert, but showed impaired coordination. In this study nystagmus, interference with memory, calculation and speech were less reliable signs of drug effect than was impaired coordination. Especially affected were: (1) the time required to tandem walk a standard line, (2) finger-hand coordination as demonstrated by the number of palmardorsal hand slaps made on the thighs, and (3) the number of sequential touches of the thumb to the four fingers performed during a measured time.

The patient who is put to sleep or grossly intoxicated by 200 mg. of pentobarbital given under the standard test conditions is assumed to have no tolerance and the likelihood of drug dependence is discounted. If he is less obviously sedated and intoxicated by the initial dose of pentobarbital, the possibility of drug dependence requiring specific treatment exists. In such a case we extend the testing period by ordering 200 mg. of pentobarbital every six hours for up to three more doses, and re-evaluate him one hour after each dose. A patient who is not put to sleep or grossly intoxicated by a total of 800 mg. of pentobarbital in this 24 hour test period has significant tolerance and will require specific treatment for his drug dependent state.

The patient whose response to the initial 200 mg. dose is to "improve" by being alert, comfortable and steady can at once be assumed to have developed a marked tolerance, probably in the range of 800 to 1000 mg. of barbiturate per day. Patients who continue to manifest signs of impending abstinence one hour after the initial 200 mg. test dose should immediately be given another 200 or 300 mg. of pentobarbital. Such a patient has extreme tolerance and probably is accustomed to taking 1200 to 1600 mg. or more of barbiturate or its equivalent per day (Table 1).

MANAGEMENT OF DRUG DEPENDENCY

Once the fact of drug dependence has been established, the patient is given enough barbiturate to keep him in a state of mild intoxication. It is essential that he receive the barbiturates on a regular around-the-clock schedule and that he be observed frequently so that appropriate adjustments in the dose can be made. For example, if excessive intoxication is seen after a dose, the next dose of pentobarbital should be reduced by 100 mg. Likewise, if objective signs of impending abstinence become apparent

266

TABLE 1

Application of Test Dose of Pentobarbital

Patient's Condition	Degree of Tolerance Demonstrated	Estimate of Habitual drug use /24 hour	Required Action
Asleep or grossly intoxicated	0	0	0
Drowsy, somewhat impaired coordination	Possible tolerance	Possibly 600-800 mg.	Continue testing with 200 mg. q6h, possibly stabilize and withdraw by 10% rule
Comfortable, steady state, fine nystagmus only	Definite tolerance	800-1000 mg.	Stabilize on q6h doses before 10% rule withdrawal
No sign of drug effects, possibly persisting signs of abstinence	Extreme tolerance	1200 mg. or more	Stabilize on q4h dose pentobarb, cautious withdrawal

between doses, the next dose will have to be increased by 100 mg. or more. Patients requiring a total daily dose of less that 1200 mg. usually do well on a schedule of medication every six hours; those requiring 1200 mg. or more daily are often managed better on a schedule of medication every four hours.

When the amount of barbiturate required to keep the patient mildly intoxicated has been established and stabilized he should be free from emotional distress and showing no signs of impending abstinence throughout the day and night. He should be sleeping and eating well. Then, and only then, one may proceed with the gradual withdrawal of the drug. The "10 per cent rule" for withdrawal is easily remembered. The rule dictates a daily reduction of the pentobarbital by no more than 10 per cent of the total 24-hour stabilization dose. Even this rate of withdrawal can be excessively rapid for a patient who has been taking 20 or more capsules daily. Such a patient initially should be withdrawn at the rate of only one capsule per day. Once started, the reduction program should proceed as evenly and regularly as possible with the bedtime dose of pentobarbital being the last to be stopped. If the clinical picture on this reduction schedule seems to vary inexplicably and without relation to the medication prescribed, it is reasonable to suspect that the patient has access to drugs other than those ordered. Additional searching of him and his possessions and restriction of visitors is then essential.

If the patient is not seen until he is already in delirium, rapid intoxication using pentobarbital is called for. This will not always immediately clear the delirium, which is much more easily prevented than cured. However it is essential to stabilize the patient with the depressant agent in the hope that this will promote the sleep without which clinical improvement rarely occurs. The use of phenothiazines is contraindicated and merely giving sodium diphenylhydantoin (Dilantin) is inadequate to prevent seizures. In our opinion there is no medication which can safely be substituted for pentobarbital in the management of barbiturate withdrawal. Dependence on other CNS depressant drugs listed earlier can conveniently and safely be managed with pentobarbital. However the physician must be alert to possible differences in the clinical picture of abstinence with some of the newer "minor tranquilizers." For example, the onset of abstinence from chlodiazepoxide may be delayed for three or four days and seizures may not occur until the eighth day after abruptly stopping large doses of that drug.[2] The familiar pentobarbital regimen is especially useful when the patient has abused combinations of CNS depressant agents showing cross tolerance with the barbiturates. This same method should be applied to the patient who has combined amphetamines and a CNS depressant drug. The amphetamines are at once stopped completely and stabilization with barbiturates, followed by gradual withdrawal according to the 10 per cent rule is applied as usual. The patient who has combined barbiturates and narcotics requires initial stabilization with both the pentobarbital and the narcotic. His barbiturate dose is maintained at the level sufficient to produce mild intoxication while the narcotics are withdrawn. After the withdrawal of the narcotics is complete, the dose reduction schedule for withdrawal of the barbiturates is begun following the 10 per cent rule.[9]

GENERAL MANAGEMENT

The management of the drug dependent patient requires close nursing supervision. The nurse should be made aware of the possibility of convulsive seizures, especially while the intoxication and stabilization process is still incomplete. General supportive measures including restoration of electrolyte balance and proper hydration, vitamins and a well balanced diet are indicated for all patients.

Ideally hospitalization should continue for a time after completion of the drug withdrawal program. Candid discussion of his drug dependency with the patient is essential. The danger of becoming dependent on other CNS depressant drugs should be emphasized. He must never rely again upon drugs to induce sleep or to allay anxiety. Following the withdrawal program, the patient may have some insomnia and attacks of irritability for several weeks or longer. We believe that these phenomena are often based on physiological factors. Oswald and Priest[7] have demonstrated that prolonged use of hypnotics produces measurable EEG and REM effects which persist for as long as five weeks after the last dose. For the patient who is insistent upon some pharmacological support during this transition period, small doses of a phenothiazine may help control his anxiety and promote sleep without the liability of beginning the drug abuse cycle over again. However our aim is to have the patient taking no drugs by the time he leaves the hospital.

Psychotherapeutic management of the patient, designed to help him find better ways of adapting to stress, coping with guilt feelings and communicating affects is begun in the hospital. Since learning to use human sources of help rather than seeking pharmacological refuge may be difficult for this patient, a long-term relationship with his physician, a psychiatrist or a mental health center is desirable. If the patient had an alcohol problem before turning to drugs, he should be encouraged to use Alcoholics Anonymous as an additional source of help. The family's enlightened cooperation is essential and it may be useful to engage the patient and the spouse in conjoint psychotherapy.

REFERENCES

1. BAKEWELL, W. E., JR., AND WIKLER, A.: Non-Narcotic Addiction: Incidence in a University Hospital Psychiatric Ward, J.A.M.A. 196:710, 1966.
2. CAFFEY, E. M., JR., HOLLISTER, L. E., KAIM, S. C., AND POKORNY, A. D.: Anti-Psychotic, Anti-Anxiety and Anti-Depressant Drugs. Vets. Admin. Med. Bull., Washington, D.C. MB-11:14, 1966.
3. CHELTON, L. G., AND WHISNANT, C. L.: The Combination of Alcohol and Drug Intoxication. Southern Med. J. 59:393, 1966.
4. EWING, J. A., AND BAKEWELL, W. E., JR.: Diagnosis and Management of Depressant Drug Dependence. Amer. J. Psychiat. 123:909, 1967.
5. HAMBURGER, E.: Barbiturate Use in Narcotic Addicts, J.A.M.A. 189:366, 1964.
6. ISBELL, H.: Abuse of Barbiturates. J.A.M.A. 162:660, 1956.
7. OSWALD, I., AND PRIEST, R. G.: Five Weeks to Escape the Sleeping-Pill Habit, Brit. Med. J. 2:1093, 1965.
8. WANGLER, J. G., EWING, J. A., AND BAKEWELL, W. E., JR.: Depressant Drug Dependency-Evaluation of Reliability of Pentobarbital Test Dose. In press.
9. WIKLER, A.: Addictions I: Opioid Addiction. In: Freedman, A. M., and Kaplan, H. I. (Eds.): Comprehensive Textbook of Psychiatry. Baltimore, Williams, and Wilkins, 1967.
10. WULFF, M. H.: The Barbiturate Withdrawal Syndrome. A Clinical and EEG Study, Electroenceph. Clin. Neurophysiol. Suppl. 14:1, 1959.

The Treatment of Acute Alcohol Intoxication and Withdrawal

by PAUL DEVENYI, M.D.

C HRONIC ALCOHOLISM is a complex, multifaceted disorder with medical, psychological and socioeconomical connotations. In spite of the often emphasized "disease concept of alcoholism," the medical profession does not regard the total problem as its exclusive responsibility. There can be little doubt, however, that the treatment of the acute alcoholic conditions is a medical obligation.[1] Acute alcoholic conditions — intoxication and the subsequent withdrawal syndrome — are fairly well defined clinical entities for which effective management is available.

ACUTE ALCOHOL INTOXICATION

The smell of alcohol on the patient's breath does not necessarily mean that all his symptoms are due to alcohol intoxication. The stuporous or comatose patient may have had only one drink, and his impaired consciousness may be due to trauma, cerebrovascular accident, or a metabolic disorder. The apparently intoxicated individual should not be brushed aside as "just drunk"; he is entitled to the same thorough differential diagnostic assessment as any other patient.

A helpful diagnostic tool is the determination of the blood alcohol level. Peculiarly, it is seldom used, possibly because of its legal implications. In our clinic we use it and keep it as confidential as any other information we learn about the patient.

A blood level higher than 0.15 per cent indicates that the patient is indeed intoxicated by alcohol. A level of 0.3 to 0.5 per cent suggests severe intoxication with endangering depressant effects on the central nervous system. If a comatose patient has a blood alcohol concentration of 0.5 per cent or more, one has a very good evidence that the coma is caused by alcohol, although other possible causes of impaired consciousness and associated injuries, should still not be overlooked. A blood alcohol level of 0.6 to 0.7 per cent is often fatal because of respiratory arrest; fortunately this seldom occurs because, usually, the patient falls asleep before he can drink enough to reach these fatal concentrations. The blood alcohol concentration is decreased by oxidation at about 0.015 to 0.02 per cent per hour. Thus, for example, a person with a blood alcohol level of 0.3 per cent will be "alcohol free" in approximately 15 to 20 hr., and one can count on the appearance of withdrawal symptoms when his blood alcohol falls below 0.15 per cent, which occurs in about 7 to 10 hr.

The average case of alcohol intoxication can be treated at home with adequate provisions for the patient's safety. The main effort should be directed toward interruption of his drinking and allowing him an opportunity to "sleep it off" under some care and supervision. One should consider hospital admission under the following circumstances:

1. It is unlikely that the patient will stop drinking and there is no satisfactory extrainstitutional facility available for him.

2. Severe withdrawal symptoms are anticipated once his drinking stops.

3. Associated or complicating illnesses or injuries are present.

4. There is extremely severe intoxication with stupor or coma and impending respiratory depression.

There are more "don'ts" than "do's" in the treatment of alcohol intoxication. The occurrence of respiratory infections, hepatic failure, peripheral neuropathy, encephalopathy, various vitamin deficiencies, head injuries, and similar complications, not infrequently seen in the acutely ill alcoholic, call for appropriate measures. In or out of hospital, the physician's main concern should be to get the intoxicated patient to bed and let him sleep. Do not attempt psychotherapy at this stage and do not argue with him. No matter how stimulated or aggressive the patient appears to be, remember that he is under the influence of a central depressant substance, and if you provide a bed he will fall asleep. Sedative drugs at this stage may potentiate the depressant effect of alcohol and induce respiratory dif-

271

ficulties; fatalities have been reported.[2] Sedatives should be avoided when the blood alcohol exceeds 0.15 per cent.

Stimulant drugs such as caffeine or the amphetamines also have no place in the treatment of alcohol intoxication. They may wake the patient up sufficiently to get him out of the hospital emergency department, but they do not aid the "sobering up" process or increase alcohol metabolism. A stimulated drunk is a more dangerous one because he may go out, continue his drinking, and operate an automobile; instead, his accumulated alcohol should be metabolized while he sleeps. The only instance where stimulants do have a place is to stimulate respiration in alcoholic coma; CO_2 inhalation or Metrazol may be needed. Unfortunately, we know of nothing that will speed up alcohol metabolism with any reliability. Several years ago, L-triiodothyronin was claimed to be effective,[3] but this has not been confirmed.[4] NAD, the naturally occurring coenzyme of alcohol metabolism, is not available in therapeutically sufficient quantities to be of practical value. The intravenous administration of glucose and insulin produces pyruvate, which can act as an accessory hydrogen acceptor, but we do not regard this of practical importance. There appears to be nothing that facilities the spontaneous reduction in blood alcohol levels beyond 0.015 to 0.02 per cent per hour.

ACUTE ALCOHOL WITHDRAWAL SYNDROME

This incapacitating, acute illness can occur in various degrees of severity and is to be distinguished from a simple hangover by (1) tremulousness (the "shakes"), (2) visual and auditory hallucinations without gross disorientation, and (3) grand mal convulsions or delirium tremens with frightening visual and tactile hallucinations, disorientation, and motor agitation. These may be regarded as a "rebound effects" in that the brain, suddenly released from the depressant effect of alcohol, swings into hyperexcitability. During intoxication there is (positional alcohol nystagmus, PAN) in which the fast component is toward the direction of the laterally positioned head (PAN I); this changes direction after alcohol has disappeared from the blood (PAN II), and will disappear or even revert to PAN I if alcohol is administered.[5]

The use of hemodialysis may speed up alcohol disappearance and prevent or alleviate withdrawal symptoms, thus suggesting that other substances responsible for the withdrawal phenomena were also dialysized.[6]

The key to effective management of the withdrawal syndrome is adequate sedation when the blood alcohol level falls below 0.15 per cent and long after it has become zero. Tremors will usually appear at the falling side of the blood alcohol curve and convulsions or delirium may also occur at the time or several days after all alcohol has disappeared from the blood. We

272

favor the benzodiazepines, particularly 50 to 100 mg of chlordiazepoxide, which is given intramuscularly (and in severe cases intravenously) for the first 12 to 24 hr. and repeated every 1 to 2 hr. as necessary. One should try to achieve a steady level of sedation rather than wait with the next dose until the patient is again ready to climb a wall.

As soon as possible, usually on the second day, we begin oral administration and reduce the dose to 50 mg, 3 or 4 times a day, and later to 25 mg, 3 to 4 times a day. Drowsiness and ataxia may be a problem in some cases, but these conditions respond to reduction of the dosage. Chlordiazepoxide has the advantage of possessing muscle relaxant as well as anticonvulsant activity, and does not produce sudden hypotension, whereas phenothiazines have been reported to increase convulsive tendencies.[7] With chlordiazepoxide we give diphenylhydantoin in a dosage of 100 mg, 3 times a day, but only to patients with a history of previous withdrawal convulsions.

Other drugs reported to be effective in alleviating withdrawal symptoms include haloperidol and chlormethiazole. Paraldehyde and barbiturates are still recommended, but we avoid them because of the frequency of associated barbiturate abuse by alcoholics. A theoretically reasonable approach would be to treat withdrawal symptoms by dosages of the causative agent, gradually tapering off in a manner similar to the treatment of opiate or barbiturate withdrawal. Alcoholics themselves do this, erratically, by treating their own withdrawal with more alcohol. Intravenous alcohol infusion has been used therapeutically for the same reason, but most centers have abandoned it. Alcohol withdrawal can be instituted "cold turkey" because substitute drugs are effective. Some authors strongly recommend magnesium salts in the treatment of delirium tremens because of magnesium deficiency in that condition.[8]

The administration of vitamin supplements is a time-honored therapy, adopted on the assumption that alcoholics eat poorly or not at all while drinking and suffer from multiple nutritional deficiencies. Components of the vitamin B complex are important coenzymes in several metabolic processes and are valuable in treatment to prevent peripheral neuropathy and Wernicke encephalopathy. However, barring a specific deficiency syndrome, the long-term administration of vitamins beyond the postacute stage is unnecessary; good food is the best nutritional therapy. We do not use ACTH or other intravenous infusions except on the rare occasion when a serious fluid and electrolyte imbalance exists.

The withdrawal syndrome, like acute intoxication, is essentially a self-limited illness; controlled observations are still necessary to determine whether drug therapy is indeed always needed.

273

The Next Step. Barring complicating illnesses, this simple treatment procedure restores most patients to fine physical health in a couple of weeks. Then what? If no preventive action is taken, they will commence their next drinking bout shortly. Unfortunately, there is no single, specific treatment for alcoholic addiction, but the alcoholic patient's desire to stop drinking is at its peak in the acute and immediate postacute period. This is the time when he will be most responsive to further suggestions, such as to take protective drugs (disulfiram or calcium carbimide), to continue psychotherapy individually or at an alcoholism clinic, and to seek vocational help.

REFERENCES

1. DEVENYI, P.: Medical Treatment and Study of Alcoholism, Addictions. 15, 4:1-19, 1968.
2. KOPPANYI, T.: Problems in Acute Alcohol Poisoning. Quart. J. Stud. Alc. Suppl. No. 1, 1961.
3. GOLDBERG, M.: Intravenous Triiodothyronine in Acute Alcoholic Intoxication. New Engl. J. Medicine, 263:1336-1339, 1960.
4. KALANT, H.: Some Recent Physiological and Biochemical Investigations on Alcohol and Alcoholism. Quart. J. Stud. Alcohol 23:52-93, 1962.
5. GOLDBERG, L.: Alcohol, Tranquillizers and Hangover. Quart. J. Stud. Alcohol Suppl. No. 1, 1961.
6. *Anon.* Dialysis: A Sobering Thought for Alcoholics. Med. World News, 10:89, 1969.
7. SERENY, G., AND KALANT, H.: Comparative Clinical Evaluation of Chlordiazepoxide and Promazine in Treatment of Alcohol Withdrawal Syndrome. British Med. J. 1:92-97, 1965.
8. NIELSEN, J.: Magnesium Metabolism in Acute Alcoholics. Danish Med. Bull. 10:225-233, 1963.

Family Therapy of Alcoholism

by JOHN A. EWING, M.D. AND RONALD E. FOX, PH.D.

V ARIOUS TYPES and manifestations of alcoholism are seen by the clinician. Family therapy is one approach which offers promise to the
alcoholic man or woman who still lives within a family setting or who shows
desire for rehabilitation back into the family. However, familial approaches
are not a panacea for all alcoholic problems. Nor can it be concluded that
the "cause" of drinking is the family. The etiology of alcoholism remains
unknown. To intervene by psychologic means such as family therapy is not
to deny the possibility of genetic, biochemic, neurologic, cultural, and
sociologic factors. At present, psychotherapeutic intervention is the main
course available to us, apart from general medical care. The use of
psychopharmacologic agents when appropriate is recommended. When the
patient has motivation for maintaining sobriety, the use of disulfiram
(Antabuse) is often of crucial assistance. However, in alcoholism there are
often major problems involving lack of insight into the existence of a drinking problem as well as absence of any genuine motivation for change. Family therapy has been particularly useful in these two areas. Successful intervention involving the whole family has often, in our experience, been a
major factor in promoting acceptance of the existence of a drinking problem
and has likewise led, more often than occurs spontaneously, to a motivation
toward change within the alcoholic himself.

Our experience has involved working with all social classes but particularly middle class patients who are suffering from gamma-type alcoholism in
the Jellinek classification.[1] The majority of our patients have been men,
although on occasion we have been able to involve some family members in
a therapeutic program designed to help a woman with alcoholism. These
patients have all had a history of 5 to 10 years of loss of drinking control.
Some have admitted this while others are still clinging to such typical
defensive statements as, "I can stop anytime I want." The excessive, uncontrolled, drinking with its characteristic damaging effects upon the patient's health, work, and family occurs typically in bouts interspersed with
periods of more or less sobriety. The patient has often been able to remain
employed even though the employer may be losing his patience. A signifi-

275

cant number have been self-employed and able to maintain their personal or family business to a surprising degree, in spite of increasing difficulties with alcohol.

In our experience the majority of these patients demonstrate major conflicts over unacceptable dependency wishes. When sober, socially acceptable defense formations predominate. Thus, the alcoholic patient may see himself and present himself as a pleasant, helpful person who cannot do enough for others and wishes to be the mainstay of his family and business. The contrast when he is drinking is very marked. At this time one cannot help being impressed with the infantile components of the personality, and it is clear that this is not lost upon the members of the family, especially the spouse. The typical spouse of the alcoholic male (when this relationship has continued over some time rather than having led to divorce) is quite adept at dealing with her husband in this regressive state, and remarkably accepting of it. Some authors claim that this "mothering" role is forced upon the alcoholic's spouse and is one which she is happy to give up whenever possible. Undoubtedly the role is required of her, but our finding from family studies is that the wife tends to have similar personality dynamics to those of her husband. Thus, she seems to cope with her own unacceptable dependency wishes by the defensive maneuver of adopting the role of the mainstay of the family, the strong partner of the marriage, and so on.

Indeed, it appears that in alcoholic marriages a homeostatic mechanism is established which resists change over long periods of time. The behavior of each spouse is rigidly controlled by the other. As a result, an effort by one person to alter his typical role behavior threatens the family equilibrium and provokes renewed efforts by the spouse to maintain the status quo.

The behavior of each partner serves both to express his own neurotic needs and to reinforce those of the spouse. Through drinking, the alcoholic is able, periodically, to give direct expression to his contained impulses. By alternating between suppression of impulses and direct expression of them, he can maintain the conflicts surrounding impulse gratification for a lifetime.

In one patient, for example, the defense of independence and maturity is dropped only when intoxication proceeds far enough to reveal the infantile strivings. Another, may be more comfortable with expressing dependent feelings while sober, and may use intoxication as the occasion to manifest a pseudomasculinity. Perhaps most often intoxication permits the release of a series of such impulses which are the focus of inner conflict. Each time the alcoholic man drinks he loses an opportunity for emotional growth. He escapes into intoxication instead of finding an alternative adaptation which might also promote change in the marriage. This cyclical pattern may serve as an expression of the alcoholic's conflicts and also fulfill one half of the

276

marital interpersonal bargain. By being passive, dependent, and sexually undemanding the alcoholic implicitly encourages his wife to be protective, nurturant, and sexually unresponsive.

When he drinks, the alcoholic's wife feels that she has no recourse other than to respond in a maternal manner, whether this is nurturant or supportive or, at times, punitive and rejecting. This completes the other half of the interpersonal bargain. It is a form of the *quid pro quo* rule which seems to govern most, if not all, enduring interpersonal relationships.[2] The behavior of each partner serves the dual purpose of satisfying his own needs and those of the mate. Thus, any possibility of change is met with dual resistances; those operating internally and those initiated by the spouse in response to the threatened loss of a critical role relationship.

Another aspect of the interpersonal bargain is that it can be kept only if it is implicit. Once the nature of the agreement is thoroughly identified it becomes difficult to maintain. There is little satisfaction in dominating someone who lets you dominate him, for then the question of who is really in control is automatically raised. The overt decision to "let" the other person behave in a particular way carries the clear implication that one can decide to do otherwise. Each person seems to feel secure only if he can force or manipulate the other into satisfying his own needs. Once this lever of manipulation is lost, other means of control must be sought. In short, the equilibrium is disturbed and another basis of homeostasis must be found.

CONCURRENT GROUP THERAPY

For over a decade, the senior author has used concurrent group therapy in the treatment of familial alcoholic problems.[3] Groups are held for one and a half hours weekly with the husbands and wives meeting at the same time but in different rooms and with different therapists. The length of treatment for couples in such groups has ranged from 3 to 30 months. A group of six or seven persons seems to work best with this form of treatment.

The treatment approach might best be described as dynamically oriented group psychotherapy in which special attention is given to the needs of the particular group under consideration. For example, the alcoholic patient typically demonstrates lower anxiety tolerance than psychoneurotic patients and it is, therefore, essential that he find support in his group early in the treatment.

Each group seems to go through predictable stages during the course of therapy. Typically, the wives show both individual and group resistance against seeing themselves as people requiring help. This resistance is manifested mainly by blaming the husbands, by acting as co-therapists, by resistance to the examination of their own motives, and by maintaining that they are in therapy only for the husbands' sake. Later, an awareness of the

277

importance of the marital interaction in the drinking pattern begins to emerge. During this stage it is possible to lead the group into an increased sensitivity to their own self-concepts. Also, an understanding of the dependency needs of both spouses is approached for the first time. It is during this phase of treatment that misgivings about the husbands' sobriety are first expressed or become obvious.

Mrs. Black was a wife who one day talked at length about a new car which she could not handle. The old automobile had been difficult to shift, but at least she knew where the fault lay. She could blame the old jalopy for any troubles that arose. That day it became clear to the group that the "new" husband was the problem for Mrs. Black.

Other wives reluctantly expressed similar ideas. "I'm getting the silent treatment; it's worse than when he's drinking," said Mrs. White. A week later, at the country club, she "accidentally" poured a shot of whiskey into her husband's iced tea while he was away from the table.

The men's group, on the other hand, is typically marked by ambivalence toward the wife's attendance. Later there is a tendency to blame the wife and to complain of her manipulation and self-righteous, martyred attitudes. It is not until the latter stages of treatment that it is possible to focus on the defenses against pregenital libidinal fixations and gain greater group awareness of previously hidden Oedipal involvements.

Some interesting reciprocal trends have been noted between the concurrent groups. Initially, there tends to be a divergence in the cohesiveness of the two groups; when one is focused on a group approach to a problem or problem area the other is often more fragmented with individual complaints about idiosyncratic problems. A related phenomenon is often noted within particular marital pairs; the husband complains about his wife at a time when she is complaining about him to her group. Frequently the behavior of an individual in the group is the exact opposite of what the spouse reports he was like during the preceding week. Thus, a husband who expressed much feeling during the week was often silent during his group meeting; or, conversely, a wife who was described as aggressive or domineering during the week would often take a more passive attitude at the following group session. As long as this "seesaw" pattern was prominent, few gains were made. However, once either member was able both to recognize and make explicit his own demands on the spouse and to discuss this with the group, considerable insight usually developed. In its more rudimentary form, the problem becomes one of learning to maintain a mature sex role identification in relation to the spouse. Typical themes during this stage of treatment would be the men describing their difficulties in feeling adequately male in relation to their wives, while the wives were discussing problems in being able to tolerate a more overtly demanding, adequate husband.

278

When it is possible to involve both spouses in concurrent group treatment, the alcoholic tends to remain in treatment longer. In addition, the likelihood of improvement in drinking and marital harmony is greatly enhanced under these conditions.

Joint Family Therapy

The interlocking and reciprocal role relationships which were mainfested during the concurrent groups have led us to the direct use of family treatment approaches. In such a setting the pattern of manipulation, resentment, and countermanipulation emerges very quickly. However, the same resistances which were noted in the groups are found in family treatment in only slightly different forms. A common defensive maneuver in this approach is the blindness to any truly reciprocal causal interaction. An example of this was provided by a husband and wife who realized only after several sessions that she always became depressed when he was sober and that he drank only when she was not depressed. Even so, both partners stoutly maintained that the wife's depression and the husband's drinking were separate problems and that it was superfluous to focus attention on the marital interaction.

Unilateral Therapy

While both concurrent groups and family therapy offer considerable promise in identifying and alleviating crippling homeostatic patterns of behavior, it is not always possible to obtain the cooperation of both spouses. In such cases it may be possible to achieve alteration in the marital equilibrium through working with one spouse.

Frequently, alcoholics are inaccessible, leaving the therapist with the alternative of working with the wife or doing nothing. It is sometimes possible to persuade the wife of an alcoholic to enter a therapeutic relationship herself. An effect of this in many instances is to initiate changes in the marriage so that stereotyped interactions are disrupted and change becomes possible.

Some wives have been seen for brief counseling where the aim was to provide the support necessary for her to make unilateral changes in her usual behavior (e.g., to stop hiding the bottle). Other wives have been seen in individual treatment or in an ongoing concurrent wives group. In these instances, the aim was to increase the wife's insight into her own dependency and into her strong needs to infantilize and protect her husband. It is important that the focus is not turned on the wife too early in the therapeutic process in order to avoid arousing her defensive denial of responsibility for the husband's behavior.

In the majority of cases in which a reasonable trial was given to the

279

recommended treatment, substantial changes in the marital interaction and the alcoholic man became apparent.[4]

Experience with marriages in which there is a significant drinking problem suggests that alcoholism can no longer be seen purely in terms of intrapsychic dynamics. The alcoholic's insight is frequently insufficient unless he is able to withstand his wife's resistance to his change and to help her find other outlets for her protective, dominating needs. Similarly, the wives of alcoholics we have treated have shown marked resemblance to each other. Appreciation of their own dependency needs and acceptance of some responsibility for the husband's drinking must accompany real changes in their marital roles. These encourage and permit reciprocal changes in the husbands and promote alleviation of the drinking problem. Individual insight must be used to highlight repetitive and self-defeating interactions with the spouse. In short, it is the family emotional homeostasis which seems to perpetuate the drinking and it is this behavior which must be changed if the drinking is to be controlled.

In our experience, changes are more likely to be maximized if both spouses are engaged in the treatment process but this is not essential. In fact, dramatic changes have been noted in alcoholics who remained inaccessible and where the entire treatment centered around the wife. Therapists should not be reluctant to gain access to the family system through whatever avenue is available.

An outgrowth of family therapy has been the oft-cited need to prevent the family from labeling any single member as the "sick" one.[5] Too rigid or naive adherence to this general principle might encourage refusal to treat an alcoholic *in absentia* especially via a spouse who insists that he is the whole problem. However, if her need to see herself as the strong member of the marriage and her drunken husband as the weak member is treated as a defense like any other, it is possible to upset the familial homeostasis and to promote a tendency to some change within the husband.

REFERENCES

1. JELLINEK, E. M.: The Disease Concept of Alcoholism. New Haven, Conn., Hillhouse Press, 1960.
2. JACKSON, DON, D.: Family rules: marital quid pro quo. Arch. Gen. Psychiat. 12:589–594, 1965.
3. EWING, J. A., LONG, V., AND WENZEL, G. G.: Concurrent group psychotherapy of alcoholic patients and their wives. Int. J. Group Psychother. 11:329–338, 1961.
4. EWING, J. A.: Unilateral Therapy of Alcoholism. N. C. J. Ment. Health 2:3–16, 1966.
5. PITTMAN, F. S., DeYOUNG, C., FLOMENHAFT, K., KAPLAN, D. M., AND LANGSLEY, D. G.: Crisis Family Therapy. In: Masserman, J. (Ed.): Current Psychiatric Therapies, Vol. 6. New York, Grune & Stratton, 1966.

Treatment of Heroin Dependence with Opiate Antagonists*

by MAX FINK, M.D., ARTHUR ZAKS, M.D., RICHARD RESNICK, M.D., AND ALFRED M. FREEDMAN, M.D.

TREATMENT OF OPIATE addiction is discouraged by the high rate of recidivism. The variety of treatment programs bespeaks the failure rate that is common to all. Some programs reduce recidivism by the careful selection of suitable patients — accepting only those with the best motivation for recovery — or by imprisonment and primitive systems of parole. The most popular new program is methadone substitution, which satisfies opiate craving by cross tolerance. Dole and Nyswander[3] and Freedman and associates,[10] have reported its effects on addiction.

Another clinical use of drugs in therapy is derived from a theory of opiate dependence. Addicts withdrawn from heroin report a craving for narcotics as soon as they return to the community in which their "habit" flourished. Their experiences lead to a theory of relapse based on a conditioning model, with emphasis on the role of subtle environmental cues and physiological components according to Wikler.[21] In these circumstances, drug dependence proceeds in several phases. In the first phase, the subject is aware of tensions or discomforts and seeks and obtains relief in narcotic use. Reinforcement of the habit occurs with each relief by drug use in a period termed *episodic intoxication*. If the drug has an addicting potential, it reduces tension or discomfort less and less efficiently, and a second state — that of physical dependence — develops. Dependence is further reinforced when the addict fails to maintain an adequate drug intake and periods of tension and discomfort increase in frequency and duration. Sooner or later the addict is withdrawn, for the supply of opiates runs out. He is admitted to a hospital or is arrested, and thus enters a phase termed *physiological disequilibrium* followed by *conditioned abstinence*. These states may probably persist for many months more than the period of simple withdrawal.

*Aided in part by grants from the USPHS MH-12567, 13003, and 13358; and from the New York State Narcotic Addiction Control Commission. Supplies of cyclazocine were made available by Sterling-Winthrop Research Laboratories, Renssalaer, New York; and naloxone was supplied by Endo Laboratories, Garden City, New York.

281

Wikler's theory[21] led to a suggestion that blockade of the relief afforded by narcotics during the period of conditioned abstinence might lead to extinction of physical dependence and conditioned drug-seeking behavior. The opiate antagonist, nalorphine, was suggested as a suitable drug for blockade, but its short duration of action and the high incidence of hallucinogenic effects limited its clinical usefulness. The development of the long-acting, related drug cyclazocine led to clinical trials reported by Martin and associates,[15] and Jaffe and Brill.[13] Cyclazocine use is associated with the agonistic effects of opiates, sometimes considered unpleasant, and clinical programs have been few. The development of a pure opiate antagonist, naloxone, has stimulated renewed interest in clinical trials, reported by us.[5,6] The reports emphasize both a test of this theory and the practical effort to provide "engagement" of the addict in a rehabilitation program.

In our studies of antagonists, randomly assigned subjects have also received other agents such as methadone[10,16,22,18] and tybamate.[20] The subjects of these studies were male opiate addicts who volunteered for admission to an inpatient treatment center in a municipal hospital in the East Harlem section of New York City. The population of this community has very low income, is predominantly Negro and Puerto Rican with low educational levels, and large numbers receive extensive welfare assistance. Their ages ranged from 17 to 54 with a mean of 26 years, and the duration of addiction is from 2 to 30 years.

Male patients applying for treatment are asked to sign a permit for an "experimental" treatment of their addiction. On admission to our study ward, the narcotic usage of each patient is estimated by inquiry. Based on their report a starting methadone dose, usually 30 to 50 mg, is defined. Methadone is given twice daily in reducing amounts for detoxification, usually within four to seven days, until the subject is drug-free. A period of observation without drugs allows medical and laboratory examinations before induction with an antagonist.

CYCLAZOCINE

Cyclazocine is an n-substituted benzomorphan derivative chemically similar to nalorphine hydrochloride. It is an active analgesic with some subjects reporting dysphoria, vivid imagery, and anxiety with its use. Cyclazocine is supplied in a liquid vehicle (0.1 mg/cc), in capsules of 0.25 mg, in tablets of 0.1 and 1.0 mg, and for intravenous use (0.5 mg/ml). The first clinical trials of cyclazocine in opiate addiction, made by Martin and associates[15] and by Jaffe and Brill,[13] defined 4.0 mg per day as an effective dose for clinical antagonism to opiates.

Induction

We first attempted to develop an induction schedule that would minimize dysphoria. In our initial study,[7] 60 patients completed detoxification and began the cyclazocine induction.[10] Of the 60 patients, 58 completed the study period, with only 2 patients beginning the active cyclazocine treatment and signing out against medical advice.

Induction was defined as achieving a daily therapeutic dose of 4.0 mg. In our first subjects, the dosage of cyclazocine was increased gradually over 40 days. To reduce this time span, groups of 4 patients each were tested in induction periods of 10, 15, 20, and 30 days. A daily increment of 0.4 mg (10-day schedule) brought forth complaints of somnolence, headache, irritability, "fuzzy thinking," illusions, and (in two instances) visual hallucinatory experiences. These symptoms were not reported on the 15-day schedule, in which dosages were divided in two increments daily, except that somnolence, weakness, and irritability appeared during the first 4 days. The 20- and 30-day induction periods were well tolerated without secondary symptoms.

Based on this experience we now use a 15-day schedule routinely. After a drug-free period of 7 to 10 days to permit laboratory tests, cyclazocine is started at 0.2 mg per day and increased 0.2 mg per day for 10 days, using the liquid vehicle form. If this is well tolerated, the dose is increased by 0.4 mg per day for 5 days. Medication is given twice daily and a maintenance dose of 4.0 mg per day is usually reached in 15 days. The medication is gradually changed to a single 4.0-mg dose on the twentieth day by giving progressively larger amounts each morning.

Recent reports that naloxone might antagonize the agonistic effects of cyclazocine prompted us to reassess a more rapid induction schedule. In an experiment now completed, patients were inducted to 4.0 mg with daily increments of 1.0 mg cyclazocine within 4 days. Initially, each patient was given 0.5 to 1.0 gm naloxone orally with each daily dose of cyclazocine. Lately, naloxone has been necessary in only a few patients, and it is now given in 0.3 to 0.6 gm at the patient's request. Twenty-four patients inducted on this rapid schedule requested naloxone only occasionally, usually during the third to sixth days.[17]

Secondary Effects

The secondary effects of chronic cyclazocine use are similar in patients with long and short induction periods. Increased libido, constipation, elation, anxiety, dizziness, headaches, restlessness, and insomnia occur occasionally during the initial four to six days of treatment, but abate during

283

the second week. In our early studies, two patients reported visual hallucinations, but these have not recurred as our experience increased.[10,11]

The secondary effects do not persist in the aftercare program when patients have received cyclazocine for more than 24 months. Some patients reported episodic drowsiness and constipation, but the effects noted during the early weeks of treatment have not been reported, even on specific inquiry.

Maintenance

Following discharge, patients are asked to return three times weekly. At each visit they are given their daily dose of cyclazocine and a supply for the intervening day or days.

The patients receiving cyclazocine report a variety of changes in behavior. Sexual activity has increased and is more satisfactory. Social activities such as dating, going to parties and dances, and spending leisure time with nonaddicts have increased. Anxiety is less and drug-seeking behavior has been curtailed. While cyclazocine serves to inhibit interest in narcotics, the use of marijuana, amphetamines, barbiturates, and alcohol has not been affected. Criminality is less and the patients' interest in vocational activities has been enhanced.

Patients report an ability to interrupt cyclazocine intake without symptoms of withdrawal. The day after taking cyclazocine they are able to experience the euphoric and sedative effects of heroin. By reinstituting cyclazocine at the full dosage, they do not become readdicted, and can continue their daily activities.

In a 1968 follow-up of patients discharged on cyclazocine a year earlier, 74 patients were traced. Of these, 15 had continued in rehabilitation from 5 to 16 months and were found to be in school or working; 11 had discontinued cyclazocine and had entered a methadone maintenance program; and 48 had resumed use of heroin.

In a more recent review of patients in our aftercare facility, 9 have continued on cyclazocine for more than 2 years; 4 for 12 to 24 months; 4 for 6 to 12 months; and 6 less than 6 months.

Heroin Challenge

To determine the duration of cyclazocine antagonism, we have used intravenous heroin "challenges" as our index.[22] During the induction phase the value of cyclazocine as an effective narcotic blocking agent is discussed in both individual and group therapy sessions with all the resident addicts. They are told that the injection of a narcotic in their usual amounts would

284

have neither euphoric nor systemic effects. To reinforce this suggestion, they are offered an opportunity for an intravenous injection of heroin in the laboratory at the same time that they receive a full daily dose of cyclazocine.[11,12] We have determined that 25 mg of heroin in 2 cc of saline solution every 2 min. elicits both the behavioral effects and EEG changes in postaddicts 7 to 10 days after a final dose of methadone. (In our earlier studies 15 to 20 mg of heroin was used.)

In patients receiving 4.0 mg of cyclazocine in single daily doses, we have observed complete blockade to 25 mg heroin in 6 hr. Of 18 patients challenged 24 hr. after receiving 4.0 mg of cyclazocine, 12 experienced no clinical effects and 6 became euphoric. These described an initial "rush" or "buzz" in their abdomen. This pleasant sensation was intense, moved to the throat, and then spread "all over," persisting for approximately 30 min. The pupils were constricted. Following this challenge, the dose of one patient was raised to 5.5 mg; there was no response to a second heroin challenge 24 hr. after a dose of cyclazocine. In 5 patients, cyclazocine was increased to 5.0 mg and in subsequent challenges they still responded with a slight and short-lasting euphoria.

Tolerance to the antinarcotic activity of cyclazocine was not observed. Patients receiving a heroin challenge up to 5 months after their first daily 4.0-mg dose of cyclazocine showed as much blockade to heroin as when the challenge was given immediately at the end of the induction period. Judging from these experiences, it is probable that the effective duration of antinarcotic activity of a single 4.0-mg dose on chronic administration is at least 20 hr. waning rapidly after 24 hr., with a peak 6 to 8 hr. after a dose of cyclazocine.[5,6]

NALOXONE

Naloxone (n-allylnoroxymorphone) is an experimental compound five to eight times as effective as nalorphine in antagonizing opiate effects in animals.[1,9,14,19] Tolerance does not develop nor does withdrawal occur on sudden cessation after two weeks of repeated administration, but its duration of action is short, less than 4 to 6 hr.

Single Administrations

We have reported two series of acute, single intravenous administration studies[8] in which 19 patient volunteers received heroin (10 to 20 mg/2 cc every 2 min.) followed after 8 to 32 min. by naloxone (0.7 to 10.0 mg/5 cc every min.). Ten subjects received two trials for a total of 29 trials. In ten patients naloxone injections were given first, followed by heroin. These studies were done in the laboratory under EEG control.

After receiving heroin, each patient reported that he was "high" (euphoric) or "floating," and exhibited nodding, pupillary constriction, and voice changes. Naloxone, even at the lowest dosage, abolished these effects within ½ to 2 min. following the injection. Subsequent to these initial studies, we routinely administered 1.0 mg of naloxone 10 to 30 min. after heroin to all "clean" subjects receiving heroin challenges. Blockade was uniformly complete. In two instances we gave 1.0 mg of naloxone to subjects receiving heroin during a period of chronic methadone use, and in both cases precipitated an intense opiate withdrawal syndrome.

When naloxone was given first, there were no effects in five patients and a feeling of coldness for 1 to 3 min. in four subjects. In subsequent trials with other subjects who had received their latest dose of methadone less than ten days before, the sensations were accompanied by irritability, gooseflesh, sweating, and other signs of precipitated-abstinence syndrome. One patient reported an "amphetamine-like" sense of stimulation. When heroin was given, eight patients felt no euphoria and two reported a mild "high," as if given an injection of weak heroin.

Chronic Oral Administration

In our first clinical study,[8] seven patients received repeated oral administrations in doses up to 100 mg twice daily. The first doses were 20 mg with increments of 30 mg daily. Heroin challenges were repeated at frequent intervals, and the dosages were increased until complete blockade was achieved. At dosages of 120 mg a full clinical reaction to heroin occurred in one patient, was partial in five, and absent in one. Complete blockade was evident in five subjects at 200 mg and in one at 160 mg. From these observations we concluded that oral naloxone was effective in blocking 20 mg heroin up to 10 hr. after a divided daily dose.

Our second series of clinical studies are in progress.[23] In these we have set single daily doses of naloxone as a practical and necessary goal for successful treatment of opiate dependence. Subjects are given increasing, single, daily doses of naloxone, and the efficacy and duration of antagonism has been assessed with challenges of 20 and 50 mg of heroin.

One subject was tested 6 hr. following daily, single, 200-mg doses of naloxone. He exhibited no effect from 25 mg heroin, but became euphoric with 50 mg. Naloxone was increased to 400 mg and this afforded blockade against 25 mg and 50 mg of heroin, but not against 75 mg.

The second subject received a daily dose of 400 mg of naloxone and was effectively blocked against the 25, 50, and 75-mg heroin injections at 6 hr.

These two subjects were rechallenged 18 hr. following drug intake. They did not evidence narcotic antagonism until naloxone was raised to 800 mg

286

daily. With this dose they were protected against both 25 and 50 mg of heroin. They were not given 75-mg challenges.

A third subject was challenged at 18 hr. postmedication. He did not demonstrate significant narcotic blockade on doses of 600, 800, or 1000 mg of naloxone. On a daily dose of 1250 mg, the 25- and 50-mg heroin challenges were blocked, but the subject became euphoric following the administration of 75 mg of heroin. At 24 hr. following a 1250-mg dose of naloxone the subject was protected against a 25-mg challenge, but reacted with an intense euphoria to 50 mg of heroin.

The fourth and fifth subjects were brought to a daily, single, oral dose of 1500 mg. They were first challenged at 18 hr., and both were protected against 25- and 50-mg doses of heroin, but experienced a euphoric reaction following the 75-mg challenge.

At 24 hr. the fourth subject demonstrated partial blockade against a 25-mg heroin injection, but became euphoric following 50 mg. The fifth subject demonstrated no narcotic blockade at 24 hr. and became "high" when given 25 mg of heroin.

Two subjects received 2400 mg and one received 3000 mg of naloxone in single, daily, oral doses. In heroin challenges after 24 hr., blockade to 25 mg and 50 mg of heroin was exhibited by the subject receiving 3000 mg of naloxone.

Secondary Effects

We have observed few secondary effects of chronic naloxone. One patient received 2.4 gm per day and reported feelings of depression and tension, and requested that the medication be stopped. The subject given 3.0 gm per day, who had received a heroin challenge without a euphoric response, suffered a grand mal seizure 7 hr. after a morning dose and 4 days after a heroin challenge. He had no prior history of seizures and no sequellae.

In no patient receiving any daily dose of naloxone did we observe withdrawal symptoms within the period of observation (up to three days).

Laboratory Investigations

Laboratory tests, which were performed weekly, were within normal limits except in two instances. One subject had an unexplained elevated white blood count between 12,000 and 18,000 wbc for seven weeks while he was on naloxone. Repeated medical examinations found no explanation. It returned spontaneously to normal.

All subjects had occasional abnormal liver-function tests, primarily SGOT and SGPT. The abnormal findings in these two tests were sporadic and bore no relation to the length of time on naloxone or to size of dosage.[2,12]

Hematological studies consisted of bleeding time, euglobulin lysis time, whole-blood coagulation time, clot retraction, quick prothrombin time, partial thromboplastin time, thrombin time, prothrombin assay, and factor V, VII, X, and XIII determinations. They were performed prior to naloxone treatment, one week following drug treatment when the subjects were on a daily dose of 200 to 500 mg of naloxone, and three to eight weeks later on a daily dose of 600 to 1500 mg. All test values were within normal limits.[23]

DISCUSSION

It has been suggested that narcotic addiction is analogous to a conditioned response; the addict responds with drug-seeking behavior[21] to stressful stimuli in his environment. According to this theory, the repeated use of heroin without the anticipated subjective effects should lead to extinction of the learned drug-seeking behavior.

This theory was first tested by the use of high dosages of methadone as maintenance treatment for addicts.[3] Because methadone is an addicting substance with euphoriant properties, these trials may not be considered an adequate test of the hypothesis. Cyclazocine, which has a length of antagonistic action greater than 24 hr., has been successfully used in the maintenance treatment of opiate dependence.[10,11,13,16] These trials are a more adequate test of the hypothesis. We have observed drug-seeking behavior to continue in these subjects. Use of opiates is markedly reduced, however, and the patients are able to maintain their social and work commitments without readdiction. In our experience we have found cyclazocine to be less effective in reducing the conditioned drug-seeking response than in providing engagement to a therapy program and preventing the development of tolerance and withdrawal.* Engagement makes possible continued job counseling, re-education, and social services, and prevention of tolerance and withdrawal allows the subject to negotiate our social system without recourse to crime.

Our studies of cyclazocine and naloxone indicate that they are safe, well tolerated, and accepted by patients and staff. Engagement with the rehabilitation program takes place rapidly and the continued contact assists community adjustment of these patients. A therapeutic optimism is engendered in both patients and staff, and this optimism is useful in the rehabilitation process, supporting the direct effects of the drugs.

In our view an ideal antagonist should have a long duration of action and a minimum of secondary effects. A short length of action requires frequent

---

*Another aspect of cyclazocine use may be its antidepressant properties.[7] Opiate-dependent subjects frequently exhibit withdrawal, retardation, and loss of drive, symptoms often associated with depressive mood.

intake of medication, a responsibility impossible for the poorly motivated postaddict to accept. It is also necessary that secondary effects be minimal, particularly on withdrawal, because patients have shown intolerance to any discomforts, even for short periods.

Cyclazocine is satisfactory as an antagonist owing to its duration of action, but its secondary effects preclude wide acceptance. Naloxone, in the oral dosages tested, is effective for more than 24 hr. and has no secondary effects, making it the ideal antagonist for therapeutic trial. The large dosages required in these trials (3.0 gm) must be confirmed, and efforts to provide alternate routes must be tested. We have assessed the possibility of investing naloxone in a silastic type of vehicle and implanting such a tube under the skin to provide continuous, sustained naloxone protection for extended periods. In theory this could be done for months because the parenteral dosage necessary for effective blockade of heroin is probably less than 1.0 mg for 4 to 6 hr.

Another theory of opiate dependence is rooted in the potential antianxiety effects of opiates. Opiates are used to reduce anxiety and tension occasioned by environmental stimuli, and from this viewpoint, an antianxiety agent should successfully reduce opiate dependence. Following the favorable reports of Feldman and Mulinos,[4] we assessed the clinical efficacy of tybamate.[20] Although daily doses of 6 to 11.2 gm per day reduced anxiety symptoms, opiate hunger remained and subjects rapidly became readdicted on their return to their community.

Summary

Based on a conditioning theory of opiate dependence, various substances have been proposed to block the euphoric effects of opiates and reduce dependence by a process of negative reinforcement. This chapter has reviewed our clinical experiences with cyclazocine and naloxone, indicating that both drugs are effective therapeutic agents.

REFERENCES

1. BLUMBERG, H., DAYTON, H. B., AND WOLF, P. S.: Counteraction of Narcotic Antagonist Analgesics by the Narcotic antagonist Naloxone. Proc. Soc. Exp. Biol. Med. 123:755-758, 1966.
2. CHERUBIN, C. E.: The Medical Sequalae of Narcotic Addiction. Ann. Int. Med. 67:23-33, 1967.
3. DOLE, V. P., AND NYSWANDER, M.: A Medical Treatment for Diacetylmorphine (Heroin) Addiction. J.A.M.A. 193:646-650, 1965.
4. FELDMAN, H., AND MULINOS, M. G.: Lack of Addiction from High Doses of Tybamate. J. New Drugs 6:354-360, 1966.

289

5. FINK, M., AND FREEDMAN, A. M.: Antagonists in the Treatment of Opiate Dependence. In: Phillipson, R. V. (ed.), Modern Trends in Combatting Drug Dependence and Alcoholism. London, Butterworth. Pp. 49-59, 1970.

6. FINK, M., FREEDMAN, A. M., ZAKS, A., SHAROFF, R. L., AND RESNICK, R.: Narcotic Antagonists and Substitutes in Opiate Dependence. In: Cerletti, A., and Bove, F. J. (eds.), The Present Status of Psychotropic Drugs, Amsterdam, Excerpta Medica, 1969, pp. 428-431.

7. FINK, M., SIMEON, J., ITIL, T. M., AND FREEDMAN, A. M.: Clinical Antidepressant Activity of Cyclazocine—A Narcotic Antagonist. Clin. Pharm. Therap. 11:41-48, 1970.

8. FINK, M., ZAKS, A., SHAROFF, R., MORA, A., BRUNER, A., LEVIT, S., AND FREEDMAN, A. M.: Naloxone in Heroin Dependence. Clin. Pharm. Ther. 9:568-577, 1968.

9. FOLDES, F. F., LUNN, J., MOORE, J., AND BROWN, I.: N-allylnoroxymorphone: A New Potent Narcotic Antagonist. Amer. J. Med. Sci. 245:23-30, 1963.

10. FREEDMAN, A., FINK, M., SHAROFF, R., AND ZAKS, A.: Cyclazocine and Methadone in Narcotic Addiction. J.A.M.A. 202:191-194, 1967.

11. FREEDMAN, A., FINK, M., SHAROFF, R., AND ZAKS, A.: Clinical Studies of Cyclazocine in the Treatment of Narcotic Addiction. Amer. J. Psychiat. 124: 1499-1504, 1968.

12. GORODETZKY, C. W., SAPIRA, J. D., JASINSKI, D. R., AND MARTIN, W. R.: Liver Disease in Narcotic Addicts. Clin. Pharm. Therap. 9:720, 739, 1968.

13. JAFFE, J. H., AND BRILL, L.: Cyclazocine, a Long Acting Narcotic Antagonist: Its Voluntary Acceptance as a Treatment Modality by Narcotic Abusers. Int. J. Addiction 1:99-123, 1966.

14. JASINSKI, D. R., MARTIN, W. R., AND HAERTZEN, C. A.: The Human Pharmocology and Abuse Potential of N-allylnoroxymorphone (Naloxone). J. Pharmacol. Exp. Therap. 157:420-426, 1967.

15. MARTIN, W. R., GORODETZKY, C. W., AND McLANE, T. K.: An Experimental Study in the Treatment of Narcotic Addicts with Cyclazocine. Clin. Pharm. Therap. 7:455-465, 1966.

16. RESNICK, R., FINK, M., AND FREEDMAN, A. M.: A Cyclazocine Typology in Opiate Dependence. Amer. J. Psychiat. 126:1256-1260, 1970.

17. RESNICK, R., FINK, M., AND FREEDMAN, A. M.: Experimental Studies of Cyclazocine, Alone and Combined with Naloxone. (In preparation.)

18. ROUBICEK, J., VOLAVKA, J., ZAKS, A., AND FINK, M.: Electrographic Effects of Chronic Administration of Methadone. (In preparation.)

19. SADOVE, M. S., BALAGOT, R. C., HATANO, S., AND JOBGEN, E. A.: Study of a Narcotic Antagonist N-allylnoroxymorphone. J.A.M.A., 183:666-668, 1963.

20. VERESS, F., MAJOR, V., FINK, M., AND FREEDMAN, A. M.: High-Dose Tybamate Therapy of Heroin Dependence. J. Clin. Pharm. 9:232-238, 1969.

21. WIKLER, A.: Conditioning factors in Opiate Addiction and Relapse. In: Wilner, D. M., and Kassebaum, G. G. (eds.), Narcotics. New York, McGraw-Hill Book Co., Inc., 1965.

22. ZAKS, A., BRUNER, A., FINK, M., AND FREEDMAN, A. M.: Intravenous Diacetylmorphine (Heroin) in Studies of Opiate Dependence. Diseases Nervous System Suppl. 30:89-92, 1969.

23. ZAKS, A., FINK, M., AND FREEDMAN, A.: Treatment of Opiate Dependence with High Dose Oral Naloxone. (In preparation.)

Recent Developments in the Therapy of Addictions

by P. H. Blachly, M.D.

Drug addiction, unlike most conditions in medicine, is characterized by three primary features: (1) the victim actively engages in his own victimization (he brings it on himself); (2) negativism, or the victim knows the usual consequences of the behavior but does it anyway; (3) a short-term reward and a long-term punishment which is probable but not certain: not every smoker gets lung cancer nor every alcoholic cirrhosis. Addiction, then, is more like gambling, crime, promiscuity, or other risk-taking behaviors than it is like pneumonia, diabetes, or cancer. The distinction is crucial in treatment, for physicians are likely to provide sympathy for the latter conditions and unhelpful moralism or rejection for the former. (The relatively rare patients with iatrogenic addiction constantly point this out to physicians as if it really makes a difference.) Treatment of addiction involves not only the identified patient, but his close contacts and the larger society. Within the identified patient it involves treatment of: (1) drug hunger and drug-seeking behavior such as heroin addiction or alcoholism, (2) the underlying tendency to solve interpersonal problems with drugs (pharmacothymia), and (3) the complications of drug abuse such as septicemia, psychosis, or cirrhosis.

Although in past times it was customary to think of persons as having a single addiction such as to opium or barbiturates, present experience indicates that patients with such single-minded devotion are exceptional, and that instead we find addicts to be omnivorous, often within the same day taking opiates, barbiturates, alcohol, stimulants, marihuana, and tobacco. Stopping or controlling one drug may have little influence on the others, or even stimulate the use of the others.

A further complication is that the doctor's allegiance is more likely to be split between patient, family, and society rather than devoted to the patient alone. Many physicians who treat addicts are government employees, and addicts are coerced into treatment. The expectations of the physician may have little resemblance to the hopes and expectations of the "patient." Unless the physician has a clear understanding of these rather general philosophical dilemmas, he may experience enough unhappiness in treatment of addicts to leave the field for more pleasant pursuits.

One must, then, clearly define at the outset two major factors: (1) What are the expectations and hopes of the patient and physician, respectively? (2) What are the resources at the disposal of the patient and physician? Obviously, the problem is entirely different if the patient is on a locked ward in a federally financed institution as opposed to seeking outpatient care from a private physician.

It is useful to consider drugs by certain classes as to the extent to which they produce physical dependence, psychological dependence, and tolerance. Table 1 gives an approximate description of this.

Taking the least serious addiction first, tobacco consumption rarely receives active treatment, and little is known about effective forms of treatment other than willpower. It is common among all users to say that they could stop smoking at any time if they really wanted to, but then ignore the factors that lead them to the belief that they do not really want to. Treatment for marihuana smoking is the same as that for tobacco smoking.

The hallucinogen user obtains treatment only when he has undesirable effects of his drug, usually in the form of a state of acute anxiety or hallucinosis. He is usually brought to the physician when psychotherapeutic efforts by his friends in the form of a "talkdown" are ineffective. The safest and most rapidly effective treatment of these conditions is droperidol (Inapsine), 2.5 to 10 mg. intramuscularly or intravenously. Droperidol has the advantage over phenothiazines that there are minimal autonomic side effects; it produces only mild sedation and is of short duration of action in the event that unpleasant extrapyramidal symptoms develop. The person who has continuing flashbacks and anxiety following use of hallucinogens may require prolonged antipsychotic drug treatment or electroconvulsive therapy. We have had one patient refractory to phenothiazines and minor tranquilizers who responded dramatically the second day to lithium carbonate.

Patients get into trouble with stimulants both while "high," when they demonstrate agitation or manic, paranoid, or aggressive behavior, and when they "crash," or have a depression following the prolonged use of stimulants. The

TABLE 1

Types	Physical Dependence	Psychological Dependence	Tolerance
Opiates	++++	++++	++++
Barbiturates and alcohol	++++	++++	++
Amphetamines	+	+++	++++
Cocaine	0	++++	0
Hallucinogens	0	++	+++
Marihuana	0	++	0
Tobacco	0	++	+

292

treatment of the "high" is the same as the treatment of acute mania, that is, titrating the patient with an antipsychotic drug such as haloperidol, droperidol, or chlorpromazine parenterally. Although the use of a depot preparation such as fluphenazine enanthate will prevent the intense "high" or paranoia resulting from the abuse of stimulants, patients are reluctant to return for treatment since treatment obviates their purpose in getting "high." The "low," depression, or "crash" following a "run" of stimulants is probably the result of depletion of norepinephrine stores in the central nervous system, and these replenish themselves spontaneously in a few days. At this time there is no effective chemical way adequately to effect the process of repletion, and the patient need only be taught that the depression is self-limited. However, a significant number of drug abusers are chronically depressed, and it remains to be tested whether a regular program of antidepressant medication might be therapeutic to some speed users.

Suicide attempts are common among drug users, and occasionally are serious, especially by users of barbiturates or alcohol. Suicidal risk is best evaluated on the basis of general competence of the patient. The better the patient's general reputation for accomplishing what he has said he is going to do, the more likely he is to complete suicide once he starts to consider it. The same impulsive tendencies which give rise to drug abuse cause patients to make frequent suicide attempts, but this is countered by their general incompetence, which often makes these attempts abortive; on balance the suicide rate is high among drug abusers.

Because of the very high rate of relapse after withdrawal from opiates in a hospital, most clinicians now prefer to put opiate addicts on a methadon maintenance program, withdrawing them very slowly on an outpatient basis when they request it and when their life has become sufficiently stable and rewarding that they can live without drugs. We use the following schedule:

For daily doses of methadon over 50 mg., decrease 10 mg per week			
then	20-50 mg.,	decrease	5 mg per week
then	8-20 mg.,	decrease	4 mg per week
then	0-8 mg.,	decrease	2 mg per week
then	orange juice for 1 week		

Thus, for the average maintenance dose of 100 mg., it will require 5 months to withdraw if everything goes well. Attempts to withdraw more rapidly are usually met with relapse to the previous opiate abused.

Methadon cannot be used for withdrawal from dependence on any other class of drugs except opiates such as heroin, codeine, Percodan, Dilaudid, morphine, and paregoric. Particularly it cannot be used for opiate antagonist analgesics such as pentazocine (Talwyn).

Barbiturates and related drugs such as glutethimide produce physical

293

dependence that may result in fatal convulsions upon abrupt abstinence. Because such addicts usually underestimate their consumption, it is important that the physician treat them with careful observation on a ward and determine their *intoxication threshold*. The intoxication threshold is that amount of pentobarbital required to produce mild intoxication manifested by slurred speech, ataxia, and nystagmus. One starts by giving 0.2 Gm. pentobarbital every 6 hours for 24 hours. If intoxication does not occur within 24 hours, increase the dose to 0.3 Gm. every 6 hours. If no intoxication occurs after another 24 hours, increase to 0.4 Gm. every 6 hours. A very few patients may even have to be raised to 0.4 Gm. every 4 hours. Once intoxication is reached, decrease the dose by 0.1 Gm. every 24 hours until the patient is stabilized. It generally requires a minimum of 1 month's hospitalization to obtain abstinence, and the relapse rate thereafter is exceedingly high.

The major problem in drug dependence is not producing abstinence, it is relapse after "cure." The simplest example is the cigarette smoker who may quit—and relapse—20 times a day. A host of environmental stimuli act as conditioning agents to increase chances for relapse—a neighborhood, certain people, a particular anxiety. As with giving up a fond romance, some persons can avoid relapse by moving to a novel environment. The physiological memory of the drug effect is harder to forget. Many of those who successfully avoid relapse admit that they nevertheless think of drugs daily. It appears that those vulnerable to drug abuse are vulnerable to a host of other impulsive destructive problem-solving maneuvers, and that to improve one, we must attempt to decrease the others simultaneously.

The treatment of the opiate withdrawal state depends upon the facilities available. The opiate abstinence syndrome has never resulted in death and hence is never a medical emergency despite the cries of anguish from the patient. It is perhaps more humane to reduce the amount of opiates gradually, but I suspect that the total amount of discomfort is the same whether one quits abruptly or gradually. Some patients prefer to have the suffering over rapidly, rather than have it drawn out. Unless the patient is on a locked ward, it is futile to attempt withdrawal. Once the patient is under observation, no medication is given until there is objective evidence of withdrawal manifested by piloerection, accompanied by muscle cramps, vomiting, and diarrhea. At that time it is useful to commence methadon, 20 mg. twice a day, and reduce it by 5 mg. per dose until the patient is off in 4 days. The persisting complaints of insomnia are best handled by reassurance that insomnia will be a problem for several months and that the patient had best grow accustomed to it.

It appears that to a large degree, *drugs are people substitutes and vice versa.* A synopsis of the reasoning behind this theory is given by the following four points: (1) people get sick over people; (2) drugs are people substitutes; (3) drug effects are more predictable than people effects; (4) people become necessary to the user only to the extent that they can provide drugs.

All the drug users I have known have been in a state of dis-ease, hurting from their interpersonal relationships at the time the drug dependency started. Such dis-ease may range from the malaise of the poverty-stricken adolescent turning to heroin, to the depression of the middle-aged professional turning to alcohol or sleeping pills, to the unsatisfied drive for achievement of the graduate student user of amphetamines. The drug used and the sociocultural background of the user may be extremely diverse. The drug first used may not be satisfactory, and the person may experiment with a variety of drugs until he either finds one that meets his needs or gives up drug seeking as a way of handling his dis-ease. But when his experience with the drug and the people from whom he obtains drugs help him to allay his discomfort, he is in a position where the probability of his repeating the use of drugs is high. Guilt for utilizing drugs for relief of dis-ease is in part allayed by the gradual development of a paranoid stance which makes him a martyr against those persons who feel that drug use is undesirable. And the *drugs will relieve* his symptoms in a variety of ways, depending on their physiological effects. If he suffers from chronic depression and anticipatory anxiety, he may find that heroin relieves these and provides a feeling of simply not caring in the presence of others. Amphetamines, by relieving fatigue and perhaps occasionally actually improving performance, may provide the ambitious person with actually increased people satisfactions. Although such an improvement is short-lived and gradually leads to deterioration, the memory of what it has done coupled with the fantasy of what it might do becomes more important to the person than the reality of his actual performance. What is most impressive to the drug user is that the drug effect, at least at first, is quite predictable; he can turn himself "on" or "off" at will. It becomes a habitual shortcut for the tedious negotiations necessary to obtain unpredictable people satisfactions. It should not be surprising that with such control over one's feelings, a delusion of omnipotence should gradually appear, for if one can turn oneself on or off, one may in fantasy also turn others on or off. Sometimes this takes the form of apparent altruism in the user giving away drugs to nonusers, in effect controlling them. Coincident with the development of the delusion of omnipotence, there may occur, sometimes for the first time, the development of a conviction about the purpose of life. This new-found purpose in life is simply to obtain drugs and repeat and perpetuate the drug experience.

As this trend develops, people gradually become mere objects to the user, needed only to supply him with drugs. He becomes increasingly condescending and arrogant, even while objectively becoming, paradoxically, most dependent on people and drugs.

Treatment of drug dependency seems to require the provision of equivalent gratification without drugs. Such treatment generally takes the form of an

295

attempt to substitute satisfying people relationships for drug relationships. For the highly addicting drugs this cannot be done while the user continues to take drugs, for the predictability and efficiency of the drugs exceeds that of the people. For this reason, total abstinence is usually essential, with the substitution of satisfying interpersonal relationships during the abstinence period. That this technique is effective for a significant proportion of drug-dependent persons is testified to by the existence of such organizations as Alcoholics Anonymous, Synanon, and Odyssey House.

On the horizon there is hope for much-improved methods of dealing with addiction. It ranges from a more intelligent appreciation by the general public of problems of drugs, to new research developments. The latter include long-acting narcotic antagonists, improved forms of methadon, and aversive conditioning procedures.

SOME RECOMMENDED SOURCE MATERIAL

Books

1. Blachly, P. H. (Ed.): Drug Abuse: Data and Debate. Springfield, Ill., Charles C Thomas, Publisher, 1971.
2. Blachly, P. H.: Seduction: A Conceptual Model in the Drug Dependencies and Other Contagious Social Ills. Springfield, Ill., Charles C Thomas, Publisher, 1971.
3. Interim Report of the Commission of Inquiry into the Non-medical Use of Drugs, Ottawa, Ontario, Canada, 1970.
4. Proceedings of the Third National Conference on Methadon Treatment, New York City, November 14-16, 1970.
5. Report of the Thirty-Third Annual Scientific Meeting of the Committee on Problems of Drug Dependence, Volume I. National Academy of Sciences–National Academy of Engineering, National Research Council, Division of Medical Sciences, Toronto, Ontario, Canada, 1971.
6. Wikler, A. (Ed.): The Addictive States. Baltimore, Williams & Wilkins Co., 1968.
7. Wittenborn, J. R., Smith, J. P., and Wittenborn, S. (Eds.): Communication and Drug Abuse (Proceedings of the Second Rutgers Symposium on Drug Abuse). Springfield, Ill., Charles C Thomas, Publisher, 1970.
8. International Journal of the Addictions.
9. Bulletin on Narcotics, World Health Organization.
10. Journal of Psychedelic Drugs.

Synanon in Drug Addiction

by ELLIOTT L. MARKOFF, M.D.

O NE OF THE MAJOR problems in the treatment of drug addiction is that
of after-care. Programs of detoxification, incarceration and compulsory treatment have been grossly inadequate to the task of modifying the
psychopathology and deficit in maturation of the addictive personality.
Withdrawal from opiates without substitution of a meaningful way of life
that is psychologically feasible for the addict promotes only a void in the
treatment process that some authors have referred to as "a refined form of
cruelty."[2] In our current treatment programs, we may be sentencing these
subjects to return, ill-fitted, to an environment hardly more likely than
before to offer any new dimensions for personal growth. A fresh approach
and a new standard of relative values may be needed before replacement
of self-identification as a "hope to die junkie" can be realized. "Involvement
with the drug and the drug-using sub-culture gives the drug addict a sense
of a personal identity, a place in society, a commitment, personal associations
based on a seemingly common purpose, a feeling of belonging to an in-group,
a vocation and an avocation and a means of filling the void in an otherwise
empty life . . . involvement with narcotics is an expression of a need for a
sense of being alive . . ."[2]

Since 1958 Synanon, a steadily expanding voluntary program for modifying and re-directing the antisocial behavior of drug addicts, has been in
operation first in Santa Monica, Calif. and in other centers in California,
Nevada, Michigan, Puerto Rico and New York. The Synanon Foundation
directs itself toward the underlying severe personality disorder, rather than
to the use of drugs alone. Drug use is prohibited, but the emptiness that this
removal could cause is filled instead by a program that is able to offer the
addict increased self-esteem, a realistic goal that is attainable and meaningful for him and a sense of involvement and participation in a social
system that accepts him without ostracism, and to which he can contribute
as a responsible, purposeful member of an open, dynamic community.
Synanon appears to be offering a segment of the addict population a vehicle
for substituting a life of purpose and performance for one of drug addiction.

297

Synanon represents an ongoing and potentially long-range program which can follow its members through graduation from the Foundation itself into the larger society, and then, through continual reinforcement and affiliation with alumni clubs, can offer a sustaining "life line" analogous to the emotional resources of one's own family. The prototype of this alumni association exists now in a Foundation concept known as the Sponsors of Synanon.

By April 1964, over 1,100 narcotic addicts had entered a Synanon facility for 24 hours or more, and not less than 25 per cent of these residents have maintained drug abstinence through a two year follow-up. This is a minimum figure since follow-up on all residents who leave Synanon is not available. Thirty-five to 45 per cent of all entrants leave prior to three months, although many seek readmission. If only those who stay at least three months rather than 24 hours are considered, the two year abstinence rate is far higher, exceeding 65 per cent.

Realistically there are no good risks in a cross-section of addicts. Addiction is notably chronic or relapsing, and even short-term abstinence is held by many workers to be a valid goal. Also, the well-intentioned addict, if such be the case, is highly ambivalent about giving up drugs and must initially be highly motivated to attempt to do so, followed by continual reinforcement of his good intentions. Most addicts see themselves as "dope fiends," hopelessly addicted for life.

PROCESS

Synanon states that it cannot waste its precious space on people who merely want to dry out, so that they can return to the streets for a fresh thrill. The applicant must become aware, as one member put it, at least of first "*wanting* to want to give up drugs." He is required to telephone for an appointment or to appear at a given time, and he is told to return another time if he appears loaded. This nonpermissive attitude has a significant effect on the addict, whose previous escapes from reality through drugs have included a pre-morbid history of unreliable or inconstant reality demands. He is here first confronted with a Synanon challenge to his abilities, and at the same time first experiences himself coping with achievement and acceptance by his peers not based on drug use. It is true, therefore, that the addict must desire to enter Synanon, and very frequently has been jailed, utterly demoralized and finally and totally rejected by his family and friends before he might consider giving up drugs. In the words of the addict, he is "smashed." However being smashed is not unique in the Synanon population compared to populations in other addict treatment efforts.

At the time of the initial interview the applicant is further smashed by a calculated effort to demolish his self-image by confronting him with his obvious lack of success and futile incompetency in living. This is done by one or more of his peers, who can have true empathy based on experience. One of the prime factors in the Synanon dynamic is the total investment of the Synanon personnel in their program, which embodies a commitment and experience far beyond that obtainable by any professional staff in an artificially structured therapeutic community. The newcomer can partially identify with the Synanon members immediately and can hope that by emulating them he too will be able to live "clean." Synanon, at this point, addresses itself to the one remaining scrap or nucleus of ego or self-esteem remaining by appealing to the individual to substitute success for failure. This success is visible all around him in the clean, former addicts who appear to be enthusiastically going places and doing things. There is a pioneer spirit, one of excitement, vitality and easy familiarity, replacing the loneliness of the street. He is also told immediately that, "Good boys and girls get good things. Bad boys and girls don't get very far." A positive, hopeful program is thus presented.

The drug addict would look for the slightest excuse and rationalization for failure and therefore has to be told only of the optimistic and positive side of his Synanon chances for success in avoiding drug use. There is a similarity here to the rearing of children, whom we spare from harsh realities until their ego mechanisms have developed further for coping with life. The first task for Synanon is attracting the entrant and then keeping him engaged long enough for the program to begin to take effect. Research criteria or statistical studies are secondary and may even be harmful to the milieu of this admission phase.

The second phase of the admission then begins. The applicant is directed to break all former associations and ties. All contact with relatives and friends is prohibited for several months. Synanon is insistent upon a minimum of contact of the new residents with non-Synanon people, because of this necessity to instill the Synanon philosophy and to prevent the easy relapse of the newcomer into his familiar patterns.

In behavioral terms, a conscious effort is made to extinguish former patterns of response. This is in accord with Wikler's[3] observations on the conditioned physical and psychological response of addicts who have been abstaining and then are exposed again to the hypodermic equipment, a former connection or source of drugs or even the street corner where they made their connections, which results in a feeling frequently described as withdrawal, accompanied by physiological signs and psychological craving for the drug. The reaction abates after about two years of abstinence. Synanon has found empirically that two years is about the least time necessary for maximum benefit in its program. In addition to drug abstinence, personality development is also seen as a result of the two year experience in Synanon.

Another difference in response, apparently related to expectations of behavior, is found in the drug withdrawal experience. Addicts at Lexington or Fort Worth may stress their discomfort and often seek to extend the period of withdrawal so as to obtain more medication. Anxiety in a hostile, i.e., anti-addiction environment, and the status derived from having a "big habit" contribute to this behavior. The withdrawal syndrome in Synanon is typically of shorter duration, and is reported to be less severe than in the individual's previous experience despite the "cold turkey" method used. This appears to be due to the emotional support offered by the members, the absolute absence of any possible offer of drugs and the status-gain of more mature behavior.

In contrast to other programs, Synanon makes itself extremely difficult to enter and extremely easy to leave; the addict therefore finds his hostility and passive-aggressive behavior no longer directed against a supposedly confining and hostile system or parental surrogate. Instead the obligation is his own, and he is forced to begin to see himself in realistic terms. He is literally out-maneuvered and can not use his psychopathic manipulations. Rather than being begged to stay, he would promptly be told to "get lost."

Another important aspect of Synanon's effectiveness relates to a quality of anti-professional and especially anti-liatric grandiosity and arrogance. Experiences of social ostracism and feelings of low self-esteem find in these postures another countervailing force. A therapeutic opportunity results from the attraction of the anti-social character to this seemingly more potent group. One's feelings of inadequacy can be compensated by a sense of strength and superiority. However when professionals present themselves as willing colleagues rather than as superior workers, they have been met with enthusiastic reception of their skills and knowledge. Perhaps some of the criticism of Synanon stems from the implied threat to our professional competence from a system that can succeed where we have failed.

Initially the individual is taught a Synanon dialectic about his progress from emotional infancy to responsible maturity, but his environment is structured to produce real rewards of greater freedom, material benefits and upward mobility that encourage him to exercise his interpersonal skills. He learns to "go through the motions" and to "act as if" until by the end of about three months he has indeed modified his asocial and isolated hedonistic behavior for something more closely approximating a healthy social response. At this point he has substituted Synanon for addiction as a behavior pattern and is, perhaps, "hooked" on Synanon.

Socially approved and reinforced status for good behavior and performance can begin to affect an alteration of the subject's low self-esteem and socially maladaptive self-image. The absurdity of his former behavior, its uselessness and needlessness, are brought home to the subject by example and experience provided in the daily Synanon dynamic. The individual finds himself helping others, doing an important job for the good of himself and the group, and in turn receives approval and support from others. In place of his former hedonistic, narcissistic behavior with its high incidence in reality of frustration and resultant rage and acting-out behavior, which could then be so easily alleviated by the illusory hedonic control represented in drug use, the individual finds workable substitutes and processes for sublimation of his former, frustrated drives.

"Addicts are emotional infants," is a fundamental statement in Synanon. From the histories obtained from many addicts, the absence in their early personality formation of clearly definable, consistent and realistic rewards or love for appropriate behavior, and the lack of healthy identifications are basic in the development of the character disorders. Drug usage has represented an illusory substitute for unconditional mother love in the addict's experience, and, typically, there has been a notable absence of a parental figure from whom the individual could experience consistent rewards for, and satisfaction in, maturation. The very discipline of addiction as a subculture or way of life in part represents a frantic attempt to secure for oneself through fantasied omnipotence the love, self-esteem and experience of achievement otherwise lacking.

We must continue to ask why the Synanon program can be acceptable to the addict when other well-conceived institutional efforts may fail. One answer is the availability of a continuum from intake to follow-up which can involve the individual in an exciting sense of significant participation. For example, in Los Angeles, Synanon runs an industrial program in a large leased warehouse, which does subcontracting work for industry at a profit to the Synanon Foundation, and operates gasoline service stations. Although this has great therapeutic value for unskilled and inexperienced young people who have seldom known the discipline of a steady job, the interest of Synanon in developing this program stems from a very real need for financial support, independence and self-reliance. Theories about the therapeutic value of industrial arts are, therefore, secondary to the immediate necessity for such a program with which every Synanon member can readily identify. Synanon's material goals are largely those of the American middle class. It holds out the tangible prospect of upward mobility and improvement for its members. This is illustrated in another Synanon saying, "If you know how to live, it's a lot better than shooting dope."

Members who have left Synanon prematurely and then returned often state that the drug experience still gave the physiological sensations but no longer seemed to gratify the psychological needs: "It wasn't real," and, "It wasn't what I wanted anymore," are frequently heard. This kind of experience first occurs for the individual somewhere around the third month of participation in the program.

Experience to date indicates that at approximately two years, the Synanon member has in effect graduated from the program and become capable of a self-sustaining existence free from drug use. Since Synanon dates only from 1958 and significant numbers of members really only go back to 1960, final evaluation of success in eliminating former patterns of destructive behavior remains for the future. In about the third year of Synanon's existence, graduation into "Third Stagers" (as those who work in the larger community and live away from Synanon are called) was held to be the most desirable goal. Those who achieved it were widely acclaimed by the Foundation. However as Synanon has expanded and found itself in desperate need of personnel who were trained and experienced to carry on the Synanon program, great efforts have been made to encourage all talented members to continue to affiliate with Synanon in staff positions after their initial transformation has been effected.

Thus there appear to be four critical stages in the progress of each individual in Synanon. The first occurs at the time of initial decision to enter Synanon and to go along with its program. At this time the newcomer experiences some feeling of relief and pleasure in the busy activity and pioneering spirit of friendly acceptance in the club.

At about three to six months, the initial novelty has worn off. A period of depression and lassitude is often seen at this time as the individual becomes increasingly introspective about the significance of his previous behavior. For many this period provides the first contemplation of self that will lead to a sustained therapeutic effort. Those who are frightened by this prospect and who feel unable to cope with reality may leave Synanon at this time. A significant number, however, will seek readmission when they recognize the inadequacy of their behavior or the disparity between their current reality situation in the larger society and the achievable goals that Synanon can offer.

For those who remain in Synanon there comes a third phase at about one year of residence characterized by a determined effort to understand oneself and the meaning of one's relationship to others. During this period many members determine for themselves their future course, whether it be as a Synanon staff member or as a worker in the larger society. There is a danger of premature over-assessment of one's capabilities at this stage, and the individual's ambitions frequently do undergo further change if he remains in the program.

The fourth phase appears after from 18 months to two years, when the individual has sufficiently stabilized and internalized his controls to become responsible, self-sufficient, and dependable. Casriel[1] writes of this process as follows: "Before any emotional growth can be obtained, the addict must be taught to live without drugs or alcohol, without acting-out antisocially and do this in an open (i.e., free to come and go) environment. The missing link in the treatment of addicts — indeed, perhaps in the treatment of all character disorders — has been the *how* of teaching the addict to mature emotionally in an *open* environment. This is the one thing an addictive personality has never learned."

ORGANIZATION

A description of Synanon's operational structure and typical weekly program will assist in understanding how the Foundation directs its procedures toward involving and re-educating the addict.

The Executive Director and Chairman of the Board of the Foundation, Charles E. Dederich, is the founder, and he appoints a Board of Staff Directors who are responsible to him for the over-all operation of the Foundation. Geographic facilities are Chapters in the Foundation assigned to a Director, who may also manage a major operation such as industries, public relations, accounting, creative arts, and Synanon schools.

Each Chapter is directly managed by an Acting Director assisted by several other directors of equal rank but of subordinate authority in the staff system. The Acting Directors are responsible for the daily operations of their respective chapters. Chapters are subdivided into departments, such as Supply, Kitchen, Maintenance, Service, Business Office, Transportation, etc. The Department Heads, in turn, have assistants and specialists as needed and supervisors who are directly responsible for the daily duties and quality of performance of their workers. Monthly individual worker progress reports are required from each supervisor. Synanon believes it can learn as much in this way about the progress of the supervisor as it can about his workers.

The Chapter's Acting Director sends a daily report to the Foundation concerning business and individual personality matters. The individual Chapters consist of many residential units and a central headquarters. Each such residence is itself placed in charge of someone of Acting Director or similar seniority level and holds a daily morning meeting to regulate its own internal operation. Each Synanon Chapter holds a daily Board meeting at which its Acting Directors and individual Department Heads, by invitation, coordinate operations and seek to solve the daily problems that arise.

The board meetings of the Chapter and the Foundation staff meetings are similar to psychiatric hospital staff meetings where operational details

303

and individual problems are considered. Transfers, living arrangements, job-assignments and evaluation of progress are subjects commonly discussed. Conferences and individual consultations are arranged with individuals who require counseling, and a resident in any Chapter may request an appointment with any Acting Director or member of the Foundation staff.

In typical Synanon style, counselors were for a time specifically appointed and titled "Wizards" to emphasize their difference from the traditional institutional model.

A newcomer in Synanon almost universally begins on the Service Crew doing janitorial duties, and works his way upwards in the organization by demonstration of competence and ingenuity. A Coordinators Department, which is responsible for communications, appointments, visitors and the mechanical details of the daily chapter operations, is representative of the increasing responsibility levels available as greater independence is earned.

A Department of Education is responsible for high school programs and other teaching efforts in the chapters. Attached directly to the Foundation staff are such divisions as Archives, a Medical Department staffed by an ex-addict physician and a Records Department. Each chapter also has its own equivalent sections. Without a further elaboration of details, one can readily appreciate Synanon's complexity and sophistication of organization.

Specific jobs and titles, known as "noise" in Synanon, are capable of rapid change. Individuals may move easily from one area to another or may function in several areas simultaneously, depending upon the needs of the Foundation. Geographic mobility is also a necessity, and the many transfers in Synanon remind one of the practice in larger business corporations.

PROGRAMS

Daily, after lunch, each Chapter and other large unit within the Synanon structure, e.g., the Industries Department, holds a one hour meeting which may be a "concepts seminar" to discuss a literary or philosophical quotation or to listen to a tape recording or a lecture, or to hold a mock speaking engagement for members to speak extemporaneously and have their topic and delivery criticized from the floor. This system of daily group meetings is a deliberate effort to inculcate habits of thinking and communication, and thereby subtly to enhance self-esteem, self-confidence and a sense of personal significance. Another important effect, the promotion of group solidarity, is apparent.

The tape sessions, consisting of previous talks or of actual interviews or interactions in the Synanon community, serve a vital function in preserving the culture and history and in transmitting this to the newcomers. Tapes are extensively used for dissemination of ideas among the chapters, so that continuity of the Synanon philosophy is maintained.

On Saturday night all Synanon chapters hold an Open House for the public. Favorable publicity and financial support are obvious goals, but another purpose is the continual exposure of the Synanon member to the larger society. This serves further to enhance his self-esteem and provides opportunities for identification with the "square" world. As a result, although several years are required for the We-They dichotomy of "squares" and "hypes" to dissipate, the member, nevertheless, finds his course of action increasingly parallels that of the larger society rather than running antithetically to it, as was his previous experience.

As part of its search for favorable publicity to gain material support, and to provide another continuing source of reinforcement and self-realization for its members, Synanon arranges civic speaking engagements. Speaker selection depends not only on the topic, but also on the developmental needs of the speaker.

The Game

The evening small *s* synanon, now called the "game," is the most structured psychotherapeutic device. In synanons, about 12 members meet three or more times weekly for the purpose of frank and direct examination of one another's attitudes and emotions. In addition special synanons are held as needed for interpersonal problem areas, and provide an excellent cultural technique for relieving tensions and hostilities and for reducing status and job differentials. They also provide critical self-evaluation for the participants and increase receptivity for new orientations and goals. The emphasis is on a here-and-now confrontation of one's behavior and feelings, often conducted with intense verbal abuse and sarcasm. Prohibition of physical violence, an absolute Synanon rule, here successfully meets its greatest challenge and through the game process helps to teach delay of impulsive action by redirection into verbal channels.

Originally there was no group leader in a synanon, and each hour and a half or two hour session was steered by that member who seemed most competent to explore the ideas of the moment. However individual talents emerged in conducting these group sessions and have resulted in the concept of the "synanist," a generally more experienced and psychologically sensitive member who serves as the group leader. Initial sessions for newcomers tend to be loud, raucous affairs, in which a great deal of yelling and cursing occur, but gradually the individual begins to seek an understanding of his relationship with his peers and with himself.

The principles of flexibility and resourcefulness are again applied by Synanon to the synanon or game situations. An individual can request placement in a given synanon because of some interpersonal problem which he wishes to discuss with a selected associate. The composition of groups is not

305

constant, but is made up for each session by a synamaster, who utilizes his knowledge of the interpersonal difficulties and needs in the chapter for the purpose of constructing a group that has some therapeutic goals. Synanon games are also often organized along homogeneous groupings, such as old people, young people, Negroes, women, "bad girls," kitchen crew, Italians or any other grouping which seems to promote better interaction and self-awareness. Members who have been in Synanon for over 18 months are encouraged to continue in synanons as leaders of these groups. However these senior members are not encouraged to enter into newcomers' games on the same emotional level, but are instead expected to provide role models and empathic participants to guide and to stimulate progress in the newer members.

The ultimate impact of the games is probably their ability to convey to each participant an awareness of personal responsibility and significance. For many it is the first experience of peer group concern for them in their lives, and serves further as a constant force to promote acceptance of group values. Thus the Synanon game is a major device for the development of more realistic self-evaluation and for the internalization of social controls.

The Trip

An example of Synanon's resourcefulness and ingenuity in maintaining contact with the current idiom is the Trip. Trips are a Synanon version of marathon group therapy that were developed to meet the need for further involvement and re-commitment of its members, after the numerical growth and physical expansion of Synanon and the increasing number of long-term Synanon members made desirable a more intensive experience to renew the original Synanon concepts and interpersonal contracts. The Trip is presented as an effort to expand man's communication into a space dimension beyond his usual experience. Participants are subjected to 36 hours of continual contact in Synanon games interrupted by planned athletic activities, swims and sometimes group dancing. Following the Trip, members of the group are expected to have several days of "debriefing" during which they have access to a quiet room for reading and contemplation and are relieved of all vocational duties in the Foundation. Interviews of the participants have indicated that the Trips are useful in achieving the renewal and strengthening of Synanon commitment and can be effective in further redirecting individual behavioral patterns.

Rituals

At the Saturday night meetings a birthday celebration of those who have completed a 12 month unit of residence is held. At this time the individual

306

so honored is called upon to make a public testimonial, which stimulates him to conceptualize what his experience in Synanon has meant to him and in what it has resulted for him; this also provides a group reinforcement for the efforts and aspirations of the other members.

Short of expulsion, there are individual reprimands known as "hair-cuts" delivered by a senior executive and "fire-place scenes", which are rarely held general meetings at which serious violators are stripped of their rationalizations and publicly reprimanded. The experienced Synanist has developed a technique wherein the individual is ridiculed and attacked for the stupidity or inappropriateness of his behavior, but in which the possibility of better performance and continued acceptance through clearly defined pathways are held open. For the person involved this effort to render his behavior ego dystonic also emphasizes the concern of the group, while to the group public reprimands are useful for vicarious super-ego reinforcement and relief of guilt.

Synanon has also adapted several religious and national holidays to its own purposes. The Jewish Passover is celebrated in Synanon with an appropriate dinner that emphasizes brotherhood and the universality of the members. Commemoration of the founding of Synanon is accompanied by such rituals as the breaking of sunglasses to represent the interruption of the addict's self-deception and the wearing of "flip-flops", a rubber sandal commonly worn by the earliest members on the beach at Santa Monica.

Another major ritual somewhat analogous to the Fourth of July celebration is the "Night of the Big Cop Out." This event represents a major breakthrough in the development of the Synanon concept when its first members broke the code of the streets by revealing one another's misbehavior to the group. A recounting of that dramatic night by some of the old-timers, replaying of historical tape recordings of the Foundation, and membership-wide rededication to the principles of honesty and responsibility for one another take place during the holiday.

CURRENT DIRECTIONS

Synanon today disavows that it is a "treatment" center for addicts. Rather it sees itself as a social movement or an educational process. A plan is envisioned for a "communiversity" where Synanon programs would be used in retraining drug abusers and non-users alike in the Synanon philosophy and style of living. To Synanon, this style is more honest and rewarding than is the social alienation of the larger society. It prefers to call its dope fiends, members or residents simply "people."

The narcissism of the organization has increased the resistance of Synanon to participation in other programs which are not Synanon directed or controlled. Former experience as social isolates and outcasts tends to increase the inherent reluctance of Synanon to broaden its activities in addict rehabilitation programs. Although former members are important leaders in other such programs, Synanon seeks to preserve itself in pure culture uncorrupted by what it regards as the dilutions and compromises of the professionally affiliated treatment efforts.

Synanon has been faulted for guiding its participants from emotional infancy up to a phase of adolescence, but in lacking channels for development of adult independence after the individual expresses adolescent rebellion. Instead the maintenance of a dependent position are seen by Synanon critics to be required for continued association with the Foundation. Perhaps the limited number of top positions in Synanon for capable members makes this criticism partially valid.

The severe impairment of early ego-formation in addicts, however, often renders them unable to function entirely independently in the general population. Instead, for many addicts, long-term support is available to them which offers a freedom of movement combined with a productive and purposeful existence. Synanon is able to offer such follow-up programs at a minimal cost to society. Whether the former addict elects to take his place individually in the general population or to continue as a worker for Synanon, doing its daily chores and participating in the rehabilitation of other addicts, his social value and personal significance have been considerably enhanced.

REFERENCES

1. Casreil, D.: So Fair a House: The Story of Synanon. New Jersey, Prentice-Hall, 1963.
2. Chein, I., Gerard, D. L., Lee, R. S., and Rosenfeld, E.: The Road to H. New York, Basic Books, 1964.
3. Wikler, A.: Conditioning Factors in Opiate Addiction and Relapse. In: Wilner, D. M., and Kassebaum, G. G. (Eds.): Narcotics. New York, McGraw-Hill, 1965.
4. Yablonsky, L.: The Tunnel Back: Synanon, New York, The Macmillan Co., 1965.

PART VIII

SUICIDE

The Prevention of Suicide

by ROBERT E. LITMAN, M.D.

D UE TO THE EXPANDING SCOPE OF PSYCHIATRIC THERAPY the problem of suicide is viewed currently with increased urgency and a change in emphasis. Formerly, for psychiatrists, suicide prevention was a matter of continuous security behind locked doors in mental hospitals. The trend toward milieu therapy, early discharge, day centers, and office practice has made psychiatrists responsible for the treatment of many suicidal patients as outpatients. Public health departments and mental health agencies in numerous cities are initiating programs for active case finding and emergency rescuing operations directed toward suicidal persons. The purpose of this article is to review these developments in relationship to psychiatric practice.

ANSWERING THE CRY FOR HELP

Retrospective investigations of deaths by suicide have revealed that in the great majority of cases suicide did not occur suddenly, impulsively, unpredictably, or inevitably, but was, on the contrary, the final step or outcome of a progressive failure of adaptation. According to this view there are, at any particular time, a relatively large number of "presuicidal" or "potentially suicidal" persons who are temporarily emotionally disturbed and are considering suicide as a possible action.

Most suicide episodes occur in the form of *crises*, discrete periods of social-psychological disequilibrium of limited duration. Suicidal persons are *ambivalent* in their motives and their goals. At the height of the suicidal crises they are emotionally mixed up and their thinking is confused. Although they feel that the present situation is untenable, unlivable, and hopeless, they also wish to be rescued, reborn, or rehabilitated into a different life situation. Even in a suicidal crisis human beings retain the human trait of *communication*. They reveal the suicidal preoccupation by certain typical symptoms or by verbal and behavioral communications ("clues to suicide"). If other persons, perceiving these

311

clues to suicide, respond with appropriate *action,* the suicidal individual may be aided to a readaptation, and the suicidal crisis is successfully surmounted.

Only a small proportion of the potentially suicidal individuals actually commit suicide. The problem of why certain people actualize their suicidal fantasies whereas most people do not requires a great deal of additional research. Often the factors for and against suicide seem for a period of time to be so evenly balanced that chance variations (whether a certain letter arrives on time, if someone answers a telephone call, the availability of a lethal weapon at a crucial moment) make the essential difference.

The concept of actively seeking out distress signals ("cries for help") from suicidal persons, even though the communications are disguised, muted, or received at second hand, in order to make a personal rescuing response, is shared by antisuicide agencies in many different cities. Such agencies have been sponsored by various professional and nonprofessional organizations including medical societies, hospitals, public health departments, churches, religious orders, individual philanthropists, and groups of citizen volunteers.[1,2] An emergency telephone number is usually the nuclear element of the service provided and frequently constitutes the entire program. Such telephone services receive large numbers of calls from or concerning persons in distress, many of whom are potentially suicidal.

Various suicide prevention services have developed somewhat different approaches and procedures. The most appropriate and useful roles for nonprofessional and professional volunteers, for paid staff workers, and for the many mental health professional disciplines have not been established with any rigidity. A complete program for emergency telephone therapy has been reported by the Suicide Prevention Center in Los Angeles.[3]

PSYCHIATRIC FIRST AID

It is remarkable how much psychotherapy can be transacted by telephone. In giving emergency psychological first aid, a telephone interviewer performs three functions which overlap. He tries to secure the line of communication, he evaluates the patient's situation, particularly the degree of danger of suicide, and he forms a treatment plan and begins to act on it.

In order to establish trust and maintain and strengthen the telephone relationship, the interviewer offers help, identifies himself clearly and honestly, looks for areas of agreement with the caller, and expresses sympathy and understanding. Seemingly inappropriate behavior by the caller

312

(joking, hostile challenges, confusion, suspiciousness, silences) are handled patiently as routine resistance attitudes covering up a helpless feeling.

The most important single element in the evaluation of suicidal danger is the patient's action plan. The when, where, how, and why of the suicide plan is investigated explicitly. It is important to learn about the symptoms of mental disequilibrium, their onset and degree. What has been the caller's usual character? What is the precipitating stress? What are his resources, personal and financial? Elements in the evaluation which carry varying weight in different contexts are age, sex, medical history, recent loss, social isolation, psychiatric history, and recent suicide attempts.

Appropriate action includes giving the caller reassurance, encouragement, and *hope*. Efforts are made to remind the caller of his usual identity which he has lost. The cooperation of family and friends is enlisted. It helps if the caller's overwhelming, giant-sized problem can be broken down into several clearly stated and logically organized small man-sized problems. The immobilized patient is stimulated toward action. For example, he is asked to make return telephone calls at a certain hour or he is given an appointment for a certain time. Persons who are recovering from suicidal states should be cautioned against prematurely resuming positions of great responsibility where initiative is required. More routine and limited tasks have therapeutic value in that they take attention away from the patient's self preoccupation and tend to create a feeling of confidence when they are successfully completed.

To function well as a telephone therapist the interviewer should have a talent for interpersonal communication, a willingness to become personally involved, and a need to rescue people in trouble. The danger of overinvolvement with patients is real. The patients' failure-prone, depressive, masochistic, and paranoid attitudes are contagious to some extent, and constitute a threat to the morale of the suicide prevention staff. In successful organizations these problems have been overcome by optimistic, forceful leadership and by frequent informal consultation between staff members with constant mutual support. I know of no successful self-help antisuicide group composed of ex-suicidal patients with Alcoholics Anonymous as a model, although there have been many unsuccessful attempts to establish suicides anonymous groups. Apparently a certain amount of psychiatric supervision and consultation is necessary for optimal functioning of a suicide prevention service.

RESISTANCE TO PSYCHIATRIC TREATMENT

Many potentially suicidal callers are referred by suicide prevention

313

services to public health facilities, family service and welfare agencies, or mental health outpatient clinics, but for the most seriously suicidal cases (about 15 per cent) the suicide prevention goal is to transfer the patient with careful haste to a psychiatric therapist, preferably in a psychiatric hospital.

A recent analysis of suicides in Los Angeles revealed that almost 15 per cent of the persons who committed suicide had received but not followed a recommendation for psychiatric treatment within a few weeks before their deaths.[7] Even with their lives at stake, most people resist psychiatric hospitalization, although facilities are now readily available (in Los Angeles), therapy is more flexible than before, and often insurance plans bear much of the cost. The patients and their families argue that hospitalization is inconvenient. For men it means a loss of earnings. They fear that the psychiatric label will make them unemployable in the future. Women fear the separation from family and children. Generally, however, the symbolic attributes of hospitalization far outweigh the reality factors. People express fear and resentment about being catagorized as psychiatric cases. Often they feel that by going to the hospital they are taking upon themselves the responsibility for what should be acknowledged as family problems. Often the resistance to hospitalization is more of a family resistance than individual resistance, and it can best be handled by family conferences in an attempt to obtain the cooperation of a number of people who are concerned.

Another important barrier to appropriate psychiatric treatment stems from attitudes of hostility and rejection directed toward suicidal persons by physicians and their assistants. It is especially unfortunate because physicians have the greatest opportunity for diagnosing and treating suicidal reactions before they become overwhelming.[8] This is particularly true for depressive disorders in relatively stable, conscientious, middle-aged persons, which category of suicides accounts for almost 40 per cent. Sometimes a physician and his psychiatric consultant hesitate about hospitalization for someone in the community who is a leading financial, political, professional, or social figure, whose image might be damaged by publicity about psychiatric illness. The outcome of such hesitation may be suicide. It is appropriate to consider sending such a notable person away to another community for hospital treatment.

Outpatient Psychotherapy

The multiplicity and complexity of the psychodynamic elements involved in suicidal states were emphasized recently in dissertations by Kubie[9] and by Grinker.[10] Less experienced therapists should be cautioned

314

against the simplistic psychodynamic cliche that suicide essentially represents hostility turned against the self ("murder in the 180th degree"), particularly if this theoretical formula leads the therapist to interpret the patient's unconscious hostility prematurely, especially against someone he loves and needs; this lowers his self-esteem, increases the regression, and activates suicidal trends. Frequently the patient breaks off contact with the therapist, and the therapeutic opportunity is lost.

The appropriate attitude for psychotherapists confronted by a genuine suicide crisis in a patient was expressed by Sigmund Freud in a 1926 letter discussing a young patient of his. Freud wrote, "What weighs on me in his case is my belief that unless the outcome is very good, it will be very bad indeed; what I mean is that he would commit suicide without any hesitation. I shall therefore do all in my power to avert that eventuality."[11]

It must be said of some suicides (about 10 per cent of the whole group) that for them self-destruction was a way of life from childhood on, so that suicide seemed inevitable. The illness of these patients might be termed "malignant masochism." They had invariably received psychiatric treatment, usually from many therapists, who reported that the patients seemed to be in love with death. Often the patients were beautiful women who stirred up intense rescuing needs in the therapists and left them feeling bereaved. The patients gave a history of a dead or absent parent as the most significant love object. Usually they had been severely abused in childhood by someone whom they felt had demanded death as the price of love. Usually they had the capacity for entering into deeply regressive symbiotic relationships with persons who were meaningful in their lives, including their therapists. The effort to work through this kind of involvement produced states of deep depression, alternating with acting out behavior which took the form of repeated suicide threats and suicide attempts.

Possibly such cases are best treated by therapy teams rather than by individual therapists. The patients seem to react badly to efforts by therapists to push them ahead and congratulate them for progress, as if the patients feel that too much is being expected of them, and they are sure to let their therapists down and have another failure. Some of these patients profit greatly from prolonged periods on the less active wards of state hospitals where their serious handicaps are recognized and little or nothing is expected of them.

A suicidal crisis may complicate office psychotherapy for many reasons. It may be due to an extraneous factor in the patient's life, such as the death of a loved one, or to some problem brought out in the therapy such as the need to separate from a parent; or it may involve an issue with the therapist, for example, his undesired vacation, or a subtle transference countertransference tension which cannot be resolved. At some point, hospitalization must be considered. There is no simple formula for this decision. It should be based upon an evaluation of a number of factors including not only the therapist and the patient but his living conditions and the people closest to him. Experience indicates that no single psychiatric procedure or technique including electric shock treatment, drugs, or psychotherapy is a guarantee against suicide. No therapist desires his patient's suicide; most therapists regard it as a highly undesirable event. Yet, if the therapist is overly anxious about suicide it will interfere with his judgment and his therapeutic attitude, and impair his usefulness to the patient. For the therapist, the two most important factors in determining whether the patient must be transferred to a psychiatric hospital are: (a) the attitude of the significant "other"— spouse, parents, etc.—whether loving and supportive or hostile and rejecting; and (b) the evolution in the patient of suicidal fantasies into an action-plan with anticipatory behavior such as buying a weapon or choosing a site for suicide and rehearsals of the suicidal act. Once made, the decision for hospitalization accentuates the crisis and any delay in carrying out the hospitalization is most hazardous.

SUICIDAL CRISES IN HOSPITALS

It is questionable whether the medical order "'routine suicide precautions" has any constructive value. Possibly it helps to reduce the psychiatrist's anxiety at the expense of the nursing staff who are invariably concerned and confused. Certainly, the suicidal patient should never be placed in an isolation room, but does the order mean that there should be a nurse or attendant with him at all moments, even in the toilet? Is the patient allowed visitors, mail, his electric shaver? I agree with Margolis and colleagues,[12] who reviewed this subject recently and recommended that each suicidal patient on a psychiatric ward should be the focus of an emergency staff conference with detailed exploration of the problem and the therapeutic roles required of all concerned— physicians, nurses, and the entire staff. The results of the conference should be incorporated into the medical chart.

Probably the most extensive study of suicide prevention in hospitals have been reported by Farberow, Shneidman and co-workers,[13] who compared charts of over 300 patients who committed suicide in Veterans Administration Hospitals with nonsuicide control cases. They recommended that suicide prevention training should be part of the education

316

of every person who works in a hospital of any type. Such training would tend to increase the sensitivity of physicians, nurses, psychologists, social workers, attendants, and aides to the overt and subtle clues which are often precursers to suicidal behavior. These experts would establish a professional climate in each ward and within each hospital that would permit easy communication from patient to aide, from aide to nurse, and from nurse to physician, thus making the problem of suicide prevention everyone's problem and everyone's responsibility. They recommend the creation in each hospital of a suicide prevention committee which would have the responsibility for continuing staff education and in addition would investigate every case of suicide that occurred in the hospital. The committee would also make recommendations for any physical changes in the hospital buildings which might be indicated.

These authors reported the predictive value of diagnosing the dependent-dissatisfied, suicidal, chronic patient. This type of patient makes demands for extra attention and reassurance—wanting to see the doctor, the nurse, the chaplain; asking for unnecessary physical examinations or dental work; requesting sedation, seclusion, therapy of various kinds, etc. In many cases, the patients made excessively self-centered demands for attention that were simply impossible to satisfy. Statements such as "Nothing is being done for me," "Other people don't like me," "I should end it all," "There is no place for me anywhere" were further indications of dissatisfaction. This demanding, time-consuming, attention-getting behavior was often irritating and disturbing to the hospital staff and to other patients as well, and these patients were occasionally referred to as hospitals pests. In handling this type of patient it was suggested that the staff be alerted to the seriousness of such behavior from the standpoint of suicidal potentiality. The excessively complaining, demanding, depressed behavior of the dissatisfied patient is an expression of desperate although excessive need for care and support. New treatments or medications often give this type of patient temporary relief and improvement.

About seven per cent of the persons who commited suicide in Los Angeles had been discharged from psychiatric hospitals within the last six months. Preparations for discharging a patient from a psychiatric hospital should include an evaluation of the suicidal potential. For this the recorded observations of the nursing staff who live with the patient around the clock are invaluable. Certain clues may alert the responsible psychiatrist. For example, some patients are extremely overdependent on the hospital. When the possibility of discharge or home visit is mentioned these patients become agitated and panicky. They commit

317

suicide on trial visits home if insufficient attention is paid to their anxious states and the type of home environment to which they are being returned. Favorable outcome after psychiatric hospitalization has been closely correlated with efforts to prepare the environment to accept the discharged patient. Often the accepting or rejecting attitudes of the most significant other person makes the difference between life and death.

Of hospital patients who will eventually commit suicide, about half do so within three months after leaving. Depressive patients tend to have at least one recurrence of symptoms after discharge.[14] Since manic depressives tend, by character, to have all-or-nothing psychological reactions they feel the transient symptoms as a total crisis. "The treatment failed. I can't stand another depression now." So thinking they take suicidal action. The nature of depressive cycles should be explained to depressive patients, and they should be warned that brief low moods are expected after discharge and do not necessarily mean the start of a new depressive period. Patients should be encouraged to call their doctors when mood swings occur. Regular outpatient follow-up consultations for at least three months after hospitalization are strongly recommended.

CONCLUSION

Although reputable authorities from all over the world sincerely believe, on the basis of clinical experience, that many persons have been influenced to refrain from self-destruction, one could not now provide strict scientific proof for the prevention of any suicide by psychiatric therapy or other means. At present the scientific study of suicide prevention measures has barely begun. Further research and exchange of information has been encouraged by the International Association for Suicide Prevention (founded in 1961), which held its Third Congress in Basel, Switzerland, September, 1965, and which will meet next in Los Angeles in 1967.

Some effects of community suicide prevention efforts are obvious. The taboos on observing and discussing suicidal behavior are reduced, and throughout the community there is increased interest and alertness concerning the clues to suicide. Will this tend to reduce the prevalence of suicide? Perhaps an attitude of guarded optimism is most appropriate.

REFERENCES

1. RESNIK, H. L. P.: Community anti-suicidal organization. Curr. Psychiat. Ther. 6:253-259, 1964.
2. McGEE, R. K.: The suicide prevention center as a model for community mental health programs. Comm. Ment. Health J. 1:162-170, 1965.

3. LITMAN, R. E., et al.: Suicide-prevention telephone service. J. Amer. Med. Ass. 192:21-25, 1965.
4. KAPHAN, M., AND LITMAN, R. E.: Telephone appraisal of 100 suicidal emergencies. Amer. J. Psychother. 16:591-599, 1962.
5. SHNEIDMAN, E. S., AND FARBEROW, N. L.: Clues to suicide. New York, McGraw-Hill, 1957.
6. FARBEROW, N. L., AND SHNEIDMAN, E. S.: Cry for Help. New York, McGraw-Hill, 1961.
7. LITMAN, R. E.: Psychiatric hospitals and suicide prevention centers. Comp. Psychiat. 6:119-127, 1965.
8. LITMAN, R. E.: Management of acutely suicidal patients in medical practice. Calif. Med. To be published.
9. KUBIE, L. S.: Multiple determinants of suicidal efforts. J. Nerv. Ment. Dis. 138:3-8, 1964.
10. GRINKER, R. R.: The psychodynamics of suicide and attempted suicide. George Washington University Symposium on Suicide, Oct. 1965.
11. FREUD, S.: Letter to Rev. Oskar Pfister. Psychoanalysis and Faith. New York, Basic Books Inc., 1963.
12. MARGOLIS, P. M., MEYER, G. G., AND LOUW, J. C.: Suicidal precautions. Arch. Gen. Psychiat. 13:224-231, 1965.
13. FARBEROW, N. L., SHNEIDMAN, E. S., AND LEONARD, C. V.: Suicide: evaluation and treatment of suicidal risk in psychiatric hospitals. Med. Bull. Veterans Admin. 8:1-11, 1962.
14. LESSE, S.: The psychotherapist and apparent remissions in depressed suicidal patients. Amer. J. Psychother. 19:436-444, 1965.

319

A Community Anti-Suicidal Organization

by H. L. P. RESNIK, M.D.

THE SUICIDAL INDIVIDUAL has been increasingly recognized as a community responsibility as well as a medical one. No longer is the suicide thought to be motivated only by disordered reason but often by a series of socio-environmental pressures. Medicine has been relatively inattentive in responding to the needs, to the pressures and to the follow-up care of these multitudes.[2,9] Consequently, it is not surprising that the medical slack[2-4] has been taken up by lay organizations such as the FRIENDS of Dade County, Florida.[6-8]

This anti-suicidal group was organized as the result of increased public sentiment following a series of emotional newspaper articles concerning the seriousness of the problem in the Miami-Miami Beach community. Resistance on the part of some service agencies and skepticism on the part of psychiatrists was the initial professional response. On the other hand, the newspaper, radio and television were more supportive. Forty-seven people initially presented themselves as workers and 26 remained following several organizational meetings during which officers were elected and approaches to the problem discussed. The community further donated the services of the telephone answering bureau, an ambulance service, a printing firm, and lastly, a meeting place in a municipal building. Contributions to the sum of $200 were utilized to maintain a post office box number, the telephone bill and mailing expenses. The telephone number chosen was FRanklin 4-3637, which spelled out F-R-I-E-N-D-S on the dial and was consequently easy to remember (fig. 1). A 24 hour duty roster was posted. Following the first several months, a training manual was evolved and utilized by the elected director of training who worked with all prospective members. Of the numerous questions that presented themselves, three appeared crucial: The foremost concerned the nature of those telephoning for help, the second, the nature of those individuals attracted to this type of work,

HELP IS AVAILABLE
24 hours of the day through Dade's suicide prevention unit.

Dial F-R-I-E-N-D-S
FR 4-3637
. . . and talk it over.

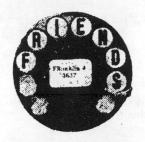

Fig. 1

and the last was whether suicidal persons will contact a wholly lay organization.

The Callers

A report card (fig. 2) containing vital statistics, personal history, and reasons for calling was completed for each caller and mailed directly to the consultant. The analysis of 602 calls during a 12-month period[7] from December 1, 1959, through November 30, 1960, indicated that two of every three callers were women, that half of the callers fell in

Given Name ______________ Case Number ________
Age ______ Sex ______ Color ______ Marital Status ________
Legal Residence ______________ Time Here ________
Occupation ______ Education ____ Religion ______ Attending? ____
Other Activities ______________ Organizations? ________
Medical Care? ________ When? ______ How Long? ________
Psychiatric Care? ________ When? ______ How Long? ________
Hospital Care? ________ When? ______ How Long? ________
Other Therapy? ________ When? ______ How Long? ________
Reason for Calling? ______________________
Considered Suicide: When? ______ Lightly? ______ Seriously? ____
Attempted Suicide: When? ______ How? ______ Seriously? ____
Suicidal Now? ______________ For How Long? ________
Date ______ Call From: Suicidal Person ______ or Other Person ____
Disposition ______________________

Fig. 2

the age ranges 30 through 49, and were from married individuals and that only 13 Negroes called. Housewives and white collar workers made up, respectively, 41 per cent and 31 per cent of the sample, Protestants 64 per cent, Catholics 22 per cent and Jews 13 per cent. About half indicated that they were suicidal at the time of the call, but only 14 per cent admitted to a previous attempt. Thirty-five per cent indicated they were drinking at the time of the call.

The Workers

Of the nuclear group of 25 workers available for calls and unselected for any variable other than their continued interest,[8] 22 were asked to complete a personal and social history form, and to undergo a series of psychologic tests.* For 19, an hour long clinical interview completed the appraisal. Of these, seven (28 per cent) were classified normal, 12 (68 per cent) neurotic, and six (24 per cent) as psychotic. A subsequent reevaluation applying criteria described by Kirkpatrick and Michael[5] for the Mid-town Manhattan Project Study resulted in some reshuffling of workers into different categories but without alteration of the findings that almost one quarter of the workers (24 per cent) fell within their severe and incapacitated group. This approximated the findings of 23.4 per cent incapacitated in the mid-town Manhattan population studied. The accumulated data were further considered in reference to the three worker categories. It was noted that normal workers handled 55 per cent of the calls, averaged a per capita case load of 45 (three times that of the neurotics, and two and a half times the psychotics) and were more flexible in their approach. The normals and neurotics coded a similar percentage of suicidal calls, 30 per cent and 28 per cent, respectively, which differed with the psychotic workers' high suicidal coding (37 per cent) and also differed with their estimation that two out of every three of their cases were serious suicide problems. The workers also reported a higher incidence of previous suicidal attempts (36 per cent) than did the callers (14 per cent). All eight of the suicidal Friends were either in the psychotic worker category (five of six workers) or in the neurotic depressive category (three out of four workers). While the latter workers did not appear to differ significantly from the total group in their management of their cases, the psychotic workers did.

---

*These consisted of the MMPI, House-Tree-Person drawings, and sentence completions administered and interpreted by Dr. Norman Reichenberg, Associate Professor of Psychology, Department of Psychiatry, University of Miami School of Medicine.

Another aspect of interest was the Friend's ability to assess the nature of the presenting call. A "Board of Experts" consisting of four third year psychiatry residents and three experienced clinical psychologists independently coded a randomly selected sample of 107 reports plus three special ones. These latter were records of successful suicides and will be discussed more fully. Of the 15 calls deemed suicidal by the Board, the Friends had correctly coded 13 of these. This strongly suggested that the Friends were not simply guessing as the probability of this occurring by chance was less than .01. Of the other 23 cases called suicidal by the workers, 14 were considered psychiatric, five personal gain, and two each social and informational; however, there was majority concurrence of the Experts and the Friends in each of the six categories.

Will Suicidal Persons Call?

A monthly list of all proper names and identifying data of callers was kept current, and regularly checked against the Medical Examiner's records for known suicides, and against the Jackson Memorial Hospital records for evidence of previous suicidal activity. The latter offered the only 24 hour emergency consultation psychiatric service and consequently most suicidal individuals were transferred there for care. The first 12 months of the operation revealed 169 persons having given proper names. Review of the Medical Examiner's 12 month total of 141 suicides revealed three persons who had called Friends prior to their act. The intervals between the call and act were 10 hours, 11 and 51 days, respectively. In effect, the organization had been contacted by 2 per cent of the reported suicides in the area.* Furthermore, the general hospital records of 91 callers out of the 169 possible names were located. These revealed that 25 or 27 per cent had been seen for an attempted suicide date *prior* to calling this organization, and that 19 (or 20 per cent) others had depressive symptomatology noted in their charts. These two categories made up almost half the sample, and did not include eight diagnosed psychotics and three alcoholics. Only 24 per cent of this traceable sample were without some prior recorded emotional difficulty.

During the first year's operation, the suicidal rate dropped from 17.11 to 16.24 per 100,000 population; however, this was in keeping with the previous year's downward trend. The most eye-catching and misleading results were those obtained by comparing 12 month periods, and these were the figures that constantly maintained the group's

---

*Personal communication from Joseph O'Lone, M.D., informed me that follow-up for 1961 revealed three callers and one worker who committed suicide.

enthusiasm. They indicated 10 less suicides or a drop of 6.6 per cent from the 151 suicides reported in the 12 months prior to the organization. Subsequent to these initial results several enthusiastic estimates must be revised.[1,2] It is when the Dade County rate is compared to the national rate that the first suggestion of FRIENDS' impact arises. For those three years prior to 1960, the change in the local rate paralleled that of the national scene. However, the first year's operation of FRIENDS was concommitant with a Miami-Miami Beach rate decrease of 0.8 per cent in the face of a continuing national rate increase of 0.09 per cent.[7]

ILLUSTRATIVE CASE REPORT

The first contact with a 75 year old man occurred with a telephone call from a parking lot attendant who had found a senile man wandering with no idea of his whereabouts, had searched his pockets for identification and had found a crumpled newspaper advertisement for FRIENDS. Another clipping 3 weeks old reported the suicide of an elderly widow. The organization was called and a Friend talked with the man who indicated that he lived alone in a small trailer and had been increasingly threatened by young hoodlums who demanded money from him. He said he did not know how to receive help or assistance and had thought of suicide by hanging most recently. During the conversation he was obviously confused. The worker took him to the Dade County Welfare Department and upon their recommendation to a nursing home and to a hospital for a preplacement physical. During this the man appeared quite relieved, was garrulous, and confided that he had a fair amount of money that he wanted his only son in New Jersey to receive. The worker suggested a will be drawn and arranged for an attorney friend to do this. The caller insisted that the Friend act as executor of the estate and he further gave him power of attorney to handle his affairs.

Approximately 1 month later the worker was informed that the man had fallen and injured himself. He summoned a physician and accompanied the ambulance to a hospital. Shortly after, the old man died of a cerebral vascular accident. The Friend then contacted the son, made funeral arrangements and attended the interring. The worker, a 65 year old retired hardware store owner, summarized the case as follows: "Everyone concerned felt very badly, but the man had spent 6 weeks at the home and those seemed to be happy ones. He confided to the other men staying there that he was very lucky and that God must have had something to do with it that he found FRIENDS and that Mr. M was the best friends he ever had."

This case is illustrative of many, although not all the facets of the FRIENDS organization. The program gradually evolved during the first year's operation, consisted of a clinical, a research, and a training and educative function. The clinical aspect of the work started with evalua-

324

tion of the suicide potential and determination of an appropriate disposition. The workers, determining the extent to which they should respond to the "cry for help" might deal completely by telephone, go to the caller's home, meet at a rendezvous, or escort the caller to the hospital emergency room. There were requests to accompany the police, and numerous referrals from the court, religious leaders and from agencies and physicians themselves. Following the initial disposition, some of the Friends retained a supportive relationship through periodic telephone calls and hospital visits. The organization, primarily through its consultant, was also in close liaison with the Dade County Medical Examiner who considered this of utmost value, thus confirming the Los Angeles experience.[1-3]

The research aspect of the program utilized some workers who did not deal with callers directly. Their work with administrative and statistical materials made it possible to offer meaningful information to those members working clinically and those active in training. The trainees were put through a long and controlled program of reading, discussion, and practical case work to prepare them for the clinical operation. Education was also community-oriented, consisting of a publicity committee to deal with the mass media in order to make known the problem magnitude and the services offered, and a lecture committee which presented the community suicidal problem before numerous groups. They also handled lectures to the police and to members of the nonprofessional hospital staffs.

The results of the FRIENDS program suggest that careful and thorough clinical evaluation of prospective workers be effected prior to their dealing directly with callers. Followup of the callers indicated that persons who were depressed and had not as yet attempted suicide, individuals with histories of previous suicide attempts, and individuals who would eventually kill themselves all have communicated with this group. The resultant effect upon the community was to increase the general awareness of the suicidal problem and to make known a group of individuals whose services were available. By the end of the first year's operation, FRIENDS of Dade County, Florida was a respected and utilized community organization.

REFERENCES

1. ELLIS, E. R., AND ALLEN, G. N.: Traitor Within, Our Suicide Problem. Garden City, Doubleday, 1961.
2. FARBEROW, N. L., AND SHNEIDMAN, E. S.: The Cry for Help. New York, McGraw Hill, 1961.

3. Fox, R.: Help for the Despairing, Work of the Samaritans Lancet, 2:1102-1105, 1962.
4. International Center of Information for Telephonic Help, 20 Promenade Saint Antoine, Geneva, Switzerland.
5. KIRKPATRICK, P., AND MICHAEL, S.: Study methods, mental health ratings. In: Srole, L. et. al. Mental Health in the Metropolis, The Midtown Manhattan Project Study, Vol. I. New York, McGraw-Hill, 1962.
6. RESNIK, H. L. P.: Observations on a Community Anti-Suicidal Organization, 'THE FRIENDS' of Dade County, Florida, Part I, The Organization (in press).
7. Ibid., Part II, The Callers (in press).
8. Ibid., Part III, The Workers (in press).
9. Ibid., Suicide and The Community, Florida Medical Society Annual Meeting, Miami Beach, Fla., 1960.

PART IX

THE AGED

Dynamic Psychotherapy of the Aged

by HAROLD HIATT, M.D.

Psychotherapy, on a dynamic basis, models itself upon the techniques of psychoanalysis. A misconception existed for many years that only the relatively young could benefit from psychotherapeutic techniques. Yet many psychiatrists and psychoanalysts,[1-11] recording their experiences in treating older patients, have reported generally good results.

The senescent patient, like the adolescent, commonly has problems in areas of independence-dependence, self-identification, difficulty with other generations, asceticism, affective disturbances, and other problems in interpersonal relationships. Often the aging patient repeats psychologically many of the personal problems that he had as a child or adolescent. This "daCapo effect" of "playing through the chorus again" of one's earlier problems is extremely common in older persons.

Twelve women and 7 men with a median age of 65 have been followed over the past 15 years by the author in outpatient psychotherapy. The average number of psychotherapy hours once or twice weekly was 10.05, the least number being 6 and the greatest being 119.

Fourteen patients had depressive reaction and the remaining 5 were in the categories of phobic, hypochondriacal, and anxiety neuroses. Busse[12] has cited the frequency of depression and hypochondriacal patterns of psychoneurosis in the aging population. The precipitating event leading to their referral for psychotherapy was a recent death of a spouse, cited in 6 instances; retirement, or retirement of a spouse, in 6; and a physical illness of a somatopsychic nature or psychosomatic variety in the remaining 6. Drugs were prescribed for 5 patients, but drug treatment was ancilliary to psychotherapy and not a primary mode of treatment.

Transference

There are two unusual features in dealing with the transference phenomenon of those beyond 60, unlikely to be seen in younger patients. First, there is the realistic fact that the therapist is likely to be 20 to 30 years younger than the patient, which has a definite impact on the transference. Second, the patient over age 60 has accrued many more key figures in his past history than is true of the younger patient. A spouse may occupy a greater span of years than a parental figure and children, who may be all that remain of the patient's family constellation. In the "replaying of the chorus" of those growing older, the therapist should try to uncover the "infantile neurosis"; however, other significant figures than the patient's parents may have an impact on the transference which the patient reflects with his physician.[13] Many important figures in one's life are symbolic representations of parents; however, the degree of emotional investment goes through some shifts as one ages.

The transference reactions of this group of 19 patients could be divided into many categories with a good deal of overlapping. There were four main transference reactions: (1) parental transference (7 patients); (2) peer or sibling transference (6 patients); (3) son, son-in-law, or grandson transference (4 patients); (4) sexual transference (2 patients).

Parental Transference. All persons who are ill, psychologically or physically, use the defense of regression to some degree. A patient who comes for treatment is asking the authority, physician, parental figure for help in the classical sense. The physician and the patient, regardless of their chronological ages, are forming a parent-child relationship.

In many instances, the aged, because of dependency needs, endow the therapist not only with parental powers, but with omnipotent powers similar to the hero worship of some children. The older person, because of the decreasing number of interested persons in his environment, may transfer to the therapist a "Godlike" trust. Perhaps it is true that the older segment of our population was reared in a "God-fearing" era, but the intensity of their faith in the therapist is in some instances frightening.[6]

A 62-year-old man was seen initially on a medical ward of a private hospital where he was convalescing from his second myocardial infarction. He had severe weeping spells as evidence of his depression. The physical illness meant weakness to him and was a severe threat to his masculinity.

In weekly psychotherapy sessions, he essentially was asking, "Show me how to be a man!" It was as though he was saying to himself, if I try to prove my masculinity by work, I fear another coronary; if I am sexually aggressive toward my wife, she will discard me. This had, in reality, been a mature, giving, dedicated man, but he needed a father figure to give him permission emotionally to be a man.

330

Peer or Sibling Transference. Six of the nineteen patients developed a transference to the therapist which has been labeled "peer transference." As the alliance in therapy developed, this put the therapist in the role of a deceased spouse, a confidant, a close colleague, or a sibling. It is true that a peer transference did not exclude a dependent, parental, or even sexual transference. But this group looked to the therapist to confirm ego reality, to help with decision making, and to share experiences of an interpersonal nature involving other members of the family. It may be somewhat startling to the therapist to have his age ignored and be transformed into a most trusted symbol of the patient's spouse, business associate, or roommate. It is felt that this type of transference reaction is unusual in psychotherapy with other age groups.

A 71-year-old widow gave as her main complaint, "My husband dropped dead right in front of my eyes." With the husband's precipitous death, the patient was left with a large amount of money, a large suburban home, and a large amount of guilt. In weekly psychotherapy, the transference was one in which the therapist was the all-powerful referee. He was to interpret and to advise her in many areas: medical problems with her internist needed to be more clearly understood; moving from a large estate to an apartment had to be negotiated; discussion with her financial advisor had to be double-checked; continuing rivalries with her daughter and sister needed to be moderated; and ambivalent questions of her spiritual devotion required discussion. The therapist was awarded the position of the husband with all of his power and omnipotence.

Son, Son-in-law, Grandson Transference. Ten of the nineteen patients made frequent references to sons, sons-in-law, or nephews in their therapeutic sessions. Four of these were considered to have this type of transference predominating. In this situation, the patient may consider himself as the teacher and the therapist as the pupil, involving a denial of dependency. Meerloo[8] refers to this as a filial transference. On the other hand, the older patient may feel impotent, weak, set back by physical illness, or financially dependent on the younger generation. This creates the "reverse oedipal" situation. This term is confusing until one realizes that the aging patient is reacting to the younger therapist in the way a child reacts to an adult. Those who have not worked through their initial oedipal feelings apparently do not do well when the roles are reversed.

An 84-year-old widow was referred by an internist who pleaded that the psychiatrist "just see her once," a frequent appeal to those interested in geriatric psychiatry. One week prior to the interview, the patient made a suicide attempt, taking a bottle of belladonna barbiturate combination prescribed, in smaller doses, to ease her persistent abdominal cramping. Transference to the therapist, on the one hand, was a clinging dependency alternating with a *"grande dame,"* intellectually superior, almost condescending position. The transference was reflected in two major themes seen in the pattern of several hours of therapy. The first was a discussion of the distant

331

past. She related, with authority, artistry, and magnetic charm, the culture, flavor, and historical significance of our fair city at the turn of the century. With validated accuracy, she described her late teens and early twenties in the social whirl of the horse-and-buggy, riverboat days of Cincinnati.

A second theme was a verbalization of anger, rivalry, and scathing indignation at her daughter and son-in-law, "the doctor." He was referred to frequently as a "dumb bastard" and an "ignorant son of a bitch," who had little class or culture and questionable professional ability.

Sexual Transference. Two patients formed an erotic or sexual transference to the therapist. Here again, one would describe dependent and peer elements in the relationship, but in the main, the response to therapy was not unlike the transference reaction seen in much younger, hysterical girls.

A 61-year-old widow described her phobia of leaving home or being alone. For the past 15 years, she had not left the city and maintained a coterie of servants including a chauffeur, a day maid, and a hired nighttime "baby-sitter" in an adjoining room. Rarely did she leave her apartment and then only with another person. In the seventh hour of a twice-a-week psychotherapy, the patient appeared in a bright pink coat, over a baby-blue dress with a pink fur hat. She protested that her fears were worse on the days of her appointment. When I pointed out that this might give some clue to the source of her fears, she associated as follows: "Thank God, it's a favorable sign; I wish I were 20 years younger [smiles at therapist]. This therapy is certainly expensive. Doctor, I have strong sensations sometimes, like a pulling at the base of the coccyx. When I was 9 or 10, I would get into the sideboard in the kitchen and take everything out, and put everything back in, and I would get a strange sensation. In grade school, when I was on a teeter-totter, I got this strange sensation. There was a boy in school, with a big hooked nose, who smelled like fish, and he told me to look and he unzipped his fly and I got that strange sensation."

Countertransference

It behooves the therapist to have a quite clear understanding of his relationship with his own parents and grandparents before treating other people's parents.[4,5,8,10,11] Countertransference reactions of oversolicitousness, idealization, and unrealistic expectations of strength on the one hand or subtle deprecations, competitive feelings, and pity on the other are commonly related to the therapist's own parents. Sometimes, the therapist feels that the older patient should be obeyed, feared, or praised, as derived from strong remnants of his own childhood. The therapist may undermine the aging persons's self-esteem if he is too condescending or patronizing.[2]

The sexual taboo with older patients is similar to the resistance met by Freud in the discovery of infantile sexuality.[8] Grotjahn[5] said that the therapist who hopes the "old person will live beyond sin and sex, like angels, is likely not to understand one of their most important sources of conflicts, guilt, and depression."

The incidence of debilitating physical illness and death is high in the aging segment of the population. Four of these nineteen patients have died, one while therapy was in progress. Countertransference reactions to this possibility must be considered. A not uncommon response by the therapist is denial and the insistence that the patient be "healthy." This may serve to counteract wishes for their death and the therapist's guilt of surviving.[9] A frightening aspect for the therapist is the deep transference of a lonely, fearful, depressed person without opportunity to form new object relationships other than that established with the therapist.[14] Rechtschaffen[14] posed the question "Does the emphasis on supportive measures for older patients in part represent a tendency to provide a less valued form of therapy for a less valued segment of the population?"

I endeavored to create a professional, peer kind of interaction with my 19 patients; however, illogical or irrational influences on countertransference appeared. They fell into four general categories:

1. *An omnipotent or unrealistic hope, with 2 patients.* A 65-year-old married woman had a reactive depression with anxiety. She had attacks of auricular fibrillation with syncope. She was seen in 31 sessions with some improvement. However, the physical decline of her arteriosclerotic heart and brain disease prevailed over psychologic treatment. In retrospect, it was unrealistic to attempt treating this patient with psychotherapy.

2. *The countertransference of feeding one's narcissism and gaining a kind of personal pleasure or personal gratification, with 8 patients.* A 68-year-old married man complained of depression and mild compulsive rituals. He was in the process of transferring his large company to his 41-year-old son, as his father had transferred the company to him. The psychiatrist was placed in the role of "superconsultant" to examine the emotional factors involved in the "changing of the guard" of a leading industrial firm. The therapist must keep close watch on his narcissistic fantasies and be careful to delineate his limited professional role to his patient and avoid the "therapist of a tycoon" role.

3. *An unreasonable anger, desire to avoid, or distinct feeling of the work of treatment, with 3 patients.* A 60-year-old married sales manager was experiencing depression with insomnia and anxiety. After 30 years of service, he became aware aware that he would never be general manager of the company. He used the therapist's support and diagnosis to gain a leave of absence with pay for 6 months and then a premature full retirement. As a crowning blow, at 2-week intervals, he submitted to the therapist forms for liberal sickness and health benefits from four different insurance companies. I had the countertransference response of "being had" by an oral aggressive patient who was acting out a plan he had devised in his many years of administrative manipulation.

4. *The feeling of pity and sorrow for a wasted life, or sympathy rather than professional empathy, with 6 of the patients.* A 61-year-old mother of five children conceived her role in life as a progressive liberal, scholar, and teacher. While in the hospital, she developed anxiety and tension of psychotic

333

proportions, after a radical breast operation. Metastatic carcinoma was demonstrated in the long bones. All of her five children had joined the "freaked-out" generation through drug ingestion and nomadism. Although they had all entered good colleges, four were dropouts. One son disappeared totally. Her psychosis cleared and she convalesced with supportive hormone treatment for terminal cancer. At this point, her husband of 34 years died of a coronary occlusion and she was left alone, though still quite mobile.

Discussion

The psychological ills of the older population seem to respond well to dynamic psychotherapy. Older patients are often wise, are full of zest (if they pace their energy), and may exhibit a degree of motivation in therapy not often seen in younger patients.

REFERENCES

1. Butler, R. N.: Intensive Psychotherapy for the Hospitalized Aged. Geriatrics 15:644-653, 1960.
2. Gitelson, M.: The Emotional Problems of Elderly People. Geriatrics 3:135-150, 1948.
3. Goldfarb, A. I.: Patient-Doctor Relationship in Treatment of Aged Persons. Geriatrics 19:18-23, 1964.
4. Goldfarb, A. I., and Turner, H.: Psychotherapy of Aged Persons. II. Utilization and Effectiveness of "Brief" Therapy. Amer. J. Psychiat. 109:916-921, 1953.
5. Grotjahn, M.: Analytic Psychotherapy with the Elderly. Psychoanal. Rev. 42:419-427, 1955.
6. Kahana, R. J.: Medical Management, Psychotherapy, and Aging. J. Geriatr. Psychiat. 1:78-89, 1967.
7. Kaufman, M. R.: Old Age and Aging: The Psychoanalytic Point of View. Amer. J. Orthopsychiat. 10:73-84, 1940.
8. Meerloo, J. A. M.: Transference and Resistance in Geriatric Psychotherapy. Psychoanal. Rev. 42:72-82, 1955.
9. Peck, A.: Psychotherapy of the Aged. J. Amer. Geriat. Soc. 14:748-753, 1966.
10. Wolff, K.: Individual Psychotherapy with Geriatric Patients. Dis. Nerv. Syst. 24:688-691, 1963.
11. Zinberg, N. W.: Psychoanalytic Consideration of Aging. J. Amer. Psychoanal. Ass. 12:151-159, 1964.
12. Busse, E. W.: Geriatrics Today—An Overview. Amer. J. Psychiat. 123:1226-1233, 1967.
13. Greenson, R. R.: The Classic Psychoanalytic Approach. In: Arieti, S. (Ed.), American Handbook of Psychiatry, Vol. II. New York, Basic Books, Inc., 1959, pp. 1399-1415.
14. Rechtschaffen, A.: Psychotherapy with Geriatric Patients: A Review of the Literature. J. Geront. 14:78-83, 1953.

The Physician's Management of the Dying Patient

by CHARLES WILLIAM WAHL, M.D.

THE FEAR OF DEATH is in many ways unique in psychic life, for unlike other fears and anxieties which owe their frightening import to the possibility only of a foreboding and dreaded circumstance, death is certain and unavoidable for all mankind. Uniquely, it is the one known fear whose referent is based on an absolutely unavoidable circumstance. In strict objectivity, it is the one inescapable fear with which we deal, based on the reality, which we often tend to ignore, that life is finite and we are finite with it. Aeschylus expressed man's plight in a very graphic way 2300 years ago:

> Alone of gods Death loves not gifts; with him
> Nor sacrifice nor incense aught avails;
> He hath no altar and no hymns of gladness;
> Prayer stands aloof from him, Persuasion fails.

While it is with awe and with pride that we survey man's fantastic progress since Aeschylus wrote these lines, with the phenomenon of Death it remains exactly as he has described it. We can postpone death, we can assuage its physical pain, but escape it we cannot.

Since the inescapable hallmark of the human estate is its finitude, then on one level the fear of death is the deliberate and rational apprehension that one day we shall cease to be. One might expect that under this condition all of us would be in a state of chronic apathy and depression; yet it is a noteworthy and remarkable paradox that while we all must die, we do not all fear death to the same degree nor in the same way.

Now this should prompt us as psychiatrists to ask several germane questions. First, does the fear of death, or thanatophobia, as it is designated in its maximal form, because of the inescapability of its referent evoke or necessitate unique methods of defensive reduction in the psychic economy? We know that the fearful concept, object or circumstance in a phobia is comparable to the manifest content of dreams, i.e., its ostensible concern only conceals another one which is more unacceptable to the self, which is latent and repressed. Is thanatophobia an exception to this rule? Can there be anything more fearful to the organism than the cessation of its being?

It is a matter not without its dynamic import that these questions, germane as they are, have never been properly addressed by psychiatry— a profession that prides itself on investigating things which others wish to shun. An entire bibliography on the subject makes very scant reading indeed. For the sad truth is that we do not have very satisfactory answers for these questions. The massive psychological defenses against death that are more fulsomely applied by mankind in the handling of this fear than in any other area of human experience have not exempted psychiatrists from their employment. The elucidation of this whole area remains one of the great tasks of our generation.

The scope of these defenses may not be immediately apparent to us without reflection. Until quite recently the very word death was taboo. Cumbersome and elaborate euphemisms were employed instead, such as "passed away" or "passed on," and the dead were referred to as the "departed." The persistence with which man has believed in an immortal state without the slightest shred of evidence that he chooses to collect in the establishment of other beliefs is noteworthy. The very word "perish" is from the Latin "perire," meaning "to pass through," an insistence that death is a transition rather than a cessation. There are those who maintain that religion can be explained as a gigantic defense against death by the guarantee of an immortal state which it is purported can be obtained by adherence to its system of belief. In addition, at gigantic cost and expressly against the tenets of the prevailing Judeo-Christian ethics, there is maintained a multibillion dollar industry, "the undertakers," to shield us from ever looking at an untreated dead person. They purvey to us an illusion, an illusion of sleep and incorruptibility. These cultural defenses are so effective that the vast majority of persons live their entire lives without ever viewing death in its pristine form.

These complex social taboos against death protect from involvement with it all segments of the population except for two groups only—the medical and the nursing professions. The physician and the nurse cannot isolate themselves from death. They see it not in its prettified form, but before the intervention of the artful hand of the embalmer. They see the deceased with his rigor mortis, agape mouth, staring eyes, and with the slack expression of the newly dead. It is the rare physician who does

336

not remember his first such contact. It is a powerful and compelling experience.

It is significant, however, that this experience rarely provokes in a physician or a nurse the fear that such an experience might presume to produce in other groups, and this seemingly has not just to do with the physician's habituation to these sights. It is appropriate for us to consider how this may be.

The usual defense against death is a precipitate of the infantile omnipotence, and this reflects itself as a complete inability to unconsciously credit or believe that the immutable self can ever cease to be. This precipitate is stronger in previously loved and cherished persons in childhood, for reasons discussed elsewhere.* And so it may be that persons who become physicians can forego the usual defenses which require separation from "memento mori" and choose a profession that brings them into contact with the dead and dying because of exceptional ego strength and feelings of magical invulnerability resultant from such childhood experiences. I am sure that oftentimes this must be so. An opposite pattern, however, also could result in the choice of medicine as a profession. I have been struck, in the physicians whom I have treated in psychotherapy for other matters, how frequently one encounters a strong antecedent fear of death of considerable proportions in their history. It would appear that the later choice of medicine as a profession sometimes may represent a counterphobic defense against death, a reaction formation to an earlier fear of it mastered by the doing of the very thing that was previously frightening. It seems sometimes to represent a kind of identification with the aggressor, a wish to be on the winning team. Just as the guilty little boy may end up as a lawyer and be comforted by being the judge rather than the judged, so the physician may handle the fear of death by identification with the profession of medicine, for by paleologic definition it is always the patient who gets sick and dies, not the doctor. In the unconscious, the M.D. degree confers immunity to all the ills and vicissitudes that beset our patients. Perhaps another indication of this is the oft-noted tendency of doctors to give sage advice that they never follow themselves. Most of us smoke and are overweight, we work too hard, we tend to ignore the rules of simple hygiene, we fail to get sufficient exercise and rest. These are of course dangerous things to do, and we would get quite angry with a patient if he did these things. It is significant that they do not evoke in us, however, the same sense of self-preservative horror. Doctors, too,

---

*Wahl, Charles W.: The Fear of Death: *In* The Meaning of Death, edited by Herman Feifel, Ph.D. New York, McGraw-Hill Book Company, 1959.

as any nurse will confirm, are notoriously bad patients when they themselves are ill. It is as if they are shocked and outraged at the wholly unbelievable fact that they themselves can be ill. In addition to this another defense for the handling of this or any fear is to learn all about it. Knowledge gives an illusion of control, and one is rarely so frightened of a thing well known to one.

These patterns of behavior have particular relevance to the physician's management of the dying or the terminally ill patient. For this antimony in the physician's character, his earlier fear of death handled by denial, reaction formation and identification with the aggressor, and his subsequent counterphobic feelings of magical omnipotence and invulnerability may result in a failure to perceive the fear of death and illness in his patients and particularly leads to mismanagement of the dying or terminally ill patient. The price of his comfort may be to remain oblivious and consequently uninvolved at a time when the patient badly needs his care.

The unconscious attitudes towards the dying which exist covertly and implicitly in our culture are often overt and explicit in more primitive cultures. Anthropologic scrutiny of these cultures helps us better to see our own subtle practices.

In many cultures the moment the process of dying begins the dying ones become an object of fear and uncanny dread. The onlookers, even the close family, respond as though contact with them may cause themselves to die. In some cultures, the dying are removed from the community to die neglected alone in the "death hut" outside the village. We do not have to look far in our hospitals to see that our dying too are often in a sense abandoned. It is not a rare sight on a ward to see a terminally ill patient alone in a room at the end of the hall with an IV rigged, the oxygen hissing, and the staff far away comforted by the feeling that they have done all they can.

In other cultures the dying person is presumed to commit a hostile act by so doing, and in one instance it is the custom to "beat him to it," so to speak, by hitting him over the head with a club. Do we ever, as physicians, feel that the patient, by perversely dying, has turned traitor, so to speak, by challenging our omnipotence, and is our detachment from him an expression of unconscious anger which the savage experiences more directly? Apropos of this, the arguments adduced in favor of euthanasia often appear to be in the service of relieving the doctor of his hostility, care and guilt rather than being such a service to the recipient. Moreover, when a patient begins to die, he is hard to love. There is a natural, though primitive, wish to free libidinal cathexis from him. It is also a common experience for the terminally ill patient to regress

338

and to become more selfish and infantile, narcissistic and demanding. We are often not prepared to face these character traits which are unpleasant, and we may respond with a vague, guilty anger. Also when a patient knows he is going to die, unconsciously he wants to punish the ones who will survive, particularly the doctor who does not save him. This may serve too to provoke the physician or the nurse to view the patient as alien, separate and frightening and justify a gradual detachment from him. These primitive practices, "anläge" of which are residual in our own unconscious, may give us clues as to how we may better help the dying patient.

Hence the most important and necessary precondition in the management of the terminally ill is that the physician have the willingness and capacity to look deeply within himself not only in scrutiny of his attitudes towards living and dying and some of the unconscious equivalences of the latter, but also an addressment to what might be called the eternal questions—"Whence came I? Whither go I?"—and have derived in terms of his own needs and understanding answers that are meaningful and significant for himself.

With this as a preludium, it is then possible to consider objectively what are the goals in managing the care of a terminally ill patient and how may this best be done. The primary goal is to assuage the terror of death and of the process of dying in the patient, not only to prevent these from adversely affecting the course of the disease, since it is quite possible to be "frightened to death," but to enable the patient, if needs be, to die with dignity and serenity in the fullest possession of his human faculties that his state permits. To this end, it is important that the patient not be deprived of hope. It is a surprising thing that the possibility of personal surcease is not resident in the unconscious. Even though the rational probabilities of survival may be slight, the individual is obdurately immune to reality testing in this area. The defense of denial in the face of death is absolute and inveterate and is persisted in even in those patients who assert that they recognize and accept this fact, and even in patients who had been categorically told so by their physicians.

The extent to which this is operative has to be seen to be believed. I recall a physician who suffered from a neoplastic disease of great malignancy. He was deeply depressed until on looking up the literature he discovered that there was a five-year survival rate of 4 per cent. He became immediately much more cheerful, convinced against logic and probability that he would be of the 4 per cent, not of the 96 per cent, and this overweening optimism persisted until his death. Las Vegas should convince us that we all, in the depths of our selves, feel immune to the laws of chance that govern others. Unconsciously, we all agree with the psalmist David who said, "A thousand shall fall at thy right hand and ten thousand at thy left, but it shall not come nigh thee." The task of the physician is to strengthen and buttress the natural and ever present defenses of denial. This small area of paleologic unreality is permitted to exist, so that the rest of the personality may be preserved reachable and intact. It must be remembered that the peculiar torture of capital punishment is not death itself (for we all must die and the death of execution itself is not a painful one), but in the fact of knowing exactly when death will occur.

The physician then, for humanitarian reasons as well as scientific ones, must never give a sentence of death and the patient is never permitted to be bereft of hope. It is my conviction that no patient should ever be told he is going to die, even if he assures his physician that he wants the "naked truth." He should be told, "You have a serious problem, but no illness is without hope and you should remember that." The patient is helped to utilize his best defenses, namely, those of denial and infantile omnipotence. To make the hope more believable it is also important not to overassure the patient or to be unduly cheerful out of context.

It is important that the patient also not be permitted to be isolated, either from friends and relatives or from the staff. The Greeks said that the most horrible of ills was not to die but to die alone. Regularity and predictability of contact with the physician implies continuity to the patient, continuity of care to the conscious, but the probability of continuity of life to the unconscious. It implies a promise, "I will see you again tomorrow at the same time and you have nothing to fear in the interim." And this dependable certainty alone has great efficacy in making the patient more comfortable. For just this reason, however, great care must be taken not to omit a promised visitation. Relatives should also be encouraged not to isolate the patient, though constant and unduly prolonged visitation should not be permitted. This implies to the patient the "death watch."

The patient is helped to make a symbolic displacement from his concern about his incurable illness to ones which are curable. He should be encouraged to be somewhat hypochondriacal and the physician should listen with interest and attention to all his complaints, particularly the physical ones and ones related to intercurrent infections, colds, skin rashes, etc. which can be treated and cured. These should be vigorously treated. The patient, by "trading up" illnesses, receives an intense reassurance and a magical relief, as though he were exchanging his fatal illness for others less lethal.

To the same end one should deliberately focus attention on the patient's "immortal physiology," such as the processes of digestion and elimination.

He should be questioned at length about these functions, and it is remarkable to see how often the obsessive–compulsive narcissistic regression of the terminally ill manifests itself in an extreme overconcern and interest in bowel movements. It represents a regressive return to infantile logic and the infantile conception of disease—"If I just avoid drafts and have a good bowel movement I can never be ill."

One should listen attentively to the patient's complaints and to the key words with which he voices them and pay particular attention to those which express a symbolic fear of death. Terminally ill patients may have a recurrence of fear of the dark, or of closed doors, or of lying recumbent or of numbness or coldness, and the wording of such phrases as "I'm deathly afraid of the dark," "I feel boxed in when the door is closed," show the primary anxiety. Recumbency may be equated with "laying down to die." All of these demands, and many of them are quite idiosyncratic, should be unobtrusively complied with. For the same reason it is not a service to the patient to utterly ablate any pain he may be experiencing. To feel nothing is to be dead, and the terror complete analgesia may produce far outweighs the advantage. The same considerations apply in the use of ataraxic or sedative drugs. These are, in my experience, rarely efficacious, particularly since the isolation and detachment from reality which they may produce cause terror in its own right. Admittedly there is a need for further experience with their use.

The patient should be touched. Not only because this assuages the fear of being "untouchable," the dying thing, a feared object, but because the touch, the caress, is the most archaic pre-verbal way we possess of communication, solace and comfort. The mother uses it long before words can solace, and to lightly pat or touch the patient who is disturbed or frightened communicates a comfort that words can never convey. Frequent backrubs and massages, therefore, not only engender physical well being, but psychic as well. Also cosmetic care of the patient should not be neglected. This is particularly important for a woman.

The patient should not be treated as if he had no future. All patients should be encouraged to plan for the future for themselves and for their relatives and children. Children are, in the unconscious, "the fruit of our loins," immortal extensions of ourselves, living defenses against the fear of being blotted out. Terminally ill patients derive comfort and satisfaction from visitation with relatives and children and in planning for them. No hospital should be organized in such a way as to prevent this contact with family members. And it is a service not only to the patient but to his survivors. Their own guilt and sadness is assuaged by opportunities to make such a service to their loved one.

Lastly, if the patient is a member of a religion that makes mandatory that he be told of any possibility of his death, this should not be done "in extremis," but should rather be done while the patient is well enough to make what plans may seem to him to be important and while he still has time to re-employ the usual denial defenses.

While the physician does not bludgeon the patient with the full and exact truth about his status, it is important that one or preferably two of his close family be informed. This is necessary for legal reasons and to enable them to have time to adjust also to the possible death of the patient.

It is remarkable to note that these simple measures, when practiced by a warm and empathetic physician, acting in concert as they do with the powerful defenses of denial, reaction formation and undoing which the seriously ill person can call upon, usually suffice in themselves to enable the terminally ill patient to cope successfully with his situation.

In a small minority of patients, however, these measures are insufficient to produce relief. In these patients the prospect of their imminent death may provoke a terror, depression or apathy that can progress to a psychotic decompensation if unchecked. The treatment of choice for these patients is intensive psychotherapy and it should begin as soon as possible after consultation.

The following is a brief enumeration of some of the factors which appear to inhere in psychotherapeutic work with the terminally ill. In the treatment of these patients it is remarkable to note, considering the seriousness and inexorability of the reality situation, how quickly the terror and depression which they have experienced is moderated and how greatly they appear to be benefited. This appears to be explained by two factors. Firstly the psychiatrist attempts to supply the patient with a unique experience in that he, in contradistinction to the other persons who surround the patient, is better able to tolerate the discussion of material frightening to him without utilizing the defensive isolation, detachment and fearful projection which others may have employed. The psychiatrist takes particular care to see the patient faithfully at the stated intervals and makes himself available to the patient at any other time he may urgently require it. Secondly, a significant difference between psychotherapy with the terminally ill and other psychoneurotic conditions is that with extraordinary rapidity a strongly positive and dependent transference to the therapist is established and very archaic aspects of ego function and interpersonal relationship are evidenced. The speed with which this archaic, regressive transference is established is not paralleled by any other treatment situation known to me. The therapist becomes in rapid order the omnipotent, primordial parent imago, and as

*Eissler, K. R.: The Psychiatrist and the Dying Patient. New York International Universities Press, Inc., 1955.

342

soon as this kind of transference is established the patient appears to have an almost complete assuagement of the terror, anxiety, depression and reality alienation that preceded treatment. The healthy usual denial defenses and the feelings of infantile omnipotence and invulnerability are then reconstituted in their pristine strength and the patient, even though consciously aware of the seriousness of his illness, and often experiencing considerable physical pain, acts as though he had "a new lease on life."

In psychotherapy with any other kind of neurosis this "transference neurosis" would be explored, studied and analyzed. In psychotherapy of the terminally ill, scrutiny of it is deliberately avoided. In addition, everything which will further reality contact and serve to limit regression to this single area of exaggerated magical relationship is done. The patient is seen, if he is ambulatory, *vis-à-vis*, and never should be worked with on the couch. The face and person of the therapist should be constantly available for testing scrutiny.

The therapist is often in a dilemma when material relating to a concomitant or antecedent neurotic problem is produced. To work with this material dynamically may in some patients produce a serious depression, since the patient unconsciously knows that he is preparing himself for better function for a future which he will not possess. And yet perhaps even more frightening to him is the thought that the therapist by so doing employs denial defenses more patently magical than his own. It is necessary to be very individualistic in the approach to the patient. Just as some persons facing certain death may be solaced by engrossing themselves in a chess game, so occasionally, after the denial defenses are re-established, the patient, with serene detachment, studies himself as though he were another. Other patients deal with quotidian experiences only or experience a second childhood which often seems to subserve the same purpose the second childhood does in the old, namely, a counterphobic reaction formation against age, death and dying, and a return to that period in life in which one was most alien and distant from the concept of death. They experience a most pleasurable revivification of early days and memories when death was far off, and this identity with one's former youthful self may persist unabated until the final moment.

It is clear, too, that another avenue of relief for the patient is based on the unconscious conception of cure—one which is described and utilized by all primitive tribes, that is, that of transference in the concrete sense— a *transfer* of the patient's ills to the therapist, as does the witch doctor who, for a fee, takes upon himself the illnesses of his clients. The dreams of the patient show decided evidence of the hope, the expectation even, that "the therapist will die instead of myself." Needless to say, this is left uninterpreted to the patient. He is instead allowed the magical lift in his

343

spirits which it produces and it is presumed that the therapist has worked through his own feelings about death and dying so that it may not be necessary for himself to feel the need to empathetically detach himself from the patient when he perceives these wishes on his part.

Finally we come to a question that perhaps you have perceived I have not dealt with previously, namely, the countertransference of the therapist and how he is affected by developing an intimate identification and relationship with a person who will soon die. I must candidly acknowledge that doing psychotherapy with the few such patients I have treated has been the most difficult and challenging professional experience of my life. Martin Grotjahn* has said that a therapist must be like the harp player in that like him he develops a callus on the tip of each finger so that he may pluck the strings without bleeding. And yet, despite this, he must have a sure and delicate touch and a consummate sensitivity to all the nuances of the strings. This is harder to achieve in psychotherapy with the dying than with any other patient; and short of one's personal psychoanalysis, I know of no experience which gives one deeper insights into oneself or others.

Perhaps this shows us that what one really does for and with a patient in this most inescapable of all life situations is to say covertly to him, "Time and Space have no representation in the unconscious. Be solaced by the knowledge that but an eyeblink of time separates my death and the death of all mankind from your own." The willingness to do this without horror or abandonment of the patient gives him a solace that one day we shall have a right to expect from another for ourselves. It will enable him and later ourselves to follow Bryant's advice in *Thanatopsis:*

> So live that when thy summons comes to join
> The innumerable caravan which moves
> To that mysterious realm where each shall take
> His chamber in the silent halls of death,
> Thou go not like the quarry slave at night,
> Scourged to his dungeon, but, sustained and soothed
> By an unfaltering trust, approach thy grave
> Like one that wraps the drapery of his couch
> About him and lies down to pleasant dreams.

*Personal communication.

REFERENCES

SHAPLEY, HARLOW, RAPPORT, SAMUEL, AND WRIGHT, HELEN: A Treasury of Science. New York, Harper and Bros., 3rd ed., revised, 1954.

WAHL, CHARLES W.: The Fear of Death. Bull. Menninger Clin. 22:214-223, 1958.

PART X

FAMILY THERAPY

Family Diagnosis and Therapy

by NATHAN W. ACKERMAN, M.D.

FOR MANY PSYCHIATRISTS schooled and trained along established paths of theory and practice, and oriented to the one-to-one relationship of doctor and patient, a method of diagnosis and therapy for the whole family signifies a radical departure from tradition. It constitutes a major shift from an exclusive focus on the manifestations of mental illness in the individual to a system of diagnosis and treatment directed to the family unit as the matrix of health. It is still relatively crude, exploratory and experimental, but is a fluid, evolving procedure.

In the purview of history, the effort to diagnose, treat, and prevent personality disorders through a family approach is propelled by several converging forces: (1) the revolutionary transformation of the family pattern, induced by social change; (2) the recognition of the principle of contagion in emotional disturbance, and the intimate connection between social and mental disorder; (3) the greater appreciation of the limitations of the conventional procedures of diagnosis, treatment and prevention that are restricted to the individual patient; and (4) specific new developments in the behavioral sciences which include a range of studies in ego psychology, small group dynamics, social psychology, anthropology and communication. Such developments, rapidly unfolding on the contemporary scene, bring a rising pressure for a method of study and therapeutic intervention in the family group as a living entity.

It is self-evident that the course and outcome of illness rest not alone on the content of unconscious disturbance, but also on the resources that can be mobilized to counteract the core of pathogenic experience. A more expanded understanding of the relations between inner and outer experience would illuminate the mechanisms of coping with conflict. It would shed light on operations of defense, homeostatic control, and on the learning and growth processes of personality.

Almost always, in discussions of contemporary mental health services, the tendency is to leap to what appears, at first glance, to be the practical side of the problem, the chronic disproportion between the limitations of available mental health facilities and the ever-mounting demand for them. Always the same outcry: more hospitals, clinics, psychiatrists, psychologists, social workers and expanded resources for professional training. But surely the quantitative insufficiency in mental health services in the present day community is not the only issue. We must face other questions. Do the conventional therapeutic procedures really cure? Are they appropriate and specific to the disorders characteristic of our time and culture? Are the goals of therapy linked to the goals of prevention? If not, why not? It is in relation to such questions that we must examine the implications of the concepts of family diagnosis and family psychotherapy.

At the family level, the procedures of diagnosis and treatment are interdependent activities. On the one hand, diagnostic judgment determines the clarity and appropriateness of the choice of therapeutic goals and the specificity of the techniques of family psychotherapy. On the other hand, it is the therapeutically oriented family interview that is itself the pathway to diagnosis.

The goals of family therapy are therefore: (1) to alleviate emotional distress and disablement and to promote the level of health, both in the family group and in its individual members; (2) to strengthen the individual against destructive forces, both within him and surrounding him in the family environment; (3) to strengthen the integrative capacity of the family. This calls for a continuous effort to enhance the homeostatic balance of both the family and the individual. It means the introduction of those influences that favorably alter the balance of forces, as between those tendencies that maintain effective health in family living and those that move toward breakdown and illness. It also signifies a concern with the level at which the family members complement one another's emotional needs, buttress one another's defenses and how this, in turn, affects the balancing and harmonizing of essential family functions.

Until now, we cannot be said to have developed a true psychotherapy of the family group, but rather only feeble and ersatz gestures in this direction. By the qualifying term 'true,' we mean a specific method of intervention that influences the family as an organismic whole, based on systematic diagnosis of family development and behavior, focused on distortion of interactional patterns, coping with the interplay between interpersonal and intrapersonal conflict, and pointing its techniques toward the relations between the emotional functioning of the family as a unit and the emotional development and destiny of any one member.

Individual therapy, or even therapy of family pairs, while exerting certain partial effects on family relations, does not of itself signify a true family therapy. Such forms of treatment concern themselves only minimally with the health functioning of the family as a whole; the effect on family relationships is indirect, secondary and non-specific. Such therapy may help or harm family relationships. It may bring family members closer together or, paradoxically, it may intensify the trend toward alienation among them. By contrast, a true family psychotherapy points its corrective influence not toward the isolated individual, but rather to the family and the relations of the family with its members.

The rationale for this method of intervention can be summed up as follows: it is a natural level of therapeutic participation in human distress. It approaches troubled persons in their usual habitat, the family and home. It defines human conflicts and disablements not in isolation, but rather in the matrix of significant relationships, the day by day intimate interchange among family members. It gives recognition to the principle that the experiences of family participation play a potent part in making or breaking the mental health of its members. These experiences may precipitate an illness, may fixate a member in illness, may reward him for staying ill, or, by contrast, motivate him for recovery.

These principles are strongly documented by clinical observation. Their validity rests on a basic axiom: mental illness by its very nature is a contagious and communicable type of disorder. The seeds of mental breakdown are passed from person to person, from one generation to the next. They exert their influence within the mind of one individual and also move between the multiple minds of family members. Over the stretch of time, the center of pathogenic conflict experience may move from one part of the family to another. It is in this sense that the chain of family relations constitutes a kind of conveyor belt of disturbance, a carrier of pathogenic foci. The contagious influence is transmitted across time and also across space. In fact, it is the organizational pattern of the family group that determines in great part how each member asserts his emotional need and which of his defenses against anxiety become operable or inoperable. To achieve his objective, the family therapist must pursue the following aims:

(1) Help the family achieve a more clear definition of the real content of conflict. The first step, in this sense, is to stir a greater accuracy of perception and a lessening of the confusion of interpretation of family conflict.

(2) Counteract inappropriate displacements of conflict.

(3) Neutralize the irrational prejudices and scapegoating that are

349

involved in the displacement of conflict. The effort here is to put the conflict back where it came from in family role relationships, that is, to reattach it to its original source and attempt to work it out there, so as to counteract the trend toward prejudicial assault and disparagement of any one member.

(4) Relieve an excessive load of conflict on one victimized part of the family, either an individual or family pair.

(5) Lift concealed interpersonal conflicts to the level of interpersonal relations, where they may be coped with more effectively.

(6) Activate an improved quality of emotional complementarity in family role relationships.

(7) Replace the lacks in the patterns of family interaction through the appropriate and selective use of the therapist's personality. This means a discriminating injection of healthy elements of emotional interaction to replace sick ones, as the alignments in family relationships shift.

In family life, disorder of emotional communication can be a serious problem. At one pole, there is the type of family in which the members hardly communicate at all; the group is fragmented and the members are alienated from one another. At the opposite pole, there is the type of family whose members have abundant contact, but they battle one another continuously in a destructive way. The distrust and the hostility are fierce. There is a strong tendency to deny and displace the blame and guilt. The members of the group argue about the wrong matters or about trivialities, and they make scapegoats of one another. Loss of emotional control is a constant threat; now and then, there may even be an outbreak of physical violence. In such families, periods of acute chaos are not uncommon, or the family alternates between phases of murderous silence and explosions of uncontrolled fighting.

In dealing with the emotional problems of family groups, the clinician fulfills the part of a parent or grandparent. He is interested; he is actively involved. He uses his therapeutic self in a special way. He activates an increasingly correct definition of the important areas of family conflict. He confronts the members with these conflicts. He elaborates their expressions, their harmful consequences, not merely for one individual, but for all members. He elucidates the failing and injurious results of the family's habitual ways of coping with these conflicts, and shares with the members his view of the deviant and destructive efforts at control and defense. He stirs an awakening to other avenues of possible solution, or at least compensation of conflict. Whenever needed, he injects into the hopper of family discussion more

350

appropriate and fitting images of family relations, with the corresponding healthier kinds of emotion.

The role of the family therapist, therefore, is an active, open, forthright one. In this situation, there can be no question of therapeutic anonymity; the therapist cannot hide his face nor can he be merely a passive listener. He pitches in with the family, implementing the emotional elements which are missing in family interaction. He acts as a kind of catalyst or chemical reagent dissolving the barriers to communication, stirring the interactional processes among the family members, shaking up the elements and promoting a realignment of family relationships toward health. He follows the movement of the center of sickness-producing disturbance from one part of the family to another. In so doing, he engages the family members in a process of working through of the elements of conflict. The core of pathogenic conflict may shift about from the mother-child pair to the husband-wife pair, and, at times, it may become concentrated in one member, such as a child, who often becomes the pawn of conflict between the parents. As the central conflict moves about from one place in the family group to another, the therapist follows along, stirring selective support now to one part of the family, now to another. He may call pointed attention to facial expressions, body postures, movements, etc.; by these means, he hopes to expand and sharpen the perception of relevant conflict experience. With discretionary use of these subverbal aspects of intercommunication, the therapist is enabled to challenge unreal and impossible demands, fruitless, vindictive forms of blaming and omnipotent destructive invasions of one member by another. Step by step, the therapist is able to activate awareness of new avenues of sharing, new kinds of intimacy, new levels of identification, and mobilize a realignment of emotional relationships toward health.

The therapist initiates the procedure of family therapy in a simple, casual manner. Regardless of the presenting complaint and regardless of which member of the group is tagged with the label of the "sick one", the therapist invites the whole family to come in and talk it over. He avoids any lengthy or complicated explanations of the family interview. He simply asks them all to join in a family conference. This approach generally brings an optimal response.

In troubled families, there is awareness of the multiplicity of disturbance and also of the contagion of such disturbance. The members know very well that the whole family is in a state of disorder. They are, therefore, receptive to a clinical approach which gives an honest recognition to this principle.

As soon as the members become invested in the live events of the

351

family interview, they show an increasing desire to participate and they then quickly lose their initial self-consciousness and restraint. The threat of personal exposure becomes less frightening, and the fundamental urge to be understood and helped becomes increasingly important. Family psychotherapy may be the method of choice; it may be the sole method, or it may be used in conjunction with individual or other therapies. On principle, family therapy has a wide range of applicability, but must, of course, be flexibly modified to accommodate different conditions. It can be helpful in those psychiatric disorders in which intrapsychic conflict is not the major problem, or where the disturbance is not of long standing. For optimal progress, all members of the family unit should be involved.

Family therapy can be of substantial value for disturbances at all periods of the life cycle—childhood, adolescence, adulthood, and old age. It is, of course, especially potent in disturbances involving the relations of the child with his family.

No method of psychotherapy is comprehensive and total; each exerts selective and differential effects on different components of human disturbance. To set one therapy in competition with another is naive and unsound. One must recognize that each psychotherapeutic method is characterized by specific strengths, but also by certain weaknesses and limitations. By way of generalization, one might say that psychoanalysis has a favored access to unconscious mental mechanisms and is useful in the resolution of those components of emotional disorder that have their origin in entrenched forms of childhood conflicts. Group psychotherapy, in turn, holds the power to modify character traits and ego defense operations. In turn, family psychotherapy possesses certain unique potentials of its own, not apparent in the other methods of therapy. The selective features of each of these methods derive from the special social structuring of the therapeutic interview. From this point of view, the application of family therapy does not preclude the use of other forms of treatment. Within this context, it is useful to think of individual therapy with specific family members, where clinically indicated, as being an auxiliary to the psychotherapy of the whole family.

Joint Psychotherapy of Marital Problems

by IAN ALGER, M.D.

S INCE the publication of Mittelman's[10] article in 1948 on the analysis of marital couples, more and more articles have appeared in the litera- ture describing concurrent, conjoint, and combined therapy with both part- ners in a marriage. Sager's[11] recent paper provides a thorough review of the topic.

Changes in theoretical understanding of the nature of neurotic symptoms have encouraged innovations in technique. If one sees all behavior as a communicative response to another person under certain conditions, then one will study the feelings that accompany it, the context within which it occurs, and the behavior of other people which precedes and follows it. New concepts in field theory, in communication theory, and in small group dynamics have encouraged experimentation in therapy with groups of people.

The natural group most easily studied in our culture is the family.[1] When a married person applies for therapy, his marriage must be under- stood as the most intimate and involving relationship in his current life.

CHOICE AND GOALS OF TREATMENT

A patient may complain of symptoms which seem to him to be unrelated to his marriage: e.g., psychosomatic dysfunctions, insomnia, or phobias. In order to engage the spouse in meaningful therapy, it is necessary to ex- plain symptomatic behavior as a way of communicating with another person under the conditions operating in that relationship. Examples of double-bind behavior, as outlined by Bateson, Jackson, Haley, and Weakland,[5] can be helpful. On the other hand, couples now frequently seek psychiatric advice because of problems in sex, finances, raising the children, or just doing any- thing together.

The goal in therapy is the achievement for each individual of the greatest possible freedom to exercise choice with fullest possible awareness of one's own feelings and ideas in relation to those of others and on society. Satir[12] and Goldfarb[6] have described patterns of excessive mutual dependency between married partners, in which both look to the other's behavior for support of their own self-esteem. This produces a kind of mutual enslavement and prevents a more mature relationship. The objective is to help each person become less paralyzingly dependent on the partner. This may either lead to separation and divorce or to a new kind of mutually satisfying and adult marriage.

When combined therapy has been agreed upon, there are still further decisions to be made, including the frequency and length of meetings, fees, and type of joint and/or individual sessions. I encourage combined therapy when one or both partners want to work on the application of insights they have had about their own behavior to other important relationships such as their work situations. Frequently, I work in joint sessions with another therapist while each marital partner is seen individually by separate therapies. In these four-way sessions, the therapists may be of the same sex, but there are also advantages in having a man and a woman therapist, as described below.

Joint sessions last 60 minutes, while the group sessions are either 1½ hours or may be extended to 4 hours. The fee for a joint session with a cotherapist is twice the cost of an individual one, and the fee for group is about half the latter.

JOINT SESSION WITH ONE THERAPIST

I still see couples in this type of session, but I increasingly prefer four-way sessions in which the couple and two therapists are present. In the three-way session, the potential for becoming caught in some of the struggles between the two partners is very great, and alliances can be formed easily and with great subtlety. They also are formed when four meet together, but can be more easily identified and dealt with than in the notoriously difficult triangular situation.

A man who presented himself to the therapist in a most forceful and self-assured way in individual sessions appeared to be shy and very tentative in those with his wife. He spoke only when she gave him a cue or when she directed him to explain a particular incident or situation. During a joint session in which he was being so directed, he began to develop one of his frequent headaches, and it was possible to associate this with a feeling of impotent rage he had towards his wife. She, in turn, became aware of her own feeling of anger towards him whenever he developed the headache, because she felt thwarted when he could not function because of the headache nor show anger when he was suffering.

Not only are reactions between the partners more clear, but the therapist inevitably must himself become more openly involved.[2] When the therapist

354

sits quietly, or when he shows some reaction in the tone of his voice, the patient in an individual session may comment on his silence or on the conveyed feeling, but the therapist can deny the patient's observation or conclusion and fall back on his therapeutic neutrality. In a joint session, however, the presence of a third person raises the likelihood that the validity of some reactions of one partner to the therapist will be supported by the other partner, making it more difficult for the therapist to avoid involvement. This trend towards greater directness and openness is important and helpful.[3]

In one joint session, I stopped the husband after he had gone on describing an episode at home and told him that I felt very bored and didn't want to hear any more. He reacted with open anger. His wife felt great relief, and said that she now realized that she often also felt bored by her husband's stories but had never before clearly pinned down the feeling. Instead, she had always listened patiently and become more and more quiet. The husband replied that when she was so unresponsive he went on at even greater length, thinking that he had left out some details and wasn't really making himself understood. In this instance, the therapist's reaction, when expressed openly in the session, allowed the wife to recognize a similar reaction in herself, and enabled the husband to understand something about the way in which he became a compulsive bore even though his own desire was to be heard and understood.

Another therapeutic technique involves a paradigmatic approach to some particular behavior of one of the patients, with the goal of so exaggerating it that other significant messages given by the behavior will become evident even to the patient.

For example, a husband related the story of an evening at home. The tone underlying the whole recital seemed to be one of his long-suffering determination to do his best in spite of his wife's "obvious" lack of concern for him. He mentioned an incident that took place one evening when his wife had dropped an egg in boiling water and some of the water had splashed into his eye, but seemed unaware of his accusing and hostile implication. At this point the therapist walked over and sat beside him and suggested that the husband play the part of the wife while the therapist would play the husband. The patient then acted out the part of dropping the egg in the water, and the therapist, in an exaggerated way, clasped his hand to his eye and went through an elaborate ritual of assuring the "wife" (played here by the husband) that it didn't hurt too badly and that he was sure the sight would be all right. The wife smiled in recognition of the situation, but the husband denied that his own actions had the same message of martyrdom that the therapist's exaggerated actions did. However, the wife said that this was exactly the message she got, and she hated it because it was so condescending and superior. They were then able to move to a new level of more direct communication with greater awareness of their own feelings which, prior to this time, had been quite covered and denied.

Each variation of joint therapy has unique aspects especially useful in selected situations. However, all the varieties have many factors in common which differentiate the general method from the usual psychotherapy in its dyadic form.

Four-way Joint Sessions

As already mentioned, the presence of two therapists[7] lessens the possibility of exclusive alliances and of a dyadic impasse. With two therapists present, each finds freedom to include his own reactions more openly in the process because he has the assurance that the other will be able to respond in a corrective manner. The very fact that the therapists are willing to expose their feelings and reactions to analysis and understanding is revealing to the patients and provides a model which many couples have never before experienced. Cotherapists work especially well together when each is attuned to a different aspect of communication: for example, when one therapist is alert to the feeling conveyed by nuance and context while the other is conceptually oriented and more sensitive to reactions communicated largely by language in a logical conceptual framework.[8]

In one session a husband in an irate manner disclosed his frustration and irritation at his wife earlier that evening when she seemed withdrawn and angry with him because he was late in getting home from work. One therapist was sensitive to the blaming quality in the wife's voice and was able to empathize with the husband's irritation. When this therapist brought his own reaction into the open, the other therapist was able to express his awareness of the wife's feeling of hurt. She felt disappointed and abandoned to all the chores of the household which had to be finished before the couple could leave for the therapy session. This combined revelation helped all four participants to see the complex interplay of feelings and allowed the couple to dispel the angry impasse.

In a session in which the cotherapist was a woman, she reacted to the husband's sarcastic and contained response to a comment she had made with an obviously angry retort that she didn't like that kind of treatment. The wife said, in some amazement, that she had often felt just the same way, but had never felt free enough to express her anger openly. The husband, in turn, felt more able to express the anger he felt towards the woman therapist. He and his wife also learned that a more direct way of dealing with their feelings could bring them closer together.

In another joint session, the woman therapist told the wife that she felt the wife had great strength as a woman. The same interpretation had been made to the patient by a male therapist in an individual session, but it did not have the same impact on the patient. Having such a comment come from another woman was very meaningful to the wife, and was not able to dismiss it as just an attempt by a man to seduce her sexually.

When two male therapists meet with a couple, the wife finds herself sitting with three men. For many a woman this is a very threatening situation, because she may feel that her needs to be understood as a woman

356

cannot be met. It is also very helpful for a wife to see how her husband can respond differently to another woman when a familiar kind of conflict situation arises, to experience the response of another woman in the therapy session, and to have her husband witness this.

COUPLE-GROUPS

Many of the advantages reviewed are also applicable here, and the widening of the therapeutic group from three or four to eight or ten can further make clear that all behavior is related to context and interaction, rendering possible a more complex group dynamic operation and more precise identifications. Markowitz[9] has described cotherapy with a man and woman therapist in a couples' group, and I have also found this a most helpful method. In an attempt to intensify the impact of the session and the involvement of the patients, sessions of four hours in length have been introduced and seem to hold promise.

VIDEOTAPE PLAYBACK

Dr. Peter Hogan and I have been using portable and relatively inexpensive videotape recordings and playback in our private practices since 1965 and have found them particularly useful in marital therapy.[4]

Briefly, the technique involves the television recording of the first 15 minutes of a joint marital session. The episodes recorded are then played back over a television monitor immediately so that all participants can stop the recording at any point to comment on their own behavior or that of others, their feeling reactions, and any discrepancies between the way they now appear and the way they remember actually feeling at the time of the original incident.

Messages are thus exchanged and reviewed at several levels and over several channels: by content of speech, tone of voice, mannerism and gesture, posture, timing, and context. In the regular course of living so much happens in a brief time that it is impossible to separate the various messages and the way in which they are delivered. With the videorecording, the same sequence can be replayed many times, and each time a new aspect may lead to new understanding. The television recording in this context is not a therapeutic method in itself but rather as a powerful adjunct to therapy.

Generally, patients have been very receptive to the recordings. No attempt is made to conceal the equipment, and when a camera operator is used he is introduced and included as part of the therapy group. At times, he may even become actively involved in the analysis and interactions of the session. Far from being reluctant to use the equipment, many patients have felt that, for the first time, they have been able to participate in therapy with a genuine equality, since both they and the therapists have

357

direct access to the objective data. A common experience on first seeing oneself has been called "image impact."

One wife commented after seeing herself that there was so great a discrepancy between the way she was feeling inside and the way her image appeared to her that she wanted to go over to "that person" and shake her. Her husband felt relief and said that he too sometimes felt like shaking her. Another husband responded to his wife in a manner that seemed petulant and, at the same time, condescendingly humble. The husband was unable to understand how his wife and the therapists had this impression, and he asked to have the recording played over several times. It was on the fourth replay that he suddenly exclaimed as he heard his wife's statement just preceding his own response that he now felt angry with her and, after another replay, was able to discern the anger in his condescending and patient tone. At that point the wife felt great relief and told how frustrated she had always felt when she was unable to explain to her husband what it was about his reaction to which she responded.

Thus, for the first time in psychiatry we have available a tool which can provide us with objective data concerning behavior in therapy and which allows us to review the data immediately and as often as we wish.

REFERENCES

1. ACKERMAN, N. W.: The family approach to marital disorders. Paper, American Orthopsychiatric Association, Chicago, 1964.
2. ALGER, I.: Joint sessions: Psychoanalytic variations, applications, and indications. In: Psychoanalysis and Marriage. New York, Basic Books, 1967.
3. ALGER, I.: The clinical handling of the analyst's responses. Psychoanal. Forum I (No. 3): 1966.
4. ALGER, I., AND HOGAN, P.: The use of videotape recordings in conjoint marital therapy in private practice: Paper, American Psychiatric Association, Atlantic City, N.J., 1966 (Accepted for publication by the Amer. J. of Psychiat.).
5. BATESON, G., JACKSON, D.D., HALEY, J., AND WEAKLAND, J. H.: A note on the double-bind, 1962. Family Proc. 2:154-162, 1963.
6. GOLDFARB, A.: Marital problems of older persons. In: Psychoanalysis and Marriage. New York, Basic Books, 1967.
7. HOGAN, P., AND ROYCE, J.: Co-therapy in a special situation. Paper, American Group Psychotherapy Association, New York, 1960.
8. HOGAN, P.: The content-context syndrome. Soc. Med. Psychoanalysts' Newsletter. IV (No. 4): 1963.
9. MARKOWITZ, M.: Analytic group psychotherapy of married couples by a therapist couple. In: Psychoanalysis and Marriage. New York, Basic Books, 1967.
10. MITTELMAN, B.: The concurrent analysis of marital couples, Psychoanal. Quart. 17:182-197, 1948.
11. SAGER, C. J.: Marriage therapy: A review. Amer. J. Orthopsychiat. 36:458-467, 1966.
12. SATIR, V. M.: Conjoint marital therapy: In: The Psychotherapies of Marital Disharmony. New York, The Free Press, 1965.

General Systems Theory and Multiple Family Therapy*

by H. Peter Laqueur, M.D.

G ENERAL SYSTEMS THEORY[1] formulates statements applying to all systems approaches in *behavioral science* as well as *general science* and deals with the properties and characteristics of *nonliving* and *living* systems.

Nonliving systems, be they open (e.g., an automatic factory, an antimissile or anti-aircraft defense system, a re-entry and recovery system in a space capsule), or closed (e.g., a watch, a thermostat, or a governor on a steam engine), are programmed for specific functions; however, growth, expansion, and self-development are not part of their existence so that they can be governed by robots and analyzed cybernetically.

Living systems have a history of (1) coming into being; (2) existing for a limited period during which they grow, expand in knowledge, skill, and capability for coping with the environment; and (3) ceasing to exist after they have fulfilled their function. In addition to a program, similar to the program of the nonliving system, the living system also has an *individual style,* which precludes full prediction of its functioning because the style contains the elements leading to creativity, spontaneity, and originality.

Every form of psychotherapy can be studied as a system with *input* (human beings and relationships accepting help), *transaction* (the therapeutic interaction taking place), and *output* (better functioning of individuals and groups, i.e., families.) General systems theory sees the individual as a subsystem of higher systems (family, kinship, community), and these in turn as parts of suprasystems (nation and the human species as a whole). Malfunction of an individual or a family can be analyzed to find the primary focus of disturbance and to devise methods for better integration of the individual and family in their environment.

*Supported by Social and Rehabilitation Service, Department of Health, Education, and Welfare, Washington, D.C.

The Multiple Family Therapy Group as a System

Multiple family therapy (MFT) was described in previous papers[2,3] and will, therefore, here be outlined only briefly as follows: Four to five hospitalized patients, mostly schizophrenics, meet together with their nearest relatives—parents, siblings, spouses—and a therapist, co-therapist, and observers in weekly sessions of 1½ hours throughout the whole period of their hospitalization for the purpose of improving mutual relationships.

MFT is a special therapeutic system comprising several subsystems: (1) the therapist, his co-therapist, and observers; (2) each family as a subsystem of the first order (within which the primary patient versus the rest of the family constitutes a subsystem of second order) within suprasystems of higher order (hospital, clinic, community).

MFT groups have the properties of a *living system* in that they come into being for a specific function and a limited time and cease to exist after they have fulfilled their function more or less successfully. They also act like living systems in the sense that they not only have a *program*, largely determined by the goals of the hospital or clinic in which they work, but also an individual *style* reflecting the personal style of the therapist. In other words, the program, i.e., *what* is to be learned by the MFT group is, essentially, a better mutual understanding of patients and their families for the purpose of assuring the patient's continued well-being after his discharge from the hospital. *How* this goal is approached is determined by the personal style of the therapist, i.e., his creativity and originality in handling new situations; his skillful readjustment of internal control and feedback system in cases of unusual malfunctions; his choice of hitherto unused pathways in critical situations; his sense of timing for scanning, probing, self-testing, and correction of probing techniques, etc. These qualities are demanded of every therapist, but to an especially high degree of the therapist of an MFT group because such a group can show all the properties of a system threatened by failure through unexpected situations, overload of information, critical events, malfunction of a subgroup, or external developments.

Mechanisms in Multiple Family Therapy

In a group of several families the therapist can use some of them in specific *"co-therapeutic"* roles. A review of some of the mechanisms operating in the MFT group will illustrate this:

1. On one level *competition,* on another *cooperation* between systems (families) produces changes in the internal power distribution of the system faster than work with a single family could do. A threat to the status of a family or an individual is felt as competition and makes the participants more receptive to messages from the therapist or other members of the

360

group. Later on, cooperation may take the place of competition and Jimmy may point out to Johnny how he and his family learned to cope with a situation similar to the one still disturbing Johnny and his family.

2. An *understanding of the total field of interaction* between subsystems (patient, family), and suprasystem (the total social environment) is attempted. This awareness of the changing surrounding field and its importance for sickness and health (based on Kurt Lewin's *Field Theory in Social Science*[4]) is one of the major assets of MFT sessions. The range and variety of therapeutic approaches available to the therapist in this field of interacting forces is much greater than in a one-way or two-way communication with single individuals or single families.

3. Perceiving the family and its components as subsystems of a larger field of interrelations, *interface problems* can be studied and dealt with in the same way as a good trouble shooter understands and repairs the component parts of a complex machine or system. Therapists seeing malfunction in a family as caused by specific malfunction of component parts or of feedback mechanisms act as *system analysts* (analyzing feedback, perception, recognition, association, and planning for response), and can then propose to the sick family new and specific possibilities for repair and restitution.

4. In our attempt to overcome the *resistance to change* of the family with a schizophrenic member or, in other words, to make the family integrate new experiences into their outlook on the world and their preparation for future behavior, we take some clues from information theory, which holds that events having the least probability of occurrence but yet occur have the highest information value. A new pattern, a new sequence of signals producing an excitation focus in the nervous system is significant information. Translated into terms of MFT, a new successful, more realistic type of behavior of one family, distinguished from their usual behavior, can act as a focus of excitation for the whole group if used skillfully by the therapist.

5. *Breaking the intrafamilial code*: To understand messages from, and to transmit information to a family, the therapist must learn the code that every family with a schizophrenic member seems to develop for their internal verbal and nonverbal communication. The help of the other families in this translation process is of priceless value. If four families are together, at least one will be able to pick up a signal from the therapist and rephrase and amplify it to make it understandable to the other three families. When problems of patient-family communication come up, schizophrenics can translate for each other often better than any therapist could do.

6. *Amplification and modulation of signals*: A sensitive patient can pick up a signal from the therapist and act as an amplifier to sensitize his family; through this first family such a signal may be further amplified and

361

modulated to other families who, without this amplification, might not yet have responded to signals from the therapist. The specific "I and Thou" relationship between therapist and first patient may through reverberating communications and feelings lead ultimately to similar warm and identifying understanding between other members of the group and give them confidence.

7. *Learning by analogy*: In a group of several families there are many opportunities for watching others respond to "analogue" conflict situations and learn from this example. The feeling of "having been there" in similar trouble helps immeasurably in learning new ways of dealing with conflicts and this feeling is more likely to occur in the MFT group with its many examples than in other forms of therapy.

8. *Learning through identification constellation*: "Fathers," "mothers," "adolescents," "married couples" form identification constellations; i.e., subsystems which learn from each other. The fellowship of experience in the MFT group, helps each to cope with existential and situational problems.

9. *Learning through trial and error*: Participants have many opportunities for trying out new behavior in the MFT group and reinforcing it through the approval of the other members of the group. New insights may be achieved through role-playing when the son of one family is asked by the therapist to play the role of the father of another family. By acting "as if" he were that parent, the actor may not only achieve for himself, but also transmit to the other children a greater understanding of the role of the parent in the given situation.

10. *Use of healthier aspects of certain families as models*: The therapist uses the healthier aspects of one family as a model and challenge for other families to change their own behavior. The participants with the most severe symptoms (the primary patients) usually improve first in MFT. The attitude of their relatives changes later when more mature behavior in the primary patients becomes manifest.

It should be noted in this context that the whole MFT group works better than a fragmented group from which many family members are absent, and certainly much better than the peer group (patients only), in which the so-called normal relatives are present only in the fantasy of the patient, but no real perspective of mutuality and reciprocity in family life can be observed and utilized.

THE THERAPIST AS SYSTEM ANALYST

Some examples of situations that may threaten the MFT group with system failure will illustrate the scope of demands on the therapist:

1. *Unexpected external events*: Such seemingly trivial events as the necessity for the group to meet in a different room than usual (because the heating

362

system broke down) can have a very disturbing influence on the group.

2. *Overload*: Several families simultaneously start violent quarrels and demand immediate arbitration of their conflicts without paying any attention to the therapist's attempt to assign priorities.

3. *Delay in feedback loop*: The therapist's timing and feedback re-input may break down when the therapist does not yet understand the intrafamilial codes and therefore cannot follow private disagreements in a family or between members of an identification constellation.

4. *Inflexibility*: If the therapist acts according to a set of rules not fitting the group, his rigidity may make him "drive through warning signs" and he may frighten and disturb patients and families rather than help them.

5. *Insufficiency of internal sensors:* Insufficient perception and sensitivity may cause some therapists to give academic psychodynamic interpretations which, although they may theoretically be correct, will increase a patient's resistance; this must be resolved or the MFT group will not succeed.

6. *Failure of external sensors*: If the therapist fails to take into account changes in the administrative climate (in ward, hospital, or clinic), he may bring members of the MFT group into conflict with the surrounding system and thus cause confusion detrimental to therapeutic progress.

7. *Breakdown of components requiring bypass or overriding or replacement:* Errors committed by co-therapists, like taking sides in a family conflict without openly saying so, or "impossible" behavior by another member of the group, may require quick face-saving correction or a change of subject before greater damage is done. Sometimes even removal of the offending member from the room or in very rare instances elimination of a whole family from the group and replacement by another family may be necessary.

The therapist is often in a dilemma: To promote freedom of expression and thereby relieve existing tensions caused by insufficient communication between family members, he must "awaken sleeping dogs" that in a more sociable setting everybody would let lie; conversely, if too much shocking information is placed at the center of the stage, some families may feel extremely threatened. It is the therapist's challenging task to avert extreme reactions and to prevent bitterness and resentment in threatened participants as much as possible so as not to delay the success of the therapeutic operation.

CAPABILITY REQUIREMENTS FOR GOAL-SEEKING, OPEN, OPTIMIZING SYSTEMS

MFT belongs to the category of systems seeking to produce desirable outputs in an efficient and effective manner under constantly varying circumstances and requiring the following characteristics to prevent system failures and breakdowns[5]:

1. Ability to probe and scan the *external* environment continuously and repeatedly with adequate sensors.

2. Ability to probe, scan, and adapt its *internal milieu* and *mechanisms faster* than the changes in external milieu occur to avoid a *lag* in system functions.

3. Ability to *change* timing, location, frequency, and direction of probing.

4. Capability for sufficient and qualitatively correct activity of *motor-output-effectors* for *reactive* and *productive* behavior.

5. Ability to *store* and *recall information* (memory).

6. Ability to *recognize* and *identify patterns* (recall and checking by comparison).

7. Ability to *feed* information *back* (to know what was done last time in analyzing a similar situation).

8. Capability for *self-stabilization* (to avoid excessive oscillations and overreactions which might throw the control system out of joint and cause it to lose balance).

9. Ability to be *more random,* i.e., flexible than the environment.

10. Ability to *adjust predictably* and to change predictions with regard to changing probabilities.

General systems theory aids in the analysis and optimum utilization of the therapist's and his co-workers' general program and style as they interact with the programs and styles of each person and family in the MFT group.

REFERENCES

1. BERTALANFFY, L.: General System Theory and Psychiatry. In: Arieti, S. (Ed.): American Handbook of Psychiatry. New York, Basic Books, 1966.
2. LAQUEUR, H. P., LaBURT, H. A., AND MORONG, E.: Multiple Family Therapy. In Masserman J. H. (Ed.): Current Psychiatric Therapies, Vol. IV. New York, Grune & Stratton, 1964.
3. ———: Multiple Family Therapy: Further Developments. Internat. J. Soc. Psychiat., Congress Issue, sect. K, 69–80, 1964.
4. LEWIN, K.: Field Theory in Social Science. New York, Harper & Row, 1951.
5. THOMAS, E. L.: Abnormal Behaviour in Non-Living Systems. Read at Tenth Annual Psychiatric Research Meeting of Group Without A Name, Cincinnati, Ohio, March 1967.

PART XI

GROUP
THERAPIES

Group Psychoanalysis

by RICHARD G. ABELL, M.D.

PSYCHOANALYTICALLY ORIENTED GROUP THERAPY, or "psychoanalysis in groups,"[1] has as its goal the treatment, alleviation and cure of mental illness through the interaction of patients in a group with each other and with a specially trained participant and observer, the therapist, using to a great extent the techniques of individual psychoanalysis. The purpose is to analyze each patient separately in a group setting. Of special importance is the analysis of the transferences, interpretations by the therapist, free and directed associations[2] and dream interpretation. Also important is the direct effect of each patient upon the others and the attitude of the analyst toward the patient. The analyst should be a devoted, interested,[3] rational but permissive authority figure with whom the patient feels free to re-enact his distorted and irrational behavior in the interpersonal situation in the group,[4] so that it can be observed and its significance pointed out initially by the analyst, and later by the group members as well as the analyst.

Neuroses have their origin, for the most part, in a family setting, and are caused to a great extent by deprivation of basic emotional needs, combined with the effects of the neurotic behavior of the parents, or other significant people, upon the infant and child. Therefore it is natural that the analysis of the patient's problems in a group setting, which represents a new family, should have a special curative value.[5] The following specific information is relevant to the formation of a group and to the actual therapeutic process.

Selection of Patients for a Group: Heterogeneous groups facilitate the working through of sexual and other problems more rapidly than homogeneous groups of either sex. My experience agrees with that of Wolf and Schwartz[1] that in general patients with the following diagnoses are suitable for treatment in groups: psychoneuroses, psychoneurotic character disorders, schizoid personalities, psychosomatic disturbances, ambulatory schizophrenia and borderline cases. The basic criterion for selecting

367

patients is their potential for relating in a manner consonant with the group process.[6]

Size and Frequency of the Group Meetings: If the group exceeds eight in size, some of the patients begin to feel inhibited and frustrated, and may be unable to speak freely even though their resistance to speaking is analyzed and they are encouraged to verbalize. Satisfactory therapy can be done in smaller groups, and some therapists work with groups as large as ten.[1] The group meets once a week (or oftener) for one and a half hours.

Analysis of Resistances which Patients Frequently have to Joining a Group

(1) First and foremost is the patient's fear of exposing his problems and intimate feelings. The patient should be reassured by telling him that he will discover that his problems are essentially like those of the other members of the group, and will form a basis for acceptance, not rejection.[1] (2) Patients frequently feel that they do not want to share the analyst with other patients. The patient believes that in a group of eight he will receive only one eighth of the therapist's attention. This misconception should be corrected by pointing out that the group process involves analyzing the transference reactions of each patient to the others at the time of their occurrence, so that far from diluting the therapy the presence of others intensifies it. Furthermore he is told that each patient should be actively associating to those events in his own background and experience which are related to the verbalizations and behavior of whatever group member is speaking, and that he should be ready to provide these associations for group interaction. Consequently each patient should be actively involved all of the time. (3) Fear of being talked about outside of the group should be met by telling the prospective patient that only first names are used and that what occurs in the group is to be kept confidential among the group members and the therapist.

Preliminary Individual Analysis

The analyst should see the patient individually for a period of time long enough to be certain that (1) the patient will benefit by being introduced into a group, (2) the patient has formed a positive attachment to the therapist which is sufficiently strong to support him during the initial anxiety-provoking meetings of the group, (3) the most dependent and infantile transferences had been worked out at least to the point of some insight,[7] and (4) the patient had become familiar with the techniques of individual analysis. The length of time may range from about 6 months to longer than a year. Patients who are referred

368

specifically for group therapy by other analysts may be introduced into a group after one interview.

Prior to the introduction of a new patient into a group I discuss with him the application of psychoanalytic techniques to the group process. He is essentially told that however mysterious his illness may seem, everything that has befallen him is related to his actual living among a relatively small number of significant people, in a relatively simple course of events,[8] and that resolution of his difficulties will depend upon his being able to modify the damaging and inhibiting effects of such persons and events upon his feeling, thinking and acting in the direction of a more realistic approach to living.

Combined Individual and Group Analysis

Many therapists[7] prefer to treat their patients privately in individual sessions once or twice a week in addition to seeing them in a group. My own experience has been that this is an excellent form of therapy and is preferable to limiting the treatment to one group session a week. However, some analysts[1] prefer to treat patients privately only in times of crisis.

Alternate Sessions: Some therapists prefer to have their groups meet once a week with the analyst and once a week without him in the "alternate session."[1] The purpose of this is to give members a chance to function in a peer group without the analyst, whom many initially see as a repressive authority figure.

After a group is started, certain patients finish therapy sooner than others. In ongoing groups, such patients are replaced by new members.

THE GROUP PROCESS

Each patient is essentially analyzed as an individual interacting in a group, in whom complicated feelings and actions are called forth by the presence of other group members toward whom he reacts initially as stereotypes of significant figures in his earlier background, and who call forth corresponding transference reactions. Patients are encouraged to tell dreams, and during the interpretation of the dream the other group members, as well as the dreamer, give their reactions. As the sessions progress, the interaction usually becomes more and more intense. Transference reactions are analyzed at the moment of their occurrence and traced to their original cause by free and directed associations. During this process the patient becomes aware of his unconscious conflicts by re-enacting them in the group under conditions which bring them to life and make them vital, intense and especially susceptible to

369

interpretation. No person who has seen a patient run out of a group in agony and vomit in the bathroom because one of the men in the group was talking to her in a loud voice which she mistook for hostile criticism, can doubt the intensity of such transference reactions. Nor can he doubt the effectiveness of their interpretation when he observes that by association she is reminded of the agony she suffered as a child from her father's loud and harsh criticisms. Nor can he doubt the curative effect of the group process when later on in therapy she says to this same man, "Why you aren't hostile, you are really a friendly person! I didn't used to see you as you are at all." Such analysis is obviously not superficial, but on the contrary, is analysis in depth.

After some experience patients become skilled in recognizing transference reactions and they are encouraged to participate in the analytic process. Becker[9] emphasizes the beneficial effects of the resolution of such transferences in releasing the patient to undergo further personality growth. In the free exchange of the group interaction patients describe exactly how they see each other. Although such confrontations are frequently distorted at first, with continued analysis and reality testing they become more and more accurate. Under the impact of direct and accurate confrontations masks are gradually dropped, defenses lowered, the members come to understand themselves in their interpersonal reactions and in consequence develop a stronger feeling of personal identity.

After some analysis the ability of patients to appraise both the negative and positive aspects of the personalities of other patients is amazingly accurate. Negative appraisals when correct are useful in helping the patient who is appraised to become more aware of those aspects of himself which other people dislike, so that he can investigate their cause and learn to replace them with better modes of interpersonal behavior. Favorable appraisals are valuable in helping patients to broaden their awareness of their own positive qualities and abilities. Accurate appraisal of the desirable qualities of one patient by the others, with re-enforcement by the analyst, is frequently a new and always a corrective experience for such patients, since it satisfies a long frustrated need for acceptance based upon recognition of real worth. In this way the important function of the therapist in personally filling the previously frustrated needs of the patient so far as this is possible[10] is diversified and multiplied in the group.

SPECIAL FACTORS OF CURATIVE VALUE

(1) Of special therapeutic value in the mixed group is the opportunity afforded members of one sex to become familiar with the real nature

of members of the opposite sex.[11] Many patients have been so infantilized by one or more key figures in their earlier background that they have no idea of how a member of the opposite sex really thinks or feels. For example, a 28 year old patient, George, who was in appearance attractive to women, had never gone out with a girl prior to beginning group therapy. He had been so emasculated by an anxious, compulsive mother that he had avoided girls because he was afraid they would dominate him; and he was, in any case, so passive that the thought of approaching a girl was foreign to him. Prior to beginning therapy he believed that all women were basically like his mother.

George had been in individual therapy for 2 years with no real breakthrough in regard to his behavior toward women. After he had been in psychoanalytically oriented group therapy for 2 years he said, "I definitely feel freer with girls now than I used to. I date. I kiss the girls goodnight and enjoy it. There's no difficulty. I didn't even used to be able to hold a girl's hand. The girls in the group had a very definite effect in bringing this about. I began to see that women have much the same problems and frailties that men do. What was a revelation to me was to hear some of the more personal things that the women in the group said. To hear how they think and react. Now I 'see' women for the first time."

(2) Patients who have been in group therapy long enough to undergo significant improvement exert a beneficial effect upon newer patients who are more disturbed. This effect seems to be due in part to the fact that the new patient regards the more advanced patient as someone who, like himself, was once more disturbed, but who during the course of therapy has improved and who therefore can serve as an example. Masserman[10] observed that a normal animal placed in a cage with one made neurotic by experimental means will exert a beneficial and curative effect upon the neurotic one, possibly by making the solution of motivational or adaptational impasse seem easier or at least attainable.

(3) Specific techniques should be directed toward bringing to the awareness of the patient those creative aspects of his personality which he selectively neglects due to the fact that they were not issues for his parents, or because his expression of them in early life called forth anxiety in his parents so that they became associated with his concept of "bad-me." Such selectively inattended, creative and positive aspects of the personality can be brought back into awareness by an accepting person,[12,13] i.e., the group analyst, who should re-enforce those aspects of the patient's behavior which show talent, ability, foresight, consideration for the feelings of others, good performance, and so on. This should

371

be done at the time the patient expresses them, often unwittingly, by his actions in the group, or recalls them from his past. In this way the effect of the original negative appraisals by the parents (or others)[14] is mitigated or corrected by a new and valid set of positive appraisals, made initially by the analyst and re-enforced by other members of the group. Thus the patient is helped to develop a new, more inclusive and more accurate sense of self.[15]

(4) The importance of giving the patient a new experience is stressed by Fromm.[16] One such new experience is the thoughtful, attentive, noncensorious, creative manner in which the analyst listens to the patient. Although always important, this takes on a special value in the group, in which the analyst is looked upon as a father figure in a new family. This attitude, combined with warmth, concern, respect for the patient's integrity and acceptance, lies at the very heart of the therapeutic process. Kenneth Appel[3] expresses this as follows: "The basic factor [in all psychotherapy] is probably the emotional relationship between the therapist and patient, the caring, loving, devotion and interest on the part of the therapist, and the faith the patient has in him." This is in agreement with Sullivan's statement that "Far more than any single action of the physician, it is his general attitude toward the patient that determines his value.[17] With continued therapy such an attitude on the part of the analyst is gradually incorporated by the group members, and their expression of it towards each other becomes an important therapeutic force during the latter stages of treatment.

(5) The analyst should participate even more directly in times of crisis, e.g., when a patient feels unbearably attacked, or during some severe crisis in his personal life. The effect upon the patient of the analyst's demonstration that he is unequivocally on the patient's side is therapeutically crucial, and its value cannot be overemphasized. This is frequently re-enforced by the supportive actions of other patients.

(6) An important therapeutic factor during psychoanalysis in groups is the immediacy of the relationship between the analyst and patient and between the group members themselves.[16,18] DeRosis[19] refers to the same phenomenon as "living a piece of experience with another," and says that once a person has done this he is forever changed. Thompson[20] emphasizes the importance of the analyst being natural and spontaneous, and states that this makes it possible for the patient to react more genuinely. Crowley[21] stresses the value of using such appropriate, unexaggerated, non-anxious and non-defensive reactions of analyst to patient to further the analytic work. An important aspect of the group process is directed toward developing such an immediacy of relationship among

372

group members by encouraging and re-enforcing free and direct expression of feelings.

TERMINATION

A patient is ready to terminate therapy when he has attained the following criteria for mental health: (1) an understanding of the dynamics of his interpersonal relations so that he can handle them appropriately; (2) the resolution of his transference reactions; (3) a diminution or disappearance of the psychological pressure of infantile and childish dependency upon the significant people in his early life, so that he is able to relate to them without too pronounced emotional reactions, as a step toward learning to deal appropriately with others in his present and future life; (4) a re-evaluation of his self-concept based upon an accurate appraisal of his real abilities; (5) the capacity to use his own talents to secure satisfaction of his current needs; (6) an expansion of his personality to include characteristics to which he was previously selectively inattentive or which were dissociated; (7) the capacity to give and receive love and to form lasting relationships of personal intimacy; (8) The patient's original symptoms and the crippling anxiety associated with them should have been effectively relieved and he should have developed a sense of competence based upon actual accomplishment.

As pointed out by Fromm-Reichmann,[2] it is not necessary that all of the patient's psychotherapeutic goals be reached during treatment. However, he must have developed an understanding of their nature and of his original difficulties and the manner of their resolution to the point where he can continue his analysis on his own subsequent to termination.

REFERENCES

1. WOLF, A., AND SCHWARTZ, E. K.: Psychoanalysis in Groups. New York, Grune and Stratton, 1962.
2. FROMM-REICHMANN, F.: Principles of Intensive Psychotherapy. Chicago, University of Chicago Press, 1950.
3. APPEL, K. E.: Religion. In: American Handbook of Psychiatry, Silvano Arieti, Editor. New York, Basic Books, 1959, pp. 1777-1782.
4. POWDERMAKER, F.: Personal communication, 1954.
5. ABELL, R. G.: Personality development during group psychotherapy: its relation to the etiology and treatment of the neuroses. Am. J. Psychoanal., 19:53, 1959.
6. KADIS, A. L., KRASNER, J. D., WINICK, C., AND FOULKES, S.: A Practicum of Group Psychotherapy. New York, Harper and Row, 1963.
7. SCHECTER, D. E.: The Integration of Group Therapy with Individual Psychoanalysis. Psychiatry: J. Study Interpersonal Proc., 22:267, 1959.

8. SULLIVAN, H. S.: The modified psychoanalytic treatment of schizophrenia. Am. J. Psychiat., 88:519, 1931-32.

9. BECKER, B. J.: Observations on the process of group psychoanalysis. Am. J. Psychotherapy., 11:345, 1957.

10. MASSERMAN, J. H.: The biodynamic approaches. In: American Handbook of Psychiatry, Silvano Arieti, Editor. New York, Basic Books, 1959, pp. 1680-1696.

11. ABELL, R. G.: Etiology and treatment of the passive male. Am. J. Psychoanal., 20:212, 1960.

12. SULLIVAN, H. S.: The Interpersonal Theory of Psychiatry. New York, W. W. Norton and Co., 1953.

13. WITENBERG, E. G., RIOCH, J. M., AND MAZER, M.: The interpersonal and cultural approaches. In: American Handbook of Psychiatry, Silvano Arieti, Editor. New York, Basic Books, 1959, pp. 1417-1433.

14. SULLIVAN, H. S.: Conceptions of Modern Psychiatry. Washington, D. C., William Alanson White Foundation, 1947.

15. ROSE, S.: A philosophy of group psychoanalysis. Am. J. Psychoanal. 16:32, 1956.

16. FROMM, E.: Personal communication, 1956.

17. SULLIVAN, H. S.: Schizophrenia: its conservative and malignant features. Am. J. Psychiat., 81:77, 1924-25.

18. MAY, R.: Theory and Methods of the Existential Psychotherapists. Paper delivered before the William Alanson White Psychoanalytic Society, May 17, 1957.

19. DeROSIS, L. E.: Group psychoanalysis as experience. J. Psychoanal. Groups, 1:107, 1962.

20. THOMPSON, C.: The Role of the Analyst's Personality in Therapy. Am. J. Psychotherapy, 10:347, 1956.

21. CROWLEY, R. M.: Human reactions of analysts to patients. Samiksa, 6:212, 1952.

Recent Advances in Transactional Analysis

by ERIC BERNE, M.D.

TRANSACTIONAL ANALYSIS IS A SYSTEM OF THERAPY based on a personality theory which recognizes three types of ego states: exteropsychic (those borrowed from parental figures); neopsychic (those oriented in an objective data-processing way toward external reality); and archaeopsychic (archaic relics from early years). These are colloquially termed Parent, Adult, and Child ego states, respectively. Transactional analysis proper attempts to diagnose which ego state in the agent gives rise to the transactional stimulus, and which ego state in the respondent controls the response. Game analysis deals with chains of ulterior, two-level transactions, and script analysis tries to uncover the unconscious life plan which forms a matrix for the ongoing games. For further information concerning this approach, the reader is referred to the basic literature on the subject.[1-5]

The discussion which follows will assume some familiarity with these terms (Parent, Adult, Child, game, and script—the only special vocabulary needed for the practice of transactional analysis). For the sake of brevity, transactional analysis will be abbreviated "TA" (referring to the system as a whole rather than to the special aspect of analyzing single transactions). Parent (P), Adult (A), and Child (C), capitalized, will be used to refer to ego states, while parent, adult, and child in lower case refer to actual people. The examples given have been skeletalized to illustrate specific points and are not offered as samples of the actual proceedings.

A. GENERAL

The use of colloquialisms has stood up well under the tests of time and extensive use in different types of facilities. In order to avoid mere intellectual exercises in the course of treatment, it is necessary to appeal to the Child as well as to the Adult of the patient. Free use of metaphor and current vernacular is one simple way to get the Child to listen, and also makes it easier for the Adult to understand what is being said. The use of basic English even in professional discussions exploits a ready-made vocabulary which enables people from different backgrounds to understand each other clearly without prolonged special training; it also helps new patients in treatment groups to become current very rapidly. Almost anyone can understand, with a minimum of preparation, the purport of such phrases as "trading stamps," "hooking the Parent," or "coming on Child."

B. Personality Structure

A great deal has been learned recently about the use of second order structural analysis. A "First Order Structural Diagram" is shown in Figure 1a; it consists simply of three circles representing the three primary ego states of any individual. It is evident, however, that at the moment the Child is fixated, the actual child already has discrete exteropsychic neopsychic, and archaeopsychic aspects. It is also evident that the Parent will sooner or later emerge in two different forms, one derived from the mother and the other from the father, although initially

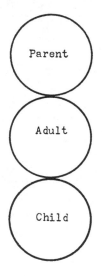

First Order
Structural Diagram

(a)

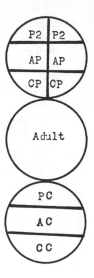

Second Order
Structural Diagram

(b)

Fig. 1.

376

one or the other is suppressed; since the real mother and father have each three ego states this must also be taken into account in advanced work. Figure 1b is a "Second Order Structural Diagram," incorporating these features of the Child and Parent. "Third Order" personality structure is so recondite that it rarely becomes of clinical significance.

1. It can be shown that the "Parents in the Parent" (P_2 in Figure 1b) are the bearers of what is commonly called "culture." The use of second order structural analysis makes possible a quite rigorous transactional treatment ("Which grandparent said what to whom?") of "cultural" factors when these are clinically significant and are not merely being used as a "wooden leg" by the patient ("What do you expect of an Indian?") or ("What do you expect of someone living in our society?"). By shifting to a transactional level, the ideological plea of "Arsisiety," for example, can be critically investigated and evaluated.

2. The Parent in the Child (PC in Figure 1b) is becoming an increasingly important area of investigation. It is colloquially known as the "electrode" because of the almost automatic responses it elicits from the individual when it becomes activated.

Genetically and functionally, the Parent in the Child often corresponds to the "bad" Freudian ogre father or witch mother, or to the introjected bad object of Melanie Klein; phenomenologically, it tends to be reacted to rather than experienced, except for its embodiment in dreams; transactionally, it functions as an automatic regulator of responses just as though it were an implanted electrode. It may equally well be a "good" introject with the same operational characteristics: in this aspect it may also produce automatic responses, but in the hope of reward rather than in fear of punishment or annihilation. Characterologically, this results in "cute kids" and "good boys."

3. The Adult in the Child (AC in Figure 1b) is colloquially known as "the professor." This is the aspect which intuitively appraises people and makes choices among them for purposes of game-playing, pseudo-intimacy, and exploitation. Clinical training is essentially a re-training of this aspect, a secondary education of the powers of appraisal which are suppressed during the socialization of the individual. The Child is given "permission" by his mentors to look at people objectively once more and to assess their potentialities intuitively. Hence this segment of his own personality is a valuable therapeutic tool of the therapist's and likewise during the course of therapy makes available to the patient his own suppressed or distorted intuitive powers. It is postulated that it was this aspect of Freud's first reported patient (Emmy von N.)[6] which taught him the fundamental rule of psychoanalysis: "Keep quiet

377

—don't talk." She said this because she was afraid of being interrupted, "because everything would then become worse": a very important principle, hence the epithet "professor" for this intelligent and perceptive system.

4. The Child in the Child (CC in Figure 1b) is colloquially called "the infant." This is an earlier point of arrest within the fixated Child ego state. In clinical terms, certain schizoid personalities or ambulatory schizophrenics ordinarily present an "immature" personality (the Child), and under stress they may suddenly or gradually regress to a still more "immature" (infantile) form of behavior: catatonia, thumb sucking, and so forth, signifying that already as children they had a locus of pathology in their personalities, which remained when the presenting (ordinarily present) fixation occurred.

C. TRANSACTIONS

The analysis of transactions has led to a fairly rigorous definition of "communication" from an objective point of view, together with some operational rules. A transaction consists of a transactional stimulus followed by a transactional response; this response, in turn, becomes a new stimulus. Communication is said to exist when the response is *appropriate* to the stimulus. A response is appropriate when its vector is parallel to that of the stimulus, as shown by a transactional diagram; such a situation constitutes a complementary transaction. Examples are found in the three commonest types of complementary transactions. (1) Adult-Adult (A-A) stimulus with A-A response (Figure 2a). This is the ordinary "work" transaction: "Pass the hammer." "Here it is." (2) Child-Parent (C-P) stimulus with P-C response (Figure 2b), or P-C stimulus with C-P response. This is a "parenting" transaction. "Mommy, I am hurt." "There, there." Or: "Here is some ice cream." "Thank you, mommy." (3) Adult-Child (A-C) stimulus with C-A response (Figure 2c), or the inverse C-A → A-C. This is a "teaching" transaction. "Hit the ball with the bat." "Like that?" Or: "Is that the way to draw a cow?" "Yes." The first rule of communication then reads: As long as the vectors are parallel, communication can proceed indefinitely.

If the vectors cross, as in Figure 3a (corresponding to a transference reaction), or as in Figure 3b (corresponding to a counter-transference reaction), communication is broken off, which in general means that the subject must be changed. If Figure 3a reads (A-A) "Where are my cuff links?" with response (C-P) "Why do you always blame me for everything?" the possibility of continuing on the subject of cuff links is remote; the situation deteriorates instantly into a game of Uproar, on the subject

378

of who blames or does not blame whom, and how and when and where. The clinical form of this, the second rule of communication, is: If communication is broken off (rather than merely terminated), look for the crossed transaction.

The third rule of communication arises from duplex transactions,

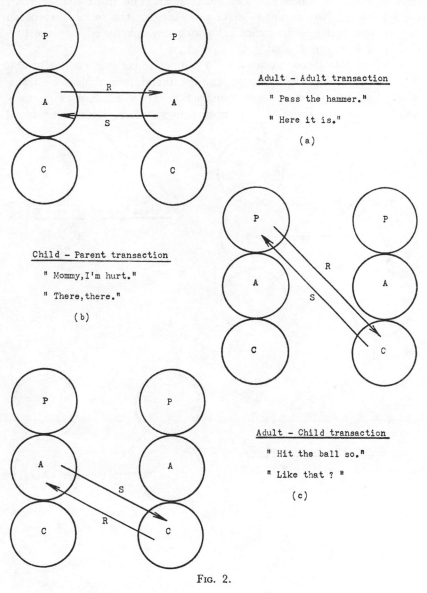

Adult – Adult transaction
" Pass the hammer."
" Here it is."
(a)

Child – Parent transaction
" Mommy, I'm hurt."
" There, there."
(b)

Adult – Child transaction
" Hit the ball so."
" Like that ? "
(c)

FIG. 2.

379

which are too complex to be described here. Briefly, these are two-level transactions. The social level is what appears on the tape or stenogram, while the psychological level deals with the "real" or ulterior purpose of the transaction. For example, the statement "I like Gauguin too" (social level) may be epithalamic, and in its context may signify a consent to sexual relations (psychological level). The third rule of communication is: No amount of data processing of the social level of an ulterior transaction will predict behavior; only a knowledge of the psychological level can do that.

The Palo Alto group[7] makes a valid distinction between congruent and incongruent double-level messages, and it is therefore incumbent on transactional analysis to recognize this distinction. There are four main channels of expression available to human beings: words, intonations, facial

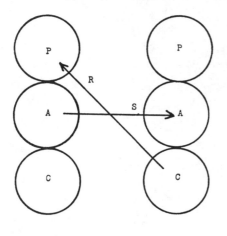

Crossed transaction type I

" Where are they? "

" Why blame me? "

(a)

Crossed transaction type II

" Where are they? "

" Don't ask questions. "

(b)

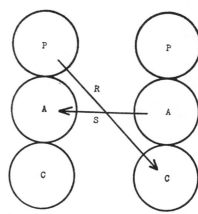

FIG. 3.

380

expression, and bodily movement and expression (actions, gestures, tics, posture, carriage). Any one ego state may capture any or all of these vehicles, or they may be split between two ego states which are simultaneously active, or a single ego state may split into natural components which express themselves independently. In the first case, all of a man may say: "I love the way she cooks!"—words, voice, face, and body. This will then be a completely congruent message. If his face frowns while the rest of him says it, it may mean: "My Child and Adult love the way she cooks, but my mother Parent frowns and says I'm not supposed to." This message is therefore incongruent. Similarly, the Parental ego states may be engaged in an activity which arouses anxiety in the Child ego state; the Parent does one thing bodily while the Child says another: "This hurts me more than it hurts you." In the third case the compliant Child may say one thing while the expressive Child taps out another, as when the woman in the therapy group says: "My marriage is perfect," but another member asks: "That is what you say, but what is your foot saying?" Here again the communication is incongruent. These examples not only illustrate congruent and incongruent communications, but by transactional analysis indicate the internal consistencies and inconsistencies which give rise to them, and tell the therapist where to look historically for the origins of inconsistencies.

D. GAMES

Here we may consider the relationships between games and "rackets." The payoff of the individual's games is determined by his racket. As an actual child, his family taught him their racket: "When the going gets tough, in our family we feel (scared), (guilty), (hurt), (inadequate), (angry), (depressed), (triumphant because we come through on top). The patient then grows up in the fear, guilt, hurt, inadequacy, anger, depression, or triumph racket. Each time he plays a game, he tries to collect the corresponding "trading stamp:" in transactional jargon, chrome, dirty brown, mauve, pink, red, blue, or gold stamps. People who collect gold stamps rarely become patients. The others save their stamps and cash them in eventually for (1) small prizes: a free drunk or masturbation; (2) toy prizes: a toy suicide; or (3) one of the big prizes: a free suicide, homicide, or psychosis. People who collect one color of stamp are generally indifferent to the others. People who collect angers let guilts go by, and people who collect fears let angers go by; and almost all disturbed people turn gold stamps back to the donor.

The ever-growing body of knowledge about games causes a continual reshuffle, reclassification, and reconsideration of games and their rela-

381

tionships to each other. Some which appeared to be variants of the same game turn out to have different origins, advantages, and payoffs. For example, First Degree Rapo (Flirtation) is closely related to the rather constructive Cavalier, while Third Degree Rapo (the false cry of "Rape"), although similar in structure to its First Degree, is more closely related to the destructive Let's You and Him Fight. Others which appeared different at first turn out to be closely related. Thus I'm Only Trying to Help You is often a variant of Let's You and Him Fight, as when the helpful person with a connection gets a car wholesale for the pigeon, and then lets the pigeon fight it out alone with the connection when the car falls apart.

Perhaps the most important advance from the clinical point of view in the area of game analysis is the demonstration that heavy drinking and the game of Alcoholic are independent variables. A female patient, diagnosed schizophrenic, was a "secret drinker." Every night she drank twelve to fourteen ounces of whiskey to help her sleep. But since this never interfered with her job, and did not involve any transactions with other people except the liquor dealer, she was not engaged in the game of Alcoholic, although she might have been classified descriptively (i.e., at a nontransactional level) as "an alcoholic." She followed many of the rules laid down for those who wish to attain this status, except those which related to transactions with other people. Thus she spent "too much" money on liquor, and may have been a "chemical" alcoholic, but she was not a "social" alcoholic because her drinking did not encroach on her relationships with others. She had never been clinically diagnosed during her hospitalizations as "an alcoholic." When she felt better, she cut down to a few ounces a day. This demonstrates that the devious transactions are what lead to the diagnosis of a clinical alcoholic and not the addiction itself.

E. Scripts

The script, or unconscious life plan, is existentially the most important of the individual's transactional sets, since it is the script which determines (or strongly tends to determine, or struggles against even enormous odds to determine) the outcome of the individual's marriage, of his occupational strivings, and of his children's upbringing. It also forms the matrix for his games. Only rarely, however, is it possible to reconstruct the script in detail from the clinical material, so that research in this area proceeds slowly. The script outcomes, or destiny choices, as originally formulated, have stood up well under the test of additional data. These are: (1) self-destruction, moral or physical; (2) destruction of others (moral or physical, including "getting rid of"); (3) flight into illness, psychic or somatic; (4) success or getting well. The childhood form of the script, the protocol, is found to correspond in each case to a primitive myth, typically a Greek myth as found in Graves or Bulfinch; the adolescent adaptation is found in a fairy tale (Little Red Riding Hood, Cinderella); the operational script as put into effect in actual living is a transparent derivative of this. Armed with this knowledge, the therapist can predict and post-dict with considerable accuracy the course of an individual's life; conversely, the study of operational scripts has shed considerable light on the structure of fairy tales. The script requires that the individual collect enough "trading stamps" to justify his election of whichever outcome he chooses. Games are played partly in order to collect the right kinds of trading stamps, according to the individual's racket. Thus mauve "hurt" stamps are collected in the game of "Why Does This Always Happen To Me." After enough stamps have been hoarded, the patient feels entitled to a free ("guilt free") suicide, which is the outcome he decided upon in his formative years. Thus games and rackets are intimately interwoven with the script which determines the final life choice.

F. Therapy

The term "group therapy" has several disadvantages for the transactional analyst. It focuses attention on the mystique of "the group," which is relevant only in a nonspecific way to the recovery of the individual patient; that is, one group is as good as another for what the presence of other people has to offer: a Boy Scout troop, the Elks Club, and a therapy group are at least equally effective insofar as "the group" has something to offer. In fact the objective evidence is that both the Boy Scouts and the Elks Club are more therapeutic in a nonspecific way than a therapy group is. Therefore it is the duty of the professional therapist to offer something specific which the others cannot. Second, the word "therapy" implies that not much is supposed to happen. Decisive interventions, such as an appendectomy, are not spoken of as "therapy," but as "treatment." The chief product of "therapy" is something called "progress." Transactional analysis has as its goal "getting well" rather than progress. Hence transactional analysis prefers instead of the term "group therapy," to substitute "group treatment," with the word "group" being used in a merely descriptive rather than in a mystical or determined way. The goal of group treatment is to get people well.[5] In transactional jargon, group therapy makes braver frogs, while group treatment attempts to change frogs into princes and princesses.

Transactional group treatment remains contractual rather than institutional. The goals are clearly stated and clearly understood between therapist and patient. Group therapy as a social institution takes the position that "Group therapy is Good," without saying explicitly what it is good for; group treatment is based on a contract which states what it is good for in each individual case as compared with all other cases.

Transactional analysis has proved to be effective in "overnight therapy," that is, continuous group meetings which last from 24 to 48 hours with time off for sleeping. The term "overnight therapy" is chosen because the decisive factor is probably the intervening period of sleep which enables the proceedings of the previous day to be assimilated by the Child in the dream work, so that the second day begins with a different emotional set. Transactional analysis appears to be an effective instrument for predicting, controlling, and understanding the proceedings and effects of such meetings. "Marathon" therapy (prolonged meetings without sleep) has not yet been studied transactionally.

In general, it is found that transactional analysts use verbs and concrete nouns where other therapists tend to use adjectives and abstract nouns. "He hit his employer in order to . . ." is preferred to "The patient exhibits aggressive impulses toward authority figures." This avoids a "demonic" implication. The patient is not regarded as "being" aggressive (passive, dependent), a kind of original sin; nor does he need an excuse: "The demon aggression is only awakened in you in response to certain stimuli." The question is not "Why is this aggressive demon in you?" nor "What did he say to awaken the aggressive demon in you?" The transactional analyst asks: "What did your Child hope to gain by hitting your employer?" The conventional approach to the incorporated object (in the sense of Melanie Klein) raises unnecessary difficulties by thinking in descriptive rather than in transactional terms. The study of adverbs is particularly interesting. "I always speak harshly to my children" is not quite the same as "I am always harsh to my children." If there is a demon, he is more likely to respond to sympathetic questions than to epithets disguised as technical polysyllables: a device he is easily able to see through.

REFERENCES

1. BERNE, E.: Transactional Analysis in Psychotherapy. New York, Grove Press, 1961.
2. BERNE, E.: Games People Play. New York, Grove Press, 1964.
3. BERNE, E.: The Structure & Dynamics of Organizations & Groups. Philadelphia, J. B. Lippincott Company, 1963.
4. BERNE, E.: Principles of transactional analysis. In Current Psychiatric

Therapies, Vol. IV, J. H. Masserman Ed. New York, Grune & Stratton, 1964.

5. BERNE, E.: Principles of Group Treatment. London, Oxford University Press (in press).

6. BREUER, J., AND FREUD, S.: Studies in hysteria. In Nervous and Mental Disease Monographs, New York, 1950.

7. SATIR, V.: Conjoint Family Therapy. Palo Alto, Science and Behavior Books, 1964.

Marathon Group Therapy: Rationale and Techniques

by IVAN B. GENDZEL, M.D.

The phrase marathon groups is frequently associated with concepts such as: transcendent experience, weekend orgy, nudity, affirmation, intimacy, precipitating psychoses, confrontation, attack, and genuineness. This presentation attempts to define what "marathon group therapy" does mean by initially comparing it to encounter groups and group therapy. The specific and unique advantages of this form of therapy are considered, and then a review of various techniques and the format of these groups is made. Finally, there is an overview of its worth in the therapeutic armamentarium, and the role of psychiatry in the marathon group movement.

Group Therapy, Encounter Groups, and Marathon Group Therapy

The use of group therapy as a therapeutic modality was initiated by Joseph Pratt about 1905 in association with his rest treatment of tuberculosis and has become an increasingly popular form of treatment, most particularly since World War II. A former consideration for the value of this experience was the ability to comprehend and experience a resolution of a transference neurosis. Factors which encouraged a movement away from this style of group therapy have included: an emphasis of ego psychology and a lessening of the relative importance of the classic and traditional analytic psychotherapies; an increasing existential and humanistic orientation; a general change in the conceptualization of mental illness with a tendency to deemphasize the medical disease model and with an increasing awareness of societal, family, and interpersonal relationships; the development of varieties of brief psychotherapies; and the desire of many for a more brief, inexpensive, and efficient form of therapy.

Under the aegis of educators and social and industrial psychologists, a separate small group movement started in 1946 during a short summer workshop and was encouraged by the subsequently formed National Training Laboratories. It emphasized the laboratory method of learning and research, and out of this movement new characteristics and philosophies of small groups have emerged.[1] These innovations and special attentions have included a here-and-now orientation, a marked emphasis on feelings and emotions, feedback procedures, interpersonal learning, and even formation of leaderless groups. Emerging from

386

this training group (or T group), and largely adapting its values and orientations, has been the encounter group movement. This has rapidly spread throughout the country so that every medium- and large-sized city, institutions of higher education, secondary schools, religious groups, and industrial organizations have had the opportunity to experience varieties of encounter groups.[2] These groups have also been called sensitivity training and human awareness, leadership training, Synanon games, psychodrama, Gestalt, nonverbal, and experiential. The particular emphasis on a style may vary, but the encounter group approach prevails. This current interest is attested to by the frequent appearance in movies, novels, newspapers, and magazines of material concerning these groups.

Time, one of the variables of any group meeting, has been adjusted so that some groups have been meeting for extended periods of time and have been labeled marathon groups. The sacrosanct 90-minute group therapy hour has been extended to include such time intervals as 6 hours, 12 hours, or more commonly 24 or more consecutive hours or several days with breaks for sleep. Early investigators have included Bach, Casriel, and Stoller,[3-11] who have helped to define the accelerated interaction said to be characteristic of this new format.

Rationale and Characteristics of Marathon Groups

Many of the general considerations concerning group therapy and encounter groups apply with equal validity to marathon groups. Confidentiality, physical restraints, no drugs or alcohol, and an attempt to present oneself honestly apply to most groups. What are the specific variables which, because of the extended-time feature, make for the unique contributions of a marathon group experience?

A marathon, unlike many open-ended groups, has two essential features:

1. A limited number of hours, usually more than 6, or perhaps 12 or 24 hours, a weekend, five 12-hour days, etc.
2. These hours are fairly consecutive and whatever momentum is built up is not allowed to dissipate during long periods when the group is apart.

The marathon group quickly becomes a world unto itself with a specific life-span. The participant is encouraged to accept the responsibility for himself and for his fate in the group. It is emphasized that there is some correlation between the paths he chooses in the group and those he chooses in the world. Importantly, he is made keenly aware that he has alternatives, and he is encouraged to risk attempting to find newer and perhaps better methods of relating with others. Change in the undesirable aspects of his presentation is acknowledged and approved by the group, thereby encouraging further attempts at change.

The time pressure helps to develop a sense of urgency and, coupled with a

387

high motivation for being in such an extended group experience in the first place, a participant is usually willing to make an attempt to change. In addition to these considerations and to the frequent impacting of meaningful and demanding experiences, over the many hours a sense of fatigue builds up which further contributes to the dropping of defensive postures and facades. The sense of urgency, the high motivation, and the increasing fatigue are the specific factors which contribute to the uniqueness of the marathon experience.

Many other features have become associated with this experience. A more relaxed, informal setting, frequently a home, and the availability of creature comforts (such as food and bathroom facilities) make for a less artificial or clinical environment. Within this universe a group life emerges which is available to the scrutiny of all. Subgrouping, whispering, or experiencing meaningfully outside of the group is strongly discouraged. Within the microcosm that emerges, less and less attention is paid to the genetic antecedents; in contrast, the "here and now" is of greatest concern. Plans for the future outside the group might also be considered, but more important are plans for the future within the group. Frequently an attempt is made to draw up a contract as to what are the changes desired during the life of the group. A participant then has the benefit of experiencing directly his own changes and the effect of these on others. He is able to discover immediately the consequences of his actions, and to consider the desire of any further change.

A sense of belonging and cohesiveness develops during the course of the group. Attempts at "instant intimacy" do not succeed as well as allowing the group to experience for itself and to deal with its inherent stresses and strains and for members to accept each other and feel related. Intensive interpersonal confrontation and most particularly expressions of intense emotions accompanied by anger and tears appear to be part of the necessary steps toward achieving the desirable and necessary cohesiveness. Given the structure of the situation, the motivations of the participants, and the highly important role of the leader, this desired goal is generally achieved.[12-14]

The role of the leader is central to the group initially in setting the structure, defining the process, establishing the contract, and organizing for the event. Of equal importance is his role within the group as an active participant, an expert in interpersonal behavior, and a model for the others. Yalom states: "The curative factors in group therapy are primarily mediated not by the therapist, but by the other members who provide the acceptance and support, the hope, the experience of universality, the opportunities for altruistic behavior, and the interpersonal feedback, testing, and learning. It is the therapist's task to help the group develop into a cohesive unit with an atmosphere maximally conducive to the operation of these curative factors."[15]

Relative to ongoing weekly groups, the role of the marathon leader, as an involved participant and a model of expected behavior, is a more vital one, and more directly revealing of himself. The meeting may even take place at his house and with other family members attending. He shares his reactions and feelings with the group and, when appropriately stimulated, may feel free to express a problem area or a dilemma of his own. These have the tendency to make him all the more human and less the blank or aloof authority. As many studies in individual therapy have shown, it is this ability of the therapist to be involved and authentic, rather than autocratic and intolerant, which serves as a model for the other participants and encourages the honest and nondefensive behavior which helps to achieve the desired group goals. Each leader must develop an approach and a style of interaction that is unique to him. He should be a person with clinical experience, but without a "clinical approach." He should be a person acceptable to himself and with a desire to help others, and a willingness to be responsible, not only for his own behavior, but for the group and its results.[16]

Techniques, Methods, and Approaches

Specific techniques, methods, or approaches vary with the nature of the individual leaders.[3,10,13,17,18] No single correct methodology can emerge, and only a few techniques are enumerated here.

Instead of the standard question of "Why are you here?" a more precise definition and contract are required. Specifically, something of the nature "What is it you want to get out of this experience?" or "How do you hope to be different at the end of the group?" may be demanded of the participants early in the meeting. An answer is satisfactory only after it is acceptable to the rest of the group. Toward the end of the therapy the contracts are reviewed, and a final opportunity to fulfill the contract is afforded, or the contract may be modified.

Developments in electronic audiovisual media have allowed for the use of a variety of sophisticated instruments. Lighting effects and music as background to what is happening have been used effectively. For instance, flashing red and white lights with loud discordant music may accentuate angry words, and music as noise may be used to force a person to speak more loudly and forcibly. Sound and video recorders allow immediate playback,[19,20] unlike that from the rest of the group. Additional personnel, familiar with the equipment and the progress of the marathon, unobtrusively operate the equipment and are available as a resource for the leader or group.

Various encounter techniques, particularly as means of starting the group, are commonly used. These range from encouraging an individual to detail either the positive or negative impressions of some or all members of the group to encouraging participants in various risk-taking activities. Significantly, there is a marked tendency for nonverbal behavior to be observed, emphasized, and interpreted, and for varieties of this behavior to be encouraged. An example

389

might be to encourage a participant physically to reach out for someone in addition to just making verbal contact with that person.

Varieties of nonverbal behavior might include the use of various art materials. The participants, either at the start or after a recess, might be asked to depict themselves by crayon or pastels on paper in any form or design in terms of how they then feel, and how they would like to feel at a later time. These drawings may then be individually presented to the group and discussed. Or two people may be asked to conduct a dialogue on paper without talking or writing any words, allowing one person to say something and the other person to respond until the conversation feels complete. At that point the two, either as a dyad or in front of the group, can discuss their "conversation" and how effective they were in communicating. Other materials, such as finger paint or clay, may be used for either individual activities, dyads, or larger groups.

The language of the body not only is listened to, but frequently is used as the major communicative form, particularly when the verbal mode becomes ineffective. For instance, two individuals who have reached an impasse and yet have not adequately resolved their situation might be asked to stand and face each other, to approach each other when ready, and then to have some variety of nonverbal interaction. The "variety" is not further specified. They are instructed to have this interaction until it feels complete and then to return to their initial place. These encounters might be very brief and involve only an exchange of an eye glance or handshake or may evolve into intense and prolonged interaction. The individuals then are asked if the encounter felt complete, particularly in terms of adequately communicating their feelings. If not, they are allowed to repeat it. The discussion that follows, both between the two participants and among the observers, lends further meaning and frequently clarifies how the verbal impasse had been reached. This interaction is particularly valuable between couples attending the meeting together. It may reveal and demonstrate to the others what could not satisfactorily be verbalized.

Another means of encouraging contact might be to ask people to stand and pair, then to face each other holding hands and closing eyes, and to try to become aware only of what the other pair of hands is "saying." The leader could then in a permissive manner encourage the hands to initially express anger, then to express warmth and affection, and perhaps even finally to explore the parts of the body to which these other hands are attached. Finally, the face could be explored and the partner helped literally "to open his eyes." The interactions would then be verbalized, initially with one another, and then with the group. This allows for an intense and significant physical contact between two participants, a chance to check the fantasied partner with the real one, and a chance to feed back to the partner the nature of the tactile impressions and how these correlate with the overall impressions of that person. A related activity might be "blind milling" when everyone, with eyes closed and arms somewhat

390

extended, moves slowly about exploring his environment. This might serve as a prelude to the "hand conversation."

Schutz has compiled many of these exercises or situations.[21] As a means of attempting to free the person of his emotional impediments and of the physical expression by the body, Schutz carefully "listens" to what the body is "saying," encourages the bodily expression of feelings, and promotes the resolution of problems by a physical reenactment within the group. Examples might include learning to trust others by falling backward into their arms, or by having an isolated and withdrawn individual forcefully "break into" other social groups.

These and many other interactions become part of the group and may be used effectively if comfortably applied by the leader at the appropriate time. The rationale for these activities is that they provide an additional means to help set a more open and intimate tone within the group and also to circumvent the usual verbal barriers. Additionally, the satisfaction of being able to meaningfully communicate on paper or by hands serves a valuable function in terms of the group's interaction and the individual sense of accomplishment. Finally, information obtained can be conceptualized and verbalized and make a contribution to the overall marathon experience.

As the final hours of the marathon approach, the sense of urgency increases, the fatigue factor becomes more important, and the cohesiveness within the group is such that there is an even more meaningful and accelerated rate of interaction. There are various "go-arounds" with one person either telling the other individuals his reactions or receiving from all the other individuals their impressions. Almost always the participants, though physically fatigued, feel exhilarated and significantly related with one another as the group ends at its predetermined time. There is frequently a reluctance to separate, and any evaluations done at this time usually reflect the positive feelings and exhilaration of the person experiencing it. There are frequent comments about "let's keep in touch," and if a follow-up meeting several weeks later has been scheduled, reference is made to this.

The participants leave the marathon meeting in a certain "high" and with various expectations of change. The intensity of involvement and the degree of intimacy, however, are not generally available when the person "reenters" his usual situation, and a sense of disappointment is commonly experienced. This depressive episode or "down" usually comes on within several days after the marathon, and lasts for several days. If there is a follow-up meeting after several weeks, the participants will then frequently question the reality and worth of their initial experience and perhaps even comment about a dreamlike quality or unreal feeling or remembrance of the experience.

In summary the marathon group experience can be said to consist of three parts. Initially, there are the many events prior to the meeting, including any individual or small trial group experiences, and the obtaining of an informed

391

consent by the participants.[22,23] Then there is the meeting itself. Finally, a follow-up meeting is usually scheduled. This is important in that it allows the participants to review somewhat more objectively and with the benefit of hindsight the intensive experience they have all been through and also allows provision for a sense of closure. Not uncommonly, relationships established during the meetings are continued subsequently, but the group as initially defined is terminated at this point.

Overview. Not every intense and emotional experience, even if it is labeled as a part of therapy, is necessarily corrective and desirable. Undoubtedly the structure of a marathon group does encourage and beget many intense emotional expressions, which hopefully benefits the participants, but this may not always be so. Attempts have been made to define what aspects of an encounter group experience are potentially most harmful, what individuals are most likely to be hurt by such an experience, and how to eliminate and "screen out" these potentially undesirable events.[22,24] Psychiatrists and inpatient units have had to care for people who have recently emerged from an intensive group experience and could not "put it all together." Here again, the ability of the leader is of paramount importance in initially screening out potential casualties, and also in evaluating and supporting such people once they are in the group. However, it has been shown that leaders are at times not as aware of the detrimental effects on a participant as are some of the other members.[24]

Whom should a psychiatrist refer for a marathon group experience? The patient might be someone "stuck" in individual or group therapy, or someone generally dissatisfied with his interaction with others or with strong neurotic tendencies which may benefit significantly from a marathon experience. However, a person with rigid or unyielding defenses or a strong need to remain isolated may be overwhelmed by these features and experience a detrimental disorganization. Though many factors enter into the selection, perhaps the most important are the motivation and informed consent of the person, and his awareness of his option to leave should he consider this desirable. (Though this is rarely exercised, the explicit awareness of this option may "permit" a person to remain and work through his anxieties.) Awareness of the opportunity to discuss this further after the group with a nonparticipant also helps to maintain a perspective on the experience and lessen the likelihood of an undesirable result.[24-26]

Are encounter groups to be considered group therapy, and is a psychiatrist in an encounter group a "therapist"? A task force of the American Psychiatric Association concluded: "In our opinion, a physician, even though he involves himself in a group nominally non-therapy in nature, still may not divorce himself from his traditional continuing responsibility to the participants whether or not they are specifically labeled his patients. [Members may join a human awareness group led by a psychiatrist because of covert expectations of a psychotherapy

392

experience.] Encounter group trainers . . . are not legally responsible for possible detrimental effects of the group on a member unless the leaders are specifically advertised as mental health experts . . . it would seem probable that the psychiatrist retains his 'mental health expert' designation even when leading a group which is not specifically labeled as therapy, but which may be a potent influence, both positively and negatively, upon the mental health of the participants."[27] This implied burden of responsibility may partially help to account for the relatively lesser participation by psychiatrists in encounter and marathon group experiences.

But some other factors may be the specific medical model and training of a physician which appears antithetical to some of the desired traits of a group leader, e.g., clinical experience but not a clinical approach. The psychiatrist's traditional role is a distant, frequently enigmatic, self-reserving one, and more in line with the classically powerful, authoritarian, and sagacious physician. The trainer or leader is more self-disclosing and personally involved, with a willingness to be less of an authority. However, there are significant variation and overlapping in various leaders' and therapists' styles, and the specific professional background may be of less importance than the leader's clinical experience and his ethics and philosophy. In addition, since fatigue and inattention are likely, a cotherapist is desirable and a harmonious relationship between the two (or more) therapists is necessary.

What then may be expected after participation in a marathon group meeting? There is certainly no basis for a claim of an enduring and permanent change in one's personality pattern from this single event. Some have suggested that people periodically attend, perhaps at monthly intervals, a number of such meetings as a method of maximizing the benefits of the experience. Others have viewed the marathon meetings as a valuable adjunct to ongoing individual or group psychotherapy, as a diagnostic situation before therapy, or as an intensive means of getting involved in either individual or group therapy. Perhaps a realistic expectation of one marathon experience is that the participant would become more aware of his own feelings, experience a sense of well-being and relatedness to others, and acquire some insight which would make for more satisfactory functioning. For those in ongoing psychotherapy, the experience could provide valuable material to be further explored. Frequently important decisions are arrived at during the intensive meeting, and a proper balance between premature and impulsive action and, hopefully, a well-thought-out and advised plan of action are achieved.

This relates perhaps most specifically to marital problems made more overt during the meeting. If the pair is present, an opportunity is given for resolution; if one spouse is not present, a tendency exists to blame the spouse, particularly in view of the feeling of approval and acceptance the participant feels from the others at the meeting. Although divorce is an occasional outcome, there is more

393

frequently a positive sense of commitment and affirmation to work constructively for fulfillment within the marriage. Most marathon participants benefit by having more of a positive sense of commitment in pursuit of their goals, particularly the interpersonal ones.

Marathon group therapy, then, offers a unique and powerful experience, the benefits and values of which are partially inherent in the structure of the group. The benefits also depend on the ability of the individual to assimilate the experiences both within the group and later, and on the skill of the therapist.

REFERENCES

1. Bradford, L. P., Gibb, J. R., and Benne, K. D.: T-Group Theory and Laboratory Method: Innovation in Re-Education. New York, John Wiley & Sons, 1964.
2. Rogers, C. R.: Carl Rogers on Encounter Groups. New York, Harper & Row, 1970, p. 9.
3. Bach, G. R.: The Marathon Group: Intensive Practice in Intimate Interaction. Psychol. Rep. 18:995-1002, 1966.
4. Bach, G. R.: Marathon Group Dynamics: I. Some Functions of the Professional Group Facilitator. Psychol. Rep. 20:995-999, 1967.
5. Bach, G. R.: Marathon Group Dynamics. II. Dimensions of Helpfulness: Therapeutic Aggression. Psychol. Rep. 20:1147-1158, 1967.
6. Bach, G. R.: Marathon Group Dynamics. III. Disjunctive Contacts. Psychol. Rep. 20:1163-1172, 1967.
7. Bach, G. R.: Group and Leader-Phobias in Marathon Groups. Voices 3:41-46, 1967.
8. Casriel, D. H., and Deitch, D.: The Marathon: Time Extended Group Therapy. In: Masserman, J. (Ed.), Therapies, Vol. 8. New York, Grune & Stratton, Inc., 1968.
9. Rachman, A. W.: Marathon Group Psychotherapy: Its Origins, Significance and Direction. J. Group Psychoanal. Process 2:57-74, 1969.
10. Stoller, F. H.: Marathon Group Therapy. Los Angeles, Youth Studies Center, University of Southern California, 1967.
11. Stoller, F. H.: Accelerated Interaction: A Time-Limited Approach Based on the Brief, Intensive Group. Int. J. Group Psychother. 18:220-235, 1968.
12. Dies, R. R., and Hess, A. K.: An Experimental Investigation of Cohesiveness in Marathon and Conventional Group Psychotherapy. J. Abnorm. Psychol. 77:258-262, 1971.
13. Gendzel, I. B.: Marathon Group Therapy and Nonverbal Methods. Amer. J. Psychiat. 127:286-290, 1970.
14. Sklar, A. D., Yalom, I. D., Zim, A., and Newell, G. L.: Time-Extended Group Therapy: A Controlled Study. Comparative Group Studies 1(4):373-386, 1970.
15. Yalom, I. D.: The Theory and Practice of Group Psychotherapy. New York, Basic Books, Inc., 1970, p. 83.
16. Rosenbaum, M.: The Responsibility of the Group Psycho-therapy Practitioner for a Therapeutic Rationale. J. Group Psychoanal. Process 2:5-17, 1969.
17. Ellis, A.: A Weekend of Rational Encounter. In: Burton, A. (Ed.), Encounter. San Francisco, Jassey-Bass Inc., 1970.
18. Mann, J.: Encounter: A Weekend with Intimate Strangers. New York, Grossman Publishers, 1970.

19. Berger, M. M., Sherman, B., Spalding, J., and Westlake, R.: The Use of Videotape with Psychotherapy Groups in a Community Mental Health Service Program. Int. J. Group Psychother. 18:504-515, 1968.
20. Damet, B. N.: Videotape Playback as a Therapeutic Device in Group Psychotherapy. Int. J. Group Psychother. 14: 433-440, 1969.
21. Schutz, W.: Joy. Expanding Human Awareness. New York; Grove Press, Inc., 1967.
22. Stone, W. N., and Tieger, M. E.: Screening for T-Groups: The Myth of Healthy Candidates. Amer. J. Psychiat. 127:1485-1429, 1971.
23. Gendzel, I. B.: Discussion of Stone and Tieger's Paper. Amer. J. Psychiat. 127:1489-1490, 1971.
24. Yalom, I. D., and Lieberman, M. A.: A Study of Encounter Group Casualties. Arch. Gen. Psychiat. (Chicago) 25:16-30, 1971.
25. A.M.A. Council on Mental Health: Sensitivity Training. J.A.M.A. 217:1853-1854, 1971.
26. Gottschalk, L. A., and Pattison, E. M.: Psychiatric Perspectives on T-Groups and the Laboratory Movement: An Overview. Amer. J. Psychiat. 126:91-107, 1969.
27. APA Task Force Report: Encounter Groups and Psychiatry. Washington, D.C., American Psychiatric Association, 1970, p. 22.

The Use of Music in Group Psychotherapy

by JOHN E. SNELL, M.D.

T HE LITERATURE DEALING WITH so-called music therapy is volumi-
nous, but much of this literature has represented the wishful
thinking of artistically inclined therapeutic dilettantes, rather than the
considered data of serious scientists. The term "music therapy" has itself
been criticized[1,2] as implying an understanding of specific effects of
music which can be therapeutically prescribed for mental illness—an
understanding which is not yet available. I am in firm agreement with
this criticism, and I would resist the employment of the term "music
therapy" to denote the use of music to be described.

This chapter will describe an application of music in group therapy
which was felt to have been useful in making possible the treatment
of a group of very severely regressed patients. The goal of the therapy
was improvement in the patient's abilities to communicate emotional
concerns.

The patients for the group were chosen from the day hospital and
inpatient services of the Massachusetts Mental Health Center, and
included men and women aged 18 to 35. All had been under treatment
an average of 6 months for variously diagnosed psychoses. Musical
training or expressed affection for music were not considered in patient
selection. The criterion for inclusion in the group was a major impairment of verbal communication, from near-mutism to almost constant
manic word-salad. The group met for 1 hour once each week, and
continued for 18 months. The number of patients ranged from 4 to 10,
with 4 patients attending for the entire duration of the group. The
author was group therapist; a nurse recorder who did not verbally
participate was always present, and an experienced hospital attendant
was usually in attendance.

The initial rationale underlying the use of such a group in treatment
of psychotics involved three assumptions: (1) psychotic speech dis-

orders may arise as defenses against recognizing and dealing with strong emotion; (2) music can be used as a stimulus to verbalization of emotions; and (3) a group setting would provide interpersonal stimulus to emotion and multiple opportunities for practice in dealing with threatening affects in interpersonal situations. The format employed follows in many respects that described by Rose, et al.[3]

Each group session was begun with the playing on a stereo-hi-fi phonograph of a short orchestral passage, usually less than 5 minutes in length but chosen for its capacity to stimulate a variety of emotions. Music of the nineteenth century Romantic movement often provided the desired variety of mood, although much modern orchestral or solo music was played also. Following the initial musical passage, the patients were instructed to talk about anything they wished. During each hour, further short passages were often played once or twice when the therapist felt that such passages might stimulate expression of specific feelings, or when the anxiety level during silences reached disruptive proportions.

Because music has the quality of stimulating emotion as well as of being an outward expression of it, it can be used flexibly to help a patient move from projection *of* to responsibility *for* feelings. The patients in the group showed a tendency to move through four discernible positions in the development of ability to discuss emotion. At first, they tended to talk about the music as entirely separate from themselves; i.e., they talked about the phonograph, asked about the recording, commented on the music's loudness, slowness, etc. Later, they began to venture comments about feelings in the music, but they still divorced the feelings from themselves, as "that is sad music, happy music," etc. In a significant jump, the patients next acknowledged that they experienced feelings, although still carefully placing responsibility upon the music: "The music makes *me* feel happy or sad." A final step was, of course, acknowledgement of internal affects by the patient with full recognition that they originated within him and that he had responsibility for them. At this stage, the patient would be engaging in the kind of honest self-observation which is a cornerstone of insight psychotherapy. With all patients functioning on this level, the music would be totally irrelevant and unnecessary, its usefulness as an emotion-stimulating focus for projection of emotion having been served.

Patients tended to return to discussion on lower levels of this progression at times of high group anxiety, apparently using the presence of the music as a "safety-valve." This allowed discussion to proceed, and, with encouragement by the therapist, the group discussion remained

397

on the higher levels for increasing periods of times as the group advanced. The use of music by patients just described seems to depend upon a quality which may be inherent in most, if not all, music, and in this sense the specificity of musical selection may be of minor importance.

A second, though related, manner in which music served this group is worth noting. Group silences were many and long, especially in the early months, and could increase the anxiety level of group members and of the therapist. The therapist often chose to modify a silence with the playing of another short musical selection. The choice of such selections was governed by the assumption that many group silences are symptomatic of the existence of strong feeling in the group which no group member is able to take responsibility for expressing. Accordingly, the therapist would offer the music as an object for projection of this feeling. An attempt was made to judge what predominant feeling was blocked from expression at the moment, and to choose a musical passage which in the therapist's opinion might stimulate that feeling.[4] It was observed that very often the brief passage would be followed by an immediate resumption of group discussion, frequently with discussion by group members of the previously unexpressed feeling, often projected onto the music.

Such attempts to apply the unique qualities of music to group psychotherapy may be valuable in their own right if they lead to improved means for working with various types of patients. The three most seriously regressed patients who were seen in the group's entire course responded with the most animation of expression, the most muscular movement, and the most verbalization following the presentation of music having the most freedom with regard to rhythm, harmony, and melodic progression. Stravinsky's "Le Sacre du Printemps" contains much of this kind of music, and the presentation of passages from this work was regularly followed by more animation and verbalization on the part of the more disturbed patients, while the less regressed patients more often expressed a dislike for it, preferring the orderly music of nineteenth century romanticism (Tschaikovsky, Brahms, Schumann, etc.). Music may therefore be potentially useful as a diagnostic tool to assay the degree of a patient's thought disorder.[5-7]

Music has always seemed to lend itself well to use in groups. There have been several main types of group application in psychiatry. Perhaps the most common has been an occupational therapy approach in which groups of patients have been organized into rhythm bands, singing groups, activity groups, music appreciation groups, etc.[8-10] Background music in the mental hospital has received some attention,[9] and

398

the industrial and marketplace adaptation of motivational background music is well known.[10] Recently, as group psychotherapy techniques have become more familiar, there has been increased interest in using music as an adjunct to group psychotherapy.[11] Weiss and Margolin presented a group therapy technique using musical stimulation.[12] Shatin and Zimet showed evidence that music could increase verbal participation in group therapy, and that "stimulating" music and "quieting" music had a differential effect upon degree and quality of participation.[13] Heckel showed that tempo has a significant effect upon operant speech levels in group therapy.[14] Lucas used "mood" music in therapy with depressed patients and showed its effect in increasing verbalization of affectual concerns.[15] Pierce described the use of music in groups in a day-care center.[16] The time may be near in which music will be seen as a powerful research and treatment tool.

REFERENCES

1. GUTHEIL, E. A.: Music as adjunct to psychotherapy. Am. J. Psychother. 8:94-109, 1954.
2. MASSERMAN, J. H.: Music and the child in society. Am. J. Psychother. 8: 63-67,1954.
3. ROSE, A. E., BROWN, C. E., AND METCALFE, E. V.: Music therapy at Westminister Hospital. Mental Hygiene 43:93-104, 1959.
4. ALTSHULER, I. M.: Four years' experience with music as a therapeutic agent at Eloise Hospital. Am. J. Psychiat. 100:792-794, 1944.
5. REINKES, J. H.: The use of unfamiliar music as a stimulus for a projective test of personality. In Proceedings of the National Association for Music Therapy. Kansas, National Association for Music Therapy, 1952, pp.224-230.
6. JENKINS, S. R.: The development and evaluation of a musical thematic apperception test. In Proceedings of the National Association for Music Therapy. Kansas, National Association for Music Therapy, 1955, pp. 101-113.
7. SIMON, B., et al.: The recognition and acceptance of mood in music by psychotic patients. J. Nerv. Ment. Dis. 114:66-78, 1951.
8. GILLILAND, E. G.: Progress in music therapy. Rehab. Lit. 23:298-306, 1962.
9. VAN DE WALL, W.: Music in Institutions. New York, Russell Sage Foundation, 1936, pp. 48-73.
10. SOIBELMAN, DORIS: Therapeutic and Industrial Uses of Music. New York, Columbia U. Press, 1948.
11. STERNE, S.: The validity of music on effective group psychotherapeutic technique. In Proceedings of the National Association for Music Therapy. Kansas, National Association for Music Therapy, 1955, pp. 130-140.
12. WEISS, D. M., AND MARGOLIN, R. J.: The use of music as an adjunct to group therapy. Am. Arch. Rehab. Ther. 3:13-26, 1953.
13. SHATIN, L., AND ZIMET, C.: Influence of music upon verbal participation in group psychotherapy. Dis. Nerv. Syst. 19:66-72, 1958.

14. HECKEL, R. V., et al.: The effect of musical tempo in varying operant speech levels in group therapy. J. Clin. Psychol. 19:129, 1963.
15. LUCAS, D., et al.: Group psychotherapy with depressed patients incorporating mood music. Am. J. Psychother. 18:126-36, 1964.
16. PIERCE, C. M., et al.: Music therapy in a day care center. Dis. Nerv. Syst. 25:29-32, 1964.

Developments in Dance Therapy

by BERNARD F. RIESS, PH.D.

ANCE THERAPY IS, in many respects the most recent arrival in the ranks of the so-called ancillary therapies. Drama, music and art are the veteran members of the group with poetry therapy as a relatively new approach. One may view the birth-order of these treatment modalities as accidental, but it is probably determined by a complex of factors ranging from early emphasis on verbal communication to the newer foci on identity, body awareness and the value of total experience. It is also obvious that dance, with its essential characteristic of movement and fluidity, requires for its scientific study more than merely technical performance skills in the art. As long as dance lacked a notational system, it raised difficulties for those who were concerned with matching behavior, change and treatment modality.

Since dance therapy is relatively new and outside the traditional techniques, the literature on its use, *raison d'être,* results and variations is sparse. In discussing developments in this field it is therefore mandatory to give the background against which it is to be viewed, outline some of the theoretical considerations which lead its proponents, and to have high hopes for its applicability and success. Some of the psychoanalytic and psychopathological studies of movement and dance will be cited along with the relatively few studies of the specific technique of dance as therapy.

The Encyclopedia Brittanica, 13th edition,[10] describes dance as "the universal human expression, by movement of the limbs and body, of a sense of rhythm which is implanted among the primitive instincts of the animal world. The rhythmic principle of motion extends throughout the universe, governing the lapse of waves, the flow of tides, the reverberations of light and sound, and the movements of celestial bodies; and in the human organism it manifests itself in the automatic pulses and flexions of blood and tissues." This is a somewhat florid view, but contemporary writing about the field seems to be in agreement that movement and dance are primitive and inevitable accompaniments of development from the undifferentiated neonate to the mature adult.

401

The viewpoint of the dance theorist can be summarized as follows.

Human movement is the organization of human energy in response to his environment. Dance movement is the rhythmic organization of human energy in response to internal drives and reactions to the environment. Movement carries with it awareness of the interaction of internal and external energies. The process of interaction is the core of all movement and the heart of dance. The most encompassing environmental factor for the human as for all organisms is space. The person, to be such, must recognize and define the differences of human and non-human objects in space with due attention to the spatial reality of his own body. The space position of the self is always central for the normally developing human.

Development should involve the awareness of the broad range of movement experiences which, in turn, affects the total movement possibilities of the body, progress in self-mastery and feelings, and percepts and emotions relating to the movement experiences.

Dance adds to the expressive qualities of movement, and the elements of discipline and order. This can happen only when the individual is able to understand his total environment and to enjoy the developmental change, which make the experiencing possible.

John Martin, a famous critic of dance, has said of Isadora Duncan:[19] "Without the benefit of formal psychology, she knew . . . that spontaneous movement of the body is the first reaction of all men to sensory or emotional stimuli. Though civilization tends to dull and inhibit this tendency, it is still the fundamental reaction of men to the universe about them. A revival of the conscious use of this faculty would mean deepening and broadening the whole range of life. If the individual becomes aware of the world in which he lives through its direct effect on his nerves and muscles, nature's fundamental perceptive mechanism, he has won his freedom from the arbitrary thou-shalts and shalt-nots which established social cults and creeds put upon him the moment he is old enough to be dominated."

To some behavioral scientists, it then becomes evident that movement and dance are, in today's world, essential therapeutic media to offset mass molding and contra-individual conformity. Wunderlich[27] points to the fact that contemporary society deprives the individual of the relatively unlimited opportunities for movement, the experience of which characterized all previous historical epochs. Since, in his words, "movement is a primordial force," deprivation leads to abnormality. Scheflen[25] makes the additional point that movement is a subtle but important medium of communication.

Psychoanalytic writers on movement have created a considerable body of literature. Deutsch writes;[8] "As psychological changes occur during treatment, the postural pattern becomes transitorily or permanently altered. . . The language of the body frequently needs no interpretation because the patient becomes aware of its meaning. . . The correlation of psychological (verbal) with postural expression shows, that in states of instinctual conflict, the defenses and the repressed emotions are readily reflected in bodily behavior. . . Postural attitudes reflect or substitute, precede or accompany the verbal expression of unconscious material. . . Movements are made in relation to fantasied objects which may include the subject himself."

Kestenberg[15,17] explains how movement correlates motor rhythms with specific patterns of discharge of anal, oral and phallic drives, tension and effort flow as indices of maturation, fixation and regression, and feeling tones as these emerge from their kinesthetic origin in infancy.

From a more experimental orientation, Freedman and Hoffman[12] classify hand movements into two general groups: those related to the outer-world of objects and those associated with the inner world of self. Wachtel[26] also points to the importance of body language in psychotherapy, and recommends video-tape records for interpreting movement.

DANCE

Doll[9] defines dance as "broadly construed to cover all types of rhythmic movement, from simple marching to complex ball-room and figure dances. Here the possibilities for gross-muscle training, strengthening of the body image, expressive release and creativity, patterned coordinated movement, social relating and group cooperation are bounded only by the imaginativeness of the instructor. . . "The cerebral palsied child, caught up in the swing of a couple dance or group movement, can sometimes unconsciously master patterns of movement which might involve months of self-defeating effort in physiotherapy. . . . For the slow learner, success on the dance floor may compensate for lack of achievement in the classroom. This often provides the needed ego-gratification for satisfactory social adjustment, while the resultant rise in self-esteem frequently reinforces the classroom situation."

Perlowitz[21] writes that social dancing represents a sublimated non-verbal abreaction in which each partner acts as a nonverbal analyst to alleviate anxiety from sexual thoughts, impulses and feelings. Blum[3] sees contemporary dances, such as the frug, as the reactions of adolescents to the current syndromes of aloneness, alienation and the counter-force of attraction.

Bender and Boas[2] in a study of Bellevue Hospital psychiatric patients, found that spontaneous dance is of special significance because of its utiliza-

403

tion of primitive motility reflex patterns, auditory reactions, visual activity and spatial relationships. By giving expression to and stimulating primitive, unconscious fantasies, it allows the patient to express both personal aims, capacities and conflicts. In addition spontaneous dance has esthetic, creative aspects which help to liberate the patient from his conflicts.[13]

DANCE THERAPY

Laban[18] has devised two methods for recording human movement: Labanotation (*what* movement is being performed) and Effort-Shape Analysis (*how* a movement is being performed). Some of the parameters of Effort-Shape Analysis are: (1) effort (the dynamics or intensity of movement), i.e., light-strong, quick-slow and direct-indirect; (2) shape (the flow or ongoingness of motion), i.e., bound-free, in towards self, and out away from self. The range of spaced used, planes of motion, and posture vs. gesture, initiation and ending constitute other parameters.

INDICATIONS

Dance therapists[5,20,23,24] see dance as of therapeutic value for: (1) schizophrenics, especially those acutely ill and regressed who may be helped because their communication is limited to "bizarre" gestures and postures similar to the movements of modern dance; (2) manic-depressives who, in the manic phase, use body action to augment verbal communication or emotional responsibility and can learn to control this fluidity by participating with the dance therapist; (3) depressed psychotics who can be helped to overcome their lethargy and (4) isolated, withdrawn patients who are given an opportunity to respond motorically to non-verbally demonstrated emotions.

Technique

Chace[5,7] summarizes her methods as follows. Patients, either individually or in groups, come to the therapy room or the therapist goes to the ward. No attempt is made to structure the session around individual patients. Where groups are involved, the procedure may start with a patient choosing a phonograph record to the music of which the patients move alone, with the dance therapist or in small groups. This warm-up establishes initial contacts and may drain off excitement and anxiety. When most of the group has been thus involved, the therapist organizes a circle in which the patients go through simple exercises, enabling the therapist to pick up individualized movement-style patterns. One such patient is then allowed or encouraged to set the rhythm for the group. The therapist then acts as a catalyst for changes in leadership. As the group moves, the verbalizations break through. Chace[6] furnished this illustration:

Mrs. C. was withdrawn from the other patients on her ward most of the time. She remained curled up in a corner of the room absorbed in her own feelings. Occasionally she was obviously responding to hallucinations. She was unable to tolerate close contact with the members of a dance session as yet.

However as the dance began a rhythmic stamping movement of her feet carried her around the room just outside of the circle of other dancers. As she stamped, she moved her shoulders forward with alternate sharp jerks reaching with her arms as she chanted, in time to the music, about her loneliness and isolation from others.

Recently she suddenly demanded, "Play that again. It is from 1920 or so." Asked if she knew the music, she stated, "It belongs to the time of my beginning." The music was repeated and she continued to dance throughout the session with intensity. At the close of the hour she relaxed heavily in her chair and in response to the question, "You are tired?" she answered, "Yes, I have just lived 20 years, and now I am here." For the first time she moved close to the other patients, chatted and laughed with them as they returned to their wards.

Dance therapy is being used with the so-called "inner city" or economically and ethnically unprivileged groups. Rogers, in New York City, has been using dance in order to bring out and capitalize on the creative potentials of deprived adolescents. During the summer of 1968, he headed a joint project of the city of New York and the state of New Hampshire in which urban and rural indigent youth lived and moved together in a total creative-arts environment in which dance played a vital role.

ANCILLARY TECHNIQUES

Razy[22] describes percussion-dance therapy at the Wiltwyck School for Boys in New York and at Childville in Brooklyn. Dance percussion therapy differs from dance therapy in that percussive media of all sorts are used to carry out rhythmic activities. Percussion can be produced not only by the usual instruments but by chairs, blackboard chalk, cans, etc. Razy gives many case illustrations of the usefulness of her approach.

At Camarillo State Hospital in California, Hering[14] describes a variant of dance therapy developed by Trudi Schoop called "body-ego technique." Less attention is given in this procedure to the social, recreational and inductive aspects, and more to abstractions such as time, force, space and structure. Freezing of bodily and hence of emotional states is felt by "body-ego" users to be the significant problem. Movement in space provides an unfreezing and releasing element. The only bond between patient and therapist is motion. Verbal interaction is discouraged.

405

Basberg[1] states that her hospital in Oslo, Norway, where a therapeutic community structure prevails, she uses jazz-ballet and folk-dancing as well as the basic dance forms commonly used in the U.S.A. She uses the expression "dance-play" to describe her current techniques.

RESEARCH

The testing of the many hypotheses advanced in dance therapy has been notably wanting. One study reported by Evangelakis and Glover[11] used 100 female in-patients, divided into five groups. Each group had a different combination of therapies, i.e., group psychotherapy, drugs or adjunctive therapy. The only group in which dance therapy was instituted showed the greatest amount of improvement.

The Committee on Research in Dance[4] and the American Dance Therapy Association are currently cosponsoring with the Postgraduate Center for Mental Health in New York City a conference on research in dance therapy.

REFERENCES

1. BASBERG, G.: Personal communication from Oslo, 1968.
2. BENDER, L., AND BOAS, F.: Creative Dance in Therapy. In: Ruitenbeck, H. M. (Ed.): The Creative Imagination. Chicago, Quadrangle Books, 1965.
3. BLUM, L.: The Discotheque and the Phenomenon of Alone-Togetherness: A Study of the Young Person's Response to the Frug and Comparable Current Dances. Adolescence, 1:351, 1966.
4. BULL, R.: (Ed.): Research in Dance: Problems and Possibilities. Proc. Com. Res. Dance, CORD. N.Y.U., New York, 1967.
5. CHACE, M.: Dance as an Adjunctive Therapy with Hospitalized Mental Patients. Bull. Menninger Clin., 17:219, 1953.
6. CHACE, M.: Use of Dance Action in Group Settings. Mimeo. copy of paper presented at the Amer. Psychiat. Ass. Convention, 1953.
7. CHACE, M.: A Psychological Study as Applied to Dance. Amer. Psychol., 12:   , 1957.
8. DEUTSCH, F.: Analysis of Postural Behavior. Psychoan. Quart., 16:195, 1947.
9. Doll, E. E.: Therapeutic Values of the Rhythmic Arts in the Education of Cerebral Palsied and Brain-Injured Children. In: Schneider, E. H. (Ed.): Music Therapy. Kansas, Lawrence Press, 1960, 1961.
10. Encyclopedia Brit.: Dance. 13th Edition: 794, 1926.
11. EVANGELAKIS, M. G., AND GLOVER, R.: De-Institutionalization of Patients. In: Schneider, E. H. (Ed.): Music Therapy. Kansas, Lawrence Press, 1960, 1961.
12. FREEDMAN, N., AND HOFFMAN, S. P.: Kinetic Behavior to Objective Analysis of Motor Behavior During Clinical Interviews. Percept. Mot. Skills, 24:527, 1967.
13. HAYS, J. C.: Effect of Two Regulated Changes of Tempo Upon Emotional Connotations in Dance. Res. Quart., 38:389, 1967.
14. HERING, D.: A Sliver of Hope, Dance Magazine, 46, May, 1965.

15. KESTENBERG, J. S.: The Role of Movement Patterns in Development. I. Rhythm of Movement. Psychoan. Quart., 34:1, 1965.
16. KESTENBERG, J. S.: The Role of Movement Patterns in Development. II. Flow of Tension and Effort. Psychoan. Quart., 34:517, 1965.
17. KESTENBERG, J. S.: The Role of Movement Patterns in Development. III. The Control of Shape. Psychoan. Quart., 36:356, 1967.
18. LABAN, R.: The Educational and Therapeutic Value of Dance. In: Sorell, W. (Ed.): The Dance Has Many Faces. New York, Columbia Univ. Press, 1966.
19. MARTIN, J.: Isadora Duncan and Basic Dance. Dance Index, 1:4, 1942.
20. OFFNER, R.: Dance as an Adjunct to Therapy with Psychotic Patients. Unpublished master's thesis, N.Y. School of Social Work. Columbia Univ., 1953.
21. PERLOWITZ, H.: Some Aspects of the Psychodynamics of Social Dancing in Relationship to Sublimation and Regressive Behavior. Psychiat. Quart. Suppl., 35:100, 1961.
22. RAZY, V.: The Value of Dance and Percussion in the Treatment of Emotionally Disturbed Children. Social Case Work, Dec., 1961.
23. ROSAN, E.: Dance Therapy for Psychotic Patients. Unpublished doctoral thesis, Teacher's College, Columbia Univ., 1956.
24. ROSAN, E.: Dance as Therapy for the Mentally Ill. Teacher's Coll. Rec. 55:215, 1954.
25. SCHEFLEN, A. E.: On the Structuring of Human Communication. Amer. Behav. Scientist, 10:8, 1967.
26. WACHTEL, P. L.: An Approach to the Study of Body Language in Psychotherapy. Psychotherapy, 4:97, 1967.
27. WUNDERLICH, R. C.: Hypokinetic Disease. Academic Therapy Quart., 2:183, 1967.

Perspectives on Work Therapy

by Leo A. Micek, M.S., and Donald G. Miles, Ed.D.

K EY[5] POINTED OUT in 1959 that in previous years there had been a proliferation of the activity therapies, each with a "professional" organization clamoring for independent status and recognition. He proposed that it was relatively unimportant what sort of activity a patient engaged in as long as all activity therapists approached him with a consistent attitude. Others[2,6,8] felt meaningful, paid work was particularly efficacious in restoring self-confidence to the patient in order that he would benefit from other therapies. Schwartz and Schwartz[9] built an argument for a variety of activity therapies to deal with the many environmental influences on patient adjustment. Denber[3] and Gurel[4] suggested that authors frequently proffered only fanciful speculation coupled with clinical intuition as a means of evaluating the substance and possible benefit of the various activity therapies. In addition to the lack of empirical evidence in assessing the utility of the various modalities, too little consideration seems to have been given to the goals of treatment.

All the major elements of everyday living should exist in some form in order that patients may develop or re-establish acceptable patterns of social behavior. Just as remunerative employment, constructive hobbies and recreational activities represent major segments of daily living, also so do industrial (work) therapy, occupational therapy and recreational therapy represent major facets of the resocialization process. The problem was to gather some evidence concerning the impact of the various treatment modalities, concentrating particularly on work as therapy.*

METHOD

As a segment of a larger NIMH-supported research project designed to evaluate the rehabilitative and therapeutic value of work for psychiatric pa-

*This study has been done in conjunction with a larger project supported in part by Grant Number 5 R 11 MH0137-04 from the National Institute of Mental Health. Some of the data were also taken from the Fort Logan Record System, supported in part by NIMH. Grant 5 R11 MH00931-06.

The authors wish to express appreciation to A. Evelyn McDonald and Joanne C. Fults for assistance with the preparation of the manuscript.

tients, approximately 1,000 adult patients at the Fort Logan Mental Health Center, Denver, Colo., were selected during 1964 and 1965 to participate in various treatment conditions and were then interviewed in their homes at various follow-up intervals after discharge or transfer to low-intensity care. Fort Logan is a relatively new state mental health facility which was designed from its inception to incorporate the concepts and philosophy of the therapeutic community.[1,7]

In accordance with the design of the larger research project from which this sample was selected, the subjects of this study were assigned, on a random basis, at the time of admission to one of three research groups. For the sake of distinction, each group was given a color designation. One of every four admissions was assigned to the "green" group for whom work therapy (W.T.) was compulsory. On a similar basis, a corresponding number of patients were assigned to the "red" group and were not permitted to participate in the W.T. program. Finally, two of every four admissions were assigned to the "yellow" group, for whom W.T. participation or nonparticipation was determined by the judgement of the clinical staff.

The workshop program operated in a building located across the street from the main Center complex. The 6,500 square feet of work space consisted of three large work rooms. All work was solicited from outside industry and brought to the workshop. Packaging, light assembly and simple wood products were the most frequent types of work available to patients, although some patients worked as supervisors and quality controllers. Wages were usually on a piece-work basis under which patients who worked at a rate competitive with outside workers would earn the minimum wage (then $1.25 an hour). However patients worked in small groups and shared equally in the earnings of the total group. Members of most of the groups were able to earn about 40 cents an hour under this system. Some form of paid work was arranged for every patient assigned to the workshop, regardless of severity of illness, and no patient was ever found to be unable to work for at least a few minutes at a time. Staff were assigned to work with the groups at a ratio of about one staff member to every 25 patients. The staff all had bachelors degrees in a behavioral science, usually psychology. Patients worked in the shop for an average of about seven hours each week. They also met once a week in small groups for an hour-long discussion of their experiences in the workshop.

Several modifications were necessary to eliminate subjects who failed to meet the predesignated criteria. The first step consisted of deleting those patients from the various color groups who had not remained in intensive care at least 20 days. This action was taken in response to the possibility that such patients were unlikely to have been hospitalized long enough to have

409

become significantly involved in any treatment program. The second procedure consisted of eliminating those patients in the green group (compulsory W.T.) who remained in W.T. less than 10 days and those in the red group (no W.T.) who had been in W.T., for various reasons, during the period of their intensive care. It was felt that this procedure might have unmatched the red and green groups, and a final modification was therefore made in an endeavor to control for certain variables which might spuriously effect the results. The green participant group was therefore matched with the red non-participant group on the variables of length of initial intensive treatment, sex, marital status, education and age. Using the same variables, a group of yellow (variable W.T.) participants was matched with a group of non-participants. The entire procedure of subject selection resulted in a total of 387 with 71 green subjects, 84 red subjects, 112 yellow W.T. participants and 120 yellow non-participants.

Within the context of the comprehensive research design, the 387 subjects of this particular portion of the study were followed-up at intervals of 3 and 12 months after discharge or transfer to low intensity treatment. Low intensity care was defined as including the treatment categories of family care, out-patient status or evening care. Since not all subjects were contacted successfully at both follow-up periods, the data from the two phases were later combined, with first priority given to use of the three-month data.

At the time of transfer to low intensity care, clinical ratings of response to treatment were made by staff who had been involved in each patient's treatment, usually a psychiatrist or a clinical psychologist. The areas rated, all on a seven-point scale ranging from "marked benefit" to "much worse," were: (1) response to group therapy, (2) response to occupational therapy, (3) response to recreational therapy, (4) response to social activity therapy and (5) response to all therapy programs. The raters were not aware that their observations were to be used as a part of this study, since such ratings are routinely made at Fort Logan for inclusion in the Center record system.

Among the many follow-up items the patients were asked by the interviewers to complete was a subjective item which asked the patient to "put a '1' in front of one of the following therapies which you think was most helpful to you while at Fort Logan." Similarly the patient was asked to "put an 'L' in front of the least helpful therapy." The following alternatives were available to the patients for rating: (1) group, (2) individual, (3) family, (4) occupational, (5) recreational and (6) work (industrial).

Results

In the analysis of rated response to the various therapies, comparing work therapy participants (greens) with non-participants (reds), Table 1 in-

410

TABLE 1

Clinical Rating of Response to
Various Therapy Programs

Therapeutic Modality	Green Group Mean	Red Group Mean	t	Level of Significance
Group	2.479	2.607	1.045	N.S. (.3)
Occupational	2.592	2.726	1.248	N.S. (.3)
Recreational	2.535	2.655	1.042	N.S. (.3)
Social Activity	2.394	2.464	.591	N.S. (.6)
Overall	2.859	3.286	3.085	.005
	N = 71	N = 84		

dicates that no significant differences were found between the two matched color groups on the first four variables, although all results were in a direction tending toward more favorable response to the treatments by the work therapy participant groups. However the category of overall response to all therapy programs was highly significant.

The results of the patients' ratings of the "helpfulness" of the various therapies, combining 3 and 12 month follow-up data, for work therapy participants (green and yellow) contrasted with non-work therapy participants (red and yellow), are indicated in Tables 2 and 3.

A comparative examination of the inter- and intra-group ratings reveals that in all instances, with the exception of the yellow participant sample, group therapy was most often rated as the most beneficial type. This rating was found to be the general consensus for both participants and non-participants in work therapy. However further consideration of the various therapy ratings indicates that members of the green group perceived work therapy as most helpful almost as frequently as they did group therapy. Further the yellow participant group most often rated work therapy as having been the most helpful of all therapies. It may also be seen that both the green and the yellow participant groups, when asked to rate the therapy which had been least helpful, infrequently designated work therapy, while often finding fault with group and recreational therapy.

Again reference to Tables 2 and 3 indicates that the various therapy ratings of the red group and yellow non-participants closely paralleled the green in most frequently stating that group therapy had been most helpful. Both groups rated recreational therapy as most helpful next most often to group therapy.

In comparing the therapies rated least helpful by all groups, striking

411

TABLE 2

Summary Table of "Green" and "Red"
Patient Ratings of Treatment Programs
3 & 12 Month Follow-up Data Combined

Green		Red	
Type of therapy	Ss	Type of therapy	Ss
Most Beneficial			
Group	13	Group	16
Work	11	Recreational	10
Individual	7	Family Group	5
Occupational	5	Individual	4
Family Group	3	Occupational	3
Recreational	2		
Not Indicated	1		
	N = 42		N = 38
Least Beneficial			
Group	13	Occupational	11
Recreational	13	Recreational	10
Occupational	9	Group	7
Work	5	Family Group	4
Family Group	2	Individual	0
Individual	0	Not Indicated	6
	N = 42		N = 38

similarities emerge. Green and yellow participants saw group therapy as having been the least beneficial, whereas the red and yellow non-participants regarded occupational therapy as having been the least helpful. The former finding is particularly interesting in view of the fact that the green and yellow participant group had also rated group therapy as first or second from the perspective of having been the most beneficial therapy. The combination of this strong positive rating coupled with an equally strong frequency of negative rating, would suggest that the greatest magnitude of controversy is cast in regard to group therapy.

DISCUSSION

Interpretation of the findings of this study is somewhat uncertain because of the nature of the ratings made by both staff and patients. The staff ratings on response to treatment were global, subjective and related only to an unspecified criterion, "improvement." It is well known that staff personnel usually consider remission of symptomatology and increased verbal ex-

TABLE 3
Summary Table of "Yellow" Patient
Ratings of Treatment Programs
3 & 12 Month Follow-up Data Combined

Yellow Ps		Yellow NPs	
Type of therapy	Ss	Type of therapy	Ss
Most Beneficial			
Work	19	Group	24
Group	16	Recreational	8
Individual	8	Individual	7
Occupational	5	Family Group	5
Recreational	5	Occupational	4
Family Group	1	Not Indicated	1
	N = 54		N = 49
Least Beneficial			
Group	17	Occupational	17
Occupational	16	Recreational	12
Recreational	7	Group	12
Work	6	Family Group	8
Individual	4	Individual	0
Family Group	3		
Not Indicated	1		
	N = 54		N = 49

pression, particularly of affective material, to be indicative of improvement. Perhaps the maintenance of an attitude of productive self-worth could be postulated as having been maintained by the work therapy participants while non-participants may have felt the loss of self-value and participation in the human community which is often observed as a side effect of unemployment. Some support for this interpretation seems to come from the patients' ratings of the various therapeutic modalities. Although patients were asked to rate the therapy according to effectiveness, it seems probable that patients actually responded by indicating the extent to which they liked or enjoyed the therapies. Since work therapy was frequently listed as "most helpful" and seldom listed as "least helpful," it would seem that some sort of personal satisfaction was derived from workshop participation. Perhaps this sense of satisfaction is sufficient to explain the behavior changes which the clinicians regarded as a better response to treatment on the part of participants. Finally some evidence seems to have been generated to support the suggestion that at least one activity therapy, work, is uniquely beneficial in a therapeutic community treatment program. The results also seem to

413

lend some support to the notion, frequently discounted, that patients are capable of recognizing the forms of therapy which will be most helpful to them. Perhaps patients should be given greater participation in the design of treatment programs.

REFERENCES

1. American Psychiatric Association Mental Hospital Service Achievement Awards, Bronze Award: The Versatile Program at the Fort Logan Mental Health Center. Ment. Hosp. 15:552, 1964.
2. AZIMA, H., AND WITTKOWER, E. D.: A Partial Field Survey of Psychiatric Occupational Therapy. Amer. J. Occ. Ther. 11:1, 1957.
3. DENBER, H. C. B.: Work Therapy in Psychiatry. In: Masserman, J. H., (Ed.): Current Psychiatric Therapies, Vol. 5. New York, Grune & Stratton, 1965.
4. GUREL, L.: Building Tomorrow's Mental Health. Unpublished paper, 1965.
5. KEY, W. H.: Coordination of the Ancillary Therapies. In: Greenblatt, M. and Simon, B. (Eds.): Rehabilitation of the Mentally Ill. Washington, D. C., American Association for the Advancement of Science, 1959.
6. KIDD, H. B.: Industrial Units in Psychiatric Hospitals. Brit. J. Psychiat. 111:1205, 1965.
7. National Institute of Mental Health: Community Mental Health Center. Washington, D.C., U. S. Government Printing Office, 1964.
8. RICHEY, R. E.: Industrial Therapy Success and Hospital Progress in a Schizophrenic Population. Dissert. Abstr. 24:3426, 1964.
9. SCHWARTZ, M. S., AND SCHWARTZ, C. G.: Social Approaches to Mental Health Patient Care. New York, Columbia University Press, 1964.

Advances in Military Psychiatry

by ALBERT J. GLASS, COL., M.C., U.S.A.

IT HAS LONG BEEN RECOGNIZED that military personnel may exhibit characteristic forms of temporary or persistent failure of adaptation as manifested by psychiatric symptoms or non-conformist behavior. These problems are especially prevalent under war-time conditions when there is a large proportion of new servicemen, a high degree of uncertainty, and a heightened exposure to deprivation and danger. It was only in this century, more specifically in World War I, that the rising efficiency of military medicine brought forth an organized effort to cope with such psychological disorders. During this conflict, by trial and error, it was demonstrated that the psychiatric casualties of battle were most effectively salvaged for duty if treated early and within the combat zone by a simplified regimen which included recuperative measures (rest, food, etc.), reassurance, strong suggestion, and a fairly prompt return to front-line duty.[1]

Curiously, this lesson of World War I was forgotten in the planning phase of World War II. Then, American civil and military medical leaders were well aware that large numbers of emotional disorders would almost certainly arise from the rapidly mobilizing military services. However, prevailing psychiatric opinion held that psychological breakdown in war mainly occurred from those participants who were vulnerable to situational stress and strain because of personality defect, or neurotic tendency, or overt mental illness. For this reason and because it was believed that psychiatrists could readily identify such predisposed persons, major reliance was placed upon psychiatric examination at induction.[2] By this means it was believed that persons with potential psychiatric and behavioral disorders would be prevented from entering the service and thus the problem could be eliminated at its source. But as the war proceeded, psychiatric screening proved to be an impractical and ineffectual procedure.[3] Hospital admissions for psychiatric disorders rose to unprecedented high levels and the military medical services were forced to find ways and means of coping with vast numbers of apparent disabling emotional conditions. Again, the early, forward treatment techniques of World War I were learned and further elaborated for employment in non-combat[4] as well as combat induced psychological disorders.[5] As a result of these World War II experiences, reinforced by further practical application during the Korean conflict, military psychiatry has become an integral part of American military medicine with distinctive methods of prevention and treatment.[6] This presentation will set forth the concepts and operational techniques of the current military psychiatry program particularly as employed by the Army Medical Service.

A primary orientation of military psychiatry revolves about an objective which necessarily includes a pragmatic concept of normality. In common with other elements of military medicine, military psychiatry endeavors to conserve the fighting or effective strength. Admittedly, normality in mental health cannot be scientifically defined. This is well stated by Redlich[7] who pointed out that "meaningful propositions on "normality" can be best made within a specific cultural context." From the standpoint of the military culture, normality in mental health is equated with adequate duty performance. While work efficiency may be considered only a narrow aspect of mental health it is of crucial importance to the military mission and one in which various indices of non-effectiveness can be readily determined such as hospital admission rates, incidence of disciplinary offenders and the like. This practical criterion of normality makes it reasonable for the military psychiatrist to concentrate his efforts upon maladjustment problems that lead to non-effective duty performance regardless of manifestations, and to discard as major objectives the relief of anxiety, unhappiness, and other somatic and psychological non-disabling discomforts which are the inevitable concomitants of many military situations.

A second major principle of military psychiatry involves an attitude or an approach toward the causality of mental disorders. Most, if not all authorities, agree upon a multifactoral causation of psychological illness or deviant behavior. Etiological factors may be considered in two categories; those which arise from the individual, and those which originate from the environment. Experiences, particularly during war, have led military psychiatrists to place emphasis upon influences external to the individual over that of intrapsychic mechanisms as being the more important determinants of behavior. From first-hand observation it became apparent that the entire milieu of the soldier was involved in adjustment which, in addition to the intensity and duration of danger and deprivation, included the support of buddies, group cohesiveness and other morale phenomena, the competency of leaders, the efficiency

416

of communication, the adequacy of training; the degree of physical fatigue, the quantity and quality of supplies and weapons, terrain, weather, and even the medical criteria and disciplinary penalties for removal from adverse situations. Personality configuration, while significant, was rarely a decisive factor in the majority of cases. Indeed, the frequency of emotional disorders was found to be more related to the characteristics of the group or the unique nature of external circumstances (combat, basic training, etc.) than the character traits of the individual.

A third basic tenet of military psychiatry derives from repeated observations of processes favorable to effective adjustment which apparently arise from the adaptational struggle of the individual in the stressful environment. The occurrence of such sustaining mechanisms was the rule rather than the exception and their failure to develop was a major cause for non-effective behavior. Also, it became evident that this beneficial reaction was responsible for the success of the forward treatment of combat psychiatric casualties. In this procedure, little was accomplished that would change individual personality or the external situation. After a brief recuperative respite along with encouragement and suggestion, psychiatric casualties were promptly returned to combat duty to provide another opportunity for the development of sustaining mechanisms or to re-establish a previously successful adjustment which had been temporarily disrupted by the vicissitudes of the battlefield. Conversely, hospitalization or any complex treatment method which necessitated prolonged withdrawal in time and space from the combat milieu made difficult, if not impossible, any initiation or restoration of the favorable adaptational process. Instead, there was produced a chronic phobic syndrome for battle situations with a consequent loss of self-esteem and crippling of function.

To explain successful adaptation under unusual circumstances, two psychological processes should be considered. First, the learning or mastery of skills or tasks not only provides self-gratification but increases one's confidence of adequately dealing with similar future dangers. Second, participation with others under adverse conditions strongly impels individuals to move closer to each other both literally and figuratively, producing what is commonly termed group cohesiveness or group identification. The emotional bond thus created serves to mitigate the effect of isolation of persons who face a difficult or hostile environment, facilitates favorable interpersonal transactions of emotional warmth, support, and even affection, and tends to subordinate individual values and needs for group mores and group standards of conduct. That this group sustaining mechanism also operates in non-combat situations such as basic

417

training has been pointed out by Bushard[8] who noted that when a trainee "commits" himself to the group objective he receives "concurrence" in the form of approval and support from his fellows and supervisors.

Recognition that non-effective military behavior is a common result of changes and difficulties in the environment or interpersonal relationships of the soldier has caused a gradual displacement of psychiatric personnel from their traditional role and location in the hospital or clinic setting to an active function in the military community. This field approach has permitted first-hand observations of maladjustment processes, has brought psychiatric personnel into working relationships with military supervisors, and has made possible the utilization of milieu as a major instrument in the development of techniques for prevention and treatment. As a result, the Army psychiatric program has developed in the following several areas of endeavor: (1) early identification and treatment; (2) prevention; and (3) milieu therapy.

EARLY IDENTIFICATION AND TREATMENT

This doctrine, sometimes termed "secondary prevention," aims at the early case finding and therapeutic management of the maladjusted soldier while he remains with his unit and is still involved in an adaptational struggle. In this approach, an operational model is utilized much like that of the "crisis" concept proposed by Caplan.[9] Emphasis is placed on understanding the natural history of maladjustment and the specific situational circumstances or interpersonal transactions which have apparently provoked non-effective behavior. Unit commanders, dispensary physicians, chaplains and other "caretaker" agencies are urged to refer problems early in the course of adjustment failure so that the short-term success gained by deviant conduct, or somatic and psychological symptoms or other evasive responses are not repeated, thereby inducing fixed patterns of disability. Also imperative is the prevention of hospitalization except for major mental disorders and the avoidance of therapeutic measures which communicate the existence of a personality defect or a basic weakness of soma or psyche, from which it might follow that failure in this or that situation was inevitable and not a responsibility of the individual. Indeed few or no attempts are made to alter personality traits. Instead, attention is pointed toward utilizing the individual's resources and assets. All efforts are directed toward encouraging or insisting that the involved person overcome or otherwise master the alleged or actual hardships, deprivations or hazards which are so obviously being accomplished by a majority of unit members. In this as well as other therapeutic endeavors, psychiatric personnel function most efficiently and

418

with high morale when they are identified with the needs and values of the military culture, for then reintegration of the alienated individual with his reference group becomes a desirable and meaningful objective.

The early identification and treatment phase of Army psychiatry is mainly carried out by out-patient units designated as Mental Hygiene Consultation Services (MHCS). These facilities have become permanent installations on all major Army posts and an integral component of all overseas divisions. The post Mental Hygiene Consultation Service located near troop concentrations, has a staff consisting of one or more psychiatrists, officer social workers and clinical psychologists, enlisted social work and psychology assistants, and clerical personnel. To insure uniformity of patient care, the senior psychiatrist heads the small psychiatric in-patient service of the local army hospital. Major mental disorders, i.e., psychoses, severe depressions, which require prolonged in-patient care are transferred to the neuropsychiatric treatment centers of Army general hospitals.

In recent years, the practices of the Mental Hygiene Consultation Services have changed in the direction of so-called field service. There have been developed, particularly in basic training centers and other large posts, techniques of sending field workers, usually mature enlisted social work assistants, to interview the problem soldier in the unit area. This intake procedure avoids the clinic atmosphere and its suggestion of illness or accentuation of dependency needs, prevents excess loss of training or duty time and facilitates the gathering of collateral information especially from military supervisors. It has also been noted that the soldier in his own surroundings can discuss personal and situational problems more freely with another enlisted man than in the more formal environment of the clinic. The field worker is strongly supported by the clinic staff and can arrange for an immediate psychiatric consultation for any referral who presents bizarre behavior or an unusual degree of depression, anxiety or withdrawal. The usual case is discussed with a supervisor, most often a social work officer, to consider the further exploration and management of the problem. Some Mental Hygiene Consultation Service units employ group therapy as the preferred method of further treatment. Others rely upon individual counseling by a social work officer or an experienced field worker supervised by an officer of the clinic staff. In all instances the field worker maintains contact with the individual referral by regular visits. Disciplinary offenders are included in the field program with intake procedures performed by field workers on all stockade inmates and subsequent counseling and treatment as stated above.

Management of routine referrals by the social work staff frees the psychiatrist to function as a consultant for the difficult and controversial cases. The psychiatrist also evaluates at the clinic those individuals with suspected organic disease, psychotic or severe neurotic symptoms and problems of serious administrative consequence. The practices and thus the effectiveness of the Mental Hygiene Consultation Services are strongly influenced by the senior psychiatrist's assertive leadership, confidence and experience with the field approach. As leader of the clinic group, the psychiatrist frequently meets informally with his staff and discusses policies and specific problems. He conducts case seminars and utilizes other means to increase the professional capacity and morale of his staff.

PREVENTION

This aspect of military psychiatry includes efforts to influence favorably the conditions under which soldiers live, work or fight so that there is less likelihood of disabling maladjustment. Preventive measures fall into two general categories.

First, there is the impact upon the involved non-commissioned and commissioned officer when psychiatric personnel deal effectively with an individual problem. Military supervisors occupy a role much like that of a foreman, or teacher, or even a parent. Thus they are in an optimum position to exert a favorable influence upon the adjustment of subordinates. When military supervisors are afforded an opportunity better to understand the causes and management of deviant or neurotic behavior, they often become more knowledgeable in the handling of personnel as well as more efficient in the early recognition of maladjustment problems.

Second, there is the more direct employment of the military psychiatrist in a staff advisory function which may influence policies, directives and regulations. Psychiatrists assigned to a major headquarters are concerned with personnel policies, such as selection criteria for induction or enlistment, assignment limitations, medical and administrative standards for retention and discharge, and procedures for the elimination or rehabilitation of personnel who exhibit unsuitable or deviant behavior. At the level of post headquarters and operational units, the psychiatrist submits recommendations relevant to local problems such as the early recognition and correction of military offenders, maladjustment of trainees, accident prevention, and morale problems of particular units. An invaluable tool of the military psychiatrist at all levels and one which offers impressive evidence to commanders is the epidemiological approach. By the use of this technique, the psychiatrist can demonstrate significant differences in the frequency of non-effective behavior among units of a post or division who are apparently exposed to the same hardships or hazards. These data raise questions which inevitably focus attention of commanders upon the important areas of leadership or situational factors which could account for such differences.

Experience indicates that the effectiveness of the psychiatrist in a staff advisory role cannot be equated with the merit or excellence of his recommendations. More important is the quality of the relationship established by the psychiatrist with commanders and other supervisory personnel which to a large extent determines whether his suggestions will receive favorable consideration. Generally, such relationships develop from the activities of the psychiatrist in his professional management of referred cases. Unrealistic recommendations for special handling or assignment without regard for the practical limitations of the military situations or the forwarding of consultation reports replete with psychiatric jargon produce a negative impression and the psychiatrist is judged accordingly. On the other hand, the psychiatrist becomes highly regarded who not only displays professional skill in the management of individual cases but renders decisions and recommendations which are meaningful and relevant from a military standpoint. The psychiatrist new to the service cannot hope to achieve military sophistication by limiting his professional activities to a traditional office or hospital practice. In order to acquire this background knowledge he must acquaint himself with the military environment, its regulations, mores, cultures and operational procedures by frequent visits to various post or unit activities usually in connection with individual case referrals.

MILIEU THERAPY

This relatively new phase of military psychiatry involves the in-patient treatment of the schizophrenic soldier in a special ward setting which is designed to utilize the milieu thus created from the group transactions of patient and staff as the major instrument of therapy. The goal of treatment is not merely to achieve a remission of symptoms but to produce sufficient beneficial change in the patient's potential for adjustment so that he can be returned to effective military duty.

The milieu therapy program was initiated by the Walter Reed Army Institute of Research under the direction of Dr. David McK. Rioch with Lieutenant Colonel Kenneth L. Artiss in charge of the project.[10] A ward of the Department of Neuropsychiatry at Walter Reed General Hospital was provided and arranged to accommodate 10 patients. The staff consisted of a single psychiatrist (Lt. Col. Artiss), one nurse, and 12 to 14 enlisted neuropsychiatric specialists (psychiatric aides), for the 24-hour care of 8 to 10 acutely schizophrenic soldier patients. Separate investigators conducted tape recorded interviews with fellow soldiers of the hospitalized patients and visited the home and community to obtain collateral information. A high level of communication was established by the staff members. The enlisted neuropsychiatric specialists recorded extensive, often verbatim notes of the patients' verbal and non-verbal behavior. Daily meetings of the staff provided for an interchange of information and permitted the planning of a coordinated therapeutic approach for this or that patient. Group therapy sessions were held each morning which were attended by the patients and all staff members. In addition a patient government group was established to make recommendations relative to pass privileges, recreational activities and the like.

The wealth of information that was obtained from the patient and significant persons in his previous military and civil life placed the psychiatrist and his staff in an optimal position to understand the major "message"[11] communicated by symptoms and behavior. In all instances schizophrenic patients were found to be deficient in social skills or acceptable modes of dealing with society. For this reason the staff endeavored by day-to-day interaction to influence, teach, or otherwise provide an opportunity for the schizophrenic patient to acquire adaptational skills and successes in social living so as to render symptomatic or deviant behavior unnecessary. The modus operandi and findings of the research group have been summarized by Artiss[12] as follows:

(1) *The schizophrenic can be understood:* This is to say that if enough trained people work with him closely enough and correlate their observations, his "major message" will become clarified and his behavioral goals known.

(2) *Understanding him helps him:* This is to say that "being understood" is a major step in the direction of successful group or social living—in that it leads to relatedness.

(3) *Working with others is a therapeutic (learning) experience for him:* This is to say that his previous attitudes have prevented his smoothly learning social skills—operationally he is found to be socially infantile and a "recover" must accumulate role-taking abilities *in groups* just as others do.

After three and one-half years of operation, the milieu therapy unit, limiting itself to six months of treatment, has returned 64 percent of its treated patients to regular duty status. Preliminary follow-up results indicate a high proportion have maintained satisfactory duty performance. Further exploratory work is underway to determine the effects of selection of patients, selection and training of staff members, and staff communication. Another pilot-type ward has been in operation at Valley Forge General Hospital for almost two years.

422

SUMMARY

Experiences of three wars have enabled military psychiatry to develop unique operational concepts and techniques. In recent years considerable progress has been made in the following areas of endeavor:

(1) the early recognition and prompt management of emotional or behavioral problems while the individual, still a member of his unit, continues the struggle to cope with his environment or situation;

(2) efforts to influence favorably the conditions under which soldiers may live, work, or fight, so that there is less likelihood of disabling maladjustment (prevention);

(3) the employment of milieu as the principal therapeutic tool for the inpatient care of schizophrenic disorders.

REFERENCES

1. The Medical Department of the United States Army in the World War, vol. X: Neuropsychiatry. Washington, D. C.: Government Printing Office, 1929.
2. Menninger, W. C.: Psychiatry in a Troubled World. New York: The Macmillan, 1948, chap. 19.
3. Ginzberg, E., et al.: The Ineffective Soldier, vol. 2: Lost Divisions. New York: Columbia University Press, 1959.
4. Perkins, M.: Preventive psychiatry during World War II. In: Preventive Medicine in World War II, vol. III. Washington, 1955, chap. VI.
5. Glass, A. J.: Psychotherapy in the combat zone. Am. J. Psychiat. 110:725-731, 1954.
6. Group for the Advancement of Psychiatry: Report No. 47, Preventive Psychiatry in the Armed Forces. New York, October 1960.
7. Redlich, F. C.: The concept of health in psychiatry. In: A. H. Leighton, J. A. Clausen, and R. N. Wilson, eds., Explorations of Social Psychiatry. New York: Basic Books, Inc., 1957. (Quoted by Hoffman): Am. J. Psychiat. 117:205-210, 1960.
8. Bushard, B. L.: The U. S. Army's mental hygiene consultation service: Symposium of Preventive and Social Psychiatry, Walter Reed Army Institute of Research, Walter Reed Army Medical Center, Washington, D. C., April 15-17, 1957, pp. 431-443.
9. Caplan, G. (Associate Professor of Mental Health, Harvard School of Public Health, Boston, Massachusetts).: Unpublished article.
10. Artiss, K. L.: Milieu Therapy in Schizophrenia. (To be published)
11. ——: The Sympton as Communication in Schizophrenia. New York: Grune & Stratton, 1959.
12. Glass, A. J., Artiss, K. L., Gibbs, J. J. ,and Sweeney, V. C.: The current status of Army psychiatry. Am. J. Psychiat. 117:673-683, 1961.

PART XII

THE COMMUNITY

Integration of Mental Health Into Public Health Programs

by W. ELWYN TURNER, M.D., M.P.H., F.A.P.H.A., DASIL C. SMITH, M.D., AND PATRICIA J. MEDLEY, M.S.W.

T HE CALIFORNIA SHORT-DOYLE ACT, passed in 1957, provided for 5C per cent state reimbursement (75 per cent after 1963) to local communities for mental health programs. To be eligible, they had to meet minimal standards for service and personnel, and could be operated as a separate governmental department if headed by a psychiatrist, a county director of medical institutions or a local director of public health. The Santa Clara County Community Mental Health Service was established within the framework of the County Health Department in 1958. Since the public health department had decentralized offices throughout the county on the basis of health districts, it appeared logical to develop mental health services in the same regions. The mental health staff then were not only physically located within the public health offices, but had frequent formal and informal contact with other public health divisions.

With the passage of Public Law 88-164, the Mental Retardation Facilities and Community Mental Health Centers Construction Act of 1963, it was possible to construct mental health centers at the same location as the public health centers. In 1965 Public Law 89-105 was passed, which provided funds to staff these new mental health programs. In 1966 Santa Clara County Health Department was successful in obtaining a substantial federal grant which not only enabled it to staff new comprehensive mental health centers but increased services at the other existing centers.

The advantages and/or disadvantages of having the local mental health program administered by the health department must be evaluated and determined locally. Among factors to be considered are population to be served, area covered, political climate, community attitudes, relationship of the health department to other county departments and to community agencies, interest of the health director and many other factors. The disadvantages would include such problems as those caused by integration of psychiatric staff into the department, the extent of the mental health pro-

427

blem, difficulty of regular health department staff in learning to communicate with the psychiatric staff, and the provision of adequate space, budget and manpower. However the advantages of having an integrated public health-mental health program appear to far outweigh any consideration of the disadvantages of such an integration.

Gains Made Through Integration

Integration of the two programs has meant that joint planning could be done more expeditiously. It has been further demonstrated that it is economical to have one administrative staff coordinate and administer the operations of both mental health and public health programs, rather than two separate administrative structures. This has meant a greater flexibility in the use of administrative resources. When the health director is responsible for both public health and mental health it provides for smooth administrative coordination and allows the mental health program chief to concentrate on overall program administration and development with less involvement in interdepartmental problems, budgetary matters and so on.

In addition the already developed close relationship of the health department with other community agencies has facilitated communication and cooperation of the mental health program with agencies not normally considered mental health agencies, such as schools, welfare agencies, police, prisons, industry-occupational health, probation, the courts and others. Health department relationships with community agencies have made it easy to contract with both voluntary and official mental health agencies. This not only provides for more service, but helps support other mental health agencies and aids in coordinating all mental health services.

The close working relationship between the mental health staff and the public health nurses has facilitated early case finding and has substantially aided in the care and treatment of the mentally ill in the community.

The recent development of community mental health strongly emphasizes the preventive aspects of psychiatry in mental health, specifically through providing mental health consultation to other professional groups within the community, such as public health nurses, teachers, welfare workers and others. This concept of prevention within mental health is indeed the basic philosophy of public health.

The close working relationship of the mental health staff and public health nurses has been of immeasurable value to both staffs in the area of preventive psychiatry. For example, public health nurses have been called upon by mental health staff to make preliminary home visits to patients who appear to be in an emotional crisis to determine the severity of the individual's condition. Upon making the home visit, they report their findings

428

to one of the mental health staff, usually a psychiatrist, and it is then determined whether the mental health staff should become involved or whether the public health nurse, with consultation from a member of the mental health staff, would continue to work with the family.

In addition to requests from mental health to public health nurses to assist in case management, the public health nurse have consulted the mental health staff about specific personal problems in their everyday activities. This has not only aided in providing them with a better understanding of the nature of emotional problems and how to deal with them, but in addition, helped them to become more aware of when to refer patients to the mental health services, as well as the kind of service which would be most appropriate for the patient, such as outpatient clinical services, emergency care or rehabilitation. By providing mental health consultation to nurses and other professional persons who are working with the community, we are indeed extending the area of psychiatry into prevention and case finding. In addition to close coordination with public health nursing, mental health staff have also offered continuing consultation services to other health department bureaus.

Examples of involvement of other health department bureaus and mental health include the following:

When it has appeared appropriate, patients seen in the Venereal Disease clinics have been referred for outpatient psychiatric service by the public health physicians. The veterinarian has become interested in exploring the effects that animals have on seriously emotionally disturbed patients and the mentally retarded. It is possible that his interest in this subject will result in a pilot research project in the future. The Division of Occupational Health has requested that the mental health staff become involved in offering consultation to industries in the community. Increasingly the medical staffs of large industries are being concerned with aspects of emotional disturbances that affect the employees' productivity and relationships to other employees.

In 1967 the mental health staff became much more involved and concerned about the use of drugs, particularly among young people. Facts became available to indicate the extent of the problem in the county and the serious effect of the drugs on the physical as well as emotional health of the individuals. Psychiatrists met with representatives of all divisions to inform them of the effects of these drugs on individuals. The concern on prevention of drug useage is seen as a total health department problem, not merely the concern of mental health.

In recent years all newly employed mental health professional staff go through a very carefully planned and complete orientation to all aspects of the public health department, including field visits with public health nurses, sanitarians, vector controls inspectors and members of the staffs of all of the other bureaus. It appears that some of the fears and anxieties that members of the public health staff could have and, in the past, did have toward mental health, have been largely removed not only because of this orientation course but because of continued contact with the mental health staff. As a result of this orientation program, several bureaus within the public health department have requested more extensive orientation of their new staff to mental health. This has allowed the staffs of both departments to become better acquainted not only as individuals but as members of a particular discipline, and requests for consultation from each of the bureaus have increased as staff has felt more comfortable with the Mental Health Bureau.

Another reason why the integration of public health and mental health has decided advantages is that this combination of the two departments appear to increase the prestige of both, but particularly of mental health, in the community. With the community already accepting the philosophy of public health in terms of prevention, early detection and treatment within the community, it is increasingly easy for mental health to move into these same areas in community psychiatry.

Recent legislation in California (the McAteer Act) has resulted in the development of comprehensive alcohol control programs within public health departments. The existence of a mental health program with the Santa Clara County Health Department, facilitated the establishment of the alcohol control program within the Bureau of Mental Health.

SIGNIFICANCE OF THE MENTAL HEALTH CENTER CONCEPT

The concept of comprehensive mental health centers throughout a community is an exciting and refreshing development in the field of psychiatry. It provides for centers offering service to patients in a wide variety of treatment modalities to meet the specific needs of the individual. It further emphasizes the preventive aspects by encouraging professional mental health staff to work with a wide variety of community groups and agency personnel who are serving families within the community around a center.

The time has come when psychiatry can no longer afford to be isolated but must become an integral part of the practice of medicine and of the community it is seeking to assist. Only in this way, with a coordinated and collaborative effort by all helping agencies, will communities be able to solve the seemingly unsolvable problems of community disorder which results from emotional disturbance.

Principles of Psychiatric Emergency Management

by SHERVERT H. FRAZIER, M.D.

T HE UNPRECEDENTED acceleration of technological advancement during the twentieth century has resulted in a proportionate increase in the human being's pace of living. This phenomenon seems concomitantly to have engendered strong potentials for psychiatric emergencies, both of an intrapsychic and an interpersonal or social character. Malfunctioning of a human being in his life situation can not only reflect, it can also precipitate an intrapsychic emergency. The concept of interpersonal or social psychiatric emergency is a fairly recent one, although the fact itself is not; it stems from the malfunctioning that develops imperceptibly from seemingly innocuous origins within a group of human beings.

The inner roots of psychiatric emergencies have generally been found to lie in inordinate dependency needs, aggression and sexuality. These give rise to a wide range of disturbances, including severe anxiety, excessive stress, confused states, psychoses, violence, unmanageable states of depression, panic and paralyzing phobias.

Suicide and homicide are almost invariably the first associations to be made with the term *psychiatric emergency*. These acts or attempts to make them are generally preceded by prolonged feelings of hopelessness and of a seemingly needless despair, which finally result in loss of aggression-control, faulty impulse-control, and sociopathy. The influences on consciousness of alcohol and drug abuse are among the other contributing causes for suicide and homicide.

DEFINITION

There appears to be no standard, comprehensive definition of what constitutes a psychiatric emergency. Primarily it is a paralysis in the sphere of reality orientation. While it usually implies some form of severe emotional or psychomotor disturbance in a patient, therefore occurring in any kind of mental illness from mental retardation to psychoneurosis, it also happens with normal persons when they are subjected to inordinate and sudden stress.[1] As the stress increases, the person goes through the stages of "alarm

431

and mobilization" (marked by a determined effort at self control) to the stage of "resistance" (with its consequent exaggeration of ego defense mechanisms), until finally the stage of "exhaustion" has been reached.[2] It is at this last stage that the psychiatric emergency becomes manifest.

The American Hospital Association[3] in a brochure published in 1965 categorized mentally ill persons requiring psychiatric emergency treatment as being: (1) persons who seek help or who will accept it voluntarily, (2) non-resistive persons who may not accept care voluntarily at first but who can be persuaded to do so (such as some senile or depressed persons) and (3) resistive persons who will not accept care voluntarily and whose behavior may be or may become actually or potentially dangerous to themselves or others. Apparently *danger* is the common denominator in the various forms of the psychiatric emergency.

The Joint Information Service of the American Psychiatric Association and the National Association for Mental Health[4] made a survey in 1965 to determine the criteria used by psychiatric hospitals and community mental health centers for defining psychiatric emergency. A total of 89 definitions was received; only three of them, however, were regarded as having been sufficiently carefully thought out to serve the purpose: (1) An emergency is any urgent psychiatric condition, functional or organic, for which immediate treatment would increase or contribute to the patient's likelihood of recovery, or would provide urgently needed protection. (2) Emergencies exist in the sphere of emotional illnesses in the same manner as they exist in the sphere of physical illness. (3) Any problem is an emergency when the responsible referring source (minister, doctor, or other person) feels incapable of handling it for even a few hours beyond the time of contacting professional help.

None of these statements, however, could really be accepted as providing an exact definition of a psychiatric emergency. Thus far it is the general consensus of the psychiatric literature that no agreement has been reached on what constitutes a psychiatric emergency.[5]

In 1959 Miller[6] defined such an emergency as having to do with any individual who has developed a sudden or rapid disorganization in his capacity to control his behavior or to carry out his usual personal, vocational and social activities. To Ungerleider,[7] any patient whose condition warranted prompt psychiatric attention for whatever reasons was an emergency. Schneidman,[8] on the other hand, stated that "there are many persons whose lethality is low but whose desperation is high," thereby focusing the effects of the emergency on the individual whose functioning has changed rather than on the individual whom his changed functioning may affect.

Another term that is used for psychiatric emergency is *crisis*, which

432

Caplan[9] described as being associated with a rise of inner tension, signs of unpleasant affect and disorganized functioning. LaPierre[10] also stated that "no circumstance, however unusual, is a crisis unless it is so defined by human beings. The individual involved must be aware of the danger which is present or he must believe that danger is present."

In 1963 Miller[11] summarized the literature on crisis as follows: (1) As to the time factor, crisis is acute rather than chronic. (2) Crisis is associated with marked changes in behavior, which usually lead to less effective functioning along customary lines. (3) The subjective aspects of crisis are characterized by a sense of helplessness and ineffectiveness. (4) Crisis produces an organismic tension, the generalized physical aspect of which is experienced and expressed in a number of ways. (5) The perception of threat in crisis is relative and unique to the individual.

Cassidy[12] in 1967 offered one of the most recent definitions of psychiatric emergency as "a sudden, serious, psychological or psycho-social disturbance which renders the individual unable to cope effectively with his life situation, his interpersonal relationships, and/or his intrapsychic conflicts."

The modern concept of psychiatric emergency differs from former definitions, which were based on the belief that only a person who was a *danger* to himself or to others constituted an emergency.[13] Today it is generally accepted that psychiatric emergencies are not limited to those who may be dangerous to themselves or to others, and that a person with disturbed behavior who is given immediate treatment and attention often responds dramatically to such care.[14]

Only a few sorts of behavior seem to be accepted consistently as constituting or implying a psychiatric emergency or crisis: suicidal behavior, whether it is meant seriously or as a gesture; assaultiveness; property destruction; extreme anxiety; panic, and bizarre action. The first three are almost invariably considered to constitute an emergency. In the majority of cases where the affected individual does not himself seek help, some friend, relative, policeman, clergyman, family physician or other agent will attempt to intervene, either directly or by calling in outside help. Whether anxiety, panic or bizarre behavior is perceived in a given situation as an emergency appears to depend on the degree to which the disturbed behavior is found threatening by or evokes fear in the beholder. Thus whether or not a given behavior is classified as a psychiatric emergency seems in large part to be contingent upon one's conception of what is a social emergency. There are, of course, many social emergencies that are not psychiatric emergencies, but virtually all psychiatric emergencies are at the same time social emergencies.

433

Homicide or suicide is a *fait accompli* and, of course, irreversible. What we need to be concerned with is the threats that are made *before the fact* by the person or persons involved or their unintended foreshadowings of their readiness to adopt either of these ultimates. Homicidal or suicidal potentials can be detected in persons with acute and chronic brain syndromes, as well as in person with psychotic and non-psychotic syndromes.

In the category of acute and chronic brain syndromes are included intoxication from alcohol and/or drugs, and delirious episodes. Psychotic syndromes are manic-depressive manifestations, manic excitement and schizophrenic turmoil. Non-psychotic syndromes include anxiety, panic, fugues, homosexual panic, postconcussive confusion and aggressive behavior. Components of acute depression and severe anxiety can be found in each of the categories, along with elements of aggressive, assaultive and bizarre behaviors. Excessive fears or phobic reactions are also found in each of these categories.

Potential Causes of Emergencies

The following are potential causes for emergency treatment.

1) Severe anxiety as seen in alcoholic dyscontrol, fatigue, hysterical behavior, infringement of rights, loss of symptom control and panic as seen in homosexual, sedational or sedative reactions.

2) Confusion associated with amnesia, brain syndromes, acute depression, dissociative phenomena leading to confusion and disorientation, fugue states (flight from reality), postconvulsion and postictal states and the turmoil of acute schizophrenia.

3) Psychosis as encountered in acute brain syndromes incidental to alcoholic intoxication, chronic ego deterioration with underlying vivid hallucinatory phenomena leading to passive carrying out of the denied wish and delirious states due to poison or intoxication with LSD, mescaline, marijuana or amphetamines. Psychosis may also be seen in electrolyte imbalance, paranoid plot, postpartum psychosis, schizophrenia and toxic metabolic states.

4) Violence may be associated with acting out for the gratification of a parent, aggressive and assaultive behavior including rape, anger, epileptic furor, catatonic or manic excitement, group aggression, homicide or suicide threats or attempts, stress and temper tantrums in small children including head-banging.

434

Types of Patients

An analysis of a psychiatric emergency consultation service in a University Hospital in Cleveland[15] was made for a six-month period ending in January, 1959. Since the publication of this analysis, it has been referred to often and has come to serve as a representative sampling of the different types of patients in such a situation. A total of 378 psychiatric emergencies was analyzed including statistics on sex, race, religion, marital status, age group and medical records.

It is interesting to note that, as recently as 1960,[16] a survey showed that 88 per cent of all the people who feel an impending "nervous breakdown" first consult their family doctor, not a psychiatrist or an emergency consultation service, and that only 4 per cent go to a psychiatrist first for help.

MANAGEMENT

Today in our social structure, which is rapidly being computerized, there is a growing feeling of depersonalization of the individual, which is providing fertile ground for an increase in psychiatric emergencies. Losing one's identity as an individual human being and becoming only a "number" in the scheme of life can be a degrading and traumatic experience, indeed. In our management of the psychiatric emergency patient, therefore, let us not forget to dignify him as a human being, a person with a name. The psychiatric emergency patient, whom it is our obligation to relieve from the pain he is suffering, is, after all, a human being in distress.

General Principles of Management

1. In the psychiatric emergency prompt action appropriate to the particular situation must be taken.

2. The disturbed, excited, panicky or unruly patient must be accepted as he is, rather than being scolded, resented, punished or avoided. A non-condemnatory attitude on the part of the physician is a requisite before he can proceed to obtain the patient's history.

3. Supportive personal and human contact should be provided for the patient by talking to him, informing him and staying with him until others are assigned to do so.

4. It is usually better to do too much rather than too little. Most patients in acute upsets have regressed to a childlike level, so that they are without the use of many of the capacities they are usually capable of demonstrating. This regression may not be recognized if the patient is well known to the physician or to the person who is with him; the usual error in such cases is to expect too much from the patient.

5. Instill into the interpersonal relationship you are creating some flavor of the concept of "tender loving care."

Appropriate Specific Treatment

Ewalt[17] thoughtfully expressed the appropriate, specific treatment of the psychiatric emergency patient in a few words: "All people, including psychiatric patients, lose control of their behavior more easily when they are fatigued. Thus while panicky escape efforts, angry outbursts and bouts of weeping may be the manifestations of ego decompensation, the required treatment in such cases is rest and food, not psychotherapy." The experience of many physicians has been that the majority of emergency patients do respond well to such supportive treatment as talking to them, encouraging them to rest, prescribing sedation when necessary and, where indicated, providing food and fluids for them.

Following the supportive treatment, such subsequent procedures can be carried out as the physical examination, the psychiatric examination, psychological testing and a mental status examination.

Aggressive Patient. Aggressive and bizarre behavior are often found as symptoms in schizophrenia, and with severely disturbed patients prompt and effective sedation is in order. General recommendations for the handling of aggressive patients include the following.

1. Those who are believed to be mentally ill and potentially dangerous, either to others or to themselves, should be dealt with by mental health professionals who are likely to have had considerable exposure to patient behavior, as well as special training in the handling of highly disturbed people.

2. Most psychiatric patients are experiencing extreme fear, even those who are docile, and therefore, they can become dangerous when confronted with ambiguous, confusing, belligerent or threatening treatment. They should be handled by people who can help provide them with a degree of clarification and assurance, such as aid them in marshalling their own resources for self-control.

3. There should be a close and friendly relationship between the emergency service and the police, through which the information and experience of each can become known to and appreciated by the other. Whenever the authority of the police is required in dealing with an aggressive patient, a mental health professional should also take part.

Anxiety and Panic. Patients who present evidence of acute anxiety and panic are more than likely to be in severe distress. Their panic is increased by their difficulty in breathing and swallowing, which in turn accentuates their anxiety and causes intense feelings of fear, accompanied by palpitations, dyspnoea, tremor, sweating and restlessness. Similar symptoms are encountered in cases of hysterical excitement; anxiety is sometimes associated with it, and experienced quite often by those with hysterical personalities when they are reacting adversely to stress.

While these acute neuroses cause considerable distress to the patient, they usually do not present undue difficulties in management, which should consist primarily of firm and calm reassurance of the patient and of those who may have accompanied him. Care is needed, however, in differentiating these conditions from other, more serious ones.[18] An anxiety attack is a disorder for which successful treatment can easily be achieved; on the other hand, it is also one in which the patient's distress may easily be reinforced.

Impulse Handling. Basically anxiety is experienced as danger to the self, arising either from within, as when the person feels in danger of being overwhelmed by his own impulses which he cannot control, or from without, as when he feels the danger to arise from some situation or event in the external environment. In either case he feels himself relatively weak and ineffective, often experiencing a loss of self-confidence that leads to a sense of the need from others for help, which need may be communicated either verbally or non-verbally. Such a state is responded to both physically and behaviorally with efforts to re-establish a more effective object relationship and thereby to strengthen the self. When the anxiety is overwhelming, this capacity for seeking an object actively (in reality or intrapsychically) is lost, and the more passive state of helplessness sets in.[19]

Self-Esteem. The psychic apparatus assumes the task of organizing perception and information in the service of anticipating and warding off such injury as may threaten from the outer environment or from the pressure or urgency of inner drives. This function includes the elaboration of an alerting and emergency system, in part represented in affects, in order to anticipate or deal with crises. It also includes the development of psychological defense mechanisms that serve to monitor, control, modify, relate, integrate or synthesize the input from the external and internal (body) environment with the data of past experience so that the conditions for living can be assured, with due regard for both external and internal reality. Conflict resolution, both intrapsychic and interpersonal, is one important aspect of this activity. It is through the defense activities of the psychic apparatus that adaptation is achieved and control established over motility in relation to the external environment.[20]

Suicide-Potential Persons. Suggested principles with regard to emergency service for potentially suicidal persons include the following.

1. The substantial evidence for suicide risk in depressed and schizophrenic

437

persons should be made known to all staff members of emergency services, as well as to all mental health personnel, and the treatment and disposition of these patients should be so planned as to reduce the suicide risk to a minimum. This would include not only setting up certain ordinary precautions while the person is in the hospital, but also acquainting his family with the implications of the illness, so that they may be alert to clues that develop after he is discharged from the hospital.

2. Persons who have been admitted to the medical and surgical wards of hospitals (or to the psychiatric ward, where that is the practice) primarily because they have inflicted injuries on themselves, should never be released without psychiatric evaluation. When the psychiatric treatment is indicated, it must be made available.

3. There are many hospitals that still prohibit the admission of psychiatric patients, whether by charter or by unwritten understanding. These hospitals should update their policies in recognition of the fact that persons who are intent on suicide are as likely as persons with manifest physical illness to be ill and to require and deserve treatment. No would-be suicide should ever be kept in jail.

4. There should be a 24-hour-a-day telephone service, manned by trained mental health personnel, to provide assistance to those who seek help for themselves and/or others who have given voice to suicidal ideas. Most appropriately this service should be a component of a comprehensive psychiatric emergency service which should in turn constitute one element of a comprehensive mental health program. This arrangement provides the advantage of immediate and direct access to treatment services when the need is indicated. Ideally the staff of the emergency service should include at least one person with special training and interest in suicidal behavior.

Prevention

It is obvious from information that has been gathered in many different areas that home visits are sometimes able to eliminate the need for hospitalizing psychiatric emergency patients. Perhaps only a facility that is better staffed than the average one is can set this as a goal of its emergency service, since repeated home visits are apparently necessary if such patients are to remain out of hospital.

Intervention during a crisis may significantly benefit the person's mental health by ensuring the healthy resolution of that crisis. It is one way of obtaining maximum results with minimal effort. Predictable crises, however, such as those that are likely to be precipitated by surgical operations, parenthood, college entry and so forth, may be handled by *anticipatory guidance*; in this the specialist helps people to rehearse ahead of time the emotional situations in which they are likely to find themselves and to begin working out in advance how to cope with their impending difficulties. Special education and training should be made available to all care-providing professionals, such as doctors, nurses, teachers and clergymen, so that they may intervene more effectively in the crises of their clients as a regular part of their everyday professional work.

The crisis of mental illness is most often preceded in a person's life by many smaller crises of lesser dimension. If these smaller crises — living troubles not illnesses — for which people seek advice, could be handled intelligently and responsibly at the proper point in time, an immeasurable amount of serious mental disruption in the making could be averted. Early detection and prevention are a necessary part of any effective mental health program.

Specific areas that require development or implementation of measures for prevention of crises are as follow.

1. All psychiatry residency training programs should include *education in the techniques and procedures* for handling psychiatric emergencies.

2. *Service should be immediately available* to all those who are already displaying sufficient disturbance to require the application of psychiatric help. Otherwise these persons are likely to deteriorate further and to become emergencies once again, if they are required to wait after the crisis resolution.

3. Every state and community should develop facilities for *follow-up* programs that will provide medication, counseling and access to rehabilitation, inasmuch as psychiatric emergencies often occur in persons who have been treated in the past for mental illness, yet are currently out of touch with a treatment program. All patients who have been professionally treated for mental illness should be informed upon remission of such a follow-up program and also encouraged to cooperate with it. Those patients who cannot or will not cooperate should be followed up by the program's personnel.

REFERENCES

1. SCHWARTZ, S. D.: Psychiatric Emergencies, Calif. Med. 88:347, 1958.
2. SELYE, H. In: WEIDER, A. (Ed.): Contributions toward Medical Psychology, Vol. 1, New York, Ronald, 1953, p. 234.
3. American Hospital Association: Psychiatric Emergencies and the General Hospital, Chicago, 1965.
4. The Joint Information Service of The American Psychiatric Association and the National Association for Mental Health: The Psychiatric Emergency, A Study of Patterns of Service, Washington, D.C., 1966.

5. COLEMAN, J. V., AND ERRERA, P.: The General Hospital Emergency Room and Its Psychiatric Problems. Amer. J. Public Health, 53:1294, 1963.
6. MILLER, A.: A Report on Psychiatric Emergencies. Canadian Hospital, 36:36, 1959.
7. UNGERLEIDER, J. T.: The Psychiatric Emergency, Analysis of Six Months' Experience of a University Hospital's Consultation Service, Arch. Gen. Practice, 3:593, 1960.
8. SCHNEIDMAN, E.: The Psychiatric Emergency, A Study of Patterns of Service; The Joint Information Service of the American Psychiatric Association and the National Association for Mental Health. Washington, D.C., 1966, p. 13.
9. CAPLAN, G.: Emotional Crises. In: Deutsch, A., and Fishbein, H. (Eds.): The Encyclopedia of Mental Health, Vol. 2. New York, Franklin Watts, Inc., 1963, p. 521.
10. LAPIERRE, R. T.: Cited by Hertzler, J. O.: Crisis and Dictatorship. Amer. Sociol. Rev. 5:157, 1940.
11. MILLER, K. S., AND ISCOE, I.: The Concept of Crisis, Hum. Org., 22:1963.
12. CASSIDY, W. J.: Psychiatric Emergencies. Henry Ford Hosp. Med. J., Vol. 15, 1967.
13. U.S. Department of Health, Education and Welfare, National Institute of Mental Health: Emergency Services, 1966, p. 1.
14. BILL, A. Z., AND SAMPLE, C. E.: The First Psychiatric Emergency. Del. Med. J. 40:115, 1968.
15. UNGERLEIDER, J. T.: The Psychiatric Emergency, Analysis of Six Months' Experience of a University Hospital's Consultation Service. Arch. Gen. Psychiat., 41, 1960.
16. GUREN, G., V. J., AND FELD, S.: Americans View Their Mental Health. New York, Basic Books, 1960.
17. EWALT, J. R., FREEDMAN, A. M., AND KAPLAN, H. I., (Ed.): Other Psychiatric Emergencies. In: Comprehensive Textbook of Psychiatry, Baltimore, Williams & Wilkins, 1967, p. 1179.
18. BRIDGES, P. K.: Psychiatric Emergencies. Postgrad. Med. J. 43:599, 1967.
19. ENGEL, G. L.: Psychological Development in Health and Disease. Philadelphia, W. B. Saunders Company, 1962, p. 126.
20. ENGEL, G. L.: Psychological Development in Health and Disease. Philadelphia, W. B. Saunders Company, 1962, p. 26.

Racial Problems in Psychotherapy

by Robert Coles, M.D.

As the Negro increasingly enters American middle class life he will probably find his way more readily to psychiatric offices and clinics. The predominant poverty that has afflicted Negroes everywhere in our country needs no documentation here; the fact that more and more Negroes are overcoming it is only slowly becoming apparent. It has been well established that the poor in general, regardless of race, are lucky to get any psychiatric care at all. When they do see a psychiatrist he may see them briefly, and with little sustained interest.

However, recent changes in our national life have already had their effect: psychiatric clinics are becoming more aware of their obligations to the poor and the exiled. Professionals in medicine, law, and education are facing the problem of communicating with impoverished people, and Negroes for the first time are emerging in significant numbers from the fearful isolation that has been their lot. It is not always a matter of white therapists seeing Negro patients; there are a good number of Negro psychiatrists, even in Southern states. In the North, Negro doctors are no strangers to white patients, although whites in the South have yet to come to that stage of acceptance.

As a white psychiatrist I have worked closely with Negro families under the stresses of desegregation in the South, as sharecroppers or migrant farm families, as participants in the sit-in movement, and in urban centers of the North, and I have come to recognize some fairly definite stages in the relationship between my colored patients and myself in practice and research. Three centuries of slavery and separate living have not enabled whites and Negroes to trust each other easily, if at all. It is best to assume that a special quality of fear and suspicion marks almost every Negro's initial attitude toward whites. This is expressed in a variety of postures: excessive ingratiation, silence punctuated only rarely and cautiously, a tell-tale politeness that never seems to turn into either explicit hostility or increasing warmth. Some white patients resort

441

to one or another of such maneuvers, but Negroes tend to demonstrate them more fixedly and regularly.

In time (it may be many months) this preliminary period gives way to one where "true feelings" are expressed—a phrase often used. Often it is not until the second year that they acquire enough confidence in a non-Negro to remark "I'm telling you the truth now," or "I'm levelling with you, giving you my real feelings." Until then many patients withhold quite conscious facts or fantasies because of profound distrust and even hate of all whites, resentment of personal hurt and exploitation, and a sense of shame for being Negro, for wishing to be white, for talking at all about such matters to a white person, and for the very fact of feeling ashamed.

The therapist who looks closely at his own feelings at this time may well discover in himself a number of racially tinged, hitherto unconscious attitudes and fantasies. Indeed it is at this critical point in treatment that the full range of symbolic associations to skin color emerge, in both patient and doctor. "Dark" skin is linked to badness and worthlessness, depression and death, to dirt, to sickness or contamination, to evidence of guilt or wrong-doing, to the mysterious, the different, the wild and the primitive, to the sexually wanton and powerful or the sexually exotic, to whatever any given person feels he is not, wishes he were not, or wishes he were. Of course each Negro patient's (or white doctor's) fantasies about the meaning of his skin color will fit into his particular life experience. Negroes share certain sets of attitudes about this, living as they do in our culture where words like "dark" or "black" are so clearly committed symbolically in our language and thinking, even apart from the specific racial prejudices so prevalent.

It has been interesting, in this regard, to observe the way different personalities accommodate themselves to the "fact" (an emotion-laden one as well as a genetic one) of their dark color. The fantasies of the hysteric may tend toward denying his condition or changing it in some dramatic fashion. Those of the obsessive-compulsive will likely center upon ways to "correct" his appearance, by making it tidy and "clean," hence ultimately white. Sexual tensions and hostilities frequently find expression in racial concerns, obviously for whites as well as Negroes. Not all Negroes for example, choose to dwell upon the weakness associated with their skin color or, for that matter, the legend of sexual prowess attached to it. Some Negroes will emphasize the harsh competitive life required of them to make a go of it, others will be more concerned with the sadness and uselessness they feel about their lot, while still others will manage to convince themselves (if not always others)

442

that there are enough substantial rewards to being colored to make any suffering encountered quite bearable.

In one of the families I studied closely in Atlanta a delinquent youth, well on his way to being a narcotics addict, remarked to me, "They say it's tough being a colored man, but if you're included out of the rat race, you can sit yourself back and live real slow and easy. . . . I watches 'whitey' rushing along taking all the pie home and giving us the crumbs; but we has our own pie, and anyway he don't know how to eat he's so worried about making it." This young man I found exceptionally bright and shrewd. The tapes of our interviews are filled with his voluble conversation, an ironic mixture of canny folk wisdom, useless generalizations, glib cliches, and sharply moving, altogether appropriate, humor.

In such cases the therapist must have a keen sense of the many-sided forms bitterness and despair can take, coupled with a willingness to work with people on their terms as well as his own. What I judged to be this youth's problem did not fit with his genuine concerns and worries. He was having a good deal of trouble with his girl friend, whereas I was concerned about his marked "antisocial" tendencies—minor stealing, taking drugs and fathering illegitimate children. "Man, you have your ideas of what's wrong with me, but I have other ideas," he once told me. In retrospect, these "anti-social" patterns ceased in the second year of therapy because I slowly and painfully learned to subordinate my interests in his.

In a number of instances I have survived enough of the risks and blind spots in treatment so that problems of racial identity were substantially diminished. This last phase of psychotherapy I have found particularly enlightening because the patient frequently has a considerable willingness to share some of the facts and feelings of his life in a spirit of earnest communication that contrasts with much of the rhetoric one hears about racial attitudes in Negroes.

For example, a young mother in New Orleans told me in one of our last interviews: "They say we hate all whites somewhere deep inside us. I don't know about anyone else, but I think I hate some in my own family more than any stranger. I think the colored are nearly twenty million, and how can you speak anything about how twenty million feel and expect it to be the real truth?. . . . When you're a Negro you have problems, just like white folks do, and then you have the added one of being a Negro; but I think it depends on each Negro what the rest of his troubles are, and that goes with how he takes being colored, too."

In our first meetings she had been utterly unable to talk about racial matters, even though her neighborhood was in the throes of a severe crisis in school desegregation, and her own daughter was caught up in it as one of the pioneering Negro children going to a nearby white school. Months after we started our conversations she seemed able to talk of little else, thereby avoiding discussion of some very significant family and personal problems as well as directing toward me her racial frustrations, anxieties, and hostilities. But one day she began by remarking, "I was thinking last night that I've given you a kind of bad hospitality the past few weeks. We've been so tired and worn with worry of late; and maybe it's because I've just never had the chance to speak my honest mind to a white. . . . To tell the truth, I didn't even know I had so much to say about how us colored people feel; but now that I've said it all, I truly think it's good to forget it for a while. Most of the time we have our problems just like anybody else. . . . I mean family troubles and the kids, or how you get along with your friends and the fights you have . . . and all that isn't a special thing, a Negro thing I mean. People all over have the same kind of things to bug them, too, just as we do."

"My headaches started three centuries ago," said another Negro patient to me; he was talking of his very real migraine headaches, but the historical background to his psychopathology must not be overlooked.

We are now living in a time specially touched by racial tensions, as a tenth of our population rises up to demand its political and social rights. Yet our psychiatric literature shows the same relative unconcern for the psychological problems facing the Negroes that the country as a whole exhibited for so long. As exceptions, the classic study of Kardiner and Ovesey[1] is only now commanding the respect and attention it deserved, and Viola Bernard's[2,3] reports of her work with Negro patients stands as another landmark in clinical and social psychiatry.[4-6]

From the meeting of blacks and whites in the clinical situation we can hopefully expect the emergence of a mutual respect that laws and changed social practices can only herald. The different strengths of the Negro and the poor will be seen in a new context and utilized in more perceptive and comprehensive therapy.

REFERENCES

1. KARDINER, A., AND OVESEY, L.: The Mark of Oppression. New York, Norton, 1951.
2. BERNARD, V. W.: Psychoanalysis and members of minority groups. J. Amer. Psychoanal. Ass. 1:2:256-267, 1953.
3. ———: Some psychodynamic aspects of desegration. Amer. J. Orthopsychiat. 26:3:459-466, 1956.
4. ADAMS, W. A.: The Negro patient in psychiatric treatment. Amer. J. Orthopsychiat. 20:305-310, 1950.
5. KENNEDY, J.: Problems posed in the analysis of Negro patients. Psychiatry 15: 313-327, 1952.
6. ST. CLAIRE, H. R.: Psychiatric interview experiences with Negroes. Amer. J. Psychiat. 108:113-119, 1951.

Home Visiting: An Aid to Psychiatric Treatment in Black Urban Ghettos

by John N. Chappel, M.D. and Robert S. Daniels, M.D.

Developments in community psychiatry during the past decade reflect increased interest in extending the locus of treatment from office and hospital to home and community. Centers reporting on the use of psychiatric home visits are enthusiastic about the technique as an adjunct to therapy.[1,2] Studies in Boston and California report over 70 percent of psychiatrists in practice making one or more home visits a year.[3,4]

The experiences reported in this chapter took place on the south side of Chicago over a period of 3 years. Early data were gained during a 3-month study of hospitalized patients from the urban community of Woodlawn.[5] This community is predominantly black and could be described as an urban slum, with high rates in most indices of social disorganization.

The authors have been involved with two psychiatric treatment programs which continue to utilize home visits. The Woodlawn Mental Health Center conducts an active aftercare program for patients with acute and chronic emotional disturbances. This program includes home visiting by psychiatrists and community mental health workers. The latter group do most of the visiting, but when difficult treatment problems are encountered, psychiatric home visits have been found valuable. The second resource is the Illinois Drug Abuse Program, which provides treatment for over 2000 narcotics addicts in the Chicago area. Home visiting by psychiatrists, nurses, and addiction specialists is used both for crisis intervention and as part of ongoing treatment.

Common Objections to Home Visiting

A number of barriers block the acceptance of home visiting by psychiatrists as a tool for improving treatment. Lip service may be paid to potential value, but there is little evidence that home visiting occupies an important role in psychiatric training or practice. The following objections are frequently raised:

445

1. Home visiting is expensive in terms of both time and money.

2. Home visiting may be difficult and dangerous, especially in ghetto slums.

3. Home visiting may interfere with treatment by providing secondary gain which leads to acting out or excessive dependence.

4. Home visiting may impose a burden on family and community by keeping an emotionally ill person at home.

5. Home visiting is not a function for psychiatrists but is more appropriately the role of nurses, social workers, or other mental health workers.

We feel that many of these objections are not always valid and may often reflect internal resistance more than external reality. The economics of home visiting should be viewed in the context of the cost of hospitalization. Mickle[2] states that home visits may prevent hospitalization. In other cases, time may actually be saved with patients who are very difficult to evaluate in the office.[1] The psychiatrist tends to be more active in the patient's home and the patient and his family are less defensive.[2]

The dangers facing psychiatrists in black urban ghettos do not appear great. No episodes of harm or violence have been reported in the literature or experienced by the authors, even in periods of civil unrest. The cost in psychic energy is offset by the change of pace which can provide an effective antidote for the loneliness which characterizes individual psychotherapy.

There is no convincing evidence that patients abuse home visits or are damaged by them. Benefit to the patient-therapist relationship is most evident with lower-socioeconomic-class patients.[6] Rather than leading to the development of dependence, the home visit often gives rise to a sense of relief that the therapist is human and cares enough to extend himself. Interpretation of behavior and limit setting can be effective safeguards against patient abuse.

Maintaining a patient in his home at any cost is not a major treatment goal. Home visiting should be evaluated in terms of its contribution to improved function, decreased symptomatic disturbance, and diminished stress for the family and community. Our experience has been that home visiting can be a source of both education and support for the patient's family. Confidence in the therapist may be increased, thus enhancing his ability to alter environmental and family forces affecting the patient.

The main reason for home visiting by the psychiatrist is that this activity can be a potent force in facilitating therapy and establishing a therapeutic alliance. Behrens[6] states that even one brief home visit helps establish rapport and avoids communication difficulties in the treatment of lower-socioeconomic-class patients. The experience in the home increases the psychiatrist's knowledge of the patient and his awareness of the nonverbal interactions that characterize the family dynamics.

446

Indications for Home Visiting

1. Crises in treatment which result in a plea for help from the family, especially if the alternative appears to be commitment, hospitalization, or imprisonment.

2. Reluctance of the patient to continue treatment, diminishing motivation, or absence from treatment in the face of a clearly continuing need for help.

3. Relapses in the course of treatment which cannot be understood in the context of the patient-therapist relationship.

4. Difficulty in communicating with or understanding the patient.

5. Transfer of a patient from one treatment modality to another, especially following discharge from hospital to an outpatient aftercare program.

6. Teaching and supervision of psychiatry residents or medical students on a treatment team.

When the indications are present and a decision has been made to visit a patient's home, the visit will be found to fall into two phases. Each phase has its own characteristics and challenges.

The Community Phase

Venturing into an urban ghetto frequently arouses anxiety in the visitor. Familiarity with the community, its residents, and others working there can do much to allay unsettling anxiety. Trust in the neighborhood grapevine and the presence of a companion known in the community help dull hackle-raising fantasy of a bullet in the back of the head. A sense of purpose and belief in the value of the visit helps raise flagging motivation.

Planning. Prearranged visits are frequently disappointing. Our experience parallels that of Meyer et al.,[7] who found that, even with patient preparation and agreement, it was not unusual to find no one home at the scheduled time. Permission for the visit is best obtained in person at the door of the home, since prior requests are often turned down. Anxiety levels and resistance to home visits may be even higher in the visited than in the visitor. One man, after learning that a visit was planned for later in the week, went so far as to move out of his hotel room without leaving a forwarding address.

The most successful time for finding ghetto dwellers at home has been late afternoon or Saturday morning. Once the visitor and his purpose have been made clear, even the most suspicious persons will usually grant permission for the visit. In every instance the authors have been admitted to patients' homes.

Attitude of the Visitor in the Community. The best protection for a visitor may be an open willingness to identify himself. We do not hesitate to ask for help from people in the street. This can be done without revealing damaging

447

information about the patient. We have yet to hear objections or to receive complaints following home visits from a psychiatrist.

Locating the Home. In deteriorating urban areas there may be no address numbers on buildings, mailboxes without names, and an absence of numbers on apartment doors. Persistent door knocking, seeking out and greeting the janitor, or stopping people may be required to locate the patient's place of residence.

In our experience ghetto dwellers with mental illness are characterized by a striking degree of social isolation. Alienation and hopelessness characterize the lives of many of our patients. Social distance seems to be part of the slum way of life. Frequently people do not know their neighbors in the next apartment.

The following case illustrates isolation, extensive pathology, and the value of persistence in pursuing community contacts.

Case 1. Mr. R. R., age 33, was a musician who had been unable to work at his profession for three years, since his marriage ended in divorce. Mrs. R., his ex-wife, had him committed when he demanded money from her, refused to leave her apartment, and lay down on the floor, making threats and delusional comments.

Mr. R. had been in intermittent treatment as an outpatient for several years. During these contacts almost nothing was learned of his life circumstances. He had sought help because he hallucinated that his skin was changing from brown to orange and because he suffered from impotence. On no occasion would he reveal his address and telephone number.

Throughout the interview in the hospital Mr. R. was suspicious and guarded. He was insistent in his wishes that the psychiatrist talk to no one about him. The psychiatrist did not agree and stressed the importance of finding better ways to deal with his problems, since past methods had not worked well.

Telephone contact with Mrs. R. led to a home visit with Mr. R.'s mother. This elderly, withdrawn woman lived alone in a small room in an old apartment building. Her husband had died shortly after the birth of Mr. R., her youngest child. The three children had been sent to a foster home when the patient was 14 months old. Contact between the mother and the children was intermittent and stormy. A few years previously the middle child, a daughter, had stabbed her mother.

The daughter had recently been admitted to Manteno State Hospital and turned out to be Mrs. K. S., another patient in the clinic, whom the psychiatrist had been unable to contact because of an incorrect address. A home visit with Mrs. S. revealed that Mr. R. had been both intelligent and talented. He had graduated in the top ten of his high school class and had shown no sign of emotional problems until he married. Mrs. S. blamed her brother's wife for his sexual problems. She did not feel that she could be of any help to her brother but expressed an interest in visiting him in the hospital. Finally, she promised to persuade him to join the aftercare program where both of them could obtain medication and group therapy.

The home visits revealed extensive family pathology that had not been evident during the long period when the patient was in outpatient treatment.

448

The family, which had previously shown no obvious interest, now agreed that help was necessary. The cooperative attitude displayed in the homes was in marked contrast to the guarded suspiciousness shown in the hospital.

The Home Phase

Once identification has been made, and double or triple locks have been opened, the second phase of the visit begins. Do not expect coffee or social amenities. There is no automatic acceptance of the psychiatrist. Deep suspicion is likely to be present regarding his motivation and interest in the patient.

Relate to the Male of the Family. The Moynihan report on the Negro family in America emphasized the absence of a man in the home and the relatively better education and earning power of women. It is our impression that the black man's current role in the family is more important than is usually apparent. Two patterns tend to emerge. Either the man expects to be avoided or ignored if he is not the patient or, less frequently, he will be authoritative, dominant, and even militant. In either case, the man's cooperation and understanding are important both to the success of treatment of family members and to support the existing family structure.

Be Alert to the Patient's Agenda. In addition to the therapist's agenda for the visit, he must be sensitive to the patient's expectations. Mutual definition of the objectives and purposes of treatment can do much to facilitate further treatment. Avoiding implied promises and dealing with hidden expectations of ongoing treatment in the home will often prevent later difficulties.

The following case illustrates both hidden agendas and hidden pathology. Hospitalization had been used for years to obscure family needs. When the needs of each family member were recognized, it became possible to terminate hospitalization without forcing the patient to return home. Appropriate help was also obtained for other individuals within the family.

Case 2. Mr. C. D., age 49, had been in the state hospital for 18 years. During most of this time he had been a "good" patient. When interviewed, his manner was bland and he displayed virtually no affect. The hospital staff felt that he had been ready for discharge for some time. They were frustrated by their inability to get Mrs. D. to come in and discuss the possibility of her husband's discharge.

Mrs. D. was visited in her apartment in a public housing project. She was an attractive, cooperative, hospitable woman who kept her home clean and well furnished. While her husband had been hospitalized she had raised the three children by herself and supported them by working as a practical nurse in a local hospital. In addition, she had taken night classes and correspondence courses, attaining the equivalent of three years of college education. It had been her practice to take any civil service examination for which she was eligible.

One year before the visit she had been appointed as a truant officer. This

449

work was done during the day in the same area in which she lived. Her two jobs created a problem in that she made too much money and had to move out of the housing project.

In this apparently benign setting the strange tale of the children was revealed. The oldest son, age 23, was a patient in Manteno State Hospital. He had been discharged from the Army the previous summer for psychiatric reasons. One month before the home visit her younger son, age 21, had been shot in a subway station where he was accused of having attempted to rape a woman. The next night the oldest son tried to get into bed with his mother. She became quite upset at this and had him committed.

The younger son was still in jail awaiting psychiatric evaluation. He had suffered from severe eczema as a child and was always depressed. Throughout adolescence he had often been in trouble and had said several times that he would die early. Most of his crimes were clumsily performed, and he was almost always caught.

The daughter, age 18, was born four weeks after her father was committed to Manteno. She had dropped out of school in grade nine and now had an illegitimate child. Eighteen months before the home visit she began breaking up everything made of glass in the apartment. She was admitted to a psychiatric ward for one week. She then left home, and there had been no repetition of the destructive behavior.

Mrs. D. made it plain that she did not want any of her family living with her, especially her husband. She felt that she had outgrown him and did not want him discharged in her care. He could live with other members of his own family. Her hope was to remarry and start a new life.

As a result of the home visit a family session was held at the hospital. Mrs. D. looked as though she had stepped out of a fashion magazine. The words she spoke to her son expressed care and concern, but her nonverbal communication was rejecting. Mr. D. remained a passive spectator and seemed oblivious to what was going on around him. Arrangements were made for Mr. D. to be discharged to live with a relative. The son returned home with his mother and was referred to an aftercare program where he could receive medication and psychotherapy.

Open All Senses. The combination of visual, auditory, olfactory, tactile, and emotional sensations provides a new context for communication with the patient. Experiencing firsthand the environment of the ghetto dweller can add another dimension to understanding his life stress. Nonverbal communication may be even more important than what is verbally offered. Do not hesitate to move around the house if invited or indicated by circumstances. Strengths in the form of alliances and support may become evident in a way that is rarely appreciated when the patient comes to a clinic or office.

It may be possible to increase the strength of family support available to the patient. The therapist may serve as a source of education and support for members of the family. Home visiting appears to increase the family's confidence in the therapist and to enhance his ability to alter environmental and social forces affecting the patient. In addition, the home experience increases the

450

psychiatrist's knowledge of the patient and his awareness of the nonverbal interactions that characterize the family dynamics. These opportunities are often missed in the hospital or clinic. Either important family members do not come to the institution or, when they do, they are too overwhelmed, inhibited, or irritated to ask the questions or express the feelings that concern them the most.

Use of a Companion. We have been impressed with the advantages of visiting with a paraprofessional colleague, such as a community mental health worker or addiction counselor who is familiar with the community. Communication is facilitated between patient, family, and therapist with less chance of mutual misunderstanding. In our experience the presence of a companion is particularly useful in developing a working relationship with paranoid or violent patients.

On two dramatic occasions men with guns had terrified their peers and family. Home visits were undertaken with a black male paraprofessional. In each case the crisis was relieved. Both men were found to be desperate. They had hoped to be killed, hurt badly, or incarcerated. This behavior was understood as a means of inflicting injury on people whom they thought no longer cared about them and also as a way of relieving guilt and shame. A profound loss of self-esteem related to job failure was present in each man. During the course of the visits violent threats dissolved into tears. Both incarceration and hospitalization were avoided. With over a year of follow-up in each case there has been no repetition of violent behavior. One of the men has become a youth counselor and has enrolled in a university mental health career program.

Conclusion

Controlled studies will be necessary to evaluate critically the role of psychiatric home visits in the treatment of black ghetto residents. Our experiences to date, however, offer some evidence that the advantages gained outweigh the disadvantages. On the basis of our experience we find support for the following statements:

1. Psychiatric home visiting is both possible and safe in a black urban ghetto.
2. Home visiting can be effective in bridging the isolation, alienation, and hopelessness found in many ghetto patients.
3. Home visiting can enlist important treatment support from family members and friends not usually encountered in clinic or office settings.
4. Home visiting can be helpful in treating violent or paranoid patients and preventing acting out which disrupts treatment and requires hospitalization or incarceration.
5. Home visiting provides an effective nonverbal way of bridging social and cultural gaps which interfere with the development of a treatment relationship between patient and therapist. The latent language of the visit provides a basis for trust and invites the patient to participate actively in treatment.

451

Many black ghetto residents feel that the institutions serving the slums are insensitive to the real needs of the people. The riots, demonstrations, and civil rights protests of recent years make it plain that black and white Americans do not understand each other and mistrust each other's motives. Visits by a white professional into a black home can help increase understanding and begin to arouse interest in addition to achieving other treatment goals.

Large segments of inner-city populations are not served by psychiatric outpatient programs. Many symptomatic individuals do not actively seek treatment but may respond well once they are involved in therapy. Programs serving urban communities must find new ways to reach this apparently unmotivated, isolated, but needy population. Home visiting provides one way of achieving such a goal.

Acknowledgments

The authors acknowledge with gratitude the helpful comments and suggestions of Dr. George Meyer, Professor of Psychiatry, University of Texas, San Antonio, and Dr. Charles Wilkinson, Professor of Psychiatry, University of Missouri, Kansas City.

REFERENCES

1. Freeman, R. D.: The Home Visit in Child Psychiatry. J. Amer. Child Psychiat. 6:279-293, 1967.
2. Mickle, J. C.: Psychiatric Home Visits. Arch. Gen. Psychiat. (Chicago) 9:379-383, 1963.
3. Brown, B. S.: Home Visiting by Psychiatrists. Arch. Gen. Psychiat. (Chicago) 7:98-107, 1962.
4. Meyer, R. E., Schieff, L. F., and Becker, A.: The Home Treatment of Psychotic Patients: An Analysis of 154 Cases. Amer. J. Psychiat. 123:1430-1438, 1967.
5. Chappel, J. N., and Daniels, R. S.: Home Visiting in a Black Urban Community. Amer. J. Psychiat. 126:1455-1460, 1970.
6. Behrens, M. I.: Brief Home Visits by the Clinic Therapist in the Treatment of Lower-Class Patients. Amer. J. Psychiat. 124:127-131, 1967.
7. Meyer, G., Margolis, P., and Daniels, R.: Hospital Discharges Against Medical Advice. II. Outcome. Arch. Gen. Psychiat. (Chicago) 8:41-49, 1963.

The Prevention of Hospitalization*

by Betty Glasser, S.M., and Milton Greenblatt, M.D.

E FFORTS ARE BEING MADE all over the country to reduce the size of our large psychiatric institutions and to reduce the stay of those patients who are admitted. Thousands of mentally ill veterans have left VA hospitals and are living in various communities with foster families or their own families. Housewives, business men, and college and high school students are being enlisted to embark upon programs aimed at rehabilitating and resocializing chronic ward inmates of mental hospitals. Today, more than ever the way is open to the development of extra-hospital facilities, family and community participation in care and treatment, and eventually the "liquidation" of the state hospital as we know it. "Community" is replacing "dynamic" as the word that most neatly characterizes psychiatry's advancing edges; ergo, one of the pivotal questions facing American psychiatry is whether or not this is the best approach to mental disorders.

At the Massachusetts Mental Health Center, the idea of a "Prevention of Hospitalization Program" evolved in the context of a growing, changing psychiatric institution that had been experimenting for years with new methods of patient-care. A small, intensive treatment, training, and research hospital operated jointly by the Commonwealth of Massachusetts and the Harvard Medical School, MMHC serves the whole State, is rich in staff and services, and enjoys a reputation as a university-teaching-research center. Demand for admission was such that in 1956 waiting might be as long as 6 weeks. After 1956, due largely to the success of a new Day Hospital facility in treating patients who would originally have been accepted for admission to the inpatient

*This work, supported by NIMH Grant MH-67, is described in full in M. Greenblatt, R. F. Morse, R. S. Albert, and Maida H. Solomon: The Prevention of Hospitalization. New York, Grune & Stratton, 1963.

service, the practice of admitting patients serially from a waiting list was challenged, based on hospital research data supporting the hypothesis that many patients are better treated on the outside.

To test this proposition, the National Institute of Mental Health sponsored a demonstration-research project at MMHC. The goal of the 3-year project, called the Community Extension Service (CES), was to discover how many persons referred for hospital care could be therapeutically managed as outpatients, and the techniques of value in such a program.

A number of other projects similar in aim and methods were studied as a background for the planning and organizing of the Prevention of Hospitalization service. In foreign countries such as Holland, where caring for the acute mentally ill in Amsterdam[1] is a civilian effort, and also in England (Worthing),[2] where there is a marked shortage of mental hospital beds, physicians do not have to overcome a tradition of an easy resort to mental hospitalization and prolonged custodial care. In some countries (e.g., Russia[3]) the beds have never existed. Here at home, coincident with plans for a community extension service at MMHC, a related project called the Home Treatment Service[4] was undertaken at Boston State Hospital. Also, Dr. Donald Coleman was servicing 170 to 200 new patients a month, averaging between two and three visits, at the Emergency Psychiatric Clinic of the Bronx Municipal Hospital Center.[5]

A common factor in all services, American and European, is that no new skills were "invented"; instead, there is a great reliance on older skills, some of which predate modern psychiatry but which are still effective in the treatment of psychiatric patients. These include firm and confident entrance into a case, and pursuit of it until some therapeutic decision has been made by an expert or by someone more aware of the problems involved than the patient or the family. All services, with the exception of the Bronx Municipal Hospital Clinic, used home visits by social workers, nurses, and psychiatrists as part of their treatment. Perhaps the most important feature is that each has succeeded in reducing the flood of admissions into the associated mental hospital and, in the process, has set up effective and flexible treatment for the nonhospitalized patient.

The Community Extension Service was established on one floor (used as a suite of offices and reception room) of an old three-story house across the street from MMHC. This location, clearly separated from the hospital, was supposed to emphasize that the CES goal was extramural treatment. At no time did the clinical staff exceed the equivalent

454

of 1½ psychiatrists, 1½ social workers, and one nurse—five individuals filling four full-time jobs. In addition to the personnel in most community mental health facilities, psychiatrist, social worker, research psychologist, and secretary receptionist, CES included a psychiatric nurse with the assumption that nursing skills would be needed to deal with acutely ill psychiatric patients and provide the same quality of care for them as was provided for inpatients.

It was decided that CES should adopt an eclectic and flexible attitude toward treatment measures and professional roles, and specifically that it should be able to offer assistance without more than a day's delay, and that it should attempt both diagnosis and treatment in the home whenever necessary. Treatment, therefore, was projected on three general levels: (1) complete and definite care entirely on an outpatient basis; (2) for those for whom hospitalization was necessary, the beginning of stages of treatment that would then be continued or intensified in the ward when a bed became available; and (3) at the very least, stop-gap services to the patient and his family, and consultative services to the referring physician that would alleviate for all parties the distress of the waiting period.

During 27 months CES provided clinical services to 128 applicants for admission to the MMHC inpatient wards and their families. The largest group was between the ages of 26 and 35. Approximately one-third of the patients were diagnosed schizophrenic; another third, depressive; and the rest as personality and psychoneurotic disorders.

The psychiatrist's role in the treatment phase was characterized by general availability and flexibility. He relied less on the patient's motivation than is customary in most outpatient clinics; he himself was often the motivating person. In addition to the usual diagnostic focus on the patient's behavior his concerns widened to include the immediate cause precipitating the request for hospitalization and the assets that could be mustered to avoid it. Psychotherapy given by CES was most often short-term, and when it did continue over a long period of time, it usually tended to be supportive.

Social diagnosis at intake was the most important and time-consuming task of the CES social worker. Casework in general was focused on helping patients into the hospital when necessary, as well as keeping them out whenever possible. The social worker, like the psychiatrist, offered both short-term contact and prolonged treatment. The goals of the short-term contacts were, generally, to get the relatives to accept the treatment plan recommended by CES and to alleviate their guilt and anxiety. Indications for extended treatment or more frequent contact were usually the greater severity of the patient's condition and/or the necessity for keeping in close touch with the home situation if prevention of hospitalization were to be accomplished.

ROLE OF THE NURSE

The psychiatric nurse, a relative stranger to the staff of a psychiatric outpatient clinic, proved to be a valuable member of the CES team. Since the patient himself became essentially the concern of the psychiatrist, and his family that of the social worker, many observers, both inside and outside of CES, wondered what there was for a nurse to do beyond administering medication.

Gradually, the differentiation in practice between the nurse's and the social worker's role became clear. Social workers are trained to provide the patient aid within the context of the resources available in the family, in the community, and in the patient himself. Nursing, on the other hand, is primarily disease-oriented. That is not to say that the nurse is not interested in health and how it is to be maintained. However, the focus of her work is the alleviation of illness and the care of the ill. Therefore, in making home visits, as in the other activities of the CES staff, the nurse's function and the services she provided were different from, though complementary to, those of the social worker.

The psychiatric nurse's clinical training and her professional ability to relate to and identify with depressed and withdrawn persons were particularly useful when home visits had to be made to reach persons who claimed they were too ill to come to the office. The nurse took part in some of the visits made by the doctor in cases in which it was necessary for him to obtain information and make a diagnostic evaluation in the home. In one such case, in which a young girl had slashed her arms on the day she had been scheduled for an office appointment, the nurse went to the patient's house to care for her until the doctor arrived. When the doctor arrived, he recommended immediate hospitalization. The nurse was able to persuade the patient to dress herself, eat a meal, and with assistance pack her bag and leave for the hospital without resistance. Meanwhile, the CES social worker, who had arrived with the psychiatrist, was talking with the distraught family to determine what might be done to help them during the time of crisis. As the nurse and the social worker became more skilled in home visits, the psychiatrist made fewer and fewer of them.

In working with chronic schizophrenics in an effort to prevent hospital readmission, we found that student nurses learned a great deal making weekly home visits and enjoyed planning an afternoon of window

456

shopping or some other diversion for the chronic patient, and that the patient in turn enjoyed the weekly visits of the student nurses, who, even though they rotated every 3 months were essentially always the same —young, friendly, cheerful, and helpful.

The Visiting Nurse Association, often used by CES, will take over a case dealing with mental illness if its assignment is clear. It obviously cannot be expected to serve as a diagnostic agency, nor can its nurse function with psychiatric patients without the supervision of a hospital or clinical psychiatric nurse or social worker. Nonetheless, the willingness of the VNA to take on the responsibility for care of mental patients, and the availabliity of its service in many communities, make it a resource which might serve most effectively in the effort to prevent hospitalization.

COMMUNITY AGENCIES

It was the belief of the CES staff that however skilled its management of a case, community agencies were often essential adjuncts. Agencies included those already tapped by the patient and his family before they arrived at CES, those called in by CES during treatment, and those to which the psychiatric team transferred the patient and/or his family at the outset or after its own treatment had ended. The community agencies thus utilized included psychiatric services, public and private, as well as those more commonly defined as social agencies. For 128 cases, a total of 191 community services were called upon. These included medical, employment, financial, care of children, educational, housing, transportation, and therapy or social service needs for relatives.

RELATIVES

CES dealt with patients who were very much involved with their families. Of the 128 patients, all but 20 lived with relatives. It was usually the family, rather than the patient, family doctor, or a source in the community that initiated the search for psychiatric treatment for the patient. Because of this important role and because the family usually participated in making the arrangements for hospitalization, its attitudes toward the patient and his illness were primary factors in all CES decisions.

A family that is emotionally dependent upon a patient, though not necessarily economically or socially so, seems to possess the most satisfactory constellation of willingness and ability to cooperate in preventing hospitalization. Families that do not feel dependent upon their patient-

457

members in any way for companionship, finances, or affection appear to be the families upon which the service can have little influence or effect.

RESULTS

After the doors of the CES had been closed to patients, the staff turned to the task of conducting 1 to 3 year follow-up interviews with the families it had served, and to an evaluation of the therapeutic activity of the experimental Community Extension Service of the Massachusetts Mental Health Center. We found that at least half of those treated by CES did not require the hospitalization for which they had been referred and could remain in the community. The personnel and procedures needed to achieve these results had been similar to those available in existing clinics and inpatient wards. Such clinics and wards can treat patients without admission if they can offer with promptness a wide variety of services, and if they are oriented to accept prevention of hospitalization as a major goal.

In the United States, staff selection of patients for admission to hospitals is not now the practice. In Europe, however, institutional psychiatrists often spend a good portion of their time seeing, in the community, patients who have been referred to them for treatment by physicians and others. Here, by contrast, in many hospitals the staff psychiatrist plays no role at all. Clearly a screening-plus-service program should be made a part of every mental hospital; admission should be a collaborative effort of social agencies and medical authorities in the community and the hospital psychiatrist.

Our cost accounting indicated that a community clinic that provides emergency and hospitalization prevention treatment probably represents a considerable saving to the state over the routine hospitalization of patients. In addition, when we consider the value to the patient and family of continued self-sufficiency, plus the patient's wages (part of which are returned in taxes), the service's value in monetary terms becomes unquestionable.

CES experience with patients—in particular, those who lacked a congenial home environment—indicated that the hospital's "halfway-out" house might well be supplemented with a "halfway-*in*" house where nonhospitalized patients could receive shelter, protection, and some care, and would not need to live in the isolation of a rented room.

Both the psychiatrists who worked on the CES staff and many physicians who came in contact with them agreed that service with a CES-type clinic might be a worthwhile addition to the second or third year of psychiatric residency training.

Another factor that is worthy of mention with regard to education is the home visit. Opportunities are rare for students to visit patients and their families in their own surroundings, become familiar with their problems, and follow them through the course of the patient's treatment. Also inherent in the community extension technic of care for the mentally ill is the attempt to bring the general practitioner closer to psychiatry. One possibility would be to offer to interested practitioners, in their own offices, expert guidance or supervision with specific patients for whom they would retain ultimate responsibility.

Implications of work in the CES point, in general, in the direction of a broader view of psychiatric practice, one that is more inclusive in a social sense. The CES processes and procedures have been widely repeated throughout the United States, and it is not inconceivable that in another decade the majority of persons headed for hospitalization could be adequately treated elsewhere, and the way thus opened for the greater community role of the large state hospital.

In discussing the concept of prevention, the goal is not the prevention of hospitalization *at any cost*. We would agree that hospitalization is usually indicated for the acutely suicidal patient, the destructive or disruptive patient, or the person with a toxic psychosis; and we would agree that it is sometimes desirable as a means of social education or of separation from a noxious environment. The concept of prevention of hospitalization is to provide an alternative to admissions that are neither indicated nor desirable. This is defined as any effective and practical extrahospital measure that will remove or diminish the forces tending to eject the patient from family or community and to necessitate his isolation in an institution, but that will involve no undue risk for either the patient or the community.

There are still many physicians who follow the familiar axiom, "When in doubt, hospitalize"; many believe that it is better to hospitalize mentally ill persons than to attempt home or community treatment. There are many professional persons who remain unimpressed with the reports of CES and similar undertakings, and unconvinced that community treatment (as opposed to hospitalization) is as (or more) effective in psychiatric disorders. There are many psychiatrists who are concerned as to whether it is best to maintain sick people in the community (they warn against saturating communities with odd-looking and bizarre-behaving persons), or once a person has been hospitalized, to return him to his family, the theory here being that the family does not want him. There is also some dissatisfaction with the end point chosen by the CES—the patient's ability to continue his life in the community without further knowledge of his impact on his social milieu. However, we believe that if the majority of professional people are oriented toward the concept of prevention of hospitalization, then eventually the stigma and shame can be disassociated from mental illness, and the day will arrive when the public will be free to feel full compassion for a human being with mental distress and social maladjustment.

REFERENCES

1. QUERIDO, A.: Cited in a Memorandum, of the Joint Commission on Mental Illness and Health, Cambridge, January 2, 1958, p. 3 (mimeographed).
   MEERLOO, J. A. M.: Emergency psycho-therapy and mental first aid. J. Nerv. & Ment. Dis. 124(6):535-45, 1956.
   LEMKAU, P. V., AND CROCETTI, G. M.: The Amsterdam Municipal Psychiatric Service: a psychiatric-sociological review. Am. J. Psychiat. 117:779-83, 1961.
   MILLAR, W. M., AND HENDERSON, J. G.: The health service in Amsterdam. Internat. J. Social Psychiat. 2(2):144, 1956.

2. CARSE, J., et al.: A district mental health service: the Worthing Experiment. Lancet 2:39-41, 1958.
   ——: Fourth Interim Report on the Worthing and District Mental Health Service together with the First Report on the Chichester and District Mental Health Service. District Mental Health Service, Worthing, England, 1958.

3. FIELD, M. G.: Approaches to mental illness in Soviet society: some comparisons and conjectures. Social Problems 7(4): 227-97, 1960.
   KLINE, N. S.: The organization of psychiatric care and psychiatric research in the Union of Soviet Socialist Republics. Ann. New York Acad. Sc. 84: 147-224, 1960, article 4.
   GILYAROVSKY, V. A.: The Soviet Union. In L. Bellak (Ed.): Contemporary European Psychiatry. New York, Grove Press, 1961, pp. 320-21.
   WORTIS, J.: Soviet Psychiatry. Baltimore, Williams & Wilkins, 1950, pp. 56-57.

4. FRIEDMAN, T. T.: Progress Report, Home Treatment Service, Boston State Hospital, July, 1961(pursuant to Grant No. OM-98 of the National Institute of Mental Health, Washington, D.C.) (Typescript.)
   ——. BECKER, A., AND WEINER, L.: The psychiatric home treatment service: preliminary report of five years of clinical experience. Am. J. Psychiat. 120(8):782-788, 1964.
   1964 American Psychiatric Association Mental Hospital Service Achievement Awards, Gold Award: The Home Treatment Service of Boston State Hospital: Mental Hospitals 15(10):545-548, 1964.

5. COLEMAN, M. D., AND ZWERLING, I.: The emergency psychiatric clinic—a flexible way of meeting community mental health needs. Am. J. Psychiat. 115:980, 1959.
   ——: Methods of psychotherapy: emergency psychotherapy. In Masserman, J. H., and Moreno, V. (Eds.): Progress in Psychotherapy. New York, Grune & Stratton, 5:78-85, 1960.

The Hospital-Affiliated Halfway House

by GEORGE J. WAYNE, M.D.

T HE HALFWAY HOUSE is one segment in the spectrum of transitional agencies for psychiatric patients. These "pathway" agencies, which also include facilities such as day hospitals, night hospitals, and sheltered workshops, facilitate the patient's progress as he moves in a graduated manner from total hospital care to his normal place in the community. For some patients the halfway house may entirely short circuit the need for hospitalization.

Transitional care is not limited to psychiatric patients. Any individual who has been disarticulated from his normal environment and activities for a prolonged period can benefit if his return is accomplished in stages. The usefulness of transitional facilities has been demonstrated for criminals released from penal institutions. Such facilities are even more urgently needed in the case of recovering psychiatric patients.

If the patient remains in the hospital after he no longer needs the hospital regimen, he has only limited opportunities to test his improving adaptive capacities. He may too willingly accept the patient role—a role which makes insufficient demand upon him so that he does not test his limits. On the other hand, if he is catapulted into the community prematurely, he often finds that his worst apprehensions about his inadequacies are swiftly realized.

There are relatively few halfway houses in this country, and fewer still have existed long enough for many generalizations to be formulated about them. Two patterns are evident among existing halfway houses. Some are totally detached from a treatment center, house a small and homogeneous group, maintain an informal, club-like atmosphere with minimal—if any—emphasis on therapy. Others are closely affiliated with a hospital and are treatment-oriented. Since the author's direct professional experience has been with a hospital-affiliated halfway house, the following discussion will be presented within that context.

When a halfway house is close to a hospital, geographically and or-

461

ganizationally, there can be constant interchange of professional and physical resources. This offers substantial advantages, both operationally and therapeutically. Economies can be affected because there is minimum duplication of personnel or physical equipment. Proximity of the parent hospital means that therapeutic support can be relinquished as the patient improves and reinstated if the patient regresses. The opportunity for rehabilitation can thus be offered to the patient whose level of recovery may be somewhat equivocal. If he does poorly, he can easily be rehospitalized. If he does well in transition, his return to home and work has been accelerated.

Both men and women are admitted to our halfway house, which can accommodate 36 guests. The age range is from 16 to 65. We find it neither necessary nor desirable to aim for homogeneity in the group. Patients with organic brain disease live side by side with persons who need little more than a temporary refuge.

An activities schedule figures importantly in the regimen of the guests. Those who are able, go to school or hold a job during the day and utilize the halfway house as a modified night hospital. Those who remain at the house during the day have the opportunity for extensive occupational and recreational therapy. None of it is mandatory nor regimented. As much as possible, the recreational activities are carried on *away* from the house. Our location in the center of a large metropolitan area makes this feasible.

Evening activities include the showing of mental health films, group discussions of topics of general interest, and social and recreational programs. Self-government is encouraged, although the extent to which this can be accomplished varies with the composition of the guest group. Patients who anticipate that their stay at the halfway house will be short-term are likely not to be interested in self-government. Older chronic patients often lack interest in the process, and the youngest of our patients rarely want to be bothered by it. But when guests at the halfway house include a number of reasonably vigorous and hopeful persons with some capacity for leadership, self-government can take on aspects of the healthy climate of open family discussions.

Our halfway house is staffed on a round-the-clock basis. The key member of the staff is the house mother, who lives on the premises and who does all the things one would expect a house mother to do: sees that the house is well run and that the people in it eat their meals, feel well, and behave themselves. It is her responsibility to enforce rules and regulations in the interest of family harmony, to be on the look-out for guests whose behavior indicates they may need prompt professional attention and to be alert to the needs and well-being of everyone in the

462

house. Such a person should be sensitive, tolerant, flexible, and non-punishing.

It is difficult to know in advance whether a patient will respond positively to the environment of the halfway house, since the milieu serves as a testing ground for individual motivation and capacity for recovery. The seemingly hopeless patient may demonstrate a capacity for expanding his limits. The ego functions of very ill persons are sometimes adaptively catalyzed in an environment which is oriented toward recovery rather than illness. Conversely, some patients who seem to be good candidates for the halfway house reveal minimum motivation when there.

The specific symptomatic ways in which a person's illness manifests itself is of great importance in assessing whether he is appropriate for the halfway house. Severe alcoholics and narcotic addicts, those whose acting-out takes sexually exhibitionistic forms, and impulse-ridden persons take a great toll in the group situation. For such patients, spending the recovery period in a homogeneous group might be more suitable. The experience with narcotics addicts at Synanon House suggests that they have a favorable course under such circumstances. In heterogeneous groups, however, the individual who indulges in antisocial behavior tends to unlock tendencies in others who may be barely managing in their struggle to conduct themselves acceptably in the halfway house community.

Persons who chronically demand or need too much attention should not remain. Quite apart from the practical problems such guests create, their insatiable demands precipitate serious sibling jealousies. The guest who surreptitiously subverts the milieu and looks on with apparent detachment while deterioration takes place should be asked to leave.

Each guest at our halfway house is required to have psychiatric supervision. Our social worker and house mother work with the patient's family. Because of the wide spectrum of psychopathology, the duration, frequency and type of therapy will vary, from token support to intensive treatment.

Psychotherapy for guests at the halfway house is in all respects the same as for persons living at home, except that the day-to-day living experiences become grist for the psychotherapeutic mill. Often these experiences catalyze movement in therapy, particularly for persons who might otherwise be isolated and withdrawn, or for those whose therapy has reached a plateau from which they cannot be budged.

Group psychotherapy is especially applicable in a halfway house, since members of the group have more ramified exposures to each other than would be true in a randomly assembled group, We observe more highly charged interactions in the therapy sessions. All group activities in the halfway house—group work, group discussions—serve a therapeutic function.

In day-to-day living, guests are very quick to register approval and disapproval of the behavior of their house-mates. This often seems like the bickering and fault-finding of a large and quarrelsome family, but its long-term effects are healthy. Strict limits are placed on the person who interminably indulges his sick needs. Guests are very outspoken in registering their impatience with behavior which is excessively narcissistic and demanding or tyrannical.

But not all peer relationships are judgmental. There are heartening instances of supportive friendships, endless encouragement as guests weather day-to-day stresses, and sometimes demonstrations of mature helpfulness when a fellow guest is physically ill and in need of care. The "Buddy System" is a spontaneous outgrowth of living within the halfway house milieu.

In the light of today's orientation to recovery from mental illness, no mental hospital is complete unless it includes a transitional facility. The facility which is most frequently established is the day hospital. Some evaluation of the comparative resources of the day hospital and the halfway house is relevant. A halfway house that is closely associated with a psychiatric hospital can offer a patient everything that a day hospital gives—and more. A greater range of patients can be accommodated at the halfway house, from those who still need intensive treatment to those who are ready to test their adaptiveness in the community. The halfway house-hospital complex offers opportunities for socializing activities, continuing psychotherapy and even somatic therapies including electrotherapy and medication which few day centers have yet been able to match.

The opportunity to leave the day hospital and return home each night is a persuasive advantage, but only for *some* patients. What of the patient with no home to go to? And what of the patient who is not yet ready to experience the stresses of his home environment? What of the family which is not ready to receive the recovering patient? Since the family situation is often a key factor in the illness, great care must be taken in preparing both patient and family for more normal transactions with each other. This can best be accomplished through family participation in halfway house activities, trial visits home, and family psychotherapy—all done at minimal risk to the patient because he has not been uprooted from the familiar and supportive halfway house environment.

On the basis of almost 4 years of continuous operation, we can advance tentative answers to the inescapable question: how much good do we do? We rarely measure progress in absolute terms. Complete recovery is a very bold goal—and too often a hollow one. We look for improvement rather than cure. We try to help each person develop a reasonable adjustment to his *individual life situation*. When we have to, we settle gratefully for partial adjustment—and, if necessary, for temporary ones. Some of our guests remain at the halfway house for only a few months; others will probably be life members. We are not prepared to say that our rapid-turnover group are our "success" stories, nor that we have failed without long-term guests.

In each individual instance, many factors have a bearing on how much help we are able to provide. The psychopathology may be of such a nature that very little improvement can be effected. Lack of motivation on the part of the patient might rigidly limit what can be accomplished. We are sometimes handicapped by the fact that the patient can afford far less psychotherapy than is indicated. In other cases, a person may be able to remain with us for only a brief period—too brief for constructive work to be done.

We can readily categorize the types of individuals whose experiences at the halfway house we consider unsuccessful: those who do not or cannot make use of the opportunities which the house offers; those who unremittingly subvert the milieu; those who are inordinate in their demands—in short, those who are destructive in their behavior.

About our successes, it is not so easy to generalize. There are favorable signs which we all recognize: the motivation to get better and the sustaining hope that one will indeed improve; the willingness to share in house activities; the ability to assume some responsibility for oneself; the readiness to offer help to others; the relinquishing of sick behavior; the courage to venture out into the community.

But there are others who do not manage to achieve this level—or, if so, not for long—yet who benefit from living in a halfway house. These include the guests who regress and have to be returned to the hospital; it includes, also, the ones who have gone as far as the halfway house and may never get beyond. Even these, in a limited way, come closer to recovery in a halfway house than in a hospital.

Current thinking with respect to hospitalized psychiatric patients stresses the advantages of having these patients treated in relatively small hospitals within the community, rather than in large hospitals in remote and isolated locations. If this is true for the hospitalized patient, it is even more urgently so for the recovering patient. The halfway house makes it possible for him to accomplish his transition exactly where he belongs—not in an atmosphere of retreat but in a setting in which he and the community confront each other and get ready to come to terms with each other.

465

Foster Home Preparation Cottage — A Transitional Program for the Chronic Mental Patient

by Aaron S. Mason, M.D. and Eleanor K. Tarpy, M.S.S.S.

THE FOSTER HOME PREPARATION COTTAGE, an approximate equivalent of a foster home in the community, was conceived to afford
a transitional program that could be structured to cope with the problem
of the large number of chronically ill patients, especially in the older
age group, who are sufficiently improved to live in a family setting but
who either have no relatives or have relatives who will not accept
them into their homes. Typically, the patient has been displaced from
the family position he occupied before admission to the hospital and his
proposed release creates a situation so threatening to relatives that they
even refuse to permit his placement in a foster home.

This group is further characterized by deep institutional dependency
resulting from many years of hospitalization and is resistant to any
change in its symbiotic existence. Within the traditional hospital structure, they find food, shelter, security and protection in return for the
passivity and compliance which constitute a crippling process that fosters
further social isolation.

The usual immediate extramural goal for this group of patients is
placement in the foster home rather than in the home of a relative. This
accounts for the creation of the foster home preparation cottage located
on the hospital grounds.* The hypothesis was that the group-living
arrangement in such a milieu would aid in the restoration of lost social
habits and in the re-establishment of more normal behavior patterns to
an extent not possible on hospital wards and would serve as a "rehearsal"
for interaction in a foster home in the community. Furthermore, it was

*The foster home preparation cottage, as described in this chapter, was
developed at the VAH, Brockton, Mass. Since then several VA hospitals have
instituted somewhat similar foster home preparation programs.

hoped that the peer-like collective living arrangement would disrupt the patients' past frames of reference, facilitate a higher level of resocialization, and thus gradually help to bridge the gap between the hospital and a community home setting.

Mode of Operation: A one-story building, formerly used as quarters for aides, was remodeled to serve as a prototype of a community home. This resulted in a dwelling with ten bedrooms, a living and dining room area, a kitchen, a hobby room, and a bathroom with a combination tub and shower. The entire cottage was furnished to reflect a warm homelike atmosphere.

A middle-aged female aide was assigned the role of foster mother, and an expatient assumed the role of the man of the household. The social-work service was delegated responsibility for the administration of the cottage, with a social worker acting as the house supervisor. The supervisor's efforts were focused on motivating the patients toward the community and guiding and supporting the foster mother with the general techniques used in a community foster-home situation.

After staff approval, new patients are escorted by the supervisor to the foster home preparation cottage. Here they are greeted by the parental surrogates, introduced to the other members, and shown their rooms where they may keep all their possessions. They are told about their responsibilities in caring for their rooms and in participating in the preparation of meals and housekeeping. Although a wide variety of formal hospital occupational therapy activities are available to them, the members set up their own activity programs centered around the house and in accordance with their interests. A re-education and retraining program provides them with the experience of foster-home living. Thus they are taught simple household repairs, the basic elements of cooking including the use of the stove and other kitchen and household appliances, and personal hygiene as practiced in a home situation.

The patient's re-introduction to the community is gradual and designed to keep separation anxiety to a minimum. Initially he accompanies the social worker during a routine call at a foster home where a former patient has been placed. During these trips, stops are made at supermarkets and shopping centers and the patient's world begins to expand. Soon, with encouragement, patients in groups of two or three will visit stores within walking distance from the hospital and shop in a more leisurely fashion.

Patients are informed about the purpose of the foster home preparation cottage and told that the length of residence will not be longer than one year. Through casework interviews, weekly group discussion periods

467

and informal daily contacts, the social worker begins to counteract the resistance toward leaving the hospital and starts motivating the patients toward community living. An effective casework technique consists of encouraging the patient to talk about the things he likes in the hospital and its advantages. Later the social worker is in the position of being able to offer identical advantages in a community situation and to reinforce these points when the patient accompanies the worker on visits to foster homes. Gradually the patient recognizes that the gap between the foster home preparation cottage and a foster home in the community is not as great as he feared, and there is a decrease in separation anxiety.

In the cottage, new identifications and group norms are formed. The foster mother, dressed in the garb of a housewife, helps the patients gradually to reacquire the social skills and techniques they will need to live in a community home. Her presence at the table during most of the meals results in a striking improvement in table manners. Through the support and encouragement she gives to the patients, she aids the social worker in developing a community orientation among the house members.

RESULTS

During the first 5 years of operation of the cottage, 60 male patients with a mean previous hospital stay of 13 years (median of 10 years) resided in the cottage for an average of 7.5 months, after which 42 (70 per cent) left the cottage to live in a community foster home. Moreover, in eight of these cases, after the patient had demonstrated a period of successful adjustment in a community foster home, relatives provided a place for him in their own families. Nine patients went to live in soldiers' homes, and six returned directly to the homes of their relatives, 4 to their wives and 2 to the homes of siblings. Three chose living arrangements such as the Y.M.C.A. or a boarding house. At the end of the 5 year period, 75 per cent of the group were still adjusting at a satisfactory level in the community. Nine patients had been rehospitalized, but seven of these again returned to the community after several months; six patients had died from intercurrent illnesses. Only five patients who had a period of residence in the cottage were returned to a hospital ward unit. During the past 2 years, an additional 40 patients have had the benefit of this program with equal success.

SIGNIFICANCE

The need for a gradual transition, rather than an abrupt relocation, for the chronic mental hospital patient has long been recognized. The foster home preparation cottage, although located on mental hospital grounds, seems to fulfill this purpose more adequately than the usual hospital ward. Factors inherent in the ward structure render it a difficult place for re-acquiring the social skills and techniques necessary for living in a home in the community. On the other hand, the cottage program more realistically provides the patient with a reintroduction to a normal extramural setting. Moreover, the continued expansion of the immediate life-space to fit the wider horizons of the community puts the accent on cognitive reality structuring to an extent not possible in a ward setting. Although clusters of patients may form social or work groups within the larger amorphous ward population, the cottage offers a group-living situation which extends to all facets of daily living. After several weeks in this reality-oriented arrangement, patients have no desire to return to the hospital ward—an indication of the disruption of their past frame of reference.

An additional advantage in the cottage program is the change in attitudes and perceptions it engenders in the patients' relatives. The families of these patients tend to believe that the staff's area of competence is confined exclusively to care and treatment within the hospital setting, whereas they are better judges of the patient's capacity to adjust to community living. When viewed by relatives and guardians, the normative social ways of life in the cottage make more of an impression on them than do the staff opinions about the restoration of the patient's social competence. The patient has an opportunity to demonstrate to his relative that he is a responsible person and can adjust in a group setting. As a result, permission may be given for the patient's placement in a foster home, whereas previously the staff faced an adamant refusal.

From the sociologic viewpoint, the basic processes of role-validation and role-commitment of the patient as a sick person are difficult to reverse on a traditional hospital ward. In the cottage, however, the altered role expectations permit an easier transition to the modes of behavior expected in the healthy community. It should be noted that the cottage program was reserved for the chronic patient deemed to have the greatest need for this transitional residence since the majority of foster home placements are effected directly from the hospital wards.

In summary, the foster home preparation cottage constitutes an effective transitional program for a large group of chronic mental patients who present great difficulties in extramural placement.

Employment of Former Mental Patients

by W. RAY POINDEXTER, M.D.

A REVIEW OF THE LITERATURE reveals that most rehabilitation efforts are directed toward helping mental patients become employable by providing opportunities to develop good work habits and regain tolerance for sustained work. The emphasis appears to be upon how the rehabilitator-therapist should go about helping the patient achieve, regain, restore, or acquire some desirable quality or ability to work that is judged to have been lost. Vocationally restorative therapies are being applied earlier in the patient's hospital stay. Sheltered Workshops and Half-Way Houses, both in and outside of the hospital, serve as transitional places for patients to work and live, and employer attitudes are becoming less rejecting of the former mental patient. Patients leaving mental hospitals today have a much better chance of being considered for employment than a few years ago.

With the vast majority of rehabilitation programs being job-oriented and financially backed by greatly increased vocational rehabilitation funds for direct aid, research and training, it can be assumed that helping the mentally ill become employed is a rewarding pursuit for those in the helping profession as well as for the clients being helped.

However, with reference to our failure to help so many people achieve sustained employment and independent living, an interesting proposition would be—"The clients who fail are being 'successful at being unsuccessful'." My own recent venture[1] in recruiting ex-mental patients as the entire work force of a private industry revealed that former mental patients who could work and wanted to work could be selected from a large group of applicants consisting of many who worked to "fail." If the success of those employed was due to the employer's job offer, a new term of "Here's a job to do" therapy would be appropriate. The employment experience concerned 110 former mental patients who applied for factory jobs in response to a newspaper want ad:

> "Help Wanted: Ten factory workers wanted for private employment. Must have a history of mental illness to qualify."

Two entrepreneuring owners of a new toy factory had agreed to employ former mental patients as their entire work force if approved by a psychiatric evaluation. This offer was relayed to various social agencies which responded enthusiastically in behalf of their many clients who "only need a job to overcome their problems." After 30 days, however, not a single client had been referred. In order to save the jobs, an advertisement was inserted in the newspapers, the editor of which was somewhat reluctant and suspicious. One hundred ten former mental patients immediately responded, and 300 eventually applied. A few brought their mothers, and a few clients appeared accompanied by their agency contacts who questioned the author sharply and critically. One said, "Why are you finding jobs for these people? That's our job." Another asked, "You know they are mental patients, don't you?"

Eleven candidates were selected for employment by the factory owners from among the 24 referred by the psychiatrist. Two of these were later found to be unsuitable because they worked too slowly. The other nine, working on the day shift, were able to equal or exceed the productivity of a group of college students on the night shift. In retrospect, the most sensitive instrument of selection was the conciseness and pertinence with which the applicants filled out their application blanks. After the first year, the employers commented of these people, "You couldn't ask for a better work force; no accidents, absenteeism was below the average rate; you could always depend on them; they were always figuring new and better ways of doing things." Only one "incident" occurred. A woman thought she heard references from the factory radio and turned it off. The foreman told her that the other workers wanted to hear the music and that if she turned it off she would be fired. She continued working with no further difficulties.

Improved manufacturing methods requiring fewer employees during the first year coincided with some of the employees being able to return to their previous occupations. As of this year, four or five of the original employees remain and eight or nine former mental patients are working two shifts to keep up with the sales demands. New toys have been introduced and the company continues to expand and prosper. Their policy of hiring the mentally recovered continues but the work force now includes other employes obtained through usual channels.

From the beginning, the primary goal was to find capable people to work for wages. We selected so-called unemployable people and depended upon them to do the job. Nine of the 11 successful applicants hired used the work opportunity to regain or maintain their health. There were no implications of research or rehabilitation—only a serious attitude of

471

"There's work to be done" was maintained. Nor were there psychiatrists or other therapists around to provide assistance.

The former patient-applicants entered into an adult contract with the employer that they would provide the help he needed for the money he was able to pay; bizarre talk or behavior would terminate the contract. It became obvious that the type, severity, and duration of the mental illness was not related to job preformance. Symptom disappearance accompanied the opportunity to perform for an employer who had confidence in his employees and whose success in business depended upon their work.

The success of the nine ex-mental patients who progressed from job applicants to successful employees revealed that there are uncomplicated practical evaluation techniques which can separate people who need only an opportunity to succeed from those who need an opportunity for failure, as well as identify those who really need the usual rehabilitation therapies. Patients were rejected mainly because their past history and attitudes during the interview suggested a specific ability to be successful in surrounding themselves with protecting benefactors. Many were so busy receiving current assistance and making arrangements to secure additional help from agencies they had no time for other work.

An interesting example of "we've got a job to do" therapy occurs in a Memorandum Report[2] on employer attitudes about former mental patient employees.

A machine shop 20 miles from Boston: "How did you come to hire your first former mental patient?", I asked the shirt-sleeved owner.

"The psychologist of a mental hospital called on me," he replied, "and noted that the machine shop's turnover was a high 36 per cent. 'When you hire off the street,' the psychologist pointed out, you don't know whom you're getting. But if you were to hire carefully screened, thoroughly qualified former mental patients, you'd know their strengths and weaknesses; you could choose those not likely to job-hop.' "

The psychologist made his points well. The owner hired one former patient; another, several more. He had such success that finally he decided to hire a man the hospital warned never would be able to work.

"This man," he recalled, "could do a fine job when he wanted to. But he'd hallucinate at his work bench. He'd tap his head against the bench and groan. I had all I was going to put up with, so one day I went up to him. 'Listen,' I said firmly, trying to sound like a strict father, 'If you want to hallucinate, that's your business. But hallucinate on your own time, not company time.' This man snapped out of it, he was so surprised. We never had any more trouble with him."

Another example of a sick patient's response to an adult statement of "Here's a job to be done" appears in Hinckley's[3] account of a patient built community center at Chestnut Lodge. Hinckley, a supervisor of recreational therapy, tells about Sam, the patient—the most persistent worker.

472

"During his first months in the hospital Sam was fed sometimes by spoon, sometimes by tube. He usually held his right arm rigid, did not talk, and rarely managed the toilet. Unless he was dressed and moved out of his room, he stayed in bed apart from the others."

"When the Kiosk construction was about to begin, I took the blueprints to his room. I identified myself in relation to the work project which had not yet begun. Having spread the plans all around him on his bed, I spoke of the broad details of the project and asked him to indicate by shaking his head one way or the other whether he would be interested in going out to look over the location. He nodded assent. On the site of the proposed construction, I talked about digging a hole for the foundation, moving the dirt for the proposed terrace, constructing wooden forms for the concrete floor, and building a 150-foot-long stone wall. Again I put some questions, asking for head-nods as answers. He assented with considerable interest that way. As we returned to the ward, the first words that he uttered in a long time were: "When do we begin?"

"At 9:30 tomorrow morning," I said, "I'll see you then."

The next morning he was ready and waiting.

Sam was the most persistent worker. He moved tons of dirt and rock and painted the building . . . . . He progressively talked and socialized and worked from 9:30 to 4:30, 5 days a week for 1 year. . . . . When the building was finished and opened, he returned to catatonia and tubefeeding. Sam didn't say what the work and its termination had meant to him.

This ability to give up an illness when there is a job to do is too infrequently observed because therapists are too busy doing all the work themselves— and the patients obligingly let them.

Until more opportunities to do a job are given to patients, the reasons for responses like Sam's will remain obscure and theoretical. A likely hypothesis might be that Sam will be as good a worker as he is a patient. When his therapist changed roles from a therapist to a builder of buildings, the patient obligingly shifted roles to become as good a worker as he had been a patient. When the builder returned to being a therapist, Sam, the worker, returned to being a patient.

Significant gains will be made in the rehabilitation of the mentally ill when more "Here's a job to do" therapy is afforded the patients and we begin to get answers from many like Sam who are trying to tell us something we are unable to understand.

"Here's a job to do" therapy is a rarely used rehabilitative approach. When applied, some patients' responses are instantaneously restorative and the therapist has free time for other patients. Among the remaining patients some obviously can't make it without further treatment assistance and a most interesting few, or perhaps many patients, who can't be bothered with such a misjudging person, leave to look for a more "understanding" (i.e., indulgent) parent.

A social psychiatric view[4] of the universe to be observed (the popula-

473

tion of the United States) reveals more and more people entering the helping professions each year to meet the needs of an increasing number of clients or patients who are variously called dependent, disadvantaged, handicapped and unemployed. Physical injury, mental illness, automation, job displacement and mendicancy are some of the reasons usually offered to explain the need for recipient aid, which is being proffered in the form of help called rehabilitation, re-training, disability payments, and unemployment compensation.

There seems to be a decreasingly proportionate number of people who take care of themselves by doing a fair day's work for a fair day's pay. This results in a large group of "successful" people taking care of or treating a large group of "unsuccessful" people with decreasing success, especially when it comes to rehabilitation of the mentally ill and chronically unemployed, many of whom are skillfully engaged in a very active aggressive game of being "successful in being unsuccessful." Eric Berne has called these people "Wooden Leg Players."* With so many professional therapists and benefactors around to provide help, sustenance and succor, the clients who need an opportunity to fail devote their lives to being helped. It's a way of life with an ulterior motive. The object is to win by being a loser.

Many rehabilitation workers are unknowingly good game partners for these clients who are succesful in being unsuccessful. The ulterior motive is a spurious contract that results in unconscious psychological gains to both parties. The contract is "I'll help you if you'll help me." When this contract is stripped of rationalization, sublimations, projections, all the other defense mechanisms and repression, the small print reads, "I'll agree to help you if you won't get well," and "I'll let you help me if you will agree not to make me well."

The transactional concept of "Games" as presented by Berne appears to be more useful in understanding the process going on between client and therapist than a repetition-compulsion theory which considers only the patient's propensities as inadequacies. The failure of rehabilitation therapists and other helping agency personnel to recognize these game-playing clients appears to be one reason for the increasing number of people in the helping and being-helped professions.[5]

Some employers have achieved remarkable results in curing patients. Not realizing that the employee needed treatment, they were able to tell

---

*Wooden Leg—an insincere plea for help is the essence of the game. When help is offered, the client's next move of "What do you expect of a neurotic" or "of a man with a bad back?" avoids work, and other efforts usually necessary for independent living.

the employee to "knock it off, we've got a job to do." The Adult ego of the employee responds and gets to work. Conversely the Child ego of the employee-patient would have complied had the employer's Parent ego offered help, thereby continuing the clientism game.

REFERENCES

1. POINDEXTER, W. R.: Screening ex-patients for employability. Mental Hosp. 14:444-447, 1963.
2. POSNER, B.: Memorandum to the Chairman: The President's Committee on Employment of the Handicapped. June 1, 1962.
3. HINCKLEY, W.: The Chestnut Lodge Kiosk. Int. J. Group Psychotherap., pp. 327-336, 1957.
4. BERNE, E.: Transactional Analysis in Psychotherapy. New York, Grove Press, 1961.
5. POINDEXTER, W. R.: Payroll Checks and Mental Illness. Transactional Analysis Bulletin, July, 1962.

Modern Approaches to Community Mental Health*

by HAROLD M. VISOTSKY, M.D.

Would you tell me, please, which way I ought to go from here?
That depends a good deal on where you want to get to.

—Lewis Carroll

IT HAS ALWAYS SEEMED to me that the conditions of intense loneliness and alienation are most characteristic of the mentally ill patient. His symptoms, and frequently his inability to cope with the world around him, set him aside and he enters a world where strange thoughts, forms, and voices disturb and haunt him. The significant people in his life — his family, his friends, and others in society — are often repulsed and confused by his symptoms and move away from him and from the stigma attached to his mental illness. Society as a whole frequently regards him with fear and with distrust, and acts to exclude him. As a rule, the mentally ill person finds himself relegated to a large state mental hospital. This usually is the most lonely and isolated of all possible worlds, peopled by others as isolated as he, and where overworked staff can spare him only a few minutes each day. The staff often are as alienated and as lonely as the patients they serve. Many patients arrive at the state hospital because they have been unable to find any alternative to hospitalization. "Many patients feel that death is the only escape for them, and some even wish for it. Ironically, the death rate for these patients is twice that for the normal population."[1] These conditions

*Presented as the Strecker Award Lecture at the Institute of the Pennsylvania Hospital, Philadelphia.

Efforts of those of my associates who played a significant role in the preparation of this article are gratefully acknowledged. They include Norris Hansell, M.D., Mrs. Anne Konar, Leo Levy, Ph.D., Hyman Pomp. Ph.D., Bernard Rubin, M.D., and Arthur Woloshin, M.D.

represented the state of service in the Illinois mental health program as it entered the 1960s.

HEALTH CARE PLANNING

Planning of services is a mechanism for bringing people together to solve problems. In Illinois a bond referendum brought together large groups of citizens organizations. Over a hundred citizens groups and organizations were represented. For the most part, these involved citizens were appalled by the many inadequacies of our mental health system. They were against neglect of people and buildings; they were against the poor systems of treatment; and they were against the ills of an overcrowded custodial warehouse for human beings. But being "against" something merely reinforces commitment and involvement — it does not provide the mechanisms for change. It is only through the efforts of professionals and skilled technicians, working together with enlightened citizens groups to move through planning, implementation, and further change, that programs are modified or created.

On the national scene we are faced with similar problems. The public is becoming more and more aware of the potential for good health. Our news media are a form of education available to all citizens, to inform them and lead them to question the health situation. With this increase in information and understanding have come increased demands by the consumer of health services. These demands are often formulated without any real understanding of the current health situation in our country, either in terms of our resources or in terms of the organization. The demands on the system create a deficiency, not in the desire to offer more and better services, but in terms of the manpower, facilities, and newer programs. We are faced with a situation in which the requirements for health services and programs are clearly in excess of the resources of the system. If the system cannot be changed, then some form of rationing and price discrimination must be practiced. This solution is unacceptable in this country, and other alternatives must be sought.

One approach to a situation in which needs and demands exceed available resources is to initiate a planning program that has the capacity to analyze the situation, explore alternative solutions to problems, and suggest priorities for the use of scarce resources. Planning is analogous to preventive medicine; it is a matter of anticipating problems and of positive action before the fact. Cries for more services, more positions, more staff, more paramedical workers are all cries for some degree of systemization in the health field. All too many people in the health field, particularly physicians, see planning as the simple prelude to centralized governmental control and decision making in everything from work hours to treatment approaches. However, our present system, which contributes little optimum care but con-

477

tributes much to spiraling costs (and thereby to public dissatisfaction and unrest), requires careful reconsideration.

Planning for community services is an action process. It requires community-wide participation that is comprehensive, coordinative, and continuous. Robert Sigmund,[2] vice president for planning at the Albert Einstein Medical Centers, lists five essential steps in the preparation of a community plan:

1. Definition and measurement of needs and requirements for comprehensive health care.

2. Inventory of existing resources.

3. Comparison of the needs and resources to identify gaps and unnecessary duplication.

4. Decisions as to which agencies should coordinate services, which agencies should expand to fill the gaps, and which agencies should contract to eliminate duplication.

5. Establishment of priority schedules for allocation of scarce resources for those operating agencies and programs which will make the greatest impact in overcoming deficiencies and achieving the goal of comprehensive health.[3]

Although these principles of planning now seem well established, the optimum patterns and methods of delivery of services according to these principles are subject to rapid change as new developments in psychiatry or in federal legislation and other pertinent areas occur.

PLANNING AND PREVENTION

All that is known about prevention in mental health today indicates that the agency which undertakes preventive measures must be community-based. It must understand the organic structure of the community and be part of it. This is why the population limits (the subzonal planning area) have been set at 200,000 people or less. We feel that a single community mental health center will have great difficulty in dealing with the totality of a complex community structure if it is larger than this number or is spread out over too great a geographical distance.

It is important for the community mental health center to understand the ecology, the social characteristics of the persons, and the institutions that comprise the community; it is only then that the center can attempt community-wide measures to reduce the incidence of mental illness. Mental health services in the near future can reasonably be expected to function differently from the way they functioned in the past. The present model pattern of service in many instances is for a community mental health center to

478

offer conventional office treatment to patients who identify themselves as being in need of treatment. It should be the function of the community mental health center to appraise systematically the various indices of mental illnesses and social disorganization through its area. It should then come to some definitive appraisal and listing of the kinds of problems that exist within the area. Among these problems, priorities should be established as to the level on which the center wishes to attack.

The center, for example, should be concerned with the identification of high-risk groups. Certain groups in the community are known on the basis of research to have a demonstrable affinity for mental illness and mental retardation. We are able to identify these people by characteristics other than the fact that they are already sick; consequently, if we can get to them before they become too ill and do something about their condition, we may be able to prevent further breakdown. Even barring the possibility of doing something about their condition before they become ill, we can at least be alerted to the fact that there is a high incidence of emotional disorder in this group and be able to establish the most appropriate program for reaching out to its members. This may mean leaving the confines of the office and actually going out into the community to work through other agencies and visit homes and neighborhoods.

These centers will be expected to invest heavily in consultation programs with firing-line personnel such as public health nurses, clergymen, general practitioners of medicine, school guidance counselors, police officers, judges, welfare workers, and a vast variety of other persons who are traditionally identified as helping and supporting persons within the community. Planning in the Illinois Department of Mental Health required the very personal involvement of our staff leadership. Recruitment of community mental health program professionals was difficult in 1963, as it is now. Our skilled clinicians were not system planners; at best they were unit or hospital planners, and they lacked the experience needed for planning on a major areawide basis. The conceptual model in community psychiatric planning must be inclusive of all mental health service levels and its personnel must have the ability to promote integration between psychiatry and all other branches of medicine and the socioeducational programs.

Programs directed against poverty, programs of prenatal care, medical care for the aged, juvenile delinquency, drug abuse, and others aimed at decreasing social disorganization within communities are all of primary interest. These programs, for example, may be directed at parents of potentially abnormal persons when such programs as genetic counseling are concerned.

A department of mental health in a state is the basic governmental unit that bears a major responsibility for the mental health of the citizens of the state. This does not imply that the department sees itself as a purveyor of services and programs. Rather, its function in the future will be to coordinate, integrate, facilitate, initiate, and finance programs for mental health regardless of their sponsorship. This pattern has taken many models in many states. The decentralization of state programs has been effectively practiced and is moving at an exciting rate in Massachusetts. The provision of services at the local level, supported by subsidy of the state, has been most creatively effected in California through the Lanterman-Petris-Short-Doyle Act; other states are moving rapidly toward variations of these models.

In Illinois the zone concept was moving to a combination of both of these models. The Department of Mental Health there offered services directly through a state hospital system and through the zone center complex. The Department made a firm commitment that mental health care for the foreseeable future would be contractually financed and would be based on the comprehensive community mental health center model whose guidelines have, in general, been described at the National Institute of Mental Health.

The System

There has been much debate and discussion on the medical versus the social model, but comprehensive community care must provide services that include both approaches. Medicine is a dynamic model incorporating knowledge from the entire field of science. The dispenser — the prime therapist — may be any one of a number of legitimate treatment professions. Psychiatry, separated or divorced from either the rest of medicine or from psychology and social sciences, becomes a specialty without an input to the system we wish to serve. The referral and treatment network thus becomes the crucial key to the effective delivery of care. A system can be designed as a large remote agency that hopefully flows downward to communities, or it can be planned as a coordinating center to which the components of community care agencies are directed upward into a flexible organization, one that did not have overlapping functions and which allowed for problems peculiar to each community. In Illinois, we chose to attempt the latter, having already partially failed with the former. We were aware that in either method the commitment and involvement of all participants, at all levels, was crucial. It was for these reasons that the referral network was so carefully considered as the keystone to the entire system.

Referral for Services

In the past, "referral" was usually limited in state systems to being "committed" or "admitted" to an institution. What is required is a mechanism

480

for a bilateral contracting for services by the patient, the department of mental health, and community resources.

In metropolitan areas, referral is highly varied, complicated, and often unreliable. This was, and still is, due in part to measures designed to reduce the evils of "case losing," unselective institutionalization, massive intrastate transferring of inpatients, and formation of back custodial wards. It was the simple result of an inadequate service delivery system's being called on to increase its performance beyond its capacity.

In planning for referral to the Department's services, there needed to be firm guarantees to the patient that

1. There be a single, permanent, easily located point of access to departmental services within the community.

2. This one point of access would be related clearly to one, relatively small, well-defined geographical territory.

3. The access involved at any one point would provide a full array of services appropriate to such an initial contact and alternative to summary institutionalization, and access to any or all departmental services would be exclusively through such a point of referral to insure proper routing for optimum services.

4. This point of referral would be responsible for, and vested with, full authority to deliver departmental services to the residents of its territory and be held accountable by the Department for the most effective delivery of those services.

5. The administration of this referral unit would be responsible for seeking out and actively encouraging the development of local public or private mental health resources.

6. The administration would make available the resources of the Department, federal funding, and resources of consultation and educational support to these community resources.

7. The administrative and service components of the system in a given territory would be an administrative unit or component of the zone system.

Zones and Zone Centers*

In planning the zone system, I became aware that a monolithic administration could not plan effectively for the variety of community components making up a large state. Although the title "administrator" for a psychiatrist seems always to require an explanatory or rationalizing note, I

_____
*Much of the work accomplished in the zone system was initiated by Dr. Francis J. Gerty, the first director of the Illinois Department of Mental Health.

grew to accept certain principles. One must delegate authority and responsibility, and make sure that accountability is part of the contract. Upon this premise we based the planning and administration of the zones in Illinois.

The zone concept developed as an important innovation in pursuing the goal of promoting better mental health. In operational terms this included the decentralization of the Department's administrative structure and the establishment of offices having regional responsibility in newly constructed mental health centers within the newly formed zones. The state was divided into eight geographic zones; by an Executive Order, (1962) public health, the youth commission, vocational rehabilitation, children and family services, and public aid accepted the same geographic boundaries for the delivery of their service programs.

The major strength of the zone concept is that it represents an important shift in style of administration. What had, in fact, transpired in the Illinois Department of Mental Health was that we followed the lead of many large organizations and successful businesses in promoting decentralization of service delivery systems. Thus the director of the Department of Mental Health vested in seven men a portion of the authority of his office and created seven district directors of mental health called "zone directors." These men were to take full responsibility for organizing and integrating mental health services throughout the area that had been designated as a zone. Currently, there are six zones downstate and one zone serving the Chicago metropolitan area. The concept of decentralization has allowed us to develop a highly flexible mental health system. It has allowed the zone director, in cooperation with the agency complex and the citizenry of his area, to work out a program of services uniquely fitted to that area.

Distributed over the state are seven new zone centers. Not all zones have a zone center, and two of the zones have two zone centers each. No zone center can be properly identified as the mental health center for a specific community simply because no zone, as drawn, can be considered to comprise a community in any reasonable sense of the word. Each zone is a conglomeration of communities with highly diversified needs, and this impairs the ability of the zone center to function optimally in terms of pursuing clinical and preventive programs in the mental health populations served, which range from 600,000 to 3½ million. The zone center, properly speaking, is an administrative hub for the organization of mental health activities in a region. It is a central point that integrates all services related to mental health, whether they are run directly by the Department of Mental Health or by private agencies which are brought into a cooperative arrangement with the Department.

The zone center also serves as a center for research and for the training of mental health professionals. It likewise serves as an ideal facility for the demonstration of new and experimental programs, which small or local community mental health centers cannot undertake. It serves as a kind of mental health intelligence unit for the area, supplying information, consultation, advice on program development, and coordinated planning for mental health activities throughout the zone. It can exercise certain evaluative and monitoring functions in terms of setting and maintaining standards for mental health services supplied throughout its area. Finally, it can serve as a backup resource for the community mental health center to handle the overflow and the special case.

Subzonal Planning

The Illinois Department of Mental Health is intent on developing true community-based mental health services. Each zone has been divided into subzonal planning areas. In the downstate area, these consist of aggregates of counties, in the townships (Chicago suburban area), and aggregates of community or neighborhood areas (Chicago metropolitan area), which contain populations of 75,000 to 200,000 persons. There are 75 subzonal planning areas.

In drawing up these subzonal planning areas, much consideration was given to the boundary lines of the areas. In the case of downstate zones, every effort was made to group the counties that exhibited a history of previous cooperative effort in the health and welfare fields. Counties were combined into a subzone if they had some natural relationship to one another and were not separated by natural barriers. Attempts were made to group together those counties that had normal trading relationships and other developed forms of social intercourse. A similar effort was made on a township basis in suburban Chicago, and within Chicago itself, to aggregate community or neighborhood areas that would work together cooperatively toward the development of a comprehensive community mental health program. In each of the subzonal areas throughout the state, we endeavored to find what we considered to be a reasonable hub city, one that was located on the main transportation routes and which could logically serve a subzonal area.

It is important to underscore the intention of the Department that the programs for the development of local community mental health services are intended to be locally controlled and, in part, locally financed. The community is expected to organize itself in consultation with the Department of Mental Health, and each hub city of each planning area must develop a comprehensive community mental health center complex. This is our first

483

line of defense against mental illness and the promotion of positive mental health. These community mental health centers in the vast majority of subzonal areas cannot develop *de novo*; they must be built on existing programs of mental health and mental retardation services currently offered by mental health clinics, day centers, psychiatric wards of general hospitals, and other community agencies.

Each subzonal planning area should have its own community mental health program, not necessarily housed in one free-standing building. The program may be an aggregate of services tied together contractually throughout the subzonal area. The community mental health center in each subzone should offer a full range of comprehensive mental health services, consisting minimally of inpatient care, outpatient care, partial hospitalization, emergency services, and consultation and education programs for the community. It is anticipated that by 1908, any patient is found to need mental health care will be able to receive this from his local comprehensive community mental health center, expeditiously and at a fee that he can afford. The zone center should stand ready to absorb patients from any subzonal area if, for one reason or another they cannot find adequate care within their subzone.

Metrozone

The Metrozone Plan being developed in the Chicago metropolitan area is an approach to a community organization model for the delivery of mental health services in a large population center. Historically, in Chicago, mental health services have been developed by voluntary sectarian and citizens organizations, and more recently by local governments. Usually, these services, although valid and much needed, were not comprehensive in scope or in their structural relationship to related community health and welfare programs. As a result, in Chicago, as in most other cities, there are large service gaps in the community, and community facilities have little relationship to state services and especially to state hospitals.

The Metrozone Plan is one that endeavors to integrate all public and voluntary mental health programs into one coherent, balanced system. It will endeavor to offer maximal service, including prevention, at the community level with state hospital inpatient service as a backup to the community services. The plan should strengthen the voluntary community services through joint funding and planning. The Metrozone Plan in the complex Chicago scene should be interpreted as a long-term plan, but it is certainly an appropriate model toward maximal utilization of its resources in the short run as well.

Outposts

A strategic feature of clinical importance is the provision of what is called an "outpost." Such a place is conceptually and concretely the key to the entire zone system and represents the point of access to the community. This is a unit within a neighborhood, which provides the referral, the access, and the follow-up to community treatment services. The salient activities in the outpost may be summarized as follows:

1. Screening, for appropriate provision or referral of services.

2. Linking, or strengthening old links with supportive, nurturant objects.

3. Planning, a total program of services with complete continuity aiming toward restoration.[3]

An outpost or service territory is a regional service entity relating to the planning areas (subzones) and the zone center. A strategic feature of its clinical importance is the outpost's provision for conferring. The fact of ready and nearby availability of an outpost allows for the more immediate attention to the mental health problem by all parties involved. It is only such an organized and locally placed unit that can convene all persons necessary to successful treatment or management of a problem. It will help any client to obtain all possible assistance from any source before resorting to hospitalization. The outpost, then, is functionally the best vehicle for the most valuable and effective use of a short-lived therapeutic community.

Experience has shown that the moment a person arrives at the source of mental health services is often the best time for corrective efforts. "It can be a time for confrontation and crisis, with all the openness and flexibility associated with this rare moment."[4] The crisis and its confrontation, as is well known, includes not only the "patient candidate," but many times an entire family also, and may even include broader elements of disturbance. The crisis may reside visibly in one person, but the problem may have social, historical, and community components. It is in the strategic management of the crisis that the key to timely and effective treatment of the problem exists.

This time of crisis is to be expeditiously and vigorously exploited if at all possible. If this opportunity for repairing the person's relationships to his family, friends, agencies, job and other life contacts is lost, it is an important and often crucial loss. There must be an attempt to involve the family and significant individuals in the patient's life during the screening process and during the entire period of mental illness. This attempt extends to the potential post-treatment load; that is, a greater effort must be made to initiate psychiatric services during the screening and planning phase as well as in the phase when the patient is returned to test his competence in his home setting. It has been the conviction of staffs in the Department of Mental Health that only an outpost type of system can ever bear effectively on the mammoth mental health problems, particularly in metropolitan areas.

An outpost, then, is a service territory that represents the first echelon of intervention relating to the planning area, or subzone, and finally to the zone center area. Its success depends upon its acceptance and implementation by all involved sectors of the mental health field and upon community understanding and support.

Target Population

It was important in planning the zone system to design a closed system in which staff who admitted patients, staff who treated patients, and staff who followed the aftercare of patients cooperated to serve a target population. Defining the target population entailed unusually careful attention to all relevant factors due to the historical, social, governmental, and economic significance of a public position on a target population. Of great importance is the large financial cost of effective services by a vast state system. It is, for example, far more costly to hospitalize than to treat a person on an outpatient basis, yet the target population must be assumed to have a high risk of institutionalization. Applying these criteria would, of course, be far less easy than defining them.[3]

Clearly, the task of a system already equipped with institutions having a large residential capacity must for the present include those persons at or near the point of hospitalization. More important, since metropolitan inpatient resources are inadequate to meet the demand, a strategic emphasis on preventing hospitalization must be effective. This requires definitive clinical judgment in the selection and outpatient treatment of seriously disordered persons whose problems require immediate attention or, if neglected, hospitalization. This early intervention as a strategy has obvious humanistic merit as well.

The clinical concept of borderline need for hospitalization encompasses four major parameters for appraisal:

1. Level of symptoms, the imminence of need.
2. Social reaction and community resources available.
3. Behavior patterns, levels of control.
4. Financial resources, personal and public.[3]

Symptoms define an index of risk of hospitalization in proportion to their severity, chronicity, number and diversity, rate of acceleration, and specifically the presence of delusions and hallucinations.

Environmental adequacy and familial resources are judged to be risk indices to institutionalization in proportion to the presence of the following findings: impulsive behavior, suicidal or homicidal compulsion, a tendency toward violence, a tendency to make poor contacts. All these findings are more severe risk markers when behavior is frequent, chronic, or accelerating in occurrence.

Financial status is a risk marker in proportion to the presence of precarious or deteriorating finances. Under this category is also rated the level and stability of employability if the person is the family breadwinner; he must have enough reserve funds to purchase food, shelter, minimal social stimulation, and minimal health and welfare services. If his finances cannot support these, they are judged to be precarious.

MODELS OF A DELIVERY SYSTEM

Daniels[5] defined community psychiatry as a developing body of knowledge and practice that relates psychiatry and social science principles to large population groups. Actually, this theory defines social psychiatry as derived from ecology, epidemiology, public health, preventive medicine, social systems theory, and community organization.[7] It has its bases in the psychological insights of the individual, small group dynamics, and understanding of family structure and organization. It has as its broad goals the establishment of programs for early diagnosis and treatment, rehabilitation, and (so far as currently possible) prevention.

Since the adoption of the Community Mental Health Centers Act, we have seen the elaboration of community mental health centers serving catchment areas of 70,000 to 200,000 persons. A good deal of criticism is directed to these free-standing institutions, and some of the disillusionment is reflected by the fact that they may not have the appropriate linkage and network connections to serve populations of the projected size, particularly when these areas represent the most difficult problems of our ghettos. Frequently, these community mental health centers are merely extensions of the state hospital into a community site. While this is an improvement over the remote state hospital, it does not provide the flexible and creative changes necessary for provision of services in a community setting.

It is important to recognize that psychiatric services cannot survive apart from the delivery of health and welfare services. They have their roots and acceptance in the school system, the health system, the legal system, and in the human services of every community. Where such services are not available, the mental health center standing alone becomes the recipient of requests for all such services. It is therefore imperative to plan such links prior to the initiation of a mental health service unit. The zone system, diagrammed in Figure 1, is one such plan.

The first echelon of care is the neighborhood outpost, which is a screen-

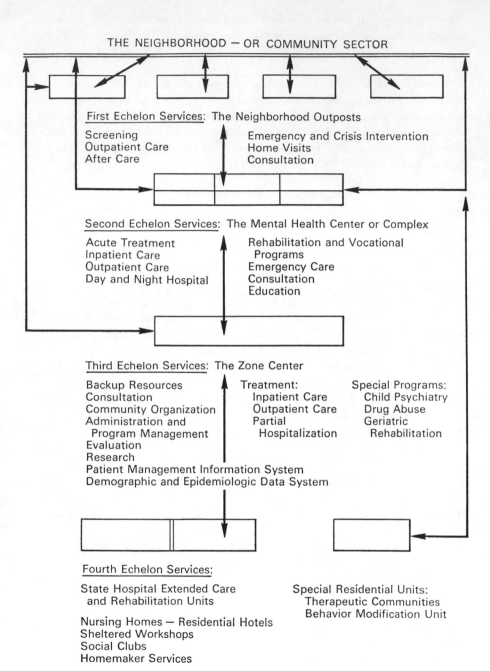

First Echelon Services: The Neighborhood Outposts

Screening	Emergency and Crisis Intervention
Outpatient Care	Home Visits
After Care	Consultation

Second Echelon Services: The Mental Health Center or Complex

Acute Treatment	Rehabilitation and Vocational
Inpatient Care	Programs
Outpatient Care	Emergency Care
Day and Night Hospital	Consultation
	Education

Third Echelon Services: The Zone Center

Backup Resources	Treatment:	Special Programs:
Consultation	Inpatient Care	Child Psychiatry
Community Organization	Outpatient Care	Drug Abuse
Administration and	Partial	Geriatric
Program Management	Hospitalization	Rehabilitation
Evaluation		
Research		

Patient Management Information System
Demographic and Epidemiologic Data System

Fourth Echelon Services:

State Hospital Extended Care
 and Rehabilitation Units

Nursing Homes — Residential Hotels
Sheltered Workshops
Social Clubs
Homemaker Services

Special Residential Units:
 Therapeutic Communities
 Behavior Modification Unit

FIG. 1. Organization of community mental health services.

ing, linking, and planning unit working with other agencies in a neighborhood. At the community and neighborhood level, with catchments serving anywhere from 25,000 to 40,000 people, we need further elaboration of the neighborhood health centers, which are early diagnostic, case-finding, treatment, and referral centers. Provision of mental health services at this level is an important link in the provision of comprehensive health care. It is at this level that certain mental health professionals (for example, social workers, psychologists, psychiatric nurses, and indigenous mental health workers), working in close collaboration with other community agents such as general health-screening teams in the neighborhood health center, can be most effective. They operate in close collaboration with other community professionals such as teachers, ministers, policemen, and general physicians. They have more extensive psychiatric treatment and consultation resources on call from the second echelon of care. The referral for more specialized treatment to the second echelon of care is part of their service program. They also provide consultation to neighborhood resources and programs of crisis intervention, as well as to those programs of primary prevention that are available.

The second echelon of care consists of a community mental health center program that can provide intensive treatment, using the modalities of individual, group, family, psychotherapy, guidance, and counseling techniques. Appropriate referral and collaborative treatment to social and family agencies, to vocational services, and to other medical health center or at the psychiatric service in a general hospital. This represents the subzonal planning area with catchments of approximately 200,000. Usually, three to six outposts are served by the second echelon of care center.

The third echelon of care is the zone center, which provides the backup resources for the community-based outpost and the related network of services, and for inpatient services to those patients who need intensive care that cannot be provided at the general hospital level or at the mental health center. The zone center provides consultant services to agencies and is the administrative hub of the echelon network. It provides special programs that cannot be provided at the neighborhood site because of their specialized nature, which requires a high degree of technical skills, or because of the scarcity or limited manpower. The zone center also provides special organizational elements such as community organization, planning, evaluation, and administration of services for this large catchment area. A zone center catchment extends to cover areas of approximately 600,000 to $3\frac{1}{2}$ million people, as in metropolitan Chicago, and backs up approximately six to eight mental health centers. It has a bed component ranging from 160 to 220 beds.

The fourth echelon of care comprises those extended care facilities of a long-term nature or those categorical programs that require a lengthy period of residence. It provides the protective, as well as the rehabilitative, treatment programs for patients who need long-term care. Included are special programs for children, such as residential centers that are linked with an appropriate educational program; services for the geriatric and the senile, and programs for the retarded who need special education over an extended period of time or who need custodial care because of the severity of their condition. State hospitals, too, can provide second echelon services for the communities in which they are embedded, and a portion of the physical plant can provide fourth echelon care supplemented by nursing homes and other facilities.

The fifth and last echelon of care is the necessary safety valve to prevent backlogs of patients in mental health centers, zone centers, and other short-term care facilities such as the psychiatric units in general hospitals. Extended care is not and must not be synonymous with custodial, back, ward care. It must represent dynamic rehabilitation care and social and psychological modification programs.

The mental health center, because of its central location, provides many advantages over the state hospital system. However, our investment in state hospital systems, if only in terms of the physical plants, requires a reorganization rather than abandonment. It is our goal to operate state facilities having no more than 1,000 beds or no less than 500 beds, and to operate these at a high standard of excellence. Our experiences have indicated a need for more ambulatory services and less bed-oriented facilities. In a closed circuit operation of echelon care, the neighborhood outpost is linked to a mental health center that has a capacity of approximately 30 to 50 beds, and has a backup resource in the zone center. Further extended-care facilities and special services are available in state hospital programs. This arrangement can provide the full component of services for approximately 250,000 to 300,000 people when intimately related to health and social services.[8]

The system of delivery must be so designed that all elements of intake, admission, screening, treatment — either in inpatient facilities or alternative care and aftercare — are linked as one continuous closed-circuit network. In the catchment areas there must be a no-decline option for providing services; that is, patients applying for services must be treated within that closed-circuit network. The system must operate on the proviso that individuals responsible for admissions share with their team the responsibility for treatment as well as aftercare. There must be an effective patient-management system of record keeping, data analysis, and registry information for effective communication among elements of this service network.

Mental Hospitals and the Community Programs

Our state mental hospitals are in a state of great flux. They are moving in the direction of better inpatient care at a rapid rate and relating themselves to the comprehensive community mental health centers that are evolving in the subzonal planning areas. There has been a sharp decline over the past 10 years (approximately 50 per cent) in the resident population of our state mental hospitals. It is expected that this decline will continue into the future, though perhaps at a slower rate.

Custodial care is necessary for only a small number of patients with mental illness and mental retardation, and with each passing year new techniques of rehabilitation are being devised, which make it more and more feasible for so-called chronic patients successfully to reintegrate with the community. The community mental health centers will have a large role in terms of aftercare. The reduction in population in our state hospitals will allow the hospitals to close down their more dilapidated and overcrowded quarters. They should be allowed to reapportion existing personnel, whose numbers are thoroughly inadequate to cope with case loads they have been called upon in the past to treat. The patients who remain will be special cases who have been refractory to every known technique known to psychiatry, but even then they will not be considered to be in terminal care. Active research programs are under way to find new ways of effecting rehabilitation. The decrease in numbers of patients will allow state hospital staffs to redeploy their efforts into other phases of mental health work. The zone center, interposed between the community and the state hospital, also will be able to circumvent a large number of inappropriate hospital admissions when different forms of treatment outside of the hospital are instituted.

Halfway Houses, Sheltered Workshops, and Foster-Care Homes

Much of our success in discharging long-term patients from our hospitals will depend on developing adequate community resources to receive and maintain them. Resettling a patient in the community from which he has been absent for many years requires special resources to aid him in the transition from hospital to community life. Availability of private homes and hotels where patients are not isolated and where interpersonal support is given is mandatory.

Similarly, the success of the rehabilitation process is heavily dependent upon reacquisition of vocational and social skills. One of the best methods to

491

accomplish this is through the sheltered workshop, where the former patient can be retrained in useful work that will enhance his self-esteem as well as his autonomy by virtue of the income derived.

In a recent mission to Russia to evaluate the mental health system there, a team of American investigators found sheltered workshops associated with mental health centers (called NP dispensaries) and with mental hospitals. These workshops provided both transitional programs to placement in specially programmed units in general industry as well as long-term sheltered workshop industries.[7]

The comprehensive community mental health center will ultimately require multiple financing through at least three levels of government: local funds, usually obtained from country tax money; state funds in the form of grants-in-aid; and federal funds, presently available only for construction and initial staffing, but in the future hopefully available for continuing operating expenses.

In the State of Illinois, forward-looking health-care legislation was passed several years ago, referred to as HB 708. This bill provided for any duly constituted political jurisdiction to levy a tax with the approval of the voters by referendum up to 1 mill per $100 of assessed property valuation. According to figures on property values throughout the state for 1966, if voters in each of the 102 counties of the state approved the levy of the 1-mill tax, close to $40 million would be allotted for mental health and retardation purposes. With matching state and federal funds, this amount could be more than doubled.

The yearly operating expenses of comprehensive community mental health services for a subzonal planning area (the mental health center area) would average $1 million. With 75 subzonal planning areas currently projected, this would mean that approximately $75 million annually would be needed to subsidize the operating expenses of such centers.

The grant-in-aid program of the Illinois Department of Health has in the past been facility-oriented. It started by funding mental health clinics, later offering matching funds to daycare centers for the retarded, and more recently allocated funds for daycare centers for the emotionally disturbed. It is considered inevitable that the Department will move aggressively in the direction of de-emphasizing grants to facilities and emphasizing block grants to planning areas to be administered by suitably appointed local boards for the provision of comprehensive mental health and mental retardation services. Block grants to planning areas for the development of com-

492

prehensive services should be made directly from general revenue on an equitable matching basis.

At the present time, 26 counties and one municipality have legislated 708 bond issues. Very few of these funding propositions have been defeated at the polls. The following is a quote from a recent speech by Mike Gorman:

I am still amazed at the local grassroots support for the centers. A recent Wall Street Journal article noted that the taxpayers in recent elections turned down more than 55% of local bond issues and in some states turned down some 75% or more bond issues to keep schools going. By the way of contrast, special bond issues to support and construct mental health centers have more than a 90% approval rate. In last November's election, for example, voters in all counties in which it appeared on the ballot in Illinois, voted for a special mill tax to underwrite community mental health costs.[8]

Of all counties in Illinois, 25 per cent are currently supporting mental health programs through passage of such bond issues. The matching formula for public-oriented programs could be one-third local effort, one-third state, and one-third continuing federal support.

Vendor Payments

Broader third-party payments by general insurance companies, Blue Cross and Blue Shield, should be encouraged. Such payments can be made either directly to hospitals, service-providing institutions, and physicians or as an indemnity to the patient himself, or both, including payment for inpatient care in a hospital and physicians' costs. Blue Cross and Blue Shield in some states (Michigan, for example) pay for treatment in extended-care facilities and for home care.

Medicare pays limited amounts for inpatient service in a psychiatric hospital, but has no special limitations if such care is provided in a general hospital. Psychiatric treatment in a general hospital is considered in the same category as any other "spell of illness." Medicaid pays a limited amount for psychiatric care on both an inpatient and an outpatient basis in a psychiatric setting, but classifies it in the general category when provided in a general hospital setting.

It would serve the public interest if vendor payments to service providers were extended beyond that of the hospital and physician. Other professions now registered or licensed under state laws should be recognized as legitimate payees for professional services rendered. Among them should be included such professionals as psychologists, social workers, and nurses. Similarly, day care and associated services should be considered eligible for payment. With national health insurance in the forseeable future, we must begin to plan the effective consortium of public and private programs.

493

According to Ivan Bennett, deputy director of the Office of Science and Technology, "The federal government is going to have to use the leverage it now has to bring about a modification of the system of health care."[9] He sees the probable shape of the future foreshadowed by community health centers of the type set up by the Office of Economic Opportunity to cope with health problems in poverty areas. These are affiliated with local hospitals and often with local medical schools. Sometimes they are sponsored by local medical societies. They should provide objective, comprehensive family care in the neighborhood. Such centers will be under local pressure to extend their services to people who do not qualify in terms of poverty. These individuals will in the future be covered by some form of universal or national health insurance.

It is primarily through effective financing of health that the private and public programs can be brought together. Effective use of community resources, financed appropriately, will allow us to move patients more effectively and economically through a spectrum of services. Both at public and private levels, patients stay too long in high-cost facilities because community-based alternatives are not available. The third-party payers are recognizing these problems and giving close attention to cost-benefit studies.

About two and one-half years ago, I initiated a program in Illinois that reimbursed private general hospitals with psychiatric units at their daily per diem rate for treatment of psychiatric emergencies within a specified geographic area if patients were confirmed as medically indigent. Under this plan, patients were hospitalized up to 21 days or, alternatively, given outpatient daily hospital care for the same term. The requirements placed upon the hospitals were that they were to exhaust all financial recovery from insurance carriers or public aid, or from the family, if it had partial ability to pay. In this way, the Illinois Department of Mental Health served as a co-insurer covering all costs that the hospital could not recover from other third-party payers.

Of the first 500 patients covered by this program, less than 5 per cent had to be sent to a state hospital or a zone center. The average stay was about 17 days, and the average cost per day was $52. When we contrast this with the patient's being removed from his community and sent to a remote state hospital, we can see significant cost benefits. The average stay for a matched group of patients was 90 days, at an average per diem rate of $10 to $12 in a state hospital, as compared with 17 days at $52 at two private hospitals. Therefore the cost of 17 days in the psychiatric unit of a general hospital, community-based, averaged about $880 to $900, as compared with approximately $900 to $1000 for a state hospital program remote from the patient's community and which was perhaps more poorly staffed and poorly programmed in providing psychiatric care.

Programmatic periods of rapid progress and growth require massive changes in attitudes, not only of individuals outside the system (for example, community understanding and acceptance) but also of rather institutionalized resistance to change.[10] If the process of combating these attitudes is successful to any degree, it creates enormous demands and expectations for service. Facilities planned today are expected to open within unrealistically short periods and to provide instant, total, and comprehensive services. These expectations are not solely limited to the public. Once the resistance of inflexible staff members is weakened, these workers lead in the demands for visible services, and become depressed and frustrated by delay. It seems to be a part of the developmental cycle for periods of rapid change to be followed by plateaus of reorganization and consolidation. Usually this serves the system in a positive fashion. Progressive management systems have time to catch up to innovational programs, and community organizations can be refined and contracts reworked with the service communities.

The task of a psychiatrist-director administering a large mental health network requires a call on all skills learned in institutions and acquired in battle. It necessitates a total commitment to and investment in a program in which the human dimension is primary. These requirements are as important in the design of zone centers as they are in training programs to combat dehumanization in the processing and treatment of patients. It means total immersion and identification with all elements of the system, even when responsibilities can be delegated. It requires the skills of an arbitrator and negotiator, not merely in dealing with labor unions, legislators, and organized special interest citizens groups, but also in leading the staff. Methods and strategies for involvement of the community participants requires political as well as sociological considerations. As in bond-issue campaigns, a piece of the action brings real commitment from community members. Services planned or given to them cannot buy the commitment evolved when they feel that they have promoted and supported their own programs. Directors must conciliate and assuage feelings of anger, pain, and disillusionment expressed by staff and supporters when their recommendations or expectations cannot be realized.

In short, community effort requires involvement with the lonely, alienated, and distressed patient through a dedicated professional staff, an aroused and committed community of supporters, and a purposeful nation. To read "trend indicators" and plan accordingly, must have an adequate public program at least five elements.

1. A health-care network, based on decentralized but well-defined service

495

echelons, each with a full spectrum of specific services that can be selected as the appropriate treatment modality for disabilities and dysfunctions. There must be appropriate alternatives to inpatient services.

2. There must be a geographic orientation of catchment areas, with manageable clientele and appropriate manpower resources. Manpower must be maximally utilized, and career ladders for personnel must be developed. The geographic catchment provides accessibility to care, prevention, education, and consultation programs.

3. Essentials of treatment must be available.

4. A psychosocial classification system must be evolved that would be useful to professional persons and agencies ranging from psychiatric services to courts, psychological diagnostics, student counseling, welfare, and other resources representing many diverse professions and professional skills. Obviously, a restricted medical or nonmedical terminology is not applicable for such varied professional groups if these interdisciplinary workers are to communicate with each other or the public on the characteristics and problems of the patients and the services rendered. For broad program planning and evaluation, uniform data are needed across agency lines. Currently, the only terminology is the diagnostic manual of the American Psychiatric Association. It serves an important reference for mental disorders, and it specifies and defines particular disorders. However, many of these definitions leave much to be desired because of multiple diagnoses and because no dynamic description or functional classification for the individual is at present operationally or prognostically useful. For this purpose, a psychosocial classification system should be designed and applied to our developing system of health care.[11]

5. Finally, a data system of patient-management information, and demographic and epidemiologic data is necessary for cost-benefit studies, evaluation, planning, and program modification.

> . . . It must be remembered that there is nothing more difficult to plan, more doubtful of success, nor more dangerous to manage than the creation of a new system. For the initiator has the enmity of all who would profit by the preservation of the old institutions—and merely lukewarm defenders in those who would gain by the new ones.[12]
>
> Machiavelli, 1469-1527

REFERENCES

1. REIDY, J.: Zone Mental Health Centers: The Illinois Concept. Springfield, Ill., Charles C Thomas, 1964.
2. SIGMUND, R.: Community Health Planning, Blue Shield Annual Program Conference, 1968.

496

3. ILLINOIS DEPARTMENT OF MENTAL HEALTH: Chicago Area Plan for Mental Health Services. 1968.

4. HANSELL, N.: Mental Health Services and Community Values: A System. (In publication.)

5. DANIELS, R.: Community Psychiatry, A New Profession: A Developing Subspecialty of Effective Clinical Psychiatry? Joint Meeting of Ohio Medical Association and Ohio Psychiatric Association, May 1965.

6. VISOTSKY, H.: Illinois Legislative Conference on Mental Health, April 15, 1968.

7. Special Report: First U.S. Mission on Mental Health to the U.S.S.R. Public Health Service Publication 1893, 1969.

8. GORMAN, M.: Comprehensive Community Mental Health Centers: Myth or Reality. Speech to Sixth Legislative Dinner, Massachusetts Association for Mental Health, February 1969.

9. BENNETT, I.: Blue Shield Annual Program Conference, 1968.

10. BERLIN, I.: Resistance to Change in Mental Health Professionals. Amer. J. Orthopsychiat. 39:1091-15, 19.

11. BAHN, A.: Need of a Classification Scheme for the Psychosocial Disorders. Public Health Rep. Vol. 80, No. 1, January 1965.

12. MACHIAVELLI. Of New Monarchies Acquired by One's Own Arms and Ability, Chapter VI.

PART XIII

INSTITUTIONAL THERAPY

The Psychiatric Unit of the General Hospital: Its Organization and Design as a Therapeutic Instrument

by Zigmond M. Lebensohn, M.D.

T HE LATE PRESIDENT KENNEDY, in his memorable message to the Congress on mental illness and mental retardation, sensed the growing importance of general hospital psychiatry when he said in 1963: "We need a new type of health facility, one which will return mental health care to the mainstream of American medicine. . . ." These health facilities, he added, "could be located at an appropriate community general hospital, many of which already have psychiatric units."

According to the latest and most reliable survey,[1] there are now somewhat less than 500 such units throughout the country. Another 500 general hospitals treat psychiatric patients on their general medical wards. Thus, a grand total of approximately 1000 general hospitals accept psychiatric patients for treatment. This figure still represents less than 20 per cent of the 5400 general hospitals in the United States, and the need for the establishment of many more psychiatric units in general hospitals is everywhere apparent.

Medical and public acceptance of general hospital psychiatry is now at an all-time high. Psychiatrists with leadership qualities and an interest in general hospital psychiatry are in brisk demand to organize and direct the new units and the new departments of psychiatry which will be springing up in general hospitals all over the country. This section is being written in the hope of giving a few guidelines regarding the organization, design, and treatment program of a psychiatric unit for the psychiatrist who has the vision and courage to enter this exciting new field.

How to Begin

Beginnings will differ from city to city and from hospital to hospital,

501

but the civic-minded psychiatrist in any city who is alert to what is going on in his own community and in his medical society will be among the first to know when a new hospital is being proposed or when an old hospital is planning to add a new wing, move to a new location, or expand its facilities. Often, the start of a building fund campaign is sufficient warning to the individual psychiatrist (or to the local psychiatric society, if there is one) to inquire whether a psychiatric unit is to be included in the new construction; and if not, why not. Such inquiries, if accompanied by genuine offers of help are warmly welcomed by most hospital Boards. If the idea of a unit is rejected, the fight must go on elsewhere or at another time. If the idea is accepted, then the work begins in earnest.

Once a chairman has been appointed, he should immediately obtain the assistance of several of his most experienced colleagues to help him draw up plans, policies, and a table of organization. It is also important to obtain the prompt support and cooperation of the local medical and psychiatric societies. With their assistance, meetings can be held to recruit psychiatrists who are interested and willing to serve on the Active or Courtesy Staff of the new department. In smaller communities with only a few psychiatrists, the psychiatrically oriented general practitioners are often willing and eager to help out in such a venture.

If there is a medical school in the area, early efforts should be made to establish the closest possible liaison with its Department of Psychiatry so that the teaching potential of the unit will be fully utilized.

Pros and Cons of the Separate Unit

Perhaps the first major decision to be made is whether to construct a separate psychiatric unit in the general hospital or to establish a Department of Psychiatry with beds distributed throughout the medical wards. Although it is possible—by using considerable initiative, ingenuity, and alertness to do a good job of treating selected psychiatric patients on a general medical ward—there are definite limitations to such an approach. Proponents of this plan point out that such an approach truly brings psychiatry closer to medicine without any of the "separateness" which has plagued psychiatry in the past. On the other hand, the range of psychiatric disorders which can be accepted becomes definitely narrowed. Consequently, its potential for rendering desperately needed services to the community becomes seriously limited, and its usefulness as a training and research area curtailed. Finally, it must be granted that the presence of an attractive and efficient psychiatric unit gives the

502

Department of Psychiatry a "locus" which enhances its status and prestige vis-a-vis the other departments in the hospital.

Designing the Unit

It goes without saying that the psychiatric unit should be designed by those who are going to use it. This includes not only the Chief Psychiatrist and his committee, but also the psychiatric nurse, who spends a great deal more time on the unit than anyone else except the patients. It is also well to discuss certain details of design with patients who are exceptionally perceptive in this regard.

Those responsible for the design should begin at the earliest possible moment to work closely with the architect and the hospital administrator. They should scour the country for ideas, visit as many hospitals as practicable here and abroad, and confer frequently to keep new ideas alive. They should try to design a setting in which all forms of accepted psychiatric treatment can be effectively practiced.

Architectural Considerations[2]

Architecturally, the psychiatric unit of a general hospital should bear the same relationship to the rest of the hospital that psychiatry itself bears to medicine; namely, it should be like the rest of the hospital in many important ways, yet different from it in certain equally important respects.

First, the similarities: The unit should occupy a wing or a floor of the main hospital building and from the outside should be indistinguishable from the medical and surgical floors. The nurses' station and examining room, although modified in design, should sufficiently resemble nursing stations in other services so that visiting surgeons, internists, and other specialists will feel "at home." Oxygen and suction should be provided in a certain number of rooms for those patients who experience serious physical complications in the course of a mental disorder, and vice versa. A patient-to-nurse call system, identical to those in other wards in the hospital, should be included with the added provision that individual units could be disconnected or removed when indicated. Obviously, the psychiatric unit should be included in the hospital call system.

Next, the differences: The first aspect which impresses the visitor as being different is the "atmosphere." The design and decor of the psychiatric unit should impart a cheerful, friendly, and home-like atmosphere which invites relaxation and diminishes anxiety. There should be no

503

frightening or unfamiliar features, such as steel bars on doors and windows, and there is certainly no need for the "antiseptic" atmosphere of the operating room. The unit should be specifically oriented to the fact (frequently overlooked) that the psychiatric patient is up and about all day long and rarely uses his bed except at night.

In 1957 Humphrey Osmond published a most provocative paper, "Function as a Basis of Psychiatric Ward Design."[3] In this he recommended that the designer keep in mind the three levels of social relationship which are required on a good psychiatric ward. These three levels are (1) personal (solitary), (2) with a limited number of people, and (3) with a larger number of people. Needs on these three levels are satisfied by providing (1) a "retreat" in the form of a small private bedroom, (2) a small parlor or alcove for small groups, and (3) a dayroom or lounge for larger group activities. Although Osmond may have had the larger mental hospital in mind, most of his ideas are highly relevant to the design of the psychiatric unit in the general hospital. Within the limitations of a predetermined overall design, we have incorporated three Osmond units in our plans at Sibley and these have proved to be eminently successful.

THE IMPORTANCE OF GOOD INTERIOR DESIGN

The pleasant and relaxing "atmosphere" to which we have referred can be achieved by the skillful use of color and texture in the walls, draperies, furniture, and floor coverings. Extreme "decorator effects" should be avoided. Most designers, however, quickly comprehend the needs of psychiatric patients once they have been explained.

Colors should be light and cheerful—pastel tones wherever possible. Traditional institutional colors should be shunned. A variety of colors is pleasing and costs little extra.

Draperies should be of a fireproof material such as Fiberglas, which comes in attractive designs and is simple to clean. Furniture should be sturdy but not institutional. Wood is preferable to steel. Despite the expense of occasional recovering, upholstered furniture in most areas should be covered in a fabric rather than plastic. Wall to wall carpeting is pleasing in appearance and very effective acoustically.

Walls should be decorated with good paintings—originals if possible, although good prints will do. No glass should be used in framing. Local artists can often be persuaded to donate paintings for a permanent or semipermanent loan collection for the hospital's use. Good art helps create a hopeful atmosphere and the expectations of respectful behavior.

504

In line with this point, I have yet to see a psychiatric patient harm or destroy a work of art in our hospital.

Size of the Unit

Perhaps no single factor is more important than unit size in determining the quality of nursing care. The number of beds on the psychiatric unit should be determined not only by the total size of the hospital of which it is an integral part, but also by local needs and availability of staff. In general, the size should be from 10 to 15 per cent of the hospital's total bed capacity. Maximum size should not be more than 25 or 30 beds. It is far better to provide two or more units of 20 to 25 beds than a single unit of 40 to 50 beds. Furthermore, two small units permit for the logical separation of patients on the basis of behavior.

Location of the Unit

There is much difference of opinion about the best location of the psychiatric unit within the general hospital. Some authorities prefer the top floor because they feel this location prevents psychiatric patients from disturbing the rest of the hospital—a rare occurrence in these days of tranquilizers. It also provides a better view for the patients and personnel. In addition, roof decks for recreation can often be provided. Other authorities prefer the ground floor to eliminate the hazard of "jumpers" and to provide easy access to the grounds. Still others prefer to sandwich the unit between other floors, apparently in an attempt to blend completely with the rest of the hospital. Local building regulations regarding the locking of fire exits, etc., must be kept in mind when selecting the final location.

Facilities for Segregating Patients

No matter how large or small the unit, there must be some effective means of segregating disturbed patients from those who are not so ill and from those who are convalescing. In a 25-bed unit, about 14 beds should be assigned to fairly cooperative patients and 11 beds to active, confused, or disturbed patients. Of these 11, two or three should be seclusion rooms with special security features for very disturbed or uncooperative patients. In a larger hospital, with two or three psychiatric units, a finer degree of segregation can be developed. This is very much to be desired.

The Problem of Security

For a variety of historical, cultural, and legal reasons psychiatric hospitals in America have been far more security conscious than their European counterparts. When security screens were introduced to replace the old-fashioned iron bars and grilles, they were hailed with enthusiasm. Thousands were installed, many of them in offices, nurses' stations, and other areas not usually accessible to patients.

I am convinced that we have overdone this business of security. Not only are security features financially expensive to install, but they are also expensive in terms of their effect on the atmosphere of the unit. They evoke a note of "differentness" the moment one enters such a unit and, when seen from the outside, they make the psychiatric unit easily identifiable to the passerby. Even in the seclusion rooms the screens should be softened by the use of easily removable draperies. In all other areas, security features, although present, should be as unobtrusive as possible. Instead of detention screens, windows of safety glass or tempered glass can be safely used, particularly if the metal window frames are of sturdy construction and if the glass panels are not too large. The total effect is one of lightness and hope and is far more therapeutic than the ubiquitous detention screen.

THE NURSES' STATION

In general it is best to have the nurses' station centrally located as it is on most medical and surgical floors. This location reduces the amount of walking; an added advantage is that plumbing, wiring, communications, etc., can be vertically stacked with those of nurses' stations on other floors. In a linear design, the nurses' station should straddle the barrier between the open and closed sections in such a way that the nurse can observe activity on both sides. In the V, Y, or snowflake design the nurses' station is best located at the bifurcation.

DINING ROOM AND SNACK BAR

The dining room may be an extension or ell of the day room and may double as an occupational therapy area. Table tops should be of durable plastic. Group dining is strongly encouraged.

A small snack bar adjacent to the dining room serves a most useful purpose in socialization. It should contain counter space, storage cabinets, a stainless steel sink, a small hot plate, and a refrigerator for milk, soft drinks, and fruit juices. Although this area remains under the control of the nurse, patients are permitted a certain amount of freedom in its use.

506

Occupational Therapy

This is playing an increasingly important role in psychiatric treatment programs in general hospitals; it may be as modest or elaborate as the staff desires. In a general hospital, occupational therapy can be practiced in one of three places: (1) at the bedside, (2) on the psychiatric unit, or (3) in a special department separate from the unit. Some such departments are quite large and are equipped with lathes, kilns, potters' wheels, and woodworking equipment. Others may use a section of the day-dining room and store equipment in a closet specially designed for this purpose.

Offices for Psychiatrists

The office is to the psychiatrist what the operating room is to the surgeon. Most psychiatric units woefully lack sufficient office space. For a 25-bed unit there should be four or five offices; two or three on the open section and two on the closed. They should be large enough to contain a small desk, two chairs, perhaps a small sofa for two, and a bookcase. Each office should be carpeted, soundproofed, and equipped with a telephone.

As the psychiatric unit of the general hospital becomes ever more important as a training ground for psychiatric residents, the need for offices for these residents will increase.

Treatment Room

The treatment room should be located on the closed section and, like most other spaces, should be designed to serve several purposes. It should be about the size of a two-bed room. A stainless steel sink, storage cabinets, a locking drug cabinet, oxygen and suction, telephone, and a large wall clock with a sweep second hand should be provided. A special mobile treatment table suitable for administering electroshock therapy and for examining patients should also be provided. A small desk and chairs are needed so that the room may also be used for examinations and interviews. The room should communicate directly with an adjacent recovery room so that a patient who has received a treatment may be wheeled there without being exposed to the gaze of other patients.

Hydrotherapy and Recovery Room

Hydrotherapy is now rarely used in American psychiatric hospitals, and yet there is some evidence that it is coming back slowly in some quarters. Our experience indicates that a multipurpose room containing one continuous tub is very useful. In addition to its sedative action in alcoholism and certain other overactive states, the tub can be used to bathe elderly and infirm patients and by those who dislike showers. If located next to the treatment room, it should be large enough to serve as a recovery room for patients receiving EST. An extra shower stall should be provided for those patients who do not have rooms with baths. Laundry tubs and drying space are also provided for patients who wish to do their personal laundry.

Clothes Lockers. The central "clothes room" typical of the state hospital has no place in general hospital psychiatry. Clothes lockers built into the walls and equipped with sliding hangers and luggage compartments should be provided in each patient's bedroom, with the exception of the seclusion rooms. The lockers should be somewhat larger than those on the medical wards because psychiatric patients bring more clothes with them than do patients confined to bed.

Telephones. For flexibility, *all* telephones should be on jacks. In the open or convalescent section telephones may remain in place, but even here, a patient confused following electroshock treatment should probably not be permitted to have a telephone until the confusion clears. With jacks, the instrument can easily be removed. In the closed section patients may make or receive telephone calls with the permission of the attending psychiatrist. At such times, an instrument may be brought in and plugged into the jack.

THE PSYCHIATRIC STAFF

Every effort should be made to staff the unit with psychiatrists of all "persuasions" so that the complete spectrum of psychiatric theory and practice can be made available. The staff should include qualified general psychiatrists, child psychiatrists, and analysts of all schools who can work together and learn from each other.

The organization of the Department of Psychiatry should follow, insofar as possible, the pattern established for other departments in the hospital. The members of the active staff should be handpicked for their professional excellence, their interest in general hospital psychiatry, their dependability, and their ability to work effectively in close collaboration with the medical staff. The active members of the department must agree to attend the monthly staff meetings with regularity. The psychiatrist on call must arrange to be immediately available during the period he is "on service." One member of the staff should be responsible for record review to ensure that all records on the psychiatric service are maintained at a high standard. Only by so doing can psychiatrists convince their medical colleagues that psychiatry is indeed a responsible and integral part of medicine.

Department Policies and Regulations

Certain general, but highly important, questions must be answered in the very beginning. Should the staff be open or closed? May patients be admitted and treated by nonpsychiatrists? Should Board certification be a prerequisite for active staff membership? What should the admission policy be? Restricted to certain diagnostic categories? Exclude certain others? Or admit all categories? Should there be a limitation to the length of stay? Should committed patients be accepted for treatment or should admission be restricted to those patients who agree to enter voluntarily and informally? Private cases only? Or a certain percentage of staff cases? The answers to most of these questions still depend largely on local hospital and community practice.

To draw up a good set of ward regulations requires the close collaboration of the chief psychiatric nurse. Such nurses are in short supply, but there is now a growing interest in psychiatric nursing in the general hospital. The psychiatric nurse plays a crucial role in setting the therapeutic tone of the unit, in training personnel, and in maintaining smooth administration.

Treatment Techniques

The psychiatric unit of a general hospital should be able to offer the whole gamut of modern psychiatric therapies, and should be geared to fast intervention in an emergency situation. Some hospitals, both here and abroad, have also established suicide units which have been of great value.

Most good hospitals lay proper stress on the establishment of a therapeutic milieu. When treatment policy for all patients is determined by the Chief of Staff, such a milieu can quickly be established, even though a dozen or so psychiatrists are treating some 25 private patients, each in his own way. Here, two factors play a prominent role: (1) the selection of a competent and congenial staff, and (2) the selection of a good psychiatric nurse.

Psychotherapy of all varieties—analytic and supportive, individual and group—is practiced daily when the psychiatrist sees his patient in his private room or in the office on the unit.

Drug therapy finds some of its most gratifying results on the psychiatric unit because the illnesses are usually acute and of short duration.

509

With a small staff working closely together it is easy to pool experience with various drugs at staff conferences. The psychiatric staff profits by learning new techniques, and the patients benefit by prompt and effective treatment.

Convulsive therapy remains one of the most rapid and effective techniques of treating the acutely depressed or acutely psychotic patient. With the use of intravenous anesthesia prior to treatment, anxiety and fear can be greatly reduced or eliminated. With the use of powerful muscle relaxants, fractures and dislocations can be avoided. Policies and staff recommendations covering the technique of electroshock therapy should be carefully written out and followed meticulously to avoid untoward complications. The psychiatrist must familiarize himself with the technique of administering oxygen before and during the treatment or arrange for a qualified anesthetist to be present. Treatments on an outpatient basis should be provided for selected patients. It is quite safe and prevents the unnecessary use of scarce bed space.

L'envoi

If the psychiatric unit maintains a broad and diverse staff and agrees to accept the entire range of psychiatric disorders, then it will come close to fulfilling its true function. It will then be able to treat schizophrenics, but not become a back ward; it will accept alcoholics, but not become a "drying out" place; it will employ electroshock therapy wherever indicated, but will not become a "shock mill"; it will use all forms of psychotropic drugs, but not become a "pill emporium"; and finally it will provide a suitable milieu for analytic psychotherapy, but not become known as a "couch haven."

In other words, the psychiatric unit must offer all acceptable modalities of treatment. In so doing, it will become one of the important nuclei from which the practice and teaching of modern psychiatry can be disseminated through the rest of American medicine.

REFERENCES

1. APA-NAMH Joint Information Service study of General Hospital Psychiatric Units (to be published March 1965).
2. This and subsequent sections dealing with architectural details are derived from my paper, Form and function in the psychiatric unit. Mental Hospitals 14(5):245-250, 1963.
3. Mental Hospitals 8 (4):23-30, 1957.

Therapy in Day and Night Psychiatric Hospitals

by ROBERT S. DANIELS, M.D.

D AY AND NIGHT PSYCHIATRIC HOSPITALS have been established in many communities in recent years. These part-time hospitals provide treatment similar in extent and intensity to the full-time hospital while the patient continues in extra-hospital functioning. This method of treatment often decreases the emotional and monetary cost of illness to the family and the community, and may reduce tendencies for the patient to become dependent on the hospital and its staff. The shame often associated with psychiatric hospitalization is diminished and self-esteem is enhanced by offering the patient an opportunity to continue in his ordinary activities through part of the day.

These part-time hospitals are intermediate between outpatient treatment and full-time hospitalization, providing some of the services of both. Ordinarily, psychiatric services are available through a variety of social and psychiatric institutions in a given community. Among these institutions may be large psychiatric hospitals, psychiatric units in general hospitals, day hospitals, night hospitals, halfway houses, mental health centers, psychiatric clinics, social agencies, and volunteer organizations. These facilities usually provide an initial evaluation service, and then make recommendations for the patient's entry into an appropriate part of the therapeutic system. In selecting an institution for treatment, the principle of minimal intervention is usually followed. A treatment program is chosen which will fulfill the patient's therapeutic needs while

511

interfering in the least way possible with the individual's ordinary functioning. As changes in therapeutic needs occur, patients may be transferred from one institution to another or from one therapy to another. Often, there is an overlap in treatment services offered. Referring sources have some choice about which institution is chosen.

The range of services and treatment provided in full- and part-time hospitals may be quite similar. The chief difference is that the full-time hospital is a more controlled and protected environment. Impulsive behavior may be dealt with more effectively; greater regression may be fostered when indicated; and the patient may be isolated from his family or other outsiders, when it is therapeutically necessary. In the part-time hospital, freedom and independence, contacts with family, and ordinary social functioning are encouraged.

Part-time hospitals vary widely in their organization, program, and patient population. Some part-time hospitals are part of a larger psychiatric or general hospital. Others have been established independently from any hospital affiliation. They may provide treatment for a full day or part of a day. Daily participation may be required, or the organization may be such that occasional supportive contacts are appropriate. The patient population may be diverse, or the part-time hospital may restrict itself to a particular age group (adolescents or old age for example), a particular diagnosis (chronic schizophrenia or alcoholism), or a particular situation (e.g., transition from full time in to full time out after a long-term hospitalization.) Treatment programs may be quite diverse. Potential types of treatment which have been included in part-time hospitals are individual psychotherapy, group psychotherapy, pharmacologic therapy, electroconvulsive therapy, activity and recreational therapy, occupational therapy and others. Many of these therapies are typical hospital treatment while some may occur in psychiatric clinics or social agencies as well. The diversity of programs, purposes and facilities make for many individual differences in part-time hospitals. However, certain treatment functions of day and night hospitals are more or less universal. It is the purpose of this communication to delineate these common treatment functions.

The treatment program on which these observations are based is the University of Chicago Service at The Illinois State Psychiatric Institute. The Service includes a full-time hospital, a day hospital and a night hospital. The full-time hospital (32 beds) occupies 2/3 of the facility. The day hospital (20 patients) and the night hospital (18 beds) occupy the remainder of the unit and share the same geographic area. This area consists of 18 single rooms, a day room, a kitchen, an adjacent

512

occupational and recreational therapy area, a nurses' station and three small offices.

The Day Hospital

The Day Hospital was established to provide a comprehensive treatment program for ambulatory psychotics, elderly patients, unemployables, and other patients not requiring full-time hospitalization. This last, somewhat vague, group has expanded as experience has increased, and currently patients in the day hospital are difficult to distinguish from typical full-time hospital patients. Homicidal or suicidal patients, patients without family or environmental supports, drug addicts, severe alcoholics, and moderate and severe organic brain syndromes have been avoided. Characteristic of the therapy program is its dynamic philosophy, its "total push" structure and its therapeutic community atmosphere. Included in the program are group psychotherapy, activity therapy, psychodrama, a patient leadership organization, and occupational, recreational and work therapies.

The Day Hospital is open 5 days a week (Monday through Friday) from 8:30 A.M. to 5 P.M. The staff meets to discuss plans and potential problems between 8:30 and 9 A.M. Patients may join this meeting, if they choose. Patients are expected to be present by 9:15, and morning coffee is used as a catalyst around which inter-action may begin. Three mornings a week each patient participates in small group psychotherapy. There are two of these groups, each being composed of about nine patients, three staff members, and a physician leader. When patients are not engaged in group psychotherapy, they are involved with on-ward recreational, occupational, and work therapies. Two mornings each week the entire patient and staff group come together for a community-wide meeting where administrative problems of mutual concern are discussed. Lunch is served family style and shared with the staff. The afternoon consists of special interest groups, psychodrama, a case conference attended by both patients and staff, and recreational activities either in the gymnasium or out of the hospital. Also, in the afternoon, patients may be interviewed for vocational training and employment counseling or they may have work assignments elsewhere in the hospital. From 4 to 4:30 the entire group meets to discuss and integrate the happenings of the day. The staff meets from 4:30 to 5:00 to deal with patient and administrative problems and to receive supervision and consultation. The staff consists of two female nurses, two male aides, an occupational-recreational therapist, a 4/5 time third year psychiatric resident, a half-time social worker, and a one-fourth time staff psychiatrist.

513

Day hospitals are of value in the following circumstances:

1. *As a definitive treatment center for many patients now treated in the full-time hospital.* Many patients do not need the protection or the limitations which occur in full-time hospitalization; indeed, total separation from their family and loss of functioning at work or elsewhere may be damaging. Full-time hospitalization interferes with capacities the patient is using effectively. The loss of the patient is difficult for his family and creates an unnecessary drain on community resources. A day hospital should be considered when there are productive aspects to the patient's environment, when the family is willing to participate actively in treatment, and when the patient is not homicidal, suicidal, or in need of external controls for acting out behavior.

2. *As a gradual transition when discharge from the full-time hospital is likely to result in increased symptoms and regression.* Some patients experience separation from the full-time hospital as a traumatic event and respond to it by an increase in symptoms and regression. In such instances a relatively brief stay in a unit which is intermediate between full time in the hospital and full time out of the hospital may be quite beneficial. Such reactions occur most frequently in individuals who are very dependent and who have been hospitalized for a long time.

3. *As a transition into the full-time hospital when patient and family cannot tolerate immediate total separation.* Occasionally during a diagnostic process, the evaluator believes that a severely ill patient should be in the full-time hospital, but recognizes that the patient and his family cannot accept this recommendation because they are involved in a symbiotic relationship. These patients and families are occasionally willing to accept treatment in a day hospital since they can reunite each evening and week end. Surprisingly, this treatment compromise is occasionally effective alone. In other instances the transitional period enables the patient and his family to accept full-time hospitalization.

4. *As a training center to re-establish work patterns and facilitate rehabilitation.* Chronic ambulatory psychotic patients often decompensate slowly over the course of years. The patient who previously worked regularly gradually withdraws as his daily routine becomes too anxiety provoking. Day hospital treatment fosters the establishment of a regular routine of activity. The patient leaves home each morning for a place where definite, but limited demands are made upon him. He is encouraged to participate with other people in a variety of activities. He is assigned responsibilities within the unit and often work elsewhere in the hospital. The creation of this job-like experience may stimulate the patterns of conflict, characteristic of his premorbid performance. A day hospital offers an opportunity for understanding and integrating these disrup-

514

tive patterns. In addition, programs of vocational rehabilitation may be started when appropriate.

5. *As a treatment center for patients who after a course of individual therapy need additional treatment emphasizing interpersonal relationships and social factors.* In the course of individual outpatient treatment, patient and therapist occasionally recognize the need for another kind of treatment experience which will provide new interpersonal relationships in a setting where these relationships are the focus of treatment. Particularly with severe neurotics, severe character disorders and borderline psychotics, the patient may reach an impasse in which he does not seem able to apply insight to acquire new and more meaningful object relationships or to increase his capacity to function generally. A day hospital provides an opportunity for multiple interpersonal relationships which can be observed, analyzed and made the focus of treatment. Group treatment may dilute a too intense transference relationship with an individual therapist or it may provide the patient with a ready made opportunity to put increased self-knowledge into operation. Individual therapy may be continued and, with effective communication between all the therapists involved, the forms of therapy may supplement and complement one another.

6. *As a treatment center where contact with family is maintained and made the focus of treatment.* With some patients, continuing intimate contact with the family is crucial to treatment. A day hospital is ideal for such patients because evenings and week ends are spent at home. The time at home provides an opportunity to continue functioning in the primary situation while undergoing treatment in a hospital environment. At the same time family members may be seen individually or in groups. Family therapy is also possible.

The Night Hospital

The Night Hospital was planned as a therapeutic experience for paday. The patient leaves for work or home each morning and returns with a living arrangement where they could continue functioning in the usual fashion during the day and on week ends. In addition, for patients who had been hospitalized full time, the Night Hospital provides continuing comprehensive treatment along with a transitional living arrangement. Thereby, patients may assume responsibility for their extra-hospital lives gradually. Included in the therapy program are group psychotherapy, social group work, activity therapy, and therapeutic use of the administrative and organizational structure.

The Night Hospital is open five nights a week, Monday through Friday. The patient leaves for work or home each morning and returns each evening to the hospital. Week ends may be spent either at home or in other suitable settings away from the hospital. Night staff and patients arrive between 4:30 and 6 P.M. The staff utilizes this time for planning, consultation, and other administrative purposes. The patients make use of the time in informal, unorganized activities, and in reintegrating themeslves into the hospital after the day away. At 6 P.M. a family style dinner is served. Following dinner two evenings a week there are one-hour periods of small group psychotherapy and social group work. The total group, consisting of a maximum of 18 patients and staff, is divided into two smaller groups for these sessions. Three nights a week there is an hour-long administrative meeting in which the entire patient and staff group participate. The purpose of this meeting is to discuss the function and operation of the unit, to analyze the difficulties which arise out of living together, and to deal with administrative matters which arise in relationship to patient care. For example, questions of passes, leaves, and discharges are discussed in this meeting and are granted or denied by the entire group after a thorough investigation and discussion. This unit is governed by the principles of the therapeutic community. Emphasized are patient responsibility, cooperation, and participation. Small group psychotherapy functions in a traditional manner. Social group work utilizes sociodrama, psychodrama, role playing, play reading, and activities. After the formal therapeutic experiences, patients and staff gather together informally for television, card playing, games, social parties, and other activities. Patients retire between 10:30 P.M. and midnight. Breakfast is served at 7:30 A.M. and the Night Hospital patient returns to work or to his home. The staff for this unit consists of two half-time third year psychiatric residents, two psychiatric nurses, two male aides and a three-quarter time social group worker. A staff psychiatrist devotes one-quarter time to the unit.

TREATMENT FUNCTIONS IN A NIGHT HOSPITAL

Night hospitals are helpful in the following ways:

1. *As a temporary intermediate residence between full-time hospitalization and total discharge.* Hospitalization is a gratifying experience for most seriously ill patients. The hospital and its staff provide lodging, food, activity, and secure interpersonal relationships while making limited demands on the patient. These gratifications are oftentimes difficult to relinquish at the time of discharge and many patients experience an exacerbation of symptoms when preparation for discharge begins. Occasionally, the separation reaction is so severe that it jeopardizes the results of the entire hospitalization. In such instances a night hospital offers the patient an opportunity to separate from the hospital and to re-establish family, social, and work patterns gradually.

516

2. *As a temporary residence for the patient who is trying to separate from his family of origin.* Gradually increasing separation from the family of origin is a treatment goal, when independence has been unduly delayed or the family's organization is intolerable and un-modifiable. Even though the decision about increased independ-ence is jointly reached by patient, family and therapist, patients and families often find it difficult to relinquish one another. A night hospital setting provides comprehensive psychiatric treatment combined with independent living and functioning during the re-mainder of the day.

3. *As a temporary residence for the patient who has no family or other environmental supports.* The patient who is physically distant from family or friends or who has alienated them so that they will not offer him help faces a realistically difficult situation at the time of his discharge from the hospital. When, in addition, he has no job, a number of reality issues are present which may prevent him from giving up the protection and security the hospital provides. A night hospital permits a gradual solution of these problems by permitting the individual to begin work while continuing to live in the hospital environment.

4. *As a treatment center where functioning at work or school may be maintained.* Some patients who require more than ordinary out-patient treatment are still able to function adequately at work or school. When psychologic symptoms do not interfere with this aspect of social functioning, encouraging continued performance increases self-esteem and discourages regression. In a night hos-pital the patient continues to function at work or school while simultaneously receiving psychiatric treatment similar to that pro-vided in the full-time hospital.

THE CHOICE OF GROUP TECHNIQUES OF THERAPY

The treatment goals for most part-time hospital patients involve re-constituting previously successful modes of coping with life as quickly as possible. Group therapy techniques are suited to these goals as they offer the opportunity to establish many intense relationships while diminishing the dependence on any individual staff member. Patients and staff share the unit's activities and these interactions may be ob-served, analyzed, and integrated in a setting closer to everyday life. Group therapy is usually reality oriented and regression is avoided. Silent patients who have difficulty relating in the intimacy of individual psychotherapy are often treated effectively in the somewhat more com-fortable psychologic distance of the group. Non-psychologically minded patients and those who express feeling states in somatic complaints may benefit from observing others examining psychologic issues in the group. For some, a group provides a protected, educational experience which supports at a time of great anxiety and prepares for more intensive therapy later.

For other patients, group psychotherapy may intensify conflict. The patient who cannot tolerate competition for the therapist's interest and attention frequently does poorly. When dependency needs are very intense a patient may not be able to participate in a sharing experience as in group forms of treatment. At such times the patient may need transfer to a unit with a different type of treatment program. Emphasis on group techniques need not exclude individual contacts when they are indicated. However, these contacts should be oriented to particular short-term goals. Attempts to prolong or to obtain repeated individual sessions should be carefully examined and often discouraged unless there are good indications for them.

Organizational and Operational Issues in Part-Time Hospitals

The establishment of a new kind of treatment facility may lead to administrative problems, particularly when that facility requires a striking departure from traditional modes of administrative and therapeutic operation. Effective leadership interprets the need for administrative flexibility and policy modifications to the already established full-time hospital and to the community. As the purposes, made of operation, and functions are clarified, one begins the educational process which will lead to adequate referral. The hospital and clinic staff need opportunities to ask questions, to express doubts, and to discuss the advantages and disadvantages of these units. As referrals begin, they have the opportunity to observe directly the effectiveness of the treatment process.

The extra-hospital community presents a somewhat different problem. Some professional and lay people become anxious when patients with severe mental illness leave the hospital for home or work daily. Such concerns must be exposed and resolved. Information about the part-time hospital's functioning and uses must be transmitted to physicians, psychiatrists, social agencies, hospitals, and other potential referral or disposition sources. Written communication is valuable; personal contacts may be necessary to insure adequate understanding. Many members of the non-hospital community greet the establishment of part-time hospital facilities with enthusiasm, but education and public relations continue to be an essential part of effective operation, even after the units are well established. Only through such educational and public relations activity will effective and frequent referrals be received.

Joint Admission of Mother and Child: a Context for Inpatient Therapy

by Henry U. Grunebaum, M.D., and Justin L. Weiss, Ph.D.

M ANY SIGNIFICANT CHANGES in the treatment philosophy of psychiatric hospitals serve the important pragmatic function of providing the patient with increased opportunities to engage in those relationships and activities which are of enduring meaning to him. Advances such as open wards, day-care plans, halfway houses, sheltered workshops, and hospital industries serve as stepping stones to the community. If there is concurrent psychotherapeutic work, the patient is ordinarily able to examine and modify his difficulties in dealing with people and in applying his abilities. These advances, then, afford the patient an opportunity for interpersonal responsibility—a context for therapy.

In this chapter we shall describe another context for therapy in which psychotic mothers under psychiatric treatment in an adult hospital ward are given the responsibility for the care of their infants and young children.

If one thinks of the many arenas in which the struggle for mastery and satisfaction in life is fought and won—or lost—*family* and *work* are the most imposing and crucial. An individual's adaptation in these two aspects of life is focal in the psychiatrist's diagnostic evaluation and therapeutic intervention. In the case of the young mother, her family *is* her work; yet it is standard psychiatric practice that mothers requiring hospitalization for mental illness be separated from their infants and young children. Recent reports from England, however, raise serious questions concerning the advisability of this separation. Douglas[1] reported in 1956 that mothers with post-partum psychotic reactions were less likely to relapse if they were given an opportunity to care for their babies in the hospital. The work of Main[4] suggests that it is similarly beneficial for mothers with neurotic depressions to have their children

519

with them in the hospital. More recently, there have been several such admissions to McLean Hospital, Waverly, Massachusetts.

Encouraged by these reports, in the fall of 1960 we began a program of "joint admission." Infants and young children were admitted to the adult wards of the Massachusetts Mental Health Center, where they have been cared for by their psychotic mothers. Our first case[2] was treated successfully, and as a result of this initial experience we have gone on to admit a total of 40 mother-child pairs over the last 3 years. The ages of the children at the time of admission ranged from 1 month to 2½ years, and they have remained in the hospital for as long as 9 months. We have described the first 12 of these cases and certain of the administrative techniques which seemed helpful.[3]

PREPARATION AND MANAGEMENT OF JOINT ADMISSIONS

We now feel confident that it is practical for even seriously disturbed women to care for their children in a mental hospital. It is of major importance, however, that the decision to bring the child in be shared by the patient, members of her family, and the participating ward staff.

The patient's immediate family, such as her husband and mother, must be included in these discussions and plans. Their viewpoint is of significance in the intake evaluation, and they customarily assume the responsibility of the care of the patient's child during her hospitalization. Their feelings about whether or not to relinquish the child to the hospitalized mother will have continuing implications for the success of the joint admission and the mother's recovery. It has been our impression that in the few cases in which the husband refused to allow his wife to care for the child in the hospital, his position reflected other difficulties in his relationship with his wife as well as with the hospital, and these patients did poorly in general.

The evaluation of which mother can usefully care for her child is not an easy one. The acute symptoms the patient manifests, her general ward adjustment, and her relationship with her therapist and the ward nurses are important. It is vital that the patient feel that the nurses on the ward understand her problems and are able and ready to help her, and that there is a meaningful alliance with the therapist in which the patient can share her feelings of anxiety, doubt, guilt, and hopelessness. Joint admission cannot be prescribed, but like any alteration of a human relationship it must be discussed and agreed on by all concerned. The decision to bring in a baby is thus reached through understanding rather than by fiat. Often the psychiatrist will suggest to the patient

520

that she consider having her baby with her, but when there are other children about the hospital she may suggest this herself.

There is not only the matter of deciding *if* the baby should come in, but also *when*. For almost all patients, admission to a mental hospital carries with it a temporary surcease from responsibility and an explicit or implicit wish to regress. The treatment program ordinarily makes certain demands upon the patient for limited responsibility while making allowances for her illness. However, joint admission presents the patient with a relatively formidable task, and her regressive tendencies must be carefully assessed and worked with. We have had a number of cases in which the agreement to bring in the baby was arrived at prematurely by the patient and doctor in the sense that the patient felt pressured by the staff and her own sense of obligation, but she was not yet personally committed to caring for the child. Such patients have usually found a way to let us know that we had failed to understand their needs at the moment through self-destructive behavior, withdrawal, regression, or postponement. We have found that if mothers are able to participate actively and responsibly in the decision to bring the child in with the father's consent and support and to make appropriate plans for the equipment necessary, only very rarely will she be unable to care for it adequately.

We have also found that the patient does better if, immediately after admission, she is given a period of time to adapt to the hospital before the child is admitted. During this time several developments take place: first, her acute symptoms may abate; second, the ward staff establishes a relationship with her; third, and most important, there is time for a careful assessment of the usefulness of joint admission for this particular patient.

This is not to say that a baby can be cared for on any ward in any hospital under any conditions. A single room should be available for the mother and child, or normal ward life will be too disrupted and the other patients may become resentful of intrusion. We have also found that mothers like to have a place for privacy with their children. Access to minimal kitchen facilities is helpful. Most of the special equipment necessary for the child's care can be brought from home by the family. Both Cassel Hospital and the West Middlesex Hospital in England have provided separate wings for joint admission, but we have neither had this opportunity nor found it necessary.

ATTITUDES OF STAFF AND PATIENTS

We have found that the attitudes of the ward personnel are the most important single consideration in introducing a joint admission. At first, the nurses were quite concerned that they would have more work on their hands than they could manage, and they feared that the other patients might abuse the baby or would be jealous of him. Many of them hoped that the plan to admit the baby would not be carried out or would fail. One of the nurses' greatest difficulties was in understanding their quasi-maternal role in relation to the baby. Having accepted some responsibility for the baby, they were not happy about sharing him with the mother and were inclined either to take over the care from her or leave her entirely on her own. Over a period of time, and with much discussion, these attitudes have changed so that the ward staff now regards having children around the hospital as a matter of course. The regulations which had hitherto prohibited the visiting of children under 16 were soon forgotten and later officially changed as children routinely came in to see their parents on the ward. This occurred with so little consequence that it was almost unnoticed, and now people wonder why this rule ever existed.

The reaction of patients on the ward is also of significance. In interviews they expressed fear that the child might be harmed, either physically or psychologically, as well as concern that the baby would deprive them of a great deal of attention and protection from the ward staff. These feelings were prominent prior to the arrival of the first baby, but patients arriving on the ward today find children already there and gain reassurance from staff and patients who recognize the unreality of these fears. There have been no observed instances of a patient harming any child.

The psychiatric residents indicate that occasionally patients have reactions of jealousy toward the baby and that other patients have feelings about their failure to mother their own children properly or wish that they had been mothered better, but that these feelings represent, as one resident put it, "grist for the psychotherapeutic mill."

Many patients seem to have derived considerable gratification and benefit from the children on the ward. As an example, a severely paranoid nursery school teacher seemed to gain considerable self-respect when she was encouraged to babysit for one of the children on the ward. In time the child's mother seemed to benefit by watching how this woman sat on the floor and participated in the baby's play, and she learned that she herself did not have to remain distant. From these and similar experiences patients gain mothering skills and confidence, not only from the hospital staff and in therapy but from the other patients on the ward.

In general, our experience with the administration of joint admission indicates that proper and successful management requires (1) a careful preliminary evaluation of the mother and the nature of her illness; (2) a working relationship with her physician and the ward staff; (3) the staff, the patient, and her family make a mutual decision to admit the baby; and (4) adequate provision for the physical needs of the child.

DEVELOPMENT OF SELECTION CRITERIA

To a considerable extent the guidelines for undertaking a joint admission will be the same as those which govern other decisions affecting patient management: control of behavior, motivation, interpersonal competence, reality testing, and so on. It is our present view that patients who benefit most from joint admission have had a reasonably successful prepsychotic adjustment and have maintained relatively close family ties. Conflicts over masculine strivings, feminine identification, and sexual guilt are prominent, and the relatively mature defenses of isolation, repression, and turning against the self, as well as projection, are in the foreground. On psychological examination they show clear signs of thought disorder with much evidence of an active internal struggle. The acute disturbance which leads to hospitalization occurs only after they have had some months of experience in attempting to adapt to parenthood and their child. It is possible that joint admission is both easier and more rewarding for them for several reasons. First, the mother has a prior relationship with the child and some experience in perceiving and satisfying its needs. In the second place, since the babies are beyond the neonatal stage they are able to show a positive response to the mother. Third, it may be (though we have no data on this point yet) that cooperation of the hospital staff and other patients is greater—and their anxiety lower—when the child is no longer a newborn.[8]

Although we feel that these observations may be useful guides in the selection of cases, we are not yet restricting our own joint admissions to patients who meet these general criteria. The matter requires further investigation.

DISCUSSION

The Effects of the Emotionally Disturbed Mother on the Development of the Child

It has long been believed that the psychotic mother represents a psychological and/or physical danger to her child. In most cases, however, the mother discharged from the hospital goes home to resume care of a child from whom she has long been separated, often without adequate support. It seems clear that the necessity for the separation of mother and child for the duration of her illness must be called into question.

We have seen no instances of physical harm to a child by its mother. There have, however, been times when a mother was temporarily less than adequate in meeting the physical and emotional needs of the child. These difficulties have been resolved either by help from the staff, or if they continued too long by removal of the child from the hospital. This latter alternative has been necessary only on rare occasions.

Sobel[6] has reported on the children of eight couples of which both mother and father had been hospitalized and diagnosed as schizophrenic. He compared the four cases in which the children continued in foster care with those who returned to their mothers, observing less satisfactory adjustment in the latter. On the other hand, Sussex et al,[7] have recently reported finding little discernible deviation in latency-age children whose psychotic mothers were in outpatient treatment. They noted that the better adjusted children were those whose mothers had considerable support from other family members, such as husband and grandmothers. These reports raise important questions concerning the influence of parental psychosis on a child: genetic factors, the amount of support which different families can provide, and the problems consequent to separation and reunion with a mother as well as those of foster home placement.

The Effect on the Child of Separation from the Mother

It is generally recognized that there must be some adverse effect on the child when it loses its mother, is cared for by a mother surrogate, and then returns after a long period of time to its own mother; yet the effects of the loss of a mothering figure twice over are dependent on the quality of care provided, the age of the child, and its coping abilities. The literature on maternal deprivation, which is by this time considerable, deals largely with institutionalization and loss of mothering. It does not usually pertain directly to the situation in which the child is cared for by a grandmother or aunt with the father still available.

Although the literature on maternal deprivation does not apply directly to the children of psychotic mothers, it may nonetheless be useful. Yarrow, reviewing the evidence for the effects of mother-child separation at various stages of the child's development, derives the hypothesis that the critical period of vulnerability to intellectual deficit (and presumably to normal ego development) is between 3 and 12 months of age.[9] If, as the evidence suggests, this is true, then there is reason to believe that before 3 months of age a mother surrogate may be more adequate than the child's own psychotic mother, since mothering rather than the mother is needed. Beyond 15 to 18 months the child seems better able to deal with his mother's loss and has the capacity to relate to other people. Since it appears from our previous work that women who are hospitalized before their child is 3 months old seem to do less well with joint admission, it may be that the needs of the mother and child coincide. The mother who cannot care for her infant in the hospital is also the mother whose child can most readily be separated from her.

Comparison of Joint Admission with Available Alternatives

When the mother of a young child requires psychiatric hospitalization, those responsible for the necessary rearrangements must consider the available alternatives for the care of the child. Relatives or friends and foster homes or institutional placement ordinarily constitute the primary resources, and the joint admission procedure should properly be compared with the alternatives families actually find and use. The most common mother surrogate is a grandmother, and it has been our experience that many patients have strong negatives feelings about having their children cared for by their own mothers or mothers-in-law. Often this disposition of the child has the effect of intensifying the patient's feelings of inadequacy. She not only feels that she has failed as a mother in comparison with her own mother, but that the hospital concurs with this view by endorsing such an arrangement.

In almost all of our cases someone else has managed the care of the baby while the mother was undergoing her initial intake and evaluation and undergoing some change in the acute symptomatic expression of her difficulties. However, since the patient, her family, and the staff are all aware of the joint admission program and consider it probable that the mother will resume the child's care as soon as she is able, these early arrangements may be made with the feeling that they are a temporary expedient rather than an assignment for an indeterminate period of time.

Pao[5] has astutely observed that the child placed in the care of others for the full term of its mother's hospitalization suffers the difficulty of separation from the mother surrogate at precisely the time that the mother is dealing with this same problem in regard to her leaving the hospital and the doctor. He points out that failure to help the mother

525

in psychotherapy with her dependent wishes and her anxiety over separation may lead to her inability to help her child, to her rehospitalization, or to both. We have felt that a significant advantage of the joint admission procedure is that it enables the mother and child to become somewhat attuned (or reattuned) to each other and helps the mother to build up some experience in the gratification of the child's dependency needs before her discharge. Stated more simply, if the mother can begin to see herself as capable of caring, she can better tolerate the loss of the hospital's day-to-day support.

REFERENCES

1. DOUGLAS, G.: Psychotic mothers. Lancet 1:124-125, 1956.
2. GRUNEBAUM, H., WEISS, J. L., HIRSCH, L. L., AND BARRETT, J.: The baby on the ward: report of a joint mother-child admission to an adult psychiatric hospital. Psychiatry 26:39-53, 1963.
3. GRUNEBAUM, H., AND WEISS, J. L.: Psychotic mothers and their children: joint admission to an adult psychiatric hospital. Am. J. Psychiat. 119:927-933, 1963.
4. MAIN, T. F.: Mothers with children in a psychiatric hospital. Lancet 7051 (2):845-847, 1958.
5. PAO, P.: Young schizophrenic mothers' initial posthospital adjustment at home. Arch. Gen. Psychiat. 2:512-520, 1960.
6. SOBEL, D.: Children of schizophrenic patients: preliminary observations on early development. Am. J. Psychiat. 118:512-517, 1961.
7. SUSSEX, J. N., GASSMAN, F., AND RAFFEL, S. C.: Adjustment of children with psychotic mothers in the home. Am. J. Orthopsychiat. 33:849-854, 1963.
8. WEISS, J. L., GRUNEBAUM, H. U., AND SCHELL, R. E.: Psychotic mothers and their children. II: Psychological studies of mothers caring for their infants and young children in a psychiatric hospital. Arch. Gen. Psychiat. 11:90-98, 1964.
9. YARROW, L. J.: Maternal deprivation: toward an empirical and conceptual re-evaluation. Psych. Bull. 58:459-490, 1961.

Work Therapy in Psychiatry*

by HERMAN C. B. DENBER, M.D.

WHEREAS HOSPITAL TREATMENT FOR MOST medical and surgical disorders is directed to an etiologically known disorder with early discharge as a goal, the situation in psychiatry is different. Much of the etiology is still shrouded in mystery. The patients are for the most part ambulatory,† and the various treatments (i.e., drugs, ECT, psychotherapy, etc.) occupy but a fraction of the day. Determined efforts have been made recently to structure the hospital day through programs aimed at mobilizing the patient's resources, preventing regression, and facilitating rehabilitation. Work therapy in this frame of reference assumes importance, since it becomes the focus of the daily activities, acting as a matrix for other psychiatric treatments.[1-3]

Historically, work and return to mental health have been interwoven, and the former was officially recognized as a treatment in France in 1839 and 1857.[4] Work therapy has been described[5] as a task involving the patient in which the therapist's energies are expended towards the accomplishment of something of use to others. Wayne,[6] reporting on work therapy in the Soviet Union, concluded that work when not characterized by an obsessive-compulsive pattern has special and lasting value. Its importance must be accepted among our therapeutic procedures as a link between the patient and his own capacities, the people around him, and the world to which he must return.

The therapeutic potentials of work have been analyzed from the psychodynamic aspects by Oseas,[7] in that work therapy simultaneously alleviated symptoms and modified maladaptive behavior. Dundas and Collins[8] pointed out that in working, a "reality confrontation" is kept in mind during the patient's treatment and rehabilitation. The thera-

---

*Some of the work upon which this paper is based was supported by Grant OM-228 from the National Institute of Mental Health, Bethesda, Maryland.
†This is not necessarily true in European institutions.

527

peutic importance of work was outlined at great length by the French Ministry of Health.[4] It was considered an important treatment adjunct, providing it was varied and adapted both to the personality and potential of each patient, with monetary gain not the primary object. Work was viewed as one aspect of the total social psychiatric treatment setting within the hospital.

Since life is represented by a series of social interaction phenomena which theoretically have precipitated, in part, the psychotic breakdown, the return to health would optimally begin with inanimate objects. It has been suggested[3] that work becomes therapeutic when it permits an elementary primitive object fixation (the work idea) which is neutral and nonthreatening in a supportive field (the group); this progresses slowly to human interpersonal relations as the patient improves. Work offers a point of fixation and well-defined boundaries in a fixed time sequence, and becomes part of the resocialization process aimed at reducing the intensity of some of the primary factors in schizophrenic disorders.

The psychiatric hospital of the past was, at best, an artifically contrived setting, primarily a holding operation until such time as the patient "regained" his prepsychotic personality and was released to the community. The patient's day, by and large, was essentially a therapeutic vacuum, with very little purposeful activity. The advent of large-scale chemotherapy with psychotropic drugs required changes in hospital procedures resulting from mobilization of previously "inert" patients. It was insufficient to use these potent drugs, group or individual psychotherapy, music, art, recreational and occupational therapies, and leave the patient "to rest" or to his own devices for the larger part of the day.

Work therapy could fill this breach, since it rested upon a fulcrum of continuous movement, had a realistic incentive (pay), took place in a group, and presented the goal of rehabilitation for the posthospital period. It would be a planned activity, making socially relevant demands on the patient.[9] Viewed as part of a total process, it became one function of a new environment which was structured to be neutral, yet warm. It had to be supportive, yet not create dependency; be permissive, but with boundaries and limits. The rules of the shop would have to be flexible (time, absences, etc.), yet be rigid enough to support the fragile psychotic ego-structure. The group process and pressures left no place for the schizophrenic to escape. Withdrawal, detachment and retirement into fantasy were difficult in a large room where movement, sound, voices, action, reality demands, and people signalled the ever-present world.

528

Work therapy for inhospital acute and chronic psychotic patients has been essentially a European method for many years, and is routine in French, Swiss, Italian, Scandinavian, and Soviet hospitals.[4,10] A distinction should be drawn between the "sheltered workshop" outside (or inside) the hospital,[11] and the inhospital factory workshop that is the subject of this paper. The former has been criticized as being "too selective, wanting only good patients," and providing only a way station to fit the needs of a small number of psychiatric patients.[12] Work therapy, as it is seen here, is a treatment for all patients. Screening devices are, therefore, unnecessary and the therapeutic potentials of work are available to all acute and chronic patients, irrespective of diagnosis.

The problems related to opening a shop within the hospital have been previously analyzed,[2,3] and are well described in other publications.[13,18] In the majority of American hospitals, considerable criticism of work therapy as opposed to "leisure-time modalities" must be overcome before one can implement such a program. The spectre of opposition by organized labor is often raised, and this may cause occasional difficulties,[14] but has never actually been a serious problem.

Where specialized personnel (i.e., those with industrial background) cannot be employed because of budget problems, ward attendants or other nonspecialized staff have been found to adapt rather easily to their new setting. European institutions frequently have a pool of artisans among their personnel who can take over many of the more specialized functions of work therapy. Nevertheless, where the workshop concept is contrary to prior ideas of patient treatment, such change in duty must be preceded by lengthy indoctrination and group discussion. Their effectiveness rests, among other factors, on their intimate knowledge and understanding of the patients' psychiatric problems. Occupational therapists would have seemed to be the most logical personnel for a workshop, but experience has not substantiated this premise. Previous training, indoctrination, and orientation seemed to have been inhibitory factors. Whether this will change with time is still an open question.

Contracts may be secured by different means. One worker can be designated to visit local industries for work suitable to the particular patient population. This individual can be hired especially for the purpose, or may already be in service but with prior business experience. In some instances, the hospital business officer designates one of his staff to handle the accounts and find contracts. The shop can also be incorporated with a Board of Directors, composed of prominent people in the community[14] who can be of considerable aid in securing contracts.

Finally, work can be contracted with sheltered workshops in the community itself.

A key problem lies in the type of work to be sought versus availability. The supply is limited by the shop's difficulty in functioning competitively in the open labor market. Generally, the type of contracts available are from those segments of industry operating on thin profit margins where labor costs are crucial. For therapeutic reasons, the work available must be varied in type, and preferably not monotonous. It must be graded in difficulty, so that it can be offered to different patients according to their degree of improvement. Practically, this is not always possible, and securing a variety of contracts will always remain a constant challenge to any shop and test the ingenuity of its leaders.

The workshop location may be either close by the actual ward, in another building on the hospital grounds, or in the nearest locality to the institution. Theoretically, it would be preferable for the patients "to go to work," and this should be done at some reasonable distance from the usual living quarters in the hospital. The hours of work should range between 4 and 5 per day.

The manner of paying patients poses only a hypothetical problem. If they work for pay, should this be deposited in their account and become subject to the same hospital rules, or should the sum be given directly to the patient? Moral and therapeutic reasons, if not legal ones as well, would indicate that a patient's earnings should be given directly to him, preferably in a "pay envelope." The feeling of having "earned" something is ego-syntonic, and patients may see this as a realistic appraisal of their worth—more as a fact of earning than the amount. If the salary goes beyond a specified level (which will vary from community to community), some contribution should be made by the patient for his hospital maintenance. Dependency has unfortunately been encouraged, perhaps unknowingly, to a greater or lesser degree in many psychiatric hospitals, and the assumption of a realistic role (paying one's bills) can be construed as a social therapeutic measure.

DISCUSSION

If work therapy is really therapeutic, the supportive evidence must be forthcoming. When questioned directly, patients state that the shop is "a good thing." They almost unanimously feel that "to work keeps you occupied, and if you are occupied, you don't think about your problems." Some feel that it permits them to channel and dissipate anxiety which otherwise might take the form of symptoms. In a number of cases, the

530

workshop represented the first stage toward rehabilitation of chronic psychotic patients. Here, the shop must be viewed as part of the overall drug and social psychiatric therapeutic program. Nevertheless, some patients vociferously object to working; this is most often a manifestation of the underlying disorder and must be treated accordingly.

The well-controlled study of Wing and Freudenberg[19] showed that "increase of working activity under active conditions of supervision was accompanied by a significant decrease in various abnormalities of behavior (immobility, mannerisms, and restlessness), although ward behavior was unaffected." After a year's activity in the hospital shop, "the average patient slept better, was less restless, talkative, or aggressive, worked with less supervision than at conventional hospital occupational therapy, and was more cooperative and friendly."[18] About 75 per cent of patients were improved by these criteria. Few patients sat by idly, and quarrels were infrequent—effects we have also observed in our own patients.

Early[15] reported that "the entire diagnostic spectrum" could benefit from the industrial therapy program. After 2 years, 23 per cent of the long-stay and long-unemployed psychiatric patients became wage earners. Another 21 per cent went into sheltered workshops, although this figure was subject to some experimental error in design.

Wing and Giddens[13] studied two groups of male schizophrenic patients hospitalized more than 2 years, one of whom entered the industrial rehabilitation unit, while the other stayed at the hospital receiving routine care. After 6 to 12 months, eight of the experimental group were working outside the institution, while none of the control group had achieved this status. Hubbs[20] selected patients because they were considered to have a potential capability for rehabilitation; a controlled study was inconclusive. Miles, et al.[21] proposed to establish a rigidly controlled experimental study to evaluate work therapy where the entire population of their hospital would be available and rating scales would be used.

Hamilton and Salmon[9] compared the psychological, clinical, and social effects of work therapy and occupational therapy in male chronic schizophrenic patients; another group had no specific treatment. Those in work therapy improved most in "social competence, clinical state, and reaction time." Financial reward did not play a crucial part in the behavioral changes, and group productivity was superior to individuals working alone. The "workshop climate" was found to be important. This was the integral part of a normal work situation, which conveyed a definite nonspecific sociopsychological climate. Workshop activities,

531

they found, may lead to significant changes in the objective assessment of reality factors.

Much of the opposition to paying patients results from unresolved staff countertransference problems. This is based, in part, on hierarchical values and the rigid tradition of roles in a psychiatric hospital. Oseas[22] did not mention the matter of realistic satisfaction through pay. It would seem reasonable to assume that the use of some concrete gratification in the highly symbolic world of the psychotic might in itself be therapeutic.

The question has been raised[9] whether the positive results of work therapy might be due to a general reactivation of patients, expressed by changes in alertness, awareness, responsiveness, and objectivity. It can be reasoned that the attention set required while working diverts and constructively channels psychomotor energy heretofore used for repression of conflict. There is a redirection of object cathexis from the inner disordered self to the structured environment. The latter becomes an external solid anchor to which the patient clings, thus replacing the inner maelstrom. The mental life now focuses upon work as a new-found "object" held in the continuously sustained matrix of the group —both staff and patients. Healthy values are given to this activity, since it is participated in and esteemed by staff and the patient's peers. The disordered motor activity, coupled with decrease in awareness and with detachment and indifference, are slowly replaced by a "return to reality." The intensive use of chemotherapy throughout this process produces a parallel progressive decrease in psychotic symptoms. Finally, there occurs a reintegrative phase in which the patient's work performance is an excellent indicator of improvement. In all probability, part of the basic effectiveness of work rests upon the fact that it is a nonformalized, socially and culturally acceptable vehicle for social interaction in groups.

REFERENCES

1. DENBER, H. C. B.: Industrial workshop for psychiatric Patients. Mental Hospitals 11:16-18, 1960.
2. ——: Work therapy for psychiatric patients. Comprehensive Psychiatry 1: 49-54, 1960.
3. ——, AND RAJOTTE, P.: Problems and theoretical considerations of work therapy for psychiatric patients. J. Canad. Psychiat. Assoc. 7:25-33, 1962.
4. Recueil des Textes Officiels. Fascicule Special No. 58-7 bis. Organisation du travail thérapeutique dans les hôpitaux psychiatriques, Paris, 1958.
5. LANDY D., AND RAULET, H.: The hospital work program. In M. Greenblatt and B. Simon (Eds.): Rehabilitation of the Mentally Ill, Publication No. 58, A.A.A.S., Washington, D.C., 1959, pp. 71-87.

532

6. WAYNE, G. J.: Work therapy in the Soviet Union. Mental Hospitals 12: 20-23, 1961.
7. OSEAS, L.: Therapeutic potentials in work. A.M.A. Arch. Gen. Psychiat. 4: 622-631, 1961.
8. DUNDAS, J., AND COLLINS, D.: Industrial work therapy versus formal occupational therapy in a large psychiatric hospital. Psychiat. Quart. Suppl. 36:278-285, 1962.
9. HAMILTON, V., AND SALMON, P.: Psychological changes in chronic schizophrenics following differential activity programmes. J. Ment. Sc. 108: 505-520, 1962.
10. DENBER, H. C. B.: Personal observations.
11. BLACK, B. J.: The protected workshop. In M. Greenblatt and B. Simon (Eds.): Rehabilitation of the Mentally Ill, Publication No. 58, A.A.A.S., Washington, D.C., 1959, pp. 199-211.
12. OLSHANSKY, S.: The transitional sheltered workshop: a survey. J. Soc. Issues 16:33-39, 1960.
13. WING, J. K., AND GIDDENS, R. G. T.: Industrial rehabilitation of male chronic schizophrenic patients. Lancet 2:505-507, 1959.
14. EARLY, D. F.: The Industrial Therapy Organization (Bristol), a development of work in hospital. Lancet 2:754-757, 1960.
15. ——: The Industrial Therapy Organization (Bristol), the first two years. Lancet 1:435-436, 1963.
16. WADSWORTH, W. V., WELLS, B. W. P., AND STOCK, R. S.: The organization of a sheltered workshop. J. Ment. Sc. 108:780-785, 1962.
17. CARSTAIRS, M.: Industrial Work as a Means of Rehabilitation for Chronic Schizophrenics. Proc. Second Internat. Cong. Psychiat., Zurich. Orell Füssli Arts Graphiques, 1:99-102, 1957.
18. Factory in a mental hospital. Foreign letters. J.A.M.A. 171:2354, 1959.
19. WING, J. K., AND FREUDENBERG, R. K.: The response of severely ill chronic schizophrenic patients to social stimulation. Am. J. Psychiat. 118:311-322, 1961.
20. HUBBS, R. S.: Rehabilitation means restoration. The sheltered workshop. Mental Hospitals 11:7-9, 1960.
21. MILES, D. G.: Personal communication.
22. OSEAS, L.: Work requirements and ego-defects. Psychiat. Quart. 37:105-122, 1963.

Progress in Hospital Community Therapy*

by MAXWELL JONES, M.D.

G ROUP INTERACTION FOR THERAPEUTIC PURPOSES has become a commonplace in modern psychiatry. Usually eight or ten patients, selected for their intelligence, motivation, ego strength, and the suitability of their problem for this type of treatment, meet at frequent, usually weekly, intervals, for about an hour for a period of time which may vary from months to years. The participants develop an awareness of their capacity to understand what lies behind behavior and analyze their own feelings for each other and how these are related to past situations with other people. Such groups are frequently run on an outpatient basis, and, theoretically at least, the patients know very little about each other in real life and meet only at the group. The leader is usually trained in psychoanalysis, and the treatment methodology has much in common with the psychoanalytic model. However, psychoanalytic methods have relatively little place in the treatment of the vast bulk of psychiatric problems; these require less specialized workers who can deal with many more patients at one time.

In America "Action for Mental Health,"[1] the final report of the Joint Commission of Mental Illness and Health, highlighted the need for complete reorganization of psychiatric hospital practice, particularly in the state institutions.

The developments in Europe, particularly Holland and Britain, had given a tremendous impetus to what was coming to be loosely called social psychiatry. Essentially the term meant the maximum use of the potentialities for treatment which were present in any one community at any one time. The term community could be applied in its intra- or extramural sense and usually meant a social subgroup such as a ward or

---

*The author wishes to acknowledge his indebtedness to Professor Reginald Revans of Manchester University and to his yet unpublished work on learning in school children.

family or, as an extended concept, a unit of the hospital or a neighborhood community. Borrowing from the now familiar model of the psychoanalytic group and from the now developing concept of social psychiatry and the behavioral sciences, community therapy has come to take many forms. It is reasonable that any group of individuals with a common problem could derive benefit by pooling their resources, yet this may lead to a heightening rather than a lessening of difficulties unless skillfully handled. This raises the whole question of the professional in community work.

The psychiatrist is seen as uniquely qualified for the role of psychotherapist and resists strenuously any attempt to undermine his authority in this area, whereas in America's war against poverty, the lack of skilled workers is being used as an opportunity to provide shortened training for unskilled and underprivileged people. The aim is to free the professional of some of his simpler, routine tasks, in order that he can apply his expertise without distraction. If we take trained social workers as one example, it is perfectly clear that there is no likelihood of having a sufficient supply. In the overcrowded and understaffed state hospital the people with skills must inevitably enlist help from whatever source available, but progress is often hampered by the rigidities of professional groups. For example, a ward may decide to have a daily community meeting of its patients and staff. The staff may include the psychiatrist, a social worker, a psychologist, and the nursing staff, but the assumption is that the psychiatrist, by virtue of his authority, is the leader in the community meeting. It may well be that his training is less adequate in this area of social interaction than either the social worker or the psychologist. In the public mind the responsibility for a sick person, inevitably, is invested in the doctor. So far, doctors have shown little tendency to delegate this authority to their peers. The emergence of analytic group psychotherapy and of community meetings inevitably raises the question of specific skills for this type of work, and it may be that the nursing profession is competing as strongly as the social workers and the psychologists for leadership in this field. Complicated problems of status, pay, and training are involved, but I am concerned here more with the problems of leadership. The psychiatrist who has not had adequate training in group work and the behavioral sciences should be less concerned about his status and professional role than about the optimum use of the social environment concerned with the treatment of patients. The same argument applies to the extramural field where the relationship between the psychiatrist and, say, the psychiatric social worker can raise problems of responsibility and authority. Psychiatrists are relative newcomers to work

535

in the outside community, and the help that they will get from the environment will in large measure depend upon their skill in handling the various professional and semiprofessional bodies along with the patients and their families.

Haylett and Rapoport[2] point out that the mental health consultant can be either a psychiatrist, a psychiatric social worker, or a clinical psychologist. "The consultant helps the consultee to clarify and find solutions for current mental health problems, either in relationship to specific clients or to programmes and practices of the consultee's organization. . . . The nature of this relationship has been described as a 'co-ordinate' one. This emphasizes the fact that the consultant has no administrative control over the consultee and that each has his own area of competence." This closely approximates what is generally understood as supervision in psychotherapy, social work, or nursing. By contrast to individual supervision, a group setting allows the group members to discuss statements made by the consultant, to examine the difference in interpretations which different individuals may put on the same statement, to interact freely with the consultant, and at times to make the consultant aware of some of his own misunderstandings, preconceptions, prejudices, and so on.

Progressive schools like those of A. S. Neil[3] at Summerhill have been practicing a system of free communications and interaction for several decades, but it is only now[4,5] that the message of these pioneers is being reinforced from the fields of behavioral science, including learning theory and group dynamics. Interaction between pupil and teacher, or patient and doctor, or inmate and correctional personnel, can be carried a stage further by invoking a neglected resource—the well-motivated and partially trained pupil, patient, or inmate. In the case of school children this resource has been utilized by Lippitt and Lohman[6] at their center for research on the utilization of scientific knowledge, University of Michigan. They have used sixth graders, working in close collaboration with their teacher, to guide, support, and instruct fourth graders in their work, play, and social interaction. To quote from their paper: "One assumption of these pilot projects has been that much of the process of socialization involves cross-age modeling by younger children after the behavior and attitudes of older children and that this process has great potentiality for planned development as an effective educational force provided that children are trained appropriately for their roles as socialization agents."

Some of the important "natural" components of this cross-age modeling process include: an older child's ability to communicate more effectively at the younger child's level than can adults; the older child's lesser likelihood of being perceived as an "authority figure," the younger child's greater willingness to accept influence when there is a greater opportunity for reciprocal effects; and, a slightly older child's providing a more realistic level of aspiration for the younger learner than does an adult. The involvement of older children in a program of collaboration with adults to help younger children will aid socialization because of (a) the important motivational significance of a trust and responsibility-taking relationship with adults around a significant task and (b) the opportunity to work through with awareness, but at a safe emotional distance, some of their own problems of relationships with sibs and peers.

Assisting in a teaching function will likewise help the "teaching student" test, internalize, and develop his knowledge, as well as help him to discover its significance. So, also the younger learners and their adult teachers will be significantly helped through the utilization of trained older children available for tutoring, drilling, listening-and-correcting, and similar "academic" functions. Finally, the child will develop a more realistic image of his own ability and present state of development and will gain a greater appreciation of his own abilities and skills if he has an opportunity (a) to help youngers to acquire skills which he already possesses and (b) to develop positive relationships with elders in which he can see himself take the necessary and next steps in the growing up process.

The foregoing remarks, based on experience in an educational setting, have much in common with therapeutic practice, whether it be carried out in a hospital, or correctional institution, a day hospital, or in the community itself. The essential ingredients are individuals with psychiatric or social problems which they are unable to cope with unaided, a staff trained in a diversity of skills related to the treatment of such problems, and the co-option of the psychiatric patient or social casualty as a resource person in the treatment process.

The use of the patient as a therapist has been developed to a greater extent than elsewhere at Henderson Hospital, near London. Here, approximately 60 patients of both sexes, diagnosed as character disorders, live in a therapeutic community without locked doors. Cases are referred from the Courts and from psychiatric clinics and usually stay from two to four months in what amounts to an intensive living-learning situation. Behavior is scrutinized in a series of groups throughout the day and the concept of two-way communication has been developed to an unusual degree. Great reliance is placed on a patient's peer group, in which older patients, who have come to a better understanding of their own

537

and other people's behavior as a result of their own group treatment, are used as culture carriers. They are more acceptable to new patients than are the "authority figures" in the form of the hospital staff. Henderson Hospital has been a therapeutic community for 18 years and has lived through an endless series of crises which have been invaluable as learning experiences as well as giving staff and patients a feeling of common identity against a relatively hostile world. Even with the general acceptance of this therapeutic community as another treatment approach the internal conflicts are of such magnitude that there is little danger of complacency, and there is a constant necessity to understand what lies behind the violent disturbances which are inevitable when a community of patients with severe character disorders live together. Much has been written about Henderson[4,7,8] but the most important single factor which impresses most visitors is the extent to which patients have succeeded in transforming their traditional egocentricity into a profound concern for each other, revelling in a group identity that affords the individual a feeling of belonging, which, in many cases, he has never experienced previously. Such a setting provides a unique opportunity for individual growth and if the first objective of all education is to develop the capacity to inquire, to become better at asking questions, or to practice how to tackle problems, then Henderson provides an excellent setting in which learning can occur. In addition, the staff have considerable skill in analytic group work and help patients to become aware of some of the factors lying behind their behavior and motivation. Authority figures trained in group dynamics and a permissive regime, which, nevertheless, sets definite limits that allow the patient to test new ways of meeting problems and of getting close to people, combine to help the patient develop the satisfactions of a useful social role. The methods used at Henderson Hospital still require a great deal of study and evaluation, but there is increasing support for its general approach from the fields of education, learning theory, group dynamics, and behavioral sciences generally. The methods used have been applied increasingly in correctional institutions, particularly in California,[8] where extensive study regarding the value of this and other approaches is being carried out.

At Dingleton, a psychiatric hospital serving the needs of 100,000 people in the Borders of Scotland, we have tried to use face-to-face confrontation for both learning and treatment purposes. Our practice has evolved from our experience in small group and ward treatment methods.[8] A crisis situation in the hospital may involve patients or staff or both, who do not ordinarily meet in the same treatment group. Moreover, there may be certain advantages in having a face-to-face confrontation set at a time

538

when the emotions are high rather than leaving it to the next day or a few days later. There is reason to think that learning may be enhanced at a time when feelings are strong, but if the level of anxiety is too high the whole process of learning may be blocked. It has been found expedient and useful to call a meeting of those involved in a crisis situation at the time when the situation is at its height. Such confrontation requires considerable skill, else the feelings may become heightened and hinder rather than help the learning situation. Constant confrontations of this kind seem to have as much validity for the training of staff personnel as for the treatment of patients.

In this discussion I have used the term "community therapy" as if it were synonymous with "sociotherapy." Neither term has general acceptance or any very specific meaning. Both terms could be applied with equal relevance to the concept of an intra- or extramural community. An essential ingredient of this approach is the optimal use of the social environment to bring about improvement in the face of social disorganization or mental illness. It is essentially an exercise in learning, and there would appear to be a continuity throughout our public life from the early home environment to the school and through further education to the whole area of social and political life. It would seem that current developments open up new possibilities for people to come to a better understanding of themselves and others. How far such concept can keep pace with the new destructive forces inherent in the atomic age must inevitably be for history to decide.

REFERENCES

1. Action for Mental Health. The Final Report of the Joint Commission on Mental Illness and Health. New York, Basic Books, 1961.
2. HAYLETT, C. H., AND RAPOPORT, L.: Handbook of Community Psychiatry. Chap. 17. L. Bellak, Ed. New York, Grune & Stratton, 1964.
3. NEIL, A. S.: Summerhill. A Radical Approach to Education. London, England, Victor Gollancz, 1964.
4. JONES, M.: The Therapeutic Community. New York, Basic Books, 1952.
5. McCORKLE, L. W., ELIAS, A., AND BIXBY, F. L.: The Highfields Story. New York, Henry Holt, 1958.
6. LIPPITT, P., AND LOHMAN, J.: A Neglected Resource—Cross-age relationships. Children 12:113, 1965.
7. RAPOPORT, R. N.: Community as Doctor. London, England, Tavistock Publications, 1960.
8. JONES, MAXWELL: Social Psychiatry. Springfield, Illinois, Charles C Thomas, 1962.

Treatment of the Hospitalized Suicidal Patient

by ALAN A. STONE, M.D.*

UCH OF THE RECENT research dealing with suicide has focused on detection of suicidal intent.[24] Evidence has been accumulated which, contrary to traditional expectation, indicates rather convincingly that most completed suicides are preceded by some communication which portends the suicidal act.[7,11,22-24] This and other related findings have led to a mental health emphasis on a variety of preventive techniques with the establishment of interdisciplinary suicide prevention centers.[8] However once serious suicidal intent has been detected and the patient hospitalized, the onerous burden of responsibility for the suicidal patient typically falls on the psychiatrist. How well do we cope with this responsibility?

It has been estimated[5,11] that approximately 100,000 people are hospitalized each year in the United States after attempting suicide. Thirty thousand of these will, within eight years, attempt suicide again, many of them within three months of discharge.[5] Studies compiled by Ettlinger[10] indicate that approximately 3 per cent to 5 per cent of those hospitalized after suicidal attempts eventually kill themselves. If one extrapolates these figures, it would appear that of the 100,000 patients admitted annually because of suicide attempts roughly 3,000 to 5,000 will eventually kill themselves after discharge. Furthermore there is convincing evidence that perhaps 20 per cent to 50 per cent of these suicides will occur within the first three months after discharge.[11,19] Some studies, e.g.,[16] have placed the subsequent suicide rate at a much higher percentage than 3 per cent to 5 per cent, and thus these extrapolated figures are meant only to suggest a rough and probably conservative approximation.

In addition suicide also occurs, though infrequently, among hospitalized psychiatric patients.‡ Although Farberow and Schneidman emphasized that

---

*Work done in collaboration with Harvey M. Shein, M.D., Assistant Professor of Psychiatry, Harvard Medical School, McLean Hospital. Cf. Amer. J. Psychiat.

‡When a suicide does occur within a hospital setting, it is not only tragic for that individual patient and family, but in addition it often has an "epidemic" effect resulting in further suicides, and causes a disastrous deterioration of staff morale.[6,28]

540

70 per cent of the in-hospital suicides occurred among schizophrenics and "many . . . were admitted by virtue of their schizophrenic symptoms in the absence of indication of any suicidal potential," they also state, "A majority (over 70 per cent) had a history of previous suicidal attempts or suicidal ideation."[11] This latter statement is compatible with our own data which suggest that in-hospital suicides are unrelated to diagnosis but almost always occur in patients known at some time to have been suicidal.[27]

The thrust of all these studies suggests that both within and without the hospital walls, a major unresolved clinical problem is managing the *known* suicidal patient rather than simply *detecting* suicidal intent. As one analyzes suicide data (now called the psychological autopsy), it is striking how often suicide occurs during a breakdown in communication between doctor and patient. This has recently been documented by Bloom[4] and is implicit in the high rate of suicide shortly after discharge. Thus at a critical point the responsible physician either misunderstands or misconstrues the patient's mental status or, perhaps more often, fails to maintain the kind of close contact in which a clinical judgment is possible.

Suicidal Intent is Conscious or Preconscious

The technique to be presented,[24] which seems justified both in light of our own data and that cited previously, is based on two crucial assumptions: (1) Suicidal intent is usually conscious or preconscious, and therefore potentially available to the psychiatrist; (2) Management of the suicidal patient within the hospital requires a kind of close monitoring which is roughly analogous to current techniques for cardiac monitoring of the acute coronary patient.

The type of monitoring which is recommended here requires an alert and informed psychotherapist who has available both actuarial data[7,11,22,23] by which one can assess dangers to the patient on a statistical basis, and also the close working relationship with the professional staff and with the patient which ensures good communication. Unless a psychiatrist or some other professional person has the kind of positive working relationship that ensures open channels of communication, the responsible physician or institution can have no reliable leverage on the suicidal patient other than that of constant observation or physical restraint. In fact suicide within the hospital usually occurs when restrictions are relaxed or the patient allowed out on visit. Clinical experience in an acute psychiatric hospital and a review of the literature indicate that as with hospitalization, the mere fact that a patient is "in psychotherapy" offers no absolute protection against suicide.[4] The safety of the patient therefore depends either on the special nature of the therapeutic alliance and of the transference, or on direct and constant surveillance. We believe that far too much reliance has been placed on the fact that the suicidal patient was in psychotherapy without specific consideration of the nature of that therapeutic relationship.[15]

The clinical method described here entails an active approach considered essential for monitoring suicidal potential. Such monitoring, at least temporarily, drastically alters the traditional approach of psychotherapy. Its goal is to ensure that the suicidal status of the patient (his suicidal intentions and his potential suicidal behavior) will remain within the focus of the therapeutic alliance, and not be lost in transference or countertransference issues.

INITIAL STEPS

The initial steps in this therapeutic approach can be outlined as follows:

1. If in doubt on a clinical or actuarial basis, the therapist should assume that suicidal thoughts are conscious and therefore express his concerns frankly, and discuss them explicitly with the patient.

2. Once the patient's suicidal thoughts are shared, it is essential that the therapist take pains to make clear to the patient that he (the therapist) considers suicidal behavior to be a maladaptive action, irreversibly counter to the patient's best interests and goals; believes such behavior arises from the patient's illness; and will do everything he can to prevent it, enlisting the rest of the staff in this effort. It is equally essential that the therapist believe in his professional stance; if not, he should simply not be treating the patient within the subtle and delicate human framework of psychotherapy.[29]

3. The therapist must directly label all suicidal ideas as crucial to any therapeutic endeavor. It is only through open and frank discussion that the patient's thoughts and fantasies concerning suicide may become objectified (in Bibring's[17] sense) as something problematic and therefore appropriate for the patient and the doctor to work on together rather than remaining a private and unexamined set of convictions. If the issues can thus be objectified, the therapist can avoid a potential danger of the patient's msiperceiving the therapist's attitude as one of moral condemnation. Weisman[29] has emphasized, with regard to the dying patient, that among the most dangerous and harmful actions of the attending doctors are those which isolate the patient further, make him feel his deliberations about dying are so embarrassing or frightening to the doctor that he dares not face them directly with the patient and work on them as on other problems. These same considerations apply with equal forcefulness to the management of the suicidal patient. If the patient is unwilling or unable to discuss his suicidal thoughts, the therapist must assume that there is no therapeutic

alliance, and must resort to continued suicidal precautions and restrictions. Since there are critical countertransference issues involved in the therapist's own fears of death and suicide,[18] it is essential that these be confronted by the therapist and other caretaking personnel in some open and systematic way (such as in staff meetings).

4. The therapist must insist that they, the patient and physician *together*, communicate the suicidal potential to important figures in the environment, both professional staff and family members. This therapeutic intervention with the family is directed against the possibility of psychosocial alienation, based typically on withdrawal by the patient and denial by the family. Suicidal intent must not be part of therapeutic confidentiality in a hospital setting.

5. The psychotherapeutic focus is not initially on past object relations, but rather on whether the patient believes his current human relationships and life situation have become intolerable. The therapist should explore by direct question, if necessary, the development and extent of such belief or conviction. Particularly important is the intensity and significance of such convictions in promoting the suicidal alternative.[3]

These five initial steps are considered essential as a form of crisis intervention. They lead on to the next phase which centers around the patient's perception of reality.

MANAGEMENT OF "REALITY CONCLUSIONS"

The initial intervention is directed at obtaining information concerning the patient's current conscious thoughts and intentions in regard to suicide. A continued monitoring approach requires that the therapist be particularly aware of his patient's reality situation and the way in which it has been understood and internalized by his patient. This becomes the central to therapeutic concern and interest but in no way minimizes the importance of dynamic and developmental factors in the etiology of suicidal potential. Psychoanalytic explanation of super-ego factors and of aggressive impulses in the dynamic unconscious to be crucial for suicide[12] is important. However it is crucial for the purpose of monitoring suicidal potential to stress that there is also *conscious* or *preconscious* evidence available in the form of the patient's convictions about "reality," since psychodynamic patterns do not have short-term predictive value for suicide.[26] This is of particular value in the initial stages since the concept of a patient's conviction about reality and his consciously intended behavior are more accessible than psychodynamic conflicts.

There are enormously varied (intrapsychic, interpersonal and situational) factors which can lead a person to relatively fixed and (to him) final convictions about reality. His reality is intolerable[25] and ungratifying; he cannot achieve those goals in life that he regards as making life worth living; there is therefore no point in any longer trying actively to achieve his goals. Not all such convictions about reality will be experienced as a rational view expressible in language. For example, in schizophrenic patients with severe ego regression, the rigid conviction about reality is experienced not in the time perspective, but in intensity of the experience and eventually in a compulsion to action.

When the hospitalized patient acknowledges such a "reality conclusion," it must be defined as such and reacted to by the therapist with immediate suicidal precautions and by enlisting help from other professionals and the patient's family. The patient must not be allowed the opportunity at this point to prove his determination, or to interpret therapeutic neutrality as rejection or a sign of helplessness in response to helplessness. Reality conclusion is used here to refer to a person's conscious attitude toward a coherent portion of this consciously apperceived (internal and external) reality which he assumes to be final and unchangeable, so that efforts to alter it are meaningless or pointless. The stress upon the person's apperception of an incapacity to alter reality in this definition of reality conclusion is consistent with Glover's[13] definition of reality testing and as the capacity to achieve essential gratifications from potentially available libidinal objects. The concept of reality conclusion is also related to Erikson's concept of actuality[9] in that both stand in contradistinction to "objective" reality. Of course, what a person apperceives as reality in this definition may be very far from consensual reality and in fact may constitute a grossly pathologic distortion of consensual reality based on unconscious factors.

For the disturbed patient who attempts suicide, there is always, in our experience, a definite point in time at which he has made a pathologically distorted organization of his internal and external reality into a rigidly maintained and encompassing picture of helplessness and hopelessness.[17] This rigid conviction is accompanied by affects characteristic of the particular patient's way of experiencing depression. These affects, though with some variation, are experienced as painful until the patient has arrived at the self-destructive "solution" to the reality conclusion. When he decides to kill himself, he may experience a wide range of more pleasurable affects (for example, relief or angry triumph) perhaps because he no longer feels helpless. This alleviation of helplessness is responsible for altering the mood and explains most examples of the paradoxical clinical phenomenon that depressed patients frequently seem improved immediately before their suicide.

The reality conclusion of an ungratifying world must be understood by the therapist and eventually by the patient in terms of object relations. Careful examination reveals that the suicidal patient no longer expects gratifying contact with new or old objects[13,21] nor does he gain sufficient sustenance from his old internalized objects (namely, his ego ideal and object representations[14]) to ward off his conclusions of helplessness and hopelessness in the fact of his human needs, limitations and aspirations.[1]

Since the patient's reality conclusions which distort his conceptions of reality into an endlessly painful situation are final, so far as he is concerned, they are frequently accompanied by negativism and withdrawal. Hence the patient may not trouble himself to communicate them in traditional therapy. He may be living and experiencing a different reality than his therapist is aware of. Unless this gap can be bridged within the context of the transference and therapeutic alliance, this is a critical and explosive time in such a patient's life; the result may be suicide. A virtue of the technique of monitoring is that there is a built-in safeguard making it almost immediately apparent that communication has failed, or indicating suicidal intention has become fixed and therefore other treatment modalities such as greater restrictions, an increase or change in drugs, and/or EST are indicated.

Many patients live for a long period (or even indefinitely) insulated against the underlying conclusion of an ungratifying reality without deciding to commit suicide. They may for example turn instead to the imaginary objects of an autistic world or oblivion provided by an addiction. An addict who loses interest in his addictive substance (typically the alcoholic) is thrown back on his underlying conviction of hopelessness and becomes a serious suicidal risk. The same is true of a schizophrenic who suddenly abandons fantasy for a reality that contains no gratifying objects. The danger is particularly great if the conclusion of a finally ungratifying reality cannot be shared with anyone; then there will be no possibility for making it less final, or for reconsidering its basis in the light of corrective reality testing. Instead this conclusion is likely to extend further into yet more distorted and ungratifying representations of reality, and to become more charged, final and tightly rationalized. Hence it eventually may precipitate the decision for suicidal action, or suicide will follow a minimal additional stress that strengthens or confirms the underlying conclusion. Furthermore when a patient has reached this point, the possibility of "opportunity" for suicide may achieve the intensity of a compulsion.

The alteration of such pathologic reality conclusions can be achieved by the patient in psychotherapy in either of two ways: (1) by identification with the more objectively realistic views of another person[20]; or (2) by mutual understanding and reconsideration of perceptions, thoughts and feelings in the context of another person's (the therapist's) views (that is, by consensual validation). Neither of these mutative situations can be achieved without the continuing presence of a meaningful object relationship. Therefore the recognition of alienation and its circumvention by the creation of a new and important relationship is crucial to the patient's survival. If the patient does not find a therapist who challenges and confronts his pathologic reality conclusion, he may turn instead, with his conviction unshaken, to suicidal action or to another suicidal patient and there find the "validation" of his conclusion that permits suicide or even a suicidal pact.

The approach of bringing these conclusions and the loneliness they imply into the open, can potentially alter alienation at least at the conscious level and permit not only the gratifying sense of sharing a "secret" with the therapist, but also can be a foundation from which alienation from other important figures can be explored and altered. The therapist's insistence on sharing his knowledge of suicidal intention with all the important family members forces a major interpersonal confrontation. Typically the important family members tend to minimize suicidal attempts. The emotional experience of this shared confrontation can open up avenues for new kinds of family interaction and thus create the possibility of changing patterns within the family. The enlistment of other professionals in the crisis protects the therapist as well as the patient since it dilutes the countertransference rescue fantasy as well as lightening the burden of responsibility, while at the same time making other treatment parameters available for the patient. New patterns of family and professional interaction can promote useful therapeutic experiences outside the limits of the therapeutic hour. Several authors have emphasized that unless specific new patterns of object relations or new ego adaptations to reality are achieved, the potential for suicide recurs.[15,16] Our experience confirms this impression and explains our emphasis in the treatment of the suicidal patient on reality considerations as opposed to analyzing complex psychodynamics.

The treatment approach we recommend is time consuming and expensive in human and financial terms. It is not meant to replace pharmacotherapy or EST. It will not work for all patients or all therapists. Therefore neither its use nor the use of other types of therapy with potentially suicidal patients can be recommended as universally applicable. However even patients who have had EST or drugs may, when returned to the community, be confronted by experiences which reevoke their convictions of a hopeless reality. It is therefore essential that psychiatrists be aware that with every suicidal patient the preservation of life may eventually depend on the possibility of a kind of communication which leads to a new human encounter.

REFERENCES

1. BIBRING, E.: The Mechanism Of depression. In: Greenacre, P., (Ed.): Affective Disorders. New York, International Universities Press, 1953.
2. BIBRING, E.: Psychoanalysis and the Dynamic Psychotherapies. J. Am. Psychoanalyt. Ass. 2:745, 1954.
3. BJERG, K.: The Suicidal Life Space: Attempts at a Reconstruction from Suicide Notes. In: Schneidman, E. S. (Ed.): Essays in Self-Destruction. New York, Science House, Inc., 1967.
4. BLOOM, V.: An Analysis of Suicide at a Training Center. Am. J. Psychiat. 123: 918, 1967.
5. COHEN, E., MOTTO, J., AND SEIDEN, R.: An Instrument for Evaluating Suicide Potential: A Preliminary Study. J. Psychiat. 122:886, 1966.
6. CRAWFORD, J. P., AND WILLIS, J. H.: Double Suicide in Psychiatric Hospital Patients. Brit. J. Psychiat. 112:1231, 1966.
7. DeLONG, W. B., AND ROBINS, E.: The Communication of Suicidal Intent Prior to Psychiatric Hospitalization: A Study of 87 Patients. Am. J. Psychiat. 117: 695, 1961.
8. DUBLIN, L. I.: Suicide: A Public Health Problem. In: Schneidman, E. S. (Ed.): Essays in Self-Destruction, Chapter 12. New York, Science House, Inc., 1967.
9. ERIKSON, E. H.: Reality and Actuality. J. Am. Psychoanal. Ass. 10:451, 1962.
10. ETTLINGER, R. W.: Suicides in a Group of Patients Who had Previously Attempted Suicide. Acta Psychiatrica Scandinavica, 40:364, 1964.
11. FARBEROW, N. L., AND SCHNEIDMAN, E. S. (Eds.): The Cry for Help. New York, McGraw-Hill, 1961.
12. FREUD, S.: Mourning and Melancholia (1917). In: Standard Edition, Vol. 14. London, Hogarth Press, 1957.
13. GLOVER, E.: Technique of Psychoanalysis. (Rev. Ed.) New York, International Universities Press, 1958.
14. JACOBSON, E.: The Self and the Object World. Psychoanalytic Study of the Child. 9:75, 1954.
15. LESSE, S.: The Psychotherapist and Apparent Remissions in Depressed Suicidal Patients. Am. J. Psychother. 19:436, 1965.
16. MOSS, L. M., AND HAMILTON, D. M.: Psychotherapy of the Suicidal Patient. Am. J. Psychiat. 112:814, 1956.
17. NEURINGER, C.: The Cognitive Organization of Meaning in Suicidal Individuals. J. Gen. Psychol. 76:91, 1967.
18. NOYES, R.: The Taboo of Suicide. Psychiat. 31:173, 1968.
19. POKORNY, A. D.: A Follow-Up Study of 618 Suicidal Patients. Am. J. Psychiat. 122:1109, 1966.
20. RAPAPORT, D.: Cognitive Structure. In: Gill, M. (Ed.): The Collected Papers of David Rapaport. New York, Basic Books, 1967.
21. RAPAPORT, D.: Edward Bibring's Theory of Depression. In: Gill, M. (Ed.): The Collected Papers of David Rapaport. New York, Basic Books, 1967.
22. ROBINS, E., SCHMID, E. H., AND O'NEAL, A.: Some Interrelations of Social Factors and Clinical Diagnosis in Attempted Suicide: A Study of 109 Patients. Am. J. Psychiat. 114:221, 1957.

547

23. ROBINS, E., GASSNER, S., KAYES, J., WILKINSON, R. H., AND MURPHY, G. E.: The Communication of Suicidal Intent: A Study of 134 Consecutive Cases of Successful Suicide. Am. J. Psychiat. 115:724, 1959.

24. SCHNEIDMAN, E. S., AND FARBEROW, N. L. (Eds.): Clues to Suicide. New York, McGraw-Hill, 1957.

25. SIFNEOS, P. E., GORE, C., AND SIFNEOS, A. C.: Psychiatric Study of Attempted Suicide as Seen in a General Hospital. Am. J. Psychiat. 112:883, 1956.

26. STONE, A.: A Syndrome of Serious Suicidal Intent. Arch. Gen. Psychiat. 3:331, 1960.

27. STONE, A. A., AND SHEIN, H. M.: Psychotherapy of the Hospitalized Suicidal Patient. Amer. J. Psychother. 22:15, 1968.

28. STOTLAND, E., AND KOBLER, A.: Life and Death of a Mental Hospital. Seattle, University of Washington Press, 1965.

29. WEISMAN, A. D., AND HACKETT, T. P.: The Dying Patient. Forest Hosp. Publ. 1:16, 1962.

PART XIV

FORENSIC
CONSIDERATIONS

Privileged Communication and Right of Privacy in Diagnosis and Therapy

by Ralph Slovenko, Ll.B. and Gene L. Usdin, M.D.

PRESENT-DAY medical privilege laws offer only a modicum of assurance that communications in psychotherapy are protected from disclosure, and the fact that many of the problems of psychiatry are virginal insofar as these laws are concerned adds to the uncertainty of the protection that they afford. With lawsuits becoming a national pastime, there is every reason to believe that hitherto disregarded potentials of litigation concerning privileged communication and confidentiality will arise with increased frequency.

Privilege: Its Meaning

Pretrial discovery and proof at a trial are governed by procedural rules called rules of evidence. One group of these rules is known as "privileges," which permit the exclusion of evidence, although relevant, on the theory that the matter is not as great as some other social value served by suppressing the evidence.[1] A privilege of non-disclosure applies in all states to communications (and observations) by a client to his attorney, to communications of husband and wife, and in some jurisdictions to communications by a penitent to his priest, by a client to his accountant, and by an informer to a newspaper reporter or to the government. While about thirty-six American states have a physician-patient privilege,[2] these statutes are so riddled with qualifications and exceptions that they do not adequately meet the needs of patients in psychotherapy.[3]

Psychiatrists, being licensed in the practice of medicine, are included within the riddled statutory privilege accorded to "physicians." Georgia in 1959 and Connecticut in 1961 enacted a specific privilege for communications between psychiatrist and patient, but these statutes, too, fail to cover many problems peculiar to psychotherapy.[4] Psychiatrists and

551

others have pointed out the great social harm that may be done to countless numbers of patients, ex-patients and future patients by even a rare subpoena of a psychiatrist to testify. Freud expressed the need for confidentiality thus: "The whole undertaking becomes lost labour if a single concession is made to secrecy."[5]

Contrary to the belief of many psychiatrists, privilege (when it exists) belongs to the patient, not to the physician. The psychiatrist therefore can be compelled to testify when his patient or ex-patient so desires. The patient is given legal control over his destiny, irrespective of other factors.[6] The patient may believe, quite unrealistically, that testimony of his psychotherapist may aid his legal position. A patient's waiver of the privilege may conceivably be a self-destructive technique; it may be an expression of hostility toward the psychiatrist; or it may be an attempted repetition of an early power struggle. An attempt even to clarify to a patient why it would be inadvisable to call upon the therapist to testify can be markedly prejudicial to effective therapy, especially when it comes at an inappropriate stage in treatment.

PROBLEMS OF PRIVILEGE

The ordinary medical statute, and classical psychoanalysis, envisions a one-to-one physician-patient relationship. Yet a one-to-one psychotherapeutic relationship is not always justified as a matter of treatment. Child therapy can never be a strictly two-person arrangement. It is increasingly accepted that the one-to-one psychotherapeutic relationship alone, analytically oriented or otherwise, does not meet the needs of the schizophrenic inpatient. The family unit and the therapeutic team have vital roles to play. However, the law has traditionally taken the position that disclosure to a person not included within the statute terminates the privilege. The law equates a disclosure to a third person with a general publication to the world. Hence, the logic has it that since "the world knows about it, why should not the court?"

With this as a background, let us consider various situations and problems that arise in the practice of psychiatry.

Domestic Cases

One area where the privilege is frequently asserted is in domestic matters, among which are cases of divorce, "alienation of affections," and custody of children.

(1) Where there is no privilege, psychiatrists in contested divorce cases could be asked to testify regarding the "fault" (e.g., adultery or brutality or criminality) of the patient-spouse. Patients involved in

marital infidelity or sexual deviation may fear litigation and consequently might not speak as freely if they suspected that the psychiatrist could be compelled to testify. It is to be recalled that most states penalize as criminal practically all sex activity other than the most conventional heterosexual act; hence, almost any clinical details of sexual material could conceivably be the start of criminal action as well as divorce proceeding against the patient.[7]

By the time spouses turn to a psychiatrist for help in working out marital difficulties, the marriage is often already in severe trouble. There are times when psychotherapy does not avert divorce, but rather ends in it. Many marriages are contracted out of neurotic purposes, and with the cure of the neurosis, separation and divorce may be a healthy solution. Those states which have lax divorce laws (such as divorce on the basis of a short period of living separate and apart) avoid allegations of fault, but in other states, where a petitioner is put to proof of fault in order to dissolve the marriage, the testimony of the psychiatrist who has treated one of the spouses would be highly pertinent (the law here out of pragmatic considerations labels one spouse as being "bad" or at "fault" and does not consider the neurotic interaction and mutual provocation which takes place between the partners).

A psychiatrist during the course of therapy may see both spouses as patients, either separately or jointly. Usually treatment of husband and wife is conducted independently by two therapists, but there are situations, such as preparatory interviews to analysis, and marital maladjustment and family problems which are not to be psychoanalyzed, in which both spouses are seen effectively by the same therapist. In such cases the legal question arises whether or not the psychiatrist can testify on behalf of the spouse who wants him to testify. The opponent spouse can apparently claim privilege as to communications obtained from him and observations made of him by the psychiatrist. Yet, by seeing the opponent spouse in therapy, the psychiatrist will naturally be affected in his evaluation and testimony on behalf of the proponent spouse.[8] No medical statute expressly covers the problem.

(2) Where there is no privilege, psychiatrists can be called upon in "alienation of affections" cases to testify whether or not a third person alienated the patient-spouse's affections away from the other spouse. In a case in Illinois, which at the time had no medical statute, counsel for Mr. X sought to question his wife's psychiatrist concerning information she had revealed during psychiatric consultations.[9] The Illinois trial court excused the psychiatrist from testifying. The decision, however, is generally considered without justification in law, as Illinois had no medical statute. In legal circles, it is generally considered that had the case

553

been appealed to a higher court, the psychiatrist would have been instructed to testify or would have faced punitive action for contempt. The fact that a trial judge and a witness take the law into their own hands is cause for concern. Rights which exist *sub rosa* do not lend dignity to the law. Yet, rather than reveal confidences, many psychiatrists claim that they would risk contempt charges.

(3) Statistically, about 40 per cent of the 400,000 divorces granted in this country each year involve children. Where there is no privilege, a psychiatrist who treats a child, or one of the spouses, may be subpoenaed to testify in a case involving custody of the child.

In child therapy especially, psychiatrists are likely to involve other members of the family in the treatment process. "Environmental manipulation" may be essential in the treatment of children. As the parents in this situation are strictly speaking not "patients," there is little assurance that the privilege under the orthodox law will be held applicable. Although there was no general publication to the world, a third person —someone other than the physician and patient—received the information and, in the eyes of the law, confidentiality has been "profaned." Under the Connecticut statute enacted in 1961, unlike under other statutes, the patient has a privilege to prevent a witness from disclosing communications between members of the patient's family and the psychiatrist.

In child custody actions, one spouse may contend that the other spouse is mentally ill and therefore incompetent to have custody.[10] Expert testimony regarding relative degrees of incompetency of the parents in borderline situations could place the psychiatrist in an omniscient, and undesirable, role. In this situation testimony could be compelled from the psychiatrist which might influence the legal decision in a way contrary to health. The psychiatrist may be required to reveal material contrary to present cultural standards but not necessarily contradictory to good parenthood.

The fact of psychiatric treatment of itself is sometimes utilized as a bargaining device against the patient-spouse in reaching a property and custody settlement. A patient-spouse, particularly one who is seeking custody of the children, is quite often willing to give in and make little or no demands, even though the conduct of the other has been outrageous. The threat of revelation of the history of psychiatric treatment, should the case be contested, often results in the patient-spouse conceding to an unfavorable agreement. Individuals are sensitive to such exposure. When divorce and custody cases are contested, attempts are made to use a history of psychiatric treatment to imply that the patient-spouse was at fault, hence not entitled to alimony or to custody of the children. The traditional medical privilege protects the content but not the fact of treatment visits.

Personal Injury Cases

In suits for personal injuries, the privilege is considered waived by the patient by virtue of his instituting the litigation. As one legal scholar has stated, the patient cannot make the medical statute both a sword and a shield.[11] The confidence of the medical consultation is considered no longer necessary, because, in bringing suit, the patient makes his physical or mental health a matter of public record. Furthermore, it is said that a good-faith claimant suing for personal injuries would not object to the testimony of any physician who examined or treated him, but rather would want the physician to testify.

The psychiatrist is sought to testify about "psychological trauma" or predisposed factors or pre-existing illness. However, therapy may be jeopardized by testimony of the treating psychiatrist; as a result, rightful causes of action may go by the board when therapy is considered more important by the patient than the outcome of the litigation. Yet, there is another way. Other evidence is usually available. Medical evidence no longer depends only upon the subpoena of the attending or treating physician. Modern court technique may make use of a non-treating medical expert. Under the Federal Rules of Civil Procedure and in states that have adopted similar rules, the trial court may order examination by a physician of a person whose mental or physical condition is in controversy.[12] The rule does not invade the confidentiality of communication. The patient is aware that he is not in a confidential relationship with the examining physician, and he retains his privilege regarding communications with his treating physician. The promise of confidentiality is essential for therapy, but not for diagnosis. It is true that cooperation with the examining psychiatrist will lead to a more reliable report. The party usually cooperates with the appointed physician; if he does not, this will come out at the trial and work to his prejudice. The psychiatrist's report will include the fact of non-cooperation. It is true that the testimony of the treating physician might be very valuable, but in considerable measure the second-best evidence of the appointed examining physician is usually adequate. There is no need to say that suit for personal injuries waives the medical privilege. Confidentiality of the treatment relationship is still essential, even though, in bringing suit, the patient makes his health a matter of public record. From the viewpoint of therapy, it would seem desirable to retain the privilege for the treating physician even in suits claiming damages for mental anguish. At the extreme, the patient might be penalized by dismissal of the case, that is, by presuming fraud on the part of the patient unless he himself waives the privilege. An automatic waiver or exception to the privilege, on the other hand, would allow opposing counsel, over the patient's objection, to put the attending psychiatrist on the stand and to require him to disclose confidences.

Will Cases

In will contest cases, the testamentary capacity of the patient is often under inquiry.[13] The rule in many jurisdictions is that death terminates the privilege. Thus, a legatee to a will in testamentary actions, or a beneficiary of a life insurance policy, cannot claim the privilege of the deceased patient, and the physician cannot insist on remaining silent.[14] As previously mentioned, the privilege belongs to the patient and not to the physician. As a result, the psychiatrist may be placed in the position of revealing scandalous conduct not only of the testator but also of family members.

Some law firms, at the time of preparation of a will, assemble proof that might be needed in the event of a will contest. Statements are taken from law witnesses who can establish, if any issue is later raised, that the testator was of sound mind. However, if a psychiatrist is called in to examine the testator, and a will contest should later occur, the argument would inevitably then be made that there must have been grave misgivings about the testator's mental competency, otherwise a psychiatrist would not have been called in.[15] To avoid suspicion, law firms can make it a matter of ordinary routine by regularly resorting to psychiatric evaluation even though the testator clearly has capacity to make a valid will.

Actions on Life and Accident Insurance Policies

Suits involving life and accident insurance policies often concern the truth of the insured's representations as to his health. Here, the insurer may desire to introduce testimony of the insured's physician to show fraud on the part of the insured in making his application. The medical privilege may be circumvented quite easily by the insurer by inserting in the application a provision whereby the insured waives his right to the privilege, for both himself and his beneficiary. As death usually terminates the privilege, a psychiatrist or any physician can be compelled to testify regarding a suicide which might affect payment of an insurance policy.

556

Personnel Screening

The law's requirement that communications relate to treatment leaves unprotected those made to a psychiatrist involved in screening persons who may be seeking employment, insurance or school admission. Furthermore, as in the case of insurance companies, business firms frequently insert in applications for employment a provision calling for waiver to the privilege, thereby opening the courtroom door to the treating physician.

Hospital Records

Mental illness, especially hospitalization in a mental institution, carries a stigma. Once a person has a record of having been in a mental hospital, the public at large, both formally in terms of employment and other restrictions, and informally in terms of day-to-day social treatment, considers him to be set apart. Public disclosure of hospitalization does not allow the patient any easy return to the community. The protection of secrecy afforded by the law in many jurisdictions leaves much to be desired.

The hospital setting is a situation where a one-to-one psychotherapeutic relationship is impossible. Indeed, every attendant and nurse in a psycho-therapeutic hospital is urged to be more than attendant or nurse—to be also a therapist. Hospital records are inevitably passed into the hands of nurses, social workers and clerks. Furthermore, treatment in a hospital requires an organized effort on the part of all members as a therapeutic team, and they must be given such information as will make their efforts meaningful and helpful. Since so many people know about the patient and have the information, courts in many states take the position that the medical privilege does not protect the record from subpoena.

In view of their possible use in court, it is important to note that hospital records are all too frequently poorly kept, due to the overload of patients, shortness of time for adequate recording, or negligence of the physician. Staff members often do not feel sufficiently confident to record, or they are too busy to record anything but acts of disobedience. Furthermore, apart from considerations of time, able psychiatrists may purposefully keep information in the record to a minimum to prevent sadistic members on the staff, attendants or nurses, from using the information to torment the patient (although an institution with such a staff is obviously not much of a hospital). As a result, physicians and other staff members when called to court have often found themselves squirming in the witness chair trying to justify or excuse an awkward, irresponsible or inadequate recording in the hospital record, on which

557

the legal profession perhaps unduly places great value.[16] Impressions derived from reading case summaries or test reports are often misleading.

Some states have provided by special statute that hospital records are privileged from public scrutiny. For example, Louisiana's statute provides: "The charts, records, reports, documents and other memoranda prepared by physicians, surgeons, psychiatrists, nurses, and employees in the public hospitals of Louisiana, public mental health centers and public schools for the mentally deficient to record or indicate the past or present condition, sickness or disease, physical or mental, of the patients treated in the hospitals are exempt [from public scrutiny], except when the condition of a patient admitted to a general hospital is due to an accident, poisoning, negligence or presumable negligence resulting in any injury, assault or any act of violence or a violation of the law".[17] The records of "public mental health centers" are considered to include records of guidance centers, mental health treatment centers, evaluation centers, and centers for the treatment of alcoholics.

Although statutes may provide for hospital records, applications for employment, insurance or school often question the applicant about previous hospitalization or treatment for mental illness. Honesty begets a truthful answer on the part of the applicant. Some may consider that such inquiry constitutes an undue invasion of an individual's right of privacy. However, the courts generally hold that a false answer constitutes misrepresentation. This is another example of the stigma of treatment for mental illness. The result is that many persons defer treatment, much to their detriment. It has been suggested that patients should receive legislative protection against injury of this type.

When information is withheld as confidential, health agencies and others complain that they cannot obtain necessary information to institute preventive health or disease control measures. In certain research, identification of the patient is unnecessary (for example, number of cases of hepatitis), but other research cannot be accomplished without names of patients and other information (for example, follow-up studies of children seen in guidance clinics). To remedy this situation somewhat, seven states have passed laws protecting members of committees and hospital groups engaged in special studies of morbidity and mortality.[18] In general, the statutes provide that all information used in the course of medical study shall be confidential; that such information shall not be admissible as evidence; and that the furnishing of such information shall not subject any person or institution to damages. [19] The statutes in effect provide that disclosures made for scientific studies are not to be considered a public disclosure which would terminate the privilege.

While the hospital record and the records of physicians or health officers are generally kept confidential, the judicial record on commitment is traditionally considered a public record and in the absence of express legislation the hearing and the resulting records are available to one and all. It is to be noted that in this country court commitment is the procedure most commonly used in the admission of patients to mental hospitals.[20] The model Draft Act Governing Hospitalization of the Mentally Ill, adopted, however, in only a few states, makes confidential the records of courts, health officers, and hospitals involved in the commitment process.[21] There is precedent for maintaining the secrecy of judicial commitment records; adoption records and juvenile records are kept private.

In those states which join hospitalization (commitment) and incompetency (interdiction) proceedings, further difficulties arise. For example, when a patient, even when discharged, proposes to sell property, prospective purchasers and title companies would have a legitimate interest in inquiring as to the patient's status (that is, whether he is on conditional release and whether the incompetency has been judicially removed). Otherwise, the purchaser's title to the property would be voidable. The Draft Act recommends complete separation of hospitalization and incompetency proceedings. It provides in effect that a person is not deprived of his right to sell or buy property, execute documents, enter into contracts, or vote because he has been hospitalized as mentally ill. A person requiring treatment in a hospital is not necessarily incapable of exercising these various rights.

Yet there are problems even when a person is not adjudicated incompetent by virtue of commitment. During the course of hospitalization, or afterwards, it may be essential to institute incompetency proceedings for the appointment of a guardian (curator). In doing so, attorneys often communicate with the hospital seeking evidence to justify the proceedings. More often than not, the proceeding is in the interest of the patient or ex-patient. It seeks to appoint someone to manage the patient's affairs, which the patient may be unable to do while hospitalized or afterwards. Not all incompetency proceedings, as the myth would have it, are maliciously instituted by members of the family to rob the patient. However, the patient on occasion does not consent to release of information; he does not want to be tagged an incompetent. The result is a begging of the question: incompetency proceedings are instituted because it is felt that the patient does not have the legal capacity to consent, yet hospital cooperation is refused because the patient declines to consent.[22]

When it exists, the privilege protects the doctor's notes, memos, appointment books, financial records, et cetera, but, as the privilege belongs to the patient, he may waive the privilege and compel their disclosure in the courtroom, just as they may be subpoenaed in states where there is no law granting privilege.

There is considerable discussion in the literature on the medical doctor's duty out of the courtroom to tell the "truth" to a patient about his illness. Hospitals encounter similar requests by patients for a copy of their records, purely for their own information. Yet there are circumstances under which the hospital or doctor cannot, for the patient's own good, tell him the "whole truth." The paranoid patient is the type of psychiatric patient that most frequently requests a copy of his record; compliance with the request would further aggravate his mental condition. While a doctor is ethically bound to do whatever is best for his patient and to avoid doing him harm, there is little or no legal authority bearing upon the right to withhold information from a patient. A patient goes to a physician for information, which he may need in planning out his life (e.g., making a will or disposing of his property). Diagnosis implies prognosis, and there are times when the information works to the detriment of the patient, as illustrated in the film "The Last Weekend," where relying on an erroneous diagnosis of a fatal disease, Alec Guinness goes out to a luxurious resort for a last fling, and is ironically killed in an automobile accident. It ought further to be considered that physicians make diagnoses with an eye toward disposition (one diagnosis is made for the court, another for Blue Cross, and so on). The Judicial Council of the AMA advises (presumably considering physical illnesses) that the decision in a non-court situation to give the contents of a report to a patient rests with the doctor who knows all the circumstances involved in the situation; but in pretrial discovery or in a courtroom, on the basis of a subpoena, the patient may require production of the records when they are pertinent to litigation.[23]

Medical records of a private physician are considered his property, but they are subject to "a limited property right" on the part of his patients with respect to the information which they contain. The patient can therefore demand disclosure, not only to himself, but also, for example, to an insurance company. Psychiatrists would argue that a different principle is needed for patients in therapy. A psychiatric record, unlike an x-ray, might reasonably be said to be the entire work product of the therapist. There is also the pragmatic consideration that psychiatric records can readily be destroyed or they may be prepared in a way unintelligible to others.

Ownership of records of patients seen in guidance centers, etc., presents a special problem. On the termination of the psychiatrist's employment with the center, the question arises as to the proper custodian of the records developed during the term of employment.[24] It has been urged that psychiatric records are the property of the psychiatrist preparing them and are not subject to "transfer" to another psychiatrist coming to the center, or to a court or social agency, unless the records were prepared in the first instance by the request of such other person or body. This argument presupposes that the center and the replacing psychiatrist will not maintain the confidentiality of the records. As we see guidance clinics in operation, physicians go and come, but the records remain; otherwise the clinic would be very much damaged by the departure of a physician. The records remain where they have always been; they are not "transferred." Patients usually return to a clinic irrespective of the presence of a particular physician. Also, taking a page from the law on self-incrimination, we might note that it has been many times held that "quasi public records" as well as "public records" are deemed to belong to the government, and the recordkeeper therefore may not object to their introduction as evidence.[25]

Psychologists, Social Workers and Counselors

Professional practitioners of psychotherapy are almost as varied as the range of persons they seek to help. The largest group of professionals trained to conduct psychotherapy are psychiatrists, numbering about thirteen thousand in this country, and they are supplemented by well over four thousand clinical psychologists and five thousand social workers. Clinical psychologists and psychiatric social workers are members of treatment teams in hospitals and clinics under psychiatric supervision, but they also practice independently in social agencies, family agencies, marriage counseling centers, and so on, and as private practitioners. In addition, a wide variety of counselors and guides (such as marriage counselors, rehabilitation and vocational counselors, parole officers, group workers, and clergymen) may use psychotherapeutic principles with their clientele. The different disciplines tend to describe their activities in different terms, as, for example, medical and quasi-medical practitioners "treat" patients, psychiatric social workers do "case work" with clients, clergymen offer "pastoral counseling", and group workers do "group work."

The medical privilege covers only the physician (the psychiatric and

561

non-psychiatric physician). The protection afforded when other members of the treatment team are involved is nil except that a few states relatively recently have adopted special statutes granting the privilege to psychologists.[26] The attorney-client privilege covers the attorney's agent,[27] but in most states the physician's agent, the nurse, is not generally included within the medical privilege, unless expressly provided by statute.[28] Likewise, psychologists, social workers, counselors and stenographers may not come within the scope of the medical privilege, even when working under psychiatric supervision. Communications to these persons may be compelled in court. This is important to the psychiatrist, who often relies on such persons.

Personnel in probation departments, welfare offices, social agencies, and child guidance clinics frequently have access to case files. Can they be trusted with confidential information? Will they gossip about what they learn from case records? If as a matter of common practice confidentiality is maintained, ought not the law allow a privilege even though there is not a one-to-one relationship? Experiences in hospitals and prisons generally have confirmed the trustworthiness of non-clinical employees (career correctional workers and welfare workers) regarding the confidential material in the case history when the importance of confidentiality has been fully explained to them. Likewise, experiences with teachers also have confirmed that with very infrequent exceptions they are, when properly prepared, as respecting of confidential material as are clinicians, lawyers, or other professional people.[29] Actually, there is no better use for case histories, so costly in their preparation, than that their findings be used by those who are involved responsibly in the care or treatment of the patient. In institutions, basic psychotherapeutic help is provided by the ordinary staff member who spends many hours with the patient or inmate, rather than by the specialist who sees him occasionally and then only briefly. The Connecticut privilege, enacted in 1961, covers communications between any persons who participate, under the supervision of the psychiatrist, in the accomplishment of the objectives of diagnosis or treatment. Other statutes, as stated, do not protect disclosures to non-psychiatric treatment personnel.

Social workers have particular problems regarding adoption and custody reports. The parent adversely affected by the report naturally wants to know the evidence. Yet, disclosure may jeopardize the relationship with the parent for further casework. Also, if reports are disclosed, no one may reveal anything to social workers. Since there is no privilege, social workers in some places resort to subterfuge. Two types of records are made.

562

Group Therapy

Patients in group therapy have transference between themselves, but legally, and strictly speaking, patients *inter se* do not constitute a physician-patient relationship. Hence, it would seem that the medical privilege does not protect against disclosure in court by a member of the group. The privilege exempts only the physician from testifying. To borrow a leaf from the husband-wife privilege, we learn that conversations held in the presence of children and other members of the family are not privileged.[30] Privileges, being derogations from the general law, are narrowly construed by the courts. The law has traditionally considered privileged communications as involving a dyadic relationship: in the case of the medical privilege, a licensed physician and a patient. It is necessary to reformulate the medical privilege in view of group therapy.[31] Given the shortage of psychotherapists, apart from the intrinsic value of group therapy, some therapists even predict a time in the near future when patients will be treated primarily in group situations.[32]

Military Cases

A privilege is not recognized in military law for communications made to medical officers and civilian physicians, although military law does recognize the privilege relationships of attorney-client, husband-wife, and priest-penitent.[33] With a disruption of the inductee's dependency equilibrium, it would appear that the need for a psychotherapy privilege exists to as great a degree in military as in civilian life. Servicemen, away from their homes, look to someone to whom they can entrust their problems and fears. They may turn to a psychiatrist as well as to a priest. In combat, the need for comfort and guidance is even more pronounced.

It might be noted that psychoneurotic and psychotic tendencies are no longer sufficient reason for draft exemption, unless it has incapacitated the individual in civilian life. The revised rules are in contrast to those applied during World War II, when more stringent requirements of emotional stability were in force. It is reported that elaborate psychiatric examinations of inductees are no longer conducted,[34] and as a result, there may be more servicemen needing psychotherapy. Today, then, with greater public acceptance of psychiatry and with more persons seeking psychiatric assistance, there is an increased need for psychiatric services in the military, and a privilege to encourage its use.[35]

There are, of course, cases of neurotic individuals in the military where psychotherapy is contraindicated, just as in the outside world.

563

There are many persons who enlist in the military service to satisfy infantile dependency needs. They are, as Erich Fromm would put it, escaping from freedom. In these cases, therapy is often inadvisable. The professional serviceman is often best left alone, leaving his compensatory system undisturbed. Homosexuals, we might mention, although they are not officially accepted in the armed forces, are found there in goodly numbers. Treatment is not sought or is ineffective where the homosexual is content with his way of life; indeed, the majority of homosexuals defend their form of sexual activity as perfectly normal (one aspect of homosexuality that is often ignored is the extreme dependency shown by homosexuals or by persons having considerable latent homosexuality). Be this as it may, psychiatry has a vital role to play in the military, particularly for the inductee.

Public Security

There are times when revelation may be necessary for the protection of society. This thorny problem was brought to the fore when two National Security Agency employees, Vernon F. Mitchell and William H. Martin defected to the Soviet Union. The psychiatrist, who had seen Mitchell, turned over his records and testified before a secret session of the House Un-American Activities Committee. He stated: "I believe a man loses his right to privileged communication if he defects. Furthermore, if the national security is threatened, I believe the rights of the Government far exceed the rights of individuals." The psychiatrist disclosed problems of family, religion and sex. He was taken to task by a number of general practitioners and psychiatrists.[36]

It is always debatable whether a disclosure can be construed as benefitting the patient or the community. However, revelation of information which is of no benefit to the patient or the community demanded by subpoena is subject to criticism, but disclosure of information without legal compulsion (as apparently happened in the Mitchell situation) is deplorable.[67] The State can ferret out its evidence, and ought to be put to its proof, without impinging on confidential relationships, such as the attorney-client, husband-wife, priest-penitent, as well as the physician-patient relationship.[38]

FBI Director Hoover at one time urged all physicians to report to the Bureau any facts relating to espionage, sabotage or subversive activity coming to their attention. Psychiatrists generally criticized the American Medical Association for cooperating with the federal police and for going even further by urging its members to help catch even the petty thief. Guttmacher attacked this suggestion with wry humor: "It is not too fantastic to predict that before long the physician's inner examining room may resemble a rural post office with its walls plastered with the mugs of wanted felons."[39]

Criminal Cases

Criminal cases are one aspect of the public security problem. A patient in therapy may have committed or may be planning to commit a crime, for example, abortion or adultery. In such cases, the psychiatrist will be in possession of highly incriminating evidence.

Psychoneurotic persons, who constitute the majority of patients in office psychotherapy, try to adapt themselves to the way of society. In general, patients in therapy are not characterized by antisocial activity or by striking inability to pursue ordinary goals. Usually the patient in psychotherapy suffers from an overly strict conscience. The criminal on the other hand has a conscience, if it can be called that, which sets few limits on his behavior. When the exceptional case of a criminal in therapy arises, psychotherapy might provide the best possibility of having the individual return to lawful and gainful pursuits. Thus, without the need of tax-supported incarceration, the goal of rehabilitation might be achieved.[40]

Lunacy Commissions

Psychiatrists and psychologists serve on lunacy commissions as officers or agents of the court,[41] and hence, not being the accused's physician, there is no privilege. Nevertheless, surreptitious psychiatric interrogation of persons accused of crime is condemned, although such persons are not "patients" and revelations are not for the purpose of therapy. Confessions elicited with the aid of hypnosis, narcosis, or other forms of partial removal of inhibitions, especially when induced by the administration of drugs, have uniformly been struck down.[42] It is contrary to medical ethics, as well as against the law, for the police to resort to the relationship of physician and patient to obtain a confession from the accused.[43] Psychiatrists examining persons on court order are cautioned to point out to the examinee that communications are not privileged, notwithstanding the possible loss thereby of valuable information.

The Connecticut statute provides that communications to a psychiatrist in the course of a psychiatric examination ordered by the court are without privilege only on issues involving the person's mental condition (that is, the psychiatrist may testify as to the accused's insanity at the time of the offense or at the time of trial, but he may not report, for example, on the validity of an alibi.)[44] It has been suggested in some quarters that even though the psychiatrist in these cases is an examining rather than a treating physician, there should be a complete privilege, otherwise there can be no effective examination, unless the psychiatrist in one way or another deludes the examinee into believing that there will be confidentiality.[45] The examiner, it is said, cannot take the absurd position of warning the accused not to give him his confidence and then expect to receive information. A complete privilege, however, would preclude cross-examination at the trial and the psychiatrist's report would sound woefully oracular, and would be ineffective.

Presentence Report

The confidentiality of a presentence investigation report of a probation department is a matter which is receiving increased attention.[46] These reports to the court often play a very influential role in the type and the length of sentence given. The issue here is not the right of the defendant to have information withheld from the court, but rather the right of the court to withhold information from the convicted defendant. The District Court of Appeal of Florida recently had an opportunity to indicate, for the first time in the jurisdiction, the status of a presentence investigation report.[47] Counsel for the defendant argued that the right to see a presentence report is basic and fundamental and that to deny him this right is to allow hearsay evidence to stand against him, depriving him of cross-examination and confrontation of witnesses. The court, however, concluded that a presentence report should be treated as a confidential compilation of information for the use of the sentencing judge, and not as a public document, and hence the defendant is not entitled to access thereto. "To strip a presentence investigation report of its confidentiality," the court observed, "would be to divert it also of its importance and value to the sentencing judge, because there might be lacking the frankness and completeness of disclosures made in confidence." Most judges feel that strict adherence to confidentiality in the use of the presentence report has made it possible for the probation officer to obtain for the court a much more accurate picture of the defendant that could be obtained if it were known that the contents of the report were going to be divulged to others. However, there is a sizeable body of opinion which feels very strongly that no presentence report should be so confidential that the defendant should not be given an opportunity to reply to any information entered in it. It would be of considerable assistance to the probation service to have this problem of confidentiality thoroughly considered in an effort to reach some sort of agreement on criteria.[48]

Prison Psychiatry

The use of psychotherapy in prison is so minimal that it hardly merits discussion. Indeed, the majority of jails and prisons, as presently constructed, and as overcrowded as they are, do not even have a suitable place in which to hold sessions. The dining room may not be available until well after the evening meal. The chapel is usually unavailable, but even when it is, smoking is not permitted, and the religious atmosphere is always there. Security precautions forbid meetings in the visiting room at most hours of the day. Attendants feel that their authority over the place is threatened by the therapist, and they resist, actively or passively. In the future, jails and prisons hopefully will change to accommodate advances in penology. In the meantime, consider the privilege of confidentiality in prison psychiatry, as theoretical as it may be.

MacCormick, a prison administrator and criminologist, has said of the prison psychiatrist's obligation of confidentiality: "Giving parole boards access to what is dug up in individual and group therapy would be opening a veritable gold mine to them. But the shaft is sealed to them and to institution administrators, and must be sealed." He maintains, however, that a prison psychiatrist is duty bound to report knowledge of new crimes being planned by the patient.[49] Freedman's viewpoint seems well taken when he retorts: "It is my personal conviction that it is not the role of the psychiatrist to uncover such information under the guise of therapy, if he expects to expose it to the warden. I cannot help feeling that disclosure under these circumstances is a sort of 'psychic entrapment'. The physician ought either to warn his patient beforehand of the reservations he has concerning confidentiality or, having committed himself to secrecy, he should maintain it."[50]

Prisoners are usually distrusting souls. They feel there is no privacy or confidence, and so they do not even want to talk to a therapist, much less talk freely with him. The therapeutic situation hopefully will demonstrate to the prisoner that not all persons are to be mistrusted. Confidentiality is of utmost importance when treating individuals who are basically distrustful of others.

Execution of Sentence and Death Penalty

It appears that termination of the trial ends the defendant's protection by the rules of evidence. As noted, a presentence investigation report relied on by judges in the imposition of sentence is usually not made available to counsel for the defense, as it is considered that information would be unavailable if it were restricted to that given in open court by witnesses subject to cross-examination.

567

An Ohio court has recently ruled that the right of an imprisoned man to counsel does not extend to psychological tests which an attorney would have an unchallenged right to obtain prior to trial.[51]

The imposition of the death penalty is an even more striking example of the principle. The prevailing law in this country on the death penalty is that an insane person, for one reason or another, may not be executed.[52] In the majority of states, the issue of post-conviction insanity may be raised only by the warden (or sheriff) having custody of the prisoner. The United States Supreme Court stated in *Solesbee v. Balkcom*[53] that the manner of procedural effectuation of exemption for insanity is a matter of grace, not of right, and hence the state is under no obligation to provide a hearing. In the *Solesbee* case, the warden refused to allow an outside psychiatrist to examine the prisoner on death's row and refused to allow counsel to inspect the prison's psychiatric records. Thus, the execution of the capital penalty lies very much in the attitude of the warden toward the penalty. A convict, waiting on death's row often for years until legal maneuvers are exhausted, is quite likely to have become psychotic, but the application of the exemption rule usually depends upon the pleasure of the warden.

Waiver of Privilege

It has been suggested that privilege should belong to the physician rather than to the patient. When an individual waives a privilege such as the attorney-client privilege, or the privilege against self-incrimination, the decision is made with full awareness of the material which will be disclosed.[54] But, in psychotherapy it may be detrimental for the patient to see, e.g., the report of projective tests which he has taken and the results of which he has not seen. When the patient waives the psychotherapy privilege, he does not know what he is waiving. It may be harmful to reveal to the patient that he is schizophrenic (whatever that might mean).[55]

The issue is whether the law should allow an individual to make an irrational decision. One clergyman, when threatened by a call to the stand upon waiver of the priest-penitent privilege, said: "It is impossible to see how anyone could or would waive his privilege of confidence in a clergyman unless he is under some kind of pressure and falls into the trap of 'selling his soul for a mess of pottage'."[56]

Competency of Testimony

Incompetency of testimony renders entirely moot the need for privileges, which are needed only to exclude competent evidence. The fundamental test of admissibility of evidence is competency, that is, its trust-worthiness.

On the basis of certain data, hereinafter set out, one might suggest that, even though the patient waives privilege and asks the psychiatrist to make disclosure, the testimony is inadmissible on grounds of incompetency. In effect, the charge is that all psychiatric testimony, especially that of the treating physician, is incompetent for courtroom purposes and of no value. Let us take note of the data:

For one thing, it is said that a therapist cannot within any reasonable degree of accuracy present to the court in a few minutes material that has been produced in years of therapy. At staff conferences, attended by persons experienced in the field, it takes considerable time to present a case report. In the courtroom, the psychiatrist faces a jury reluctant to accept psychiatric theories and unable to evaluate the testimony, particularly when it must be done in summary fashion. Indeed, non-psychiatric physicians complain that psychiatrists talk in gobbledygook and have developed a private jargon of their own, a tower of Babel, resulting in a communication gap between psychiatrists and other physicians.

Second, it is said that "the art of psychiatry outweighs the science." At the 1962 American Psychiatric Association meeting, Dr. Robert Stotler and Dr. Robert H. Geertsma of UCLA related the results of an experiment showing that expert psychiatrists can differ widely in their clinical evaluation of a single case. The two California researchers pointed out that psychiatrists were unable to agree on the diagnosis, prognosis, etiology and other aspects of a case which all had observed equally. Psychiatrists, it is said, make their diagnoses in form of camouflaged social value judgments. It has been suggested that a new system of psychiatric classification is needed, based on the patient's reaction to the therapeutic situation rather than on the standard (and inadequate) clinical nosology. Some say consequently that as long as psychiatry is so much an art and there is so much confusion, psychiatric testimony lacks value for the court.[57]

Third, it might be said that data from free association, fantasies, or memories are not reliable for use in court as they represent the way the person experienced an event, and not necessarily how the event occurred. They are not "facts." Psychic reality is not the same thing as actual reality. In fantasy life, a patient may tell of hidden treasures; its correspondence in reality is not of crucial importance in treatment. A classic example is Freud's case of the young girl whose fantasied sexual traumatic relationship with her father affected her personality, although her father had had no overt sexual contact with the child. As the material revealed in psychotherapy does not deal with reality of the outer

569

world, it would make poor, even prejudicial evidence. The material is often of childhood fantasies and not germane to current activities of the patient.[58] A 13-year-old girl in our culture who claims that she is having sexual relations with every male member of the family is sick whether or not it is the fact of the matter. The therapist is not compelled to check on the outer reality. Furthermore, the therapist does not cross-question his patient. In therapy, the important thing is how the patient looks at herself and the world. But, in the courtroom, in a criminal case, e.g., involving incest or contributing to the delinquency of a minor, it makes a world of difference whether the allegation is in the realm of fantasy or reality. Reik states that psychoanalysis has no contribution to make to evidence of guilt, as it is concerned with mental reality rather than material reality.[59]

There are times when the psychotherapist deliberately participates in the psychosis of a patient by entering the fantasy and from that position attempting to pry the patient loose from his psychosis (John Rosen and Milton Wexler are among the notable exponents of this practice). The procedure, however, has been reported to get out of control. Lindner reported that, as one patient was losing his delusion, larger and larger areas of Lindner's mind were being taken over by the fantasy.[60] Counter-transference and identification with the patient results in a loss of objectivity.

Our reply, in brief, to the suggestion of incompetency of psychiatric testimony:

(1) It is a mistake to restrict the above observation, on the need to summarize, to the psychiatric witness. Every person asked to testify wonders, "How can I possibly report what happened in so short a time?". The practical administration of justice sets limits on the detail which can be required of the testimony of any witness. The court, unlike the scientist, is hampered by limitations of time. It is, therefore, incumbent upon every witness to present his testimony clearly and concisely. It is the task of every expert witness to distill in a few minutes information and knowledge acquired over the years. Indeed, one might say that this is the heart and substance of an expert witness. It is interesting to note, however, that when the psychiatrist avoids his jargon and uses the language of the law, he is admonished not to talk like a lawyer.[61]

(2) As far as the "art of psychiatry outweighing the science" goes, let us refer to one judge who analyzed the value of evidence and the adversary courtroom procedure in this way: "All the witnesses are lying, and everybody knows it, but somehow justice comes out of it." The judge, of course, did not mean to say that witnesses are guilty of perjury, but rather that subjective elements (memory and perception,

feeling and will, attention and thought) are involved in the observation of "facts". In the courtroom, as in science and in every other mode of experience, subjective factors are operative and cannot be eliminated.[62] Furthermore, a single witness is not expected to carry the entire burden of proof. IIe is expected simply to further the inquiry.

(3) It is true that a psychotherapist does not make use of a corps of investigators; a psychotherapist is sedentary, he does not pursue his practice in the homes of his patients or in their places of business. External facts if obtained might in truth, blind him to the inner reality of the patient. Further, a search for evidence may jeopardize the therapist's confidential relationship with the patient. Yet, a psychotherapist is soon able to feel a difference in reports that have no basis in outer reality. Thus, a report of rape keeps changing when there is no correspondence with outer reality. The fact that Lindner was finaly able to write about the delusion as a delusion shows that he was able to get outside of it.

PROBLEMS OF THE RIGHT OF PRIVACY

Privileges, as pointed out, exempt certain confidential communications from the law's command to disclose. When the law does not require disclosure, an individual who breaches confidentiality out of the courtroom may be subjected to a suit for damages for an invasion of privacy (or for defamation). According to the AMA Law Department, one out of seven AMA members have been the target of a malpractice suit or claim.[63] Fortunately for psychiatrists, but unfortunately for patients who learn of breach of privacy, legal suits against psychiatrists for this or other grounds have not as yet occurred with the frequency that they could.[64] Psychiatrists are usually not sued for breach of privacy because patients do not want further to make their life a public spectacle or are not aware that they have a cause of action.

Social Affairs and Corridor Conversation

The First Amendment of the Constitution, protecting free speech, ordains that we are a "public opinion" state. We talk freely about politics, and also about our activities, and we love to gossip. Work constitutes a major part of our life, and many of us find little else to talk about. It is not surprising then to find a tendency among psychotherapists to discuss their patients outside the office, at home, at the club, and at cocktail parties. Sometimes, patients' names are used, and ofttimes the discussion degenerates into mere chatter. Some serious difficulties, for example, have arisen in the treatment of patients in clinics as a result of open discussion of patients in hallways. As a result,

571

patients overhearing the discussion become quite upset and threaten to terminate therapy. There is a clear violation of the patient's right of privacy when treatment material is not kept confidential.[65]

Jeopardy to Patients or Others

It sometimes happens, as pointed out above, that to keep the confidence may jeopardize the patient or society. There may be danger, for example, that the patient will commit suicide. There is danger in an epileptic patient driving a bus, unless his employer is notified. There is danger in an airplane pilot who should be grounded because of mental illness, but who, fearful of losing his job, does not tell his employer. There is harm to the family of a patient who is dissipating, without their knowledge, all of the family's funds and property.

Under the law there is no duty to come to the aid of third parties, but the psychiatrist may act in emergencies. The physician may reveal a confidence when it becomes necessary in order to protect the welfare of the patient or the community. In such situations, the revelation is made only to avert the catastrophe; as the revelation is with just cause, the psychiatrist would not be liable in damages for invasion of privacy.[66] The general public, prospective patients and patients in therapy will not lose faith in the psychiatrist as a keeper of secrets when in cases of emergency he acts contrary to strict and absolute confidentiality. Sooner or later, the patient frequently realizes that the psychiatrist has acted in his interest (which is just the contrary when an opposing party in litigation compels the psychiatrist to testify). However, situations of real emergencies necessitating disclosure are rare.

Child Treatment

"Environmental manipulation," as pointed out, may be essential in the treatment of children. With some children, it is particularly desirable to involve the child's parents in the treatment process. Therapeutic gains with the child himself will often be short-lived unless the parents are also able to change. A meaningful relationship with the psychiatrist often depends upon cooperation. The psychiatrist may find sensitive teachers who may be able, in consultation with the psychiatrist, to contribute effectively to the child's treatment through the teacher-pupil relationship.

The broad treatment approach, however, does not forsake the confidentality of the child's revelations. The psychiatrist, as a matter of good practice, makes clear to both the child and his parents the type of rapport he will have with each. Confidentiality, realistically speaking, is maintained. There is no publication to the world. The psychiatrist is in

572

this situation working with persons who are directly responsible for the patient and who can assist in the treatment.

There are times, however, when it may be necessary to write off the parents. There are various situations: the parents and/or the child may or may not be in treatment. All physicians have encountered psychotic parents who deny treatment to an acutely ill child or who are devastating to the child.

It is reported that physical assaults on children may be "a more frequent cause of death than such well-recognized and thoroughly studied diseases as leukemia, cystic fibrosis and muscular dystrophy, and it may rank with automobile accidents."[67] The percentage of mental assaults can well be imagined to be multifold that number. There is growing support for a law requiring doctors and hospitals to report cases of suspected abuse of children.[68] It is felt by many physicians, however, that such a law would be useless without a clause protecting doctors and hospitals from retaliation by irate parents who are investigated.[69] It may occur, however, that abusive parents may not bring their child to therapy out of fear of a report, or they may take their child out of therapy should abuse be reported.

Political and Other Candidates

We often find individuals running for political office who are extremely sick. Our century has had its share of pathological individuals at the head of government. By running for public office, it might be suggested that an individual is no longer entitled to keep his life and motivations in private, out of the public gaze. It might be said that the community has a right to know. It will be recalled that Senator Wayne Morse, in the course of his fight against the confirmation of Clare Boothe Luce as Ambassador to Brazil, asked Mrs. Luce's doctor if she ever had been under psychiatric treatment. It is occasionally proposed that potential leaders can be scientifically chosen.[70] Seemingly, psychiatrists and psychologists would be first to shun such an omniscient and apparently anti-democratic role. Suppose, among other things, that the individual refuses to submit to examination. Mind-tapping, as Szasz has called it,[71] without consent and cooperation would be a clear violation of constitutional rights. Psychiatrists are already accused of presumptuous interference in political, social, and cultural matters which are not directly pertinent to their medical province, the relief of individual suffering.

Personality tests have inspired the wrath of, among others, Martin L. Gross, whose recent book "The Brain Watchers" has already received wide notice. Gross attacks personality tests on two grounds: first, that the "brain-watching" system is a violation of human rights; and second, that it fails to isolate the qualities which its practitioners (quite wrongly) suppose to be the best. This is apparently a reaction to an overemphasis in past years of the value of psychological testing. It is true that psychological testing leaves something to be desired in measuring an individual's coping mechanisms, therefore the difficulty in predicting performance; however, the fact remains that psychological testing can tell us a great deal about the individual's pathological conflicts.

Yet the uncompromising moralist will say that all individuals, irrespective of whether they are candidates for public office or applicants for employment of school admission, should not even be asked to submit to mind-tapping.[72] As Justice Brandeis put it, in another connection, there is a right "to be let alone." The social values here are claimed to outweigh the objective evidence. A judicial or political decision after all does not rest solely on scientific evidence. It is interesting to recall the 1946 California decision holding that Charlie Chaplin was the father of Miss Berry's child, notwithstanding findings of blood-grouping tests; Chaplin, out of social considerations, was held to bear a responsibility to the girl.

Teaching and Writing

Scientific teaching and writing post a unique and difficult problem for the psychiatrist. This is an area where psychiatrists are especially vulnerable to suit. Non-psychiatric physicians in this regard usually have no difficulty; the configuration of the body can be discussed without anyone recognizing the patient. Psychiatrists are obliged to disguise their clinical data to avoid the recognition of the patient even though it involves detriment to the scientific value of the material.[73] The psychiatrist, more than anyone else, runs the risk of being charged with professional indiscretion. The doctrine of privacy prohibits the public use of identifying characteristic of any individual unless his prior consent has been obtained. The law of privacy makes available significant protection to the patient against the disclosure of intimate facts of his life.

Campus Psychiatry

A number of universities have appointed psychiatrists as part of their health services to examine disciplinary cases and to counsel or treat students. Some colleges, it is believed, require a report on some non-referral as well as on referral students. Campus psychiatry is beset with many problems.

In cases of physical illness, a surgeon operates on a minor only with the consent of the parent (or guardian) except in emergencies. However, in psychotherapy, a minor for one reason or another may not wish that contact be made with his parents. The requirement that a college or a psychiatrist notify the parents of all minors who consult the psychiatrist would destroy service at once. As a consequence, university health services treat students as though they were adults. Although the parents may afford private treatment, university clinics treat students on a long-term basis at a nominal fee when they do not wish to contact their parents. Good practice would require that no one is told about treatment unless the student's permission is obtained or there is a problem involving suicide, potential homicide, or some kind of behavior which is going to handicap markedly the student or his parents. In any case, no action is taken without letting the student know, except in instances of acute psychoses or danger to life.[74]

Some university health services, quite appropriately, notify students of exceptions to confidentiality in the following manner: (1) when a student's mental condition is such that immediate action must be taken to protect the student or others from serious consequence of his illness; and (2) when a student is referred for evaluation and an opinion or recommendation is requested.[75] In the first situation, immediate voluntary or involuntary hospitalization may be arranged and in such cases the college administration and parents are notified as quickly as possible. Cases in the second exception are called administrative referrals and in such situations the student is informed initially that a report will be made to the referring individual or agency, but the actual interview itself remains confidential as far as content is concerned.

Thus, we see that the prevailing practice on notification of parents in the case of treatment of minors for mental illness is, curiously enough, just the opposite of the procedure generally followed, and approved by the law, in the case of treatment of minors for physical illness. In the former case, notification is made only in emergencies; in the latter case, lack of notification in emergencies is legally excused. Of course, the usual reason for the distinction is the element of time.

Communications Between Doctors and Treatment Centers

Proper and efficient care of patients often requires communications between various physicians and hospitals. However, a release of information to other doctors interested in the patient should be cleared, preferably in writing, with the patient. If not handled properly, the physician may be sued for breach of confidentiality.[76]

In the majority of states, hospital records are not as readily available

575

to clinics as they should be, and vice versa, resulting in considerable delay and duplication of effort. There is also marked need for improvement in exchange of information among clinics treating various members of a family. A coordinated mental health program requires the development of a record system that places patient and family history at the finger tips of physicians, clinics and hospitals. A record system similar to medical records of the military has been suggested. Under such a system, records would go with the patient from the hospital to the clinic in his community. If commitment is again necessary or there is a transfer between hospitals, the record would go along with the patient.[77]

The trend, however slow, is toward interrelated medical centers and central medical records. The trend is not only toward interrelated medical institutions, but also collaboration with nursing homes and other institutions. To what extent does a patient by undertaking treatment impliedly give permission to other physicians, and to researchers, recorders and others, to view the records? Apart from legal considerations, exchange and transfer of information should have the approval of the patient, otherwise the therapeutic relationship might be impaired. It is unlikely that a patient will protest a procedure designed to facilitate proper treatment.

Communications with Non-Medical Persons

When making application of one type or another, the patient may be asked and he may acknowledge that he is seeing or has seen a physician or psychiatrist.[78] As a result, the psychiatrist may receive requests for information from an employer, parole board, credit-rating organization, insurance company,[79] welfare department,[80] military,[81] schools or others. An insurance company inquires if the patient feels "insecure"; the football coach asks if the boy has "a sense of belonging"; the police want to know whether a driver's license should be taken away. The patient may regard the therapist as a potential spy or informer even though the information is furnished with his written consent. It is to be noted, as Hollender has pointed out, that the psychiatrist's traditional function has been oriented to treatment and not to public service; the physician's traditional job has been to treat the sick, not to prepare historical reports or explanatory documents.[82]

Fee Collection

In early law physicians could not maintain an action to recover fees for medical services. Fees were regarded as honorable, and not demandable of right. Times have changed. Patients sue now physicians for malpractice; physicians sue patients for payment of their bills. In some states the physician is allowed not only a cause of action, but also a ranking over other creditors.[83]

Yet, even in our "age of commercialism," the roles of creditor and debtor, issues of fairness of charges, promptness of payment—especially at times of emotional tension—are generally considered not to promote "warm human relations" or "mutual confidence." The psychiatrist is peculiarly sensitive about his standing in the community. He has special problems in enforcing his claim for payment of his bill; he is reluctant to engage the services of a bill-collecting agency or to bring the matter to court.

The Report of the Group for the Advancement of Psychiatry (GAP) states: "Psychiatrists are less likely to use such services since they tend to discuss financial matters with their patients more fully and reach agreements more often than do other physicians. While we will not argue the pros and cons of using such service, it should be pointed out that under some circumstances, when an account is turned over to an agency for collection, it may be a breach of the confidential relationship in that a patient should be able to control who knows he is in psychotherapy. This matter should be considered before such a step is taken."[84] However, it has traditionally been held in the law on privileges that confidentiality goes out the window in litigation between the parties.[85] Thus, when a patient sues a physician for malpractice, the physician may discuss diagnosis and treatment. By bringing suit, the patient waives his secrecy privilege. The same principle applies in a suit brought by the physician for the patient's failure to perform his obligation under the contract, to wit, to pay for services rendered. The fact that the privilege belongs to the patient does not prevent the physician from claiming payment in court for his services. The privilege precludes a third person from calling the physician as a witness against the patient; it is not applicable in suits between physician and patient (and similarly, between attorney and client).

Furthermore, it is to be noted that the medical privilege applies only to the communication itself, and not to the fact that a communication was made. Thus, under the orthodox medical privilege, the fact of the physician-patient relationship, that the person was under treatment, the number of visits, and the duration of treatment, are not privileged areas.[86] This may be all the information that may be needed to uphold a claim for payment. There may be no need to reveal the content of the sessions.

Be that as it may, the dynamics of behavior underlying failure to pay a bill surely are not to be ignored. Money has important meanings to

577

everyone, on many different levels of psychic functioning. The pattern of giving and receiving money is symbolic of many interpersonal transactions. Lack of punctuality in the payment of fees may be a manifestation of temporary financial shortage, a problem in the patient related to money or to giving, an identification of money with "vulgarity," or an indication of resentment toward the therapist and of a desire to frustrate him. Likewise, counter-transference manifestations may reflect themselves in the therapist's attitude toward payment of fees. Conscious and unconscious conflicts may influence the therapist in determining his fee policy. Unlike most other medical specialities, as GAP points out, a fee in psychotherapy is usually agreed upon at the outset. A patient's disregard of a bill for a considerable period may indicate that the therapist himself is negligent in failing to bring to the patient's awareness possible avoidance of a responsibility which is part of the reality situation. Payment of fees is part of the reality situation which therapists supposedly impose on patients.

Combined Individual and Group Therapy

A patient who is in combined individual and group therapy may state that material discussed in the individual setting should not be brought to the group. This is, of course, a defensive mechanism on the part of the patient and a denial of the group process, but nonetheless it might be suggested that a breach of confidence would invade his right of privacy. As a matter of law, such a holding is unlikely. It might be said that the patient cannot complain when he voluntarily takes part in combined therapy, or it might be said that the therapist has in fact acted in his interest and there has been no damage.

Case Presentations

Patients treated by medical students, interns or residents are frequently presented at case conferences. Individuals beginning psychotherapy at an educational institution usually agree in advance to appear at a conference. Conferences are explained as a part of the educational program, designed to help the patient as well as the therapist. Presentation before a conference can be helpful not only for the training of the therapist, but also for the health of the patient. Conference presentation may result in a corrective emotional experience. The patient may derive a genuine sense of acceptability not only by the therapist but also by members of the group. In some institutions, a patient who is reluctant about appearing before a group, whether or not behind a one-way mirror, is not presented. The presentation of a patient behind a mirror, without his knowledge, might be said to violate his right of privacy.

A patient usually comes to the therapeutic situation with a fear that unauthorized persons may learn of his disclosure. This fear may be reduced by assurance that information given will not be passed on. The therapist must make good on this assertion. The maintenance of confidentiality, however, is a matter of considerable delicacy in view of the prevailing law on the medical privilege.

Connecticut in 1961 enacted a specific statute for the psychiatrist-patient relationship which has been recommended as a model for all states by GAP, following its abandonment of an earlier recommendation. The Connecticut statute is quite detailed in its provisions,[87] yet, as we have attempted to show, there are a number of situations which strictly speaking fall outside even its protection. Clauses might be added to the already complicated statute to cover these matters, but the fundamental solution must come by full and fair acceptance by the courts of the need of confidentiality even in the courtroom. Otherwise, the best of statutes will come to naught. The example that psychiatrists themselves show in maintaining the privacy of the patient might best convince the courts, and the general public, of the merit of a privilege. The fundamental guidepost is that no information about a patient should be released without authorization by the patient or his legally designated guardian.

A communication of whatever type is a bond between two people. The teller becomes part of the hearer's life, and vice versa. A relationship is established that is sacred in nature. A patient in psychotherapy especially expects an inviolable "a therapist who never tells anything", in fact as well as in law.

The problem in the law is where to draw the line separating the privileged from the unprivileged. The desideratum for all privileges, we would suggest, is that a communication made in reasonable confidence that it will not be disclosed, and in such circumstances that disclosure is shocking to the moral sense of the community, should not be disclosed in a judicial proceeding.[88] Many of the problems presented in this paper can fairly be resolved by the application of such an over-all principle. The alternative is cumbersome legislation to cover specifically every conceivable situation.

ACKNOWLEDGMENT

Thanks are due to Dr. Jay Katz of Yale University, Dr. Zigmond M. Lebensohn of Washington, D. C., and Dr. Philip Q. Roche of Conshohocken, Pennsylvania, for reading over the final draft and for their suggestions.

579

1. "The search for truth is the basic aim of our law. Truth, like motherhood, should be sacrosanct. Yet the law, in many of its rules of evidence, treats the search for truth in a cavalier fashion and as being far from sacred. Many rules of evidence result in the suppression rather than in the ascertainment of the truth. Nowhere is this better demonstrated than in the field of the testimonial privileges afforded several relationships. Every testimonial privilege afforded a party or witness necessarily and inevitably results in the suppression of material and relevant, and in some cases of basic, facts. Thus any testimonial privilege constitutes a legislatively created barrier to the search for truth. The public policy behind some of these privileges is so apparent and basic that it outweighs the public policy behind the unfettered search for the truth. But as to other testimonial privileges and public policy behind them is not so apparent or basic. The existence or continuance of such privileges presents a highly debatable and controversial question." Judge Peters, Book Review. Calif. L. Rev., 47:783, 1959.

   The following quotation from 8 Wigmore on Evidence (3rd ed.) §2192, pp. 64, 67, is an excellent statement of the law: "For more than three centuries it has now been recognized as a fundamental maxim that the public (in the words sanctioned by Lord Hardwicke) has a right to every man's evidence. When we come to examine the various claims of exemption, we start with the primary assumption that there is a general duty to give what testimony one is capable of giving, and that any exemptions which may exist are distinctly exceptional, being so many derogations from a positive general rule. . . . The investigation of truth and the enforcement of testimonial duty demand the restriction, not the expansion, of these privileges. They should be recognized only within the narrowest limits required by principle. Every step beyond these limits helps to provide, without any real necessity, an obstacle to the administration of justice."

   Opponents to privileges argue that privileges give first consideration to the individual client or patient, doctor or lawyer, as against the public interest or the welfare of the community as a whole. See, e.g., Baldwin, Confidentiality between physician and patient. Md. L. Rev., 22:181, 1962. But why identify a trial with the public interest and privileges with individual interest? It is just as logical to say that a trial concerns only the immediate litigants, and that a privilege concerns a broad class of persons (all patients and all clients).

2. Jurisdictions recognizing the physician-patient privilege are (with citation to statutes): Alaska (58-6-6), Ariz. (12-2235-36, 13-801-02), Ark. (28-607, 43-2004), Calif. (CCP §1881, Penal Code §1321), Colo. (153-1-7-1-8, 39-7-13), Dist. of Col. (14-308), Hawaii (222-20), Idaho (9-203, 19-2110), Ill. (51-5-1), Ind. (2-1714, 9-1602), Iowa (622.10, 782.1), Kan. (60-2805, 62-1413), Mich. (27.911, 28.945, 28.1045), Minn. (595.02), Miss. (§1697), Mo. (491.060), Mont. (93-701-4, 94-7209), Neb. (25-1206-07), Nev. (48.080), N.Y. (C.P.A. §352, 354), N.D. (31-0106-07), Ohio (2317.02, 2945.41), Okla. (12-385, 22-702), Ore. (44,040, 136.510), S.D. (34.3631, 36.0101-03), Utah (77-44-1,-2, 78-24-8), Wash. (5.60.060, 10.52.020, 10.58.010), Wis. (325.21), and Wyo. (1-139). Some other states have limited privileges, protecting only a narrow class of information. Kentucky (213.200) limits its privilege to vital statistics. Louisiana's privilege (15:

476) applies only in criminal cases. New Mexico (20-1-12) limits the privilege to cases of venereal disease and workmen's compensation claims. North Carolina (8-53) and Virginia (8-289-1) demand disclosure when it is necessary to "a proper administration of justice". Pennsylvania's privilege (28-328) extends only to information which tends to blacken the character of the patient. Virginia's privilege (8-289-1) is limited to civil cases. West Virginia's privilege (§4992) is available only before justices of the peace. Federal courts in civil cases adopt the rules of evidence of the state in which the trial is held: hence, the medical privilege exists in some federal courts and not in others; furthermore, in criminal cases, the privilege is disallowed in all federal courts. Jurisdictions without a physician-patient privilege are Ala., Conn., Del., Fla., Ga., Me., Md., Mass., N.H., N.J., R.I., S.C., Tenn., Texas, and Vt. Connecticut and Georgia recently enacted a special privilege for communications between psychiatrist and patient. See *infra* note 4.

3. As a result of adverse criticism, the physician-patient privilege, where it exists, has been narrowly construed by the courts. As one court put it, there has been "considerable criticism of physician-patient privilege statutes in recent years, on the ground that such statutes [have] but little justification for their existence and that they [are] often prejudicial to the cause of justice by the suppression of useful truth, 'the disclosure of which ordinarily [can] harm no one.'" Van Wie v. United States, 77 F. Supp. 22 (N.D. Iowa 1948). The legislative and jurisprudential restrictions on the medical privilege are enumerated in Slovenko, J. of La. State Med. Soc. 110:39, 1958.

4. The Georgia statute creates a privilege for "communication between psychiatrist and patient." The statute however sets out no guides, leaving the extent of protection to case-by-case determination by the courts. Ga. Code Ann. §38-418 (Supp. 1960). The GAP model statute proposed protection on the same basis as confidential communications between attorney and client (GAP Report No. 45, 1960), but it soon became clear that this proposal was inadequate, and in its stead GAP suggested the recently enacted Connecticut statute. The Connecticut statute is discussed in detail in Goldstein and Katz, Psychiatrist-Patient Privilege: The GAP Proposal and The Connecticut Statute, Am. J. of Psychiat. 118:733, 1962. The Connecticut statute is divided into three sections: the first creates the privilege; the second defines principal terms; the third sets out the conditions under which the privilege ends. Conn. Stat. Ann. §52-146a (Supp. 1961). The statute provides:

"§1. *Psychiatrist-Patient Privilege.* In civil and criminal cases, in proceedings preliminary thereto, and in legislative and administrative proceedings, a patient, or his authorized representative, has a privilege to refuse to disclose, and to prevent a witness from disclosing, communications relating to diagnosis or treatment of the patient's mental condition between patient and psychiatrist, or between members of the patient's family and the psychiatrist, or between any of the foregoing and such persons who participate, under the supervision of the psychiatrist, in the accomplishment of the objectives of diagnosis or treatment.

"§2. *Definitions.* As used in this act, 'patient' means a person who, for the purpose of securing diagnosis or treatment of his mental condition, consults a psychiatrist; 'psychiatrist' means a person licensed to practice medicine who devotes a substantial portion of his time to the practice of psychiatry, or a person reasonably believed by the patient to be so qualified; 'authorized representative' means a person empowered by the patient to assert the privilege and, until given permission by the patient to make disclosure, any person whose communications are made privileged by §1 of this act.

"§3. *Exceptions.* There is no privilege for any relevant communications under this act

"(a) when a psychiatrist, in the course of diagnosis or treatment of the patient, determines that the patient is in need of care and treatment in a hospital for mental illness;

"(b) if the judge finds that the patient, after having been informed that the communications would not be privileged, has made communications to a psychiatrist in the course of a psychiatric examination ordered by the court, *provided* that such communications shall be admissible only on issues involving the patient's mental condition;

"(c) in a civil proceeding in which the patient introduces his mental condition as an element of his claim or defense, or, after the patient's death, when said condition is introduced by any party claiming or defending through or as a beneficiary of the patient, if the judge finds that it is more important to the interests of justice that the communication be disclosed than that the relationship between patient and psychiatrist be protected."

A bill proposing privilege of communications between psychiatrists and their patients has been prepared for introduction at the 1963 session of the Maryland General Assembly. Item 117 before the 1961 Maryland Legislative Council. A Joint Committee is now working on a draft for a communication bill for Pennsylvania.

5. Freud, Collected Papers, vol. 2, p. 356 (Basic Books 1959).
6. In former times all personal rights were cast in terms of property rights.
7. Slovenko and Phillips, Psychosexuality and the Criminal Law, Vand L. Rev. 15:797, 1962. On occasion the physician is called upon to advise the single person about his sexual behavior. Without making a value judgment on premarital coitus, the fact remains that fornication may be a healthy milestone in the life of a person. Inasmuch as fornication by unmarried people is prohibited in all states except ten, the physician could theoretically be considered an accessory to the crime. There are also problems in giving advice to married couples (consider birth control advice). The privilege against self-incrimination of crime is available to the physician as well as to the patient.
8. See generally Brody, Simultaneous Psychotherapy of Married Couples, in Masserman, ed., Current Psychiatric Therapies, vol. 1, p. 139 (1961). In recent legislation, Louisiana has provided that whenever the parties to a separation or divorce proceeding effect a reconciliation prior to rendition of judgment, all pleadings and testimony can be separated from other court records and maintained in a confidential status. La. R.S. 13:4687 (Act 421 of 1962).
9. Binder v. Ruvell, Harry Fisher, Judge, Civil Docket 52C2535, Circuit Court of Cook County, Illinois, June 24, 1952, reported in A.M.A.J. 150:1241, 1952, and commented upon in Nw. U.L. Rev. 47:384, 1952.

10. Grosberg v. Grosberg, 269 Wis. 165, 68 N.W.2d 725 (1955) (child custody case in which testimony of a psychologist was used to establish the neurotic condition of the mother).

11. Chafee, Privileged Communications: Is Justice Served or Obstructed by Closing the Doctor's Mouth on the Witness Stand?, Yale L.J. 52:607, 1943.

12. Fed. R. Civ. P. 35; Ganes, The Clinical Psychologist as a Witness in Personal Injury Cases, Marq. L. Rev. 39:329, 1955; Hare. Medical Testimony: Doctors and Lawyers Cooperate, J. Am. Jud. Soc. 41:78, 1957.

13. Usdin, The Psychiatrist and Testamentary Capacity, Tul. L. Rev. 32:89, 1957.

14. Rhodes v. Metropolitan Life Ins. Co., 172 F.2d 183 (5th Cir. 1949). In some states, the heir can claim or waive the secrecy privilege. The Connecticut statute provides that when a deceased patient's mental condition is introduced by any party claiming or defending through or as a beneficiary of the patient, there is no privilege should the judge find "that it is more important to the interests of justice that the communication be disclosed than that the relationship between patient and psychiatrist be protected." Conn. Stat. Ann. §52-146a (Supp. 1961).

15. Proceedings of the Institute on Law and the Mind, p. 28 (U. of Wis. Extension Law Dept., 1961).

16. Radauskas, Kurland and Goldin, A Neglected Document—The Medical Record of the State Psychiatric Hospital Patient, Am. J. of Psychiat. 118: 709, 1962. Consider the following court opinion of a hospital record: "There is good reason to treat a hospital record entry as trustworthy. Human life will often depend on the accuracy of the entry, and it is reasonable to presume that a hospital is staffed with personnel who competently perform their day to day tasks. To this extent at least, hospital records are deserving of a presumption of accuracy even more than other types of business entries." Thomas v. Hogan, 308 F.2d 355 (4th Cir. 1962).

17. La. R.S. 44:7(A).

18. Calif., Conn., Ill., Mich., Minn., S. Dak., and Neb.

19. Regulations of the Food & Drug Administration, effective October 1962, concerning investigational stage of new drugs, require complete records of the disposition of the drug and case histories of the patients, and that adequate reports be furnished to the sponsor, and that these records be open to inspection by the Food & Drug Administration on request. The records must include "characteristics of patients by age, sex and condition."

20. Ross, Commitment of the Mentally Ill: Problems of Law and Policy, Mich. L. Rev. 57:945, 1959; Slovenko and Super, Commitment Procedure in Louisiana, Tul. L. Rev. 35:705, 1961, and J. of La. State Med. Soc. 113: 463, 1961. The new Ohio Mental Health Law provides that patient records, including hospital and court records, shall be kept confidential except under certain circumstances. An exception is made for court journal entries and docket entries, apparently for the benefit of those concerned with property and contract problems of patients since judicial hospitalization in Ohio still results in incompetency. Records may be disclosed upon consent of the patient and approval of the request by the hospital or court; when necessary in court proceedings; and when necessary to carry out the provisions of the mental health law. Ohio Rev. Code, chap. 5122, §§5122:31, 5122.36; Haines

and Myers, Hospitalization and Treatment of the Mentally Ill: Ohio's New Mental Health Law, Ohio State L.J. 22:659, 1961.

21. U. S. Public Health Service, Publication No. 51 (rev. ed. 1952). A brief summary of the act, by one of its authors, appears in Felix, R.: Hospitalization of the Mentally Ill, Am. J. of Psych. 107:712 (1951).

22. "Confidential medical information about a patient should not be released without the consent of the patient, if he is competent, or someone authorized to consent for him, if he is not competent, unless the disclosure is required by law or is vitally necessary for protection of the public interest. Where a court commits a patient to a mental hospital, authority to act for the patient will be granted either to a guardian appointed for that purpose or to a public official. This guardian or public official is subject to the control of the court. He is required to act in the best interest of the patient in all matters, including the release of information." AMA News, Sept. 17, 1962.

23. In the case of physical illness, the courts have held, for example, that an X-ray film belongs to the physician in the absence of a specific agreement to the contrary, but the patient may require the production of the X-ray in court. See McGarry v. Mercier Co., 272 Mich. 501, 262 N.W. 296 (1935). In Wallace v. University Hospitals of Cleveland, 171 Ohio St. 487, 172 N.E.2d 459 (1961), the Supreme Court of Ohio dismissed a former patient's suit for an injunction to compel a hospital to furnish him with a copy of his hospital record because, while the appeal was pending, the hospital furnished him with a photostatic copy of his record. As a consequence, the Court said, the case was moot and it felt bound to dismiss the case, which it did "reluctantly."

On whether a patient (treated for physical illness) is entitled to a copy of his medical report, the Judicial Council of the AMA states that, "Whether the contents of the medical report are to be given to the patient rests with the decision of the doctor who knows all the circumstances involved in the situation." The Judicial Council also points out that, "The records are medical and technical, personal and often informal. Standing alone they are meaningless to the patient but of value to the physician and perhaps to a succeeding physician. The patient, however, or one responsible for him, is entitled to know the nature of the illness and the general course or regimen of therapy employed by his physician. The extent to which the physician must advise his patient may be limited by the nature of the illness and the character of the patient. The physician in advising his patient must always act as he would wish to be treated were he in a like situation." AMA News, April 30, 1962. See also Physician's Legal Brief, Jan. 1963.

Records of a deceased physician cannot be sold because the information they contain is confidential (and therefore they are not inventoried as property in the estate of the physician). It is recommended that records of a deceased physician which might be pertinent to any litigation in which a patient may be involved should not be destroyed without prior notice to the patient. AMA News, Dec. 11, 1961, p. 14, col. 2.

24. Hospital records are exclusively the hospital's property. A few states apparently hold that clinical records are the property of the hospital and *also* the physician's property. Menninger, A Manual for Psychiatric Case Study, p. 35 (2d ed. 1962). In the Veterans Administration, the clinical records belong, not to the hospital, but to the Veterans Administration.

25. See Amato v. Porter, 157 F.2d 719 (10th Cir. 1946); Comment, Harv. L. Rev. 68:340, 1954. In a recent controversy in Wisconsin, Dr. Hertha Tarrasch, psychiatrist, claimed records and files relating to patients who availed themselves of psychiatric services offered at the Rock County Guidance Clinic upon a public basis. Dr. Tarrasch and social workers and psychologists under her direction and control compiled the records. Upon the termination of employment with Rock County, Dr. Tarrasch claimed the records, alleging (1) a proprietary interest in the records as constituting her work product and (2) a right to the records as being privileged confidential communications. The case was compromised. The parties agreed that the records and files would be placed under Dr. Tarrasch's exclusive control until 1970 but that their physical location would be determined by the court in its discretion.

26. Eleven states privilege the psychologist-client relationship, to wit, Ark., Cal., Colo., Ga., Ky., Mich., N.H., N.Y., Tenn., Utah, and Wash. The first psychologist-client privilege was enacted in 1948 in Kentucky. No jurisdictions privilege communications to social workers or marriage counselors as such.

  When specially protected, psychologists need not be concerned whether they fall under the medical statute as an agent of the physician. In recent years there has been an increase in the number of non-medical people engaged in psychotherapy, either privately or in an institutional setting or both. Psychologists, social workers, and even nurses conduct private or largely independent practices. See Jerome Frank, Persuasion and Healing (1961); Fischer, Nonmedical Psychotherapists, A.M.A. Archives of Gen. Psychiat. 5:7, 1961; Health Manpower Chart Book (1955).

27. Where there is no medical privilege, there is the important holding that the attorney-client privilege protects a report made by a doctor to the lawyer when the lawyer asked the patient to see the doctor. Lindsay v. Lipson, 116 N.W.2d 60 (Mich. 1962); City & County of San Francisco v. Superior Court, 231 P.2d 26 (Cal. 1951); Comment, Yale L.J. 71:1226, 1962.

28. First Trust Co. of St. Paul v. Kansas City Life Ins. Co., 79 F.2d 48 (8th Cir. 1935); Leusink v. O'Donnell, 255 Wis. 627, 39 N.W. 675 (1949). Physicians treating physical illnesses are frequently confronted with the situation where the patient is brought to the office by a housekeeper-companion who is present during the examination. In many states, courts hold that both the physician and third person can be called on to testify about the communications. Some states, however, hold that communications between the patient and physician are privileged when the third party is serving either as an assistant to the physician or as an interpreter between the physician and patient. Ostrowski v. Mockridge, 242 Minn. 265, 65 N.W.2d 185 (1954).

29. Fenton, Group Counseling—A Preface to Its Use in Correctional and Welfare Agencies (Institute for Study of Crime and Delinquency, Sacramento, Calif.); Fenton and Wallace, State Child Guidance Service in California Communities (1938).

30. Hopkins v. Grimshaw, 165 U.S. 342 (1897); Wolfe v. United States, 291 U.S. 7 (1934); 58 Am. Jur., Witnesses §381. Cf. Freeman v. Freeman, 238 Mass. 150, 130 N.E. 220 (1921) (discretion of judge to determine minor child's comprehension of parent's conversation).

Consider also the attorney-client privilege. If any of the attorney's or client's documents or verbal statements are disclosed to third parties (anyone other than the attorney or the client), then those documents or statements are no longer regarded as confidential. In the language of the old common law, the confidence has been "profaned" and the privilege terminated. Such "profanity" could occur either at the source or point of origin of the information, or it could take place later on. At common law the client's or attorney's necessity of having immediate office personnel permitted access to documents without destroying their confidential nature is accepted and approved.

The rulings on the medical privilege vary from state to state. Some courts allow the privilege when the third party is related to the holder of the privilege insofar as the testimony of the physician is concerned but not, oddly, as to the third party. The court in Denaro v. Prudential Ins. Co., 154 App. Div. 840, 139 N.Y.S. 758, 761 (1913) said: "[W]hen a physician enters a house for the purpose of attending a patient, he is called upon to make inquiries, not alone of the sick person, but of those who are about him and who are familiar with the facts, and communications necessary for the proper performance of the duties of a physician are not public, because made in the presence of his immediate family or those who are present because of the illness of the person. *Of course, the persons who are present are not denied the right to testify.* It is only the physician who is bound by the rule." (Emphasis added.)

31. Furthermore, in this day of highly sophisticated eavesdropping devices, it is practically impossible to assure privacy. Possibly the only way to be sure remarks remain private is not to make them. See Dash, Schwartz and Knowlton, The Eavesdroppers (1959).

32. Schecter, The Integration of Group Therapy with Individual Psychoanalysis, in Masserman, ed., Current Psychiatric Therapies, vol. 1, p. 145 (1961). "Group psychotherapy is booming." Time, Feb. 8, 1963, p. 38.

33. Oldham, Privileged Communications in Military Law, Military L. Rev. July 1959.

34. Perhaps this is a reaction to the earlier overemphasis on the importance of psychological testing. Too much was expected, yet now it is said that "the efforts to weed out personality risks from the armed forces during World War II was a complete fiasco." Review of Gross, The Brain Watchers, by Parkinson, Genius by the Yard, Sat. Rev., Oct. 13, 1962, p. 32.

35. See Glass, Artiss, Gibbs and Sweeney, The Current Status of Army Psychiatry, Am. J. of Psychiat. 117:673, 1961; Glass, Advances in Military Psychiatry, in Masserman, ed., Current Psychiatric Therapies, vol. 1, p. 159 (1961).

36. Washington Post Sept. 22, 1960, p. 1.

37. The report of the House Committee on Un-American Activities said Martin was "sexual abnormal: in fact, a masochist." It said Mitchell had "posed for nude color slides perched on a velvet-covered stool." AP News-Release, Aug. 14, 1962.

38. The image of the physician *qua* physician is little enhanced by divulgence of information. In the words of Dr. Victor W. Sidel:
". . . The doctor's duty to heal the sick . . . includes a duty to keep others from getting sick. Therefore, when he faces a food handler with

typhoid fever who refuses to recognize the danger of his disease to others, he sees no break in ethical principles in promptly reporting the danger to the appropriate authority. Again, the doctor's duty to the sick includes a duty to keep others from getting injured. When a patient, therefore, tells a physician that he plans to commit a crime of violence—for example, 'I'm going to murder the mayor at noon tomorrow'—the physician takes steps to see that the mayor is protected. Furthermore, such a patient is almost always really saying, 'I have a terrible urge (or very vivid fantasies involving the urge) to kill the mayor. Please protect me from my urge.' This is usually true also of the patient who tells the doctor that he plans to commit suicide. The doctor will not hesitate to make appropriate revelations to prevent violence, either self-inflicted or inflicted on others, because in so doing he is furthering his professional goals for his patient and for his community.

Sidel, Confidential Information and the Physician, New Eng. J. Med. 264: 1133, 1961; see also Sidel, Medical Ethics and the Cold War, Nation 191: 325, 1960.

39. Guttmacher, The Mind of the Murderer 215 (1960).

40. "[As a class], patients willing to express to psychiatrists their intention to commit crime are not ordinarily likely to carry out that intention. Instead, they are making a plea for help. The very making of such pleas affords the psychiatrist his unique opportunity to work with patients in an attempt to resolve their problems. Such resolutions would be impeded if patients were unable to speak freely for fear of possible disclosure at a later date in a legal proceeding." Goldstein and Katz, Psychiatrist-Patient Privilege: The GAP Proposal and the Connecticut Statute, Am. J. of Psychiat. 118: 733, 1962.

41. People v. Hawthorne, 293 Mich. 15, 291 N.W. 205 (1940); United States v. Chandler, 72 F. Supp. 230 (1947).

42. However, an old conviction was upheld when a drug administered to an addict in custody, to alleviate narcotic addiction withdrawal pains, rendered the arrested person talkative enough for production of a confession. Mueller, The Law Relating to Police Interrogation: Privileges and Limitations, in Sowle, ed., Police Power and Individual Freedom 131 (1962); Sheedy, Narcointerrogation of a Criminal Suspect, J. Crim. L., C. & P.S. 50:118, 1958.

43. In the case of Leyra v. Denno, 347 U.S. 556 (1954), the defendant, after being questioned by the state police for the greater part of four days concerning the murder of his aged parents, complained of an acutely painful attack of sinus. The police promised to get a doctor. They got a psychiatrist with a considerable knowledge of hypnosis. Instead of administering medical aid, the psychiatrist, working in a room which was wired, "by subtle and suggestive questions simply continued the police effort" to get the accused to admit guilt. The United States Supreme Court threw out the evidence.

In Oaks v. People, 371 P.2d 443 (Colo. 1962), it was held that a psychiatrist could not testify to what he had been told about the defendant, whom he examined for the state (before charges had been brought) on the basis that under the guise of psychiatric examination, the psychiatrist had obtained information on guilt.

In McDonough v. Director of Pataxent Institution, 183 A.2d 368 (Md. 1962), the defendant, a delinquent, refused a psychological examination on

587

the basis of the Fifth Amendment, but the court found no violation of his constitutional rights.

44. *Supra* note 4. Compare People v. Bickley, 22 Cal. Rptr. 340 (1962), where the trial court allowed a psychiatrist to testify even after an insanity plea for an accused murderer had been withdrawn. The accused had not been compelled to give the psychiatrist any information but did so voluntarily. The California Supreme Court affirmed the trial court's ruling, holding that the accused's constitutional rights were not violated by allowing the psychiatrist's testimony, which was held relevant on the issue of penalty. The Court also ruled that the psychiatrist was qualified to testify that the accused had a character defect and was not susceptible to rehabilitation.

45. Haines, The Future of Court Psychiatry, vol. 2, no. 1 (1957), reprinted in Nice, ed., Criminal Psychology, p. 268 (1962).

46. Guttmacher, The Mind of the Murderer, chap. 19 (1960).

47. Morgan v. State, Fla. App., June 13, 1962.

48. Observation made by Louis J. Sharp, Chief, Division of Probation, Administrative Office of the United States Courts, at the Sentencing Institute and Joint Council for the Fifth Circuit, May 9, 1961. See 30 F.R.D. 185 (1962). Mr. Justice Black's opinion in Williams v. New York, 337 U.S. 241 (1948) seems to be authority for confidential treatment, although as noted there is controversy about the point. Sharp, The Confidential Nature of Presentence Reports, Catholic U. L. Rev. 5:127, 1955.

49. MacCormick, A Criminologist Looks at Privilege, Am. J. of Psychiat. 115: 1079, 1959.

50. *Ibid.* Our observations *supra* in the section on criminal cases on reporting of crimes is *a propos* here.

51. Holmes, The Sheppard Murder Case (1962).

52. Hazard and Louisell, Death, The State, and the Insane: Stay of Execution, U.C.L.A. L. Rev. 9:381, 1962.

53. 339 U.S. 9 (1950).

54. Silving, Testing of the Unconscious in Criminal Cases, Harv. L. Rev. 69: 683, 1956.

55. Hollender, The Psychiatrist and the Release of Patient Information, Am. J. of Psychiat. 116:828, 1960.

56. In the $1,000,000 Van Sant alienation-of-affections suit in 1961 in Delaware, which did not have a priest-penitent privilege, counsel made a motion asking that the Rev. Percy F. Rex be compelled to answer any and every question put to him. Rev. Rex, asking the court to be excused, said: "In all kinds of pastoral counselling the clergyman seeks information from all sides. His usefulness depends upon his impartiality and therefore he refrains from being judgmental, and seeks to reconcile the parties to each other and to the God of all mankind. To be forced to testify for public record in a court would tend to destroy his impartial position as a reconciler of person to person and persons to God."

Answer to Motion to Compel Answer, Civil Action No. 154, Superior Court, Wilmington, Del. The suit was finally settled out of court, and the Delaware Legislature shortly thereafter passed a privileged communication statute for clergymen.

57. Furthermore, it is often said: "Many medical men find it difficult to think and feel about psychiatrists as they do about other physicians. Psychiatry

appears to them strange, unfamiliar, and unlike other medical specialties."
Bartemeier, American Medicine and the Development of Psychiatry, J.A.M.A.
163:95, 1957, quoted in Taylor, The Psychiatrist and the General Practitioner, A.M.A. Archives of Gen. Psychiat. 5:1, 1961. Sociologists make the
claim that psychiatrists differ from their fellow physicians in "technical
skills, conceptual systems, scientific orientation, historical background, and
(attitudes toward) problems of confidentiality." Smith, Psychiatry in Medicine: Intra- or Interprofessional Relationships?, Am. J. Sociol. 63:285, 1959.

58. Slovenko, Psychiatry and a Second Look at the Medical Privilege, Wayne L.
Rev. 6:175, 1960, revised version, Slovenko and Usdin, The Psychiatrist
and Privileged Communication, A.M.A. Archives of Gen. Psychiat. 4:431,
1961.

59. Reik, The Unknown Murderer (1930), reprinted in part one of The Compulsion to Confess (1959).

60. 50-Minute Hour ("The Jet-Propelled Couch").

61. Commenting on the testimony presented in the case of Briscoe v. United
States, 248 F.2d 640 (D.C. 1957), rev'd, 251 F.2d 386 (D.C. 1958), Wat-
son observed: "[This case] involved a psychologist, a psychiatrist and a couple
of lawyers, each of whom jumps their role. The judge talks like a psychiatrist; the psychologist talks like a lawyer; the psychiatrist jumps back and
forth between both. The end result is that the only one who made the right
diagnosis was the original policeman on the case and he, listening to the
confession in a case of arson, said the man was nuts." Proceedings of the
Institute on Law and the Mind, p. 77 (U. of Wis. Extension Law Dept.,
1961).

62. Munsterberg in his *On the Witness Stand,* a work of note on the psychology
of testimony, reports an automobile accident case wherein one witness testified that the road was dry and dusty while another witness stated that it had
rained and the road was muddy. In another case, where it was essential to
determine whether at a certain disturbance the number of guests in the
auditorium was greater than the forty who had been invited to attend, Munsterberg reports that there were witnesses who insisted that there could not
have been more than twenty persons present, and others who maintained that
they saw more than a hundred. He points out that these were not cases of
intentional deception or of mental disease. The witnesses were highly re-
spectable persons who did not have the slightest interest in changing what
they had observed. Moreover, these were cases in which every layman was
prepared to give his impressions; these were not cases which demanded professional or technical knowledge. Munsterberg, On the Witness Stand (1927).
See further Slovenko, The Opinion Rule and Wittgenstein's Tractatus, U.
Miami L. Rev. 14:1, 1959.

63. Review of Medical Professional Liability Claims and Suits, J. of A.M.A.,
May 10, 1958, p. 227. According to a study of the California Medical Association, "The malpractice suit is a symptom of the breakdown in the doctor-patient relationship." Blum, Malpractice Suits—Why and How They
Happen: A Summary of a Report to the Medical Review and Advisory
Board of the California Medical Association, p. 4 (1958). It is also said
that the courts are "tightening up" on the doctor's responsibility to his patient, Medical World News, Oct. 26, 1962, p. 37.

64. Legal suits in general are rare against psychiatrists. Bellamy, Malprac-

tice Risks Confronting the Psychiatrist: A Nationwide Fifteen-Year Study of Appellate Court Cases, 1946 to 1961, Am. J. of Psychiat. 118:769, 1962. Thus far anything goes on the couch; the ready defense: "That's my type of treatment." See Wittenberg, Common Sense About Psychoanalysis (1961).

65. The development of the law of privacy, which has been called the "right to be let alone," is often said to have come about largely because of one man's fury. The Boston socialite Samuel Warren became outraged at the depth of detail the local newspapers were printing about himself and his family in connection with the forthcoming marriage of his daughter. Warren felt that there ought to be a law against it. With his former law partner, Louis Brandeis, who was later to become one of the great justices of the Supreme Court, he turned out a challenging article which appeared in the Harvard Law Review in 1890. It laid the groundwork for the development of the law of privacy as we know it today. Hauser, The Right of Privacy, Sat. Rev., Nov. 11, 1961, p. 74.

66. In the case of A.B. v. C.D., 7 F. (Scott) 72 (1905), a physician who revealed to patient's spouse that the patient was suffering from a venereal disease was held not liable. Likewise, no liability was imposed on a physician who, after warning the patient to vacate a hotel, reported to the owner that his "guest" probably was afflicted with a "contagious disease." Simonsen v. Swenson, 104 Neb. 224, 177 N.W. 831 (1920). However, the Maryland court recently recognized "the right to redress for wrongful invasion of privacy" by unwarranted verbal disclosure of information which resulted in the patient's loss of employment. Carr v. Watkins, 227 Md. 578, 177 A.2d 841 (1962).

67. A.M.A. Journal quoted in Flato, Parents Who Beat Children, Sat. Eve. Post, Oct. 6, 1962, p. 30.

68. California at present is the only state that requires physicians and hospitals to report child abuse to law-enforcement agencies. The Children's Bureau has drafted a model law, based largely on the California statute, for submission to state legislatures.

69. "The key to solving the child-maltreatment problem," says St. Vincent's Dr. Fontana, "in the final analysis is in the hands of our lawmakers. Only they can protect the physician testifying in such cases from libel and malpractice charges. Only they can give the medical profession the means of preventing thousands of cases annually of permanent disability and death." Quoted in Flato, op. cit. supra note 67.

Under the law, parents have an obligation to care for their young in sickness and health. An infant is made a ward of the court, invading the parents' custody, where the life or health of the child is endangered by the medical neglect of its parents, such as where the parents are members of a faith healing group and refuse to consent to a blood transfusion or a surgical operation for their child. See People v. Labrenz, 411 Ill. 618, 104 N.E.2d 769 (1952).

70. On testing of judges and jurors, see Frank, Courts on Trial 250 (1949); Forer, Psychiatric Evidence in the Recusation of Judges, Harv. L. Rev. 73: 1325, 1960; Redmount, Psychological Tests for Selecting Jurors, Kan. L. Rev. 5:391, 1957.

71. Szasz, Mind Tapping: Psychiatric Subversion of Constitutional Rights, Am. J. of Psychiat. 119:323, 1962.

72. In a recently enacted statute, Massachusetts prohibits an employer from establishing the polygraph examination as a condition of employment, or continued employment. One might speculate whether such a law is an unconstitutional limitation on the rights of employers. Some attorneys are skeptical about its constitutionality, but apparently a test case has not yet occurred. The General Counsel of the National Labor Relations Board has ruled that a company was within its rights to require applicants for employment to sign an agreement consenting to submit to polygraph examination as a condition of employment, or continued employment. Case No. SR-57, Aug. 6, 1959. See also Christal v. Police Commission, 33 Cal. App.2d 564 (police officer required to submit to polygraph examination when accused of attempting to commit a felony).

73. Consider one example of many, Wille's *Case Study of a Rapist: An Analysis of the Causation of Criminal Behavior,* J. of Social Therapy, vol. 7, no. 1, 1961. For the sake of preserving the anonymity of the persons involved, a good deal of the most vital data were deleted when Wille's article was arranged in its final form. Freud in his case history "Notes Upon a Case of Obsessional Neurosis" pointed out that it was not easy to compose, not only because of the inevitable compression, but also because of the need for greater discretion in print. The patient being well known in Vienna, it taxed his powers of presentation to the full. "How bungling are our attempts to reproduce an analysis; how pitifully we tear to pieces these great works of art Nature had created in the mental sphere." In his opening remarks Freud explained how it is that intimate secrets could be more easily mentioned than the trivial details of personality by which a person could be readily identified, and yet it is just these details that play an essential part in tracing the individual steps in an analysis. Freud, Collected Papers, vol. 3, p. 293 (Basic Books 1959); Jones, The Life and Work of Sigmund Freud, vol. 2, p. 262 (1955).

74. Farnsworth and Munter, The Role of the College Psychiatrist, in Blaine and McArthur, eds., Emotional Problems of the Student, p. 1 (1961); Peabody, Campus Psychiatry, in Masserman, ed., Current Psychiatric Therapies, vol. 1, p. 1 (1961).

75. Policy of Tulane University Health Center, publicized in student newspaper.

76. Berry v. Moench, 8 Utah 2d 191, 331 P.2d 814 (1958). In the case of Alexander v. Knight, 197 Pa. Super. 79, 177 A.2d 142 (1962), the court sharply rebuked a physician for giving a medical report on a patient, without consent, to another physician employed by attorneys who represented an opponent in the litigation. The court said: "We are of the opinion that members of a profession, especially the medical profession, stand in a confidential or fiduciary capacity as to their patients. They owe their patients more than just medical care for which payment is exacted; there is a duty to total care; that comprehends a duty to aid the patient in litigation, to render reports when necessary and to attend court when needed. That further includes a duty to refuse affirmative assistance to a patient's antagonist in litigation. The doctor, of course, owes a duty to conscience to speak the truth; he need, however, speak only at the proper time."

77. Davis and Silva, Proposal for a Statewide Mental Health Program (unpublished paper, Louisiana Department of Hospitals). A recent development in

591

the processing of records is the "Social Service Exchange," which acts as a clearing house for participating social agencies. GAP Report No. 45, Confidentiality and Privileged Communication in the Practice of Psychiatry (1960).

78. E.g., Hague v. Williams, 37 N.J. 328, 181 A.2d 345 (1962).

79. There is the requirement for medical certification of disability in order to qualify for workmen's compensation or other type of disability insurance benefits. The disabled patient finds it to his advantage to obtain such certification from his doctor.

80. Welfare departments question the physician about indigent patients that he has treated. The welfare authorities need a report to learn the extent of attention the patient requires. By requesting and accepting welfare medical care, it is considered that the patient waives his right to secrecy. However, there should be no disclosure of facts that might reflect on the patient's character. Physicians are cautioned to furnish information to organizations such as the Red Cross and the Cancer Society only upon written release from the patient. Eaton, When to Violate a Patient's Confidence, Medical Economics, Mar. 12, 1962, p. 147.

81. In one case the U.S. Air Force requested information from a physician concerning one of his patients whose work record in civilian life showed considerable absenteeism. Although superficially the cause could be ascribed to upper respiratory infections the physician knew the patient was an alcoholic. The physician wrote to the Air Force offering his opinion that the patient's poor work record was primarily due to alcoholism. After his discharge the patient sued the physician for breaching the physician-patient privilege. While saying that "a patient's illness has long been thought of as a protected professional confidence upon which every patient may rely," the court however found that the physician's "right, if not his duty, to his government to make a full disclosure of the facts superseded his duty to his patient to remain silent." However, this holding has been contested by medical authorities in other cases. Physician's Legal Brief, Aug. 1962, vol. 4, no. 8.

The medical privilege has been held inapplicable to investigations of the physician's books by the internal revenue. See Note, Syracuse L. Rev. 5:288, 1954.

82. Hollender, The Psychiatrist and the Release of Patient Information, Am. J. of Psychiat. 116:828, 1960. Szasz in a recent article discusses the matter of inquiries by psychoanalytic institutes to training analysts concerning analysands who are applying for admission to the institute. The institutes ask questions not only about the applicant's qualifications for analytic work, but also about his personality and his analysis. See Szasz, The Problem of Privacy in Training Analysis, Psychiatry 25:195, 1962.

83. La. Civil Code Art. 3191 (Slovenko ed.).

84. GAP Report No. 45, Confidentiality and Privileged Communication in the Practice of Psychiatry, p. 105 (1960).

85. In Yoder v. Smith, 112 N.W.2d 862 (Iowa 1962), a former patient had a good paying job, but was long past due on his bill, and showed no inclination to pay anything on the debt. The doctor resorted to a collection agency, which wrote the employer of the debtor for help in collecting the debt. The debtor thereupon sued, unsuccessfully, charging that his privacy

had been invaded. The court held that contacting the debtor's employer was a reasonable way for the creditor "to pursue his debtor and persuade payment, although the steps taken may result in some invasion of the debtor's privacy." In Patton v. Jacobs, 118 Ind. App. 358, 78 N.E.2d 789 (1948), the court denied a claim of invasion of privacy where a collection agency used by the physician notified the patient's employer of the bill owing the physician for medical services. However, unwarranted disclosure of indebtedness may be (and has been) treated as an invasion of privacy. See, e.g., Brents v. Morgan, 221 Ky. 765, 299 S.W. 967 (1927); Trammell v. Citizens News Co., 285 Ky. 529, 148 S.W.2d 708 (1941). It might be noted that the usual approach employed by collection agencies is "to instill anxiety and yet remain on friendly terms with the debtor." Black, Buy Now, Pay Later, p. 53 (1961).

See Crawfis, The Physician and Privileged Communications as They Relate to Mental State, Ohio State Med. J. 46:1082, 1950; Hassard, Privileged Communications: Physician-Patient Confidences in California, Calif. Med. 90:411, 1959. See also Wolberg, The Technique of Psychotherapy 663 (1954).

86. Compare United States v. Summe, 208 F. Supp. 925 (E.D. Ky. 1962), where an attorney, who had been called to appear at an investigation concerning the income tax returns of two of his clients, was asked certain questions concerning the preparation of the returns. The Court held that the investigating special agents did not have unlimited authority to examine the attorney but were, rather, limited to questions which did not violate the attorney-client privilege.

87. *Supra* note 4.

88. See the dictum by Judge Edgerton in Mullen v. United States, 263 F.2d 275, 281 (D.C. 1958).

PART XV

REVIEWS
AND
INTEGRATIONS

The Art of Psychotherapy

by Francis J. Braceland, M.D.

> God opens one book to physicians that a good many of you don't know about—The Book of Life. That is none of your dusty folios with black letters between pasteboard and leather but it is printed in bright type and the binding of it is warm and tender to every touch. They reverence that book as one of the Almighty's infallible revelations.
>
> —*Oliver Wendell Holmes—Elsie Venner*

THE ART OF MEDICINE is based on the skillful use of human relationships as well as the skillful application of scientific knowledge. Evidence abounds that while the emotions, attitudes and expectations of patients are of great importance in their response to treatment, the emotions, attitudes and expectations of the physician are equally important. It has been suggested that the practice of medicine flourishes best when doctors think most highly of their functions. There is truth in this statement if we assume that objectivity and scientific perspective are not lost in the process. Therapeutic optimism is a powerful force for good, despite the occasional occupational hazard known as *furor therapeuticus*. To believe that we can help our patients in some manner, no matter what their condition may be, and that it is our obligation to try is an indispensable professional attitude for the true physician.

The observant doctor hardly needs a scientific treatise to know that it is not always *what* he does that helps the patient, but rather *how* he does it. Nor can he help noticing that now and then a patient recovers when he, the doctor, has been at a complete loss as to what to try next. Psychotherapists observe the same phenomenon and have sometimes referred to it as the sudden transference cure. They have also noted that inadvertent breaks in technique seem to facilitate more constructive work with certain patients. They are even witnesses to spontaneous recoveries. Here, presumably, the patient has an experience which makes something fall into place for him and he is able to make sense of something that had eluded him before.

The understanding and manipulation of social forces is a major ingredient of the art of medicine. Not only do the ideas that people have about illness in general, or about a particular illness, influence their manifestations; such ideas also influence the course and outcome and even the response to etiological treatment. What the patient ascribes the illness to and believes it to mean, his notions of treatment, his cooperation or lack of it, his will to recovery or the reverse, the confidence or lack of confidence he has in the physician and in physicians in general—all of these factors make their contribution to the presenting problem. Some patients need symptoms. If they are unable to keep the ones they have, they may summon up others far worse. For patients with serious personality disorders, physical symptoms may channel off anxiety that would otherwise be dealt with more drastically.

Psychiatrists deal with many of the people who have resorted to the more drastic solutions. Psychiatric problems are many and complex, and so are the possible causes. However, disturbed human relationships are usually important in the chain of causation as well as in the persistence of a psychiatric disorder, and corrective experience in the doctor-patient relationship is necessary. All forms of psychotherapy stress the quality of this relationship. The therapist himself is a therapeutic force. His use of himself matters more than the doctrine or method he follows. In this relationship there must be something akin to faith. Jerome Frank reminds us that faith, hope, eagerness and joy are healing emotions and that the therapist should never underestimate their importance.

The art of psychotherapy involves the creation of the proper atmosphere from the start. The therapist seeks to mobilize the patient's expectation of help, even though the patient may deny that he needs it. To gain the patient's trust often calls for great resourcefulness and even a large degree of self-sacrifice. Unquestionably it is easier to help patients who seek psychotherapy on their own than it is to help those who come unwillingly. But the real test of the therapist is to overcome the distrust and estrangement of the patient he is privileged to treat.

The doctor's attitude will be as important as any verbal communication. He must have the courage to be himself and be prepared to accept the patient as he is. He needs to be relaxed and quiet and at ease with the patient and never lose sight of the fact that there is more to understand than is first apparent. It is a commonplace to say that a great part of the medical art is in knowing how to listen. There are many individuals who need little more than the opportunity to talk and to verbalize their thoughts and feelings. Ideas and feelings which cannot be discussed are extremely threatening to many people. Once spoken, however, they can be examined and reduced to their proper proportions. For others, the problem is essentially that they have not had any opportunity to express themselves before and no one has had time to listen. Relief follows swiftly when these persons encounter a trained and sympathetic listener.

In too many cases, unfortunately, matters are not as simple as noted. Patients require an extended period of therapy before the experience becomes corrective. The therapist must arrive at emotional as well as intellectual understanding. Emotional understanding presupposes mutuality, an appreciation of what the emotions under observation mean to the patient, an identification. Identification is the basis of all emotional understanding, and it depends less on conscious effort than on a desire to understand and an ability to sympathize. To identify, the therapist must be able to feel, if only briefly, that he is the other person. To do this, he must be able to dispense with his awareness of himself. In this way, there arises a mutual experience. Michael and Enid Balint describe this aspect of psychotherapy as biphasic. The psychotherapist must first identify, and then withdraw from the identification and become an objective professional person again. They submit that this is one of the ways a professional relationship differs from a private relationship.

Another major difference is the expert knowledge of the physician. In addition to having the ability to identify in the right setting while having only a limited involvement with his patient, the doctor has at his fingertips special knowledge and skill as the result of his training and experience. He uses this knowledge as he listens and observes. He uses it with discrimination, not rigidly or automatically as the untrained person coversant with theoretical knowledge would tend to do.

The art of psychotherapy is concerned with the dynamics of communication, including all the nuances, allusions and non-verbal cues which may be of significance. The therapist needs to be in command of himself at all times, remaining alert not only to changes in the patient's tensions, feelings and behavior but also to the changes being produced in himself. Self-understanding is of major importance. The therapist must not act out his own immature impulses and needs in the treatment situation. He must not reject the patient because he is difficult or not easy to love or because he is hostile and uncooperative. He has to

599

endure frustration, to remain cool under personal attack, and to master fear, however formidable the patient happens to be.

There are levels of communication. Even silence can be communication. The confidence which grows out of companionable silence may pay important dividends later. If the therapist is free from anxiety he will more readily determine the proper form of contact with the patient. Such a consideration is of great importance in dealing with psychotic patients.

The psychiatrist's ability to help a patient depends in part on his training and on the image the patient has of him as a physician, but it also has something to do with his really caring about the patient's welfare and the physician's ability to bear a great burden of responsibility on the patient's behalf. To be therapeutic, he may have to change himself, to sacrifice certain feelings and attitudes which bring him satisfaction. He will have to guard against the rise of unwonted zeal— the need to imbue the patient with the doctor's own philosophy of proprieties in feeling and behavior, against the need to cure quickly and completely, against the need to prescribe and instruct and interfere in ways that do more harm than good. The inexperienced therapist may be tempted to do these busy things. Although the therapist must maintain his own identity and his own privacy, he can never be a stranger to his patient. He cannot help revealing what he is and what he believes in. He shows this in countless ways. He must therefore believe in the methods he uses, for if he believes in them, the patient is more likely to accept them. It is also incumbent upon him to believe in the inherent capacity of even the most regressed patient to attain, with help, a better solution of his difficulties. There can be no giving up in the face of apparent failure or of painfully slow progress interspersed with relapses. The long-term view is required. Even an imperfect result is a source of satisfaction to the dedicated psychotherapist.

What the doctor has to do, as the Balints see it, is to accept the whole of the muddle presented by the patient. In some treatments, what he has to do is "to accept the illogical, irrational parts of his patients, take them seriously, and even though they are only fairy-tale-like wishes or fears, not deny their importance and power." The therapist himself must accept the fantasies of the patient before he can ask the latter to test and accept reality.

Today the deteriorating patients common in the past are much less in evidence in psychiatric hospitals. This happy situation is due to drug therapy, to vastly improved hospital atmosphere, to improved psychotherapeutic programs and other factors. Certainly there has been encouraging progress in treating psychotic patients by psychotherapeutic means. Intensive psychotherapeutic work with psychotic patients has brought new insights. For the psychotic patient, the essential factor in his response to psychotherapy is the feeling of having been understood by the therapist.

C. Mueller notes that the literature over the years reveals the diversity of paths by which the therapist may be able to establish contact with the patient and provide the stimulation necessary for a return to reality. The decisive element of success is always difficult to establish and it varies from patient to patient. The particular school of psychiatric thought to which the therapist adheres seems to be less important than his ability to be creative, to use himself as a therapeutic tool, to respond to the patient's requirements in the here and now and to change his approach as the situation warrants. There can be no absolute positions in psychotherapy. Flexibility is indispensable. This is especially the case when we are dealing with psychotic patients. The method of approach will depend on the condition of the patient. Some therapists address themselves to the non-psychotic portions of the personality in an effort to establish a working relationship. Others meet the patient on his own ground, entering into his psychotic world in order to reach him. Some therapists become adept in paraverbal or non-verbal communication with psychotic patients. They do so on the basis that ordinary language has little if any communicative value in working with some of these patients. According to Mueller even when language is intact, the therapist may be unable to bridge the gap between himself and the patient by verbal means for nothing he can say has as much impact on the patient as the patient's own thoughts and images, his cosmic experiences and his whole allegorical world. To reach him, the therapist has to learn his language and understand the fascination of his internal experience. The doctor-patient relationship may then afford the patient the opportunity of recapturing the lost "thou" and the "we" within the threatening "you" and "they" of his own distorted universe.

More gratification must be afforded the psychotic than the neurotic patient. The psychotic patient cannot tolerate much frustration. When it is necessary to impose a limit on aggressiveness, the therapist should attempt to do so by his own person rather than by restraints or by retaliation. The rational, objective attitude is unbearable to the patient, and so is the passive attitude of benevolent neutrality. The belief that the psychotic patient is incapable of transference is no longer tenable. However, the transference is likely to be on a very archaic and undifferentiated level. In the schizophrenic, for example, it is intense, stormy and rapidly fluctuating, demanding much and accompanied by violent rages and aggressive behavior. In his delusional ideas the patient moves constantly from one extreme to the other. He himself incarnates both good and evil, and the same ambivalence is apparent in the transference. As the therapist emerges increasingly from his non-existence for the patient, the more ambivalent the transference becomes.

At the same time, appearances may be deceiving. The patient may be insulting, rejecting or physically abusive because he is afraid. The therapist has assumed for the patient the evil, perhaps seductive aspects of the patient's own personality. This is a role which the therapist must accept before the patient may come to recognize and to accept as his own these repressed, distorted aspects of himself. It is important that the psychotherapeutic experience provide a relationship different from the patient's expectations, different indeed from the relationship he has tried to provoke by his usual maneuvers.

Countertransference is more difficult with psychotics than with neurotics. Yet it is an extremely important factor in their treatment. Savage calls it the therapist's biggest asset and his biggest stumbling block. Countertransference is more massive, chaotic and fragile with psychotic than with neurotic patients. There is an element of fear to be dealt with, along with any narcissistic tendencies disturbing to the relationship. While an element of magical omnipotence is almost indispensable, as Savage puts it, it can lead to serious errors. If the patient's progress is slow, the therapist may lose interest, or he may put more pressure on the patient than the patient can tolerate, or he may overestimate the patient's progress. If the therapist wishes to prove something by his treatment, if he is looking for something to verify some pet theory, the patient may be lost forever, at least to him. If he needs to be successful, to be a healer against all odds, the result may be disastrous for all concerned.

In sum, the processes of recovery in psychotic patients take place in the dynamic framework of transference and countertransference. Progress during therapy depends in a certain sense on the self-discipline of the therapist, indeed on self-sacrifice. Sometimes the patient recaptures his forces and profits from therapy at the very moment the physician is enduring almost unbearable frustration or sense of failure. It is as if he had to part with something himself before the patient could even start on the road to recovery.

In clinical medicine, cure usually means to return the patient to the status quo ante. To say that the patient "is as good as he ever was" is a cause for universal rejoicing. This criterion is not valid in psychiatry. The premorbid state represented by this anterior status is the source of the patient's difficulties; if he is simply returned to this condition, he remains vulnerable. The personality is still weak and fragile; the disturbance may recur with the advent of the slightest frustration or temptation. The goal in psychiatry is to improve the status quo ante, hence to reinforce and strengthen the personality. It is not easy. There is much more to learn of the art of using the human personality in an infinite number of ways to create different psychological effects and to make the bond between patient and therapist a surer instrument of healing.

There is no universal blueprint for the psychotherapist. There is only a task. Of this task the Balints have this to say: "The therapist must never forget that he is a professional and that his task is not to love or to be strict or to make good the deprivations in the patient's past or present, but to listen attentively to what is said and to understand it in a professional capacity, and in particular never to forget that there is always something new to understand. What he must be on the lookout for are not faults in the patient's environment or history, but misunderstandings, exaggerations, painful contradictions, and omissions, which characterize and color the patient's present wishes, hopes and vision."

All of this constitutes the fusion of the scientist and the healer and this constitutes the true art of medicine. Like all great art, the art of psychotherapy is the skillful and creative application of scientific knowledge to a human problem. Ruskin wrote, "Fine art is that in which the hand, the head and the heart of man go together."

REFERENCES

BALINT, M., AND BALINT, E.: Psychotherapeutic Techniques in Medicine. Springfield, Ill., Charles C Thomas, 1962.
MUELLER, C.: Les therapeutiques analytiques des psychoses. Rev. franc. psychan., 22:575, 1958.
SAVAGE, C.: Countertransference in therapy of schizophrenics. Psychiatry, 24:53, 1961.
FRANK, J. D.: The dynamics of the psychotherapeutic relationship; determinants and effects of the therapist's influence. Psychiatry, 22:17, 1959.

Patients' Expectations in Psychotherapy: Their Effects on Results

by STANLEY LESSE, M.D.

M ANY PSYCHOTHERAPISTS BELIEVE that the positive results they obtain in a given patient are due to the specific intended techniques they have employed, while failures are often considered to be due to nonspecific or unintended phenomena. However, both intended and unintended factors determine the process and results of psychotherapy.

I have elsewhere equated unintended effects with placebo reactions and have demonstrated how they apply to the process and outcome of psychotherapy.[1,2] Placebo effect as employed here is defined as "the psychologic, physiologic, or psychophysiologic effect of any procedure or medication given with therapeutic intent which is independent of or minimally related to the specific effects of the medication, and which operates through a psychologic mechanism." Placebo reactions may magnify or negate specific positive or adverse therapeutic reactions, and a negative placebo effect may even cancel out a positive placebo effect. Positive and negative reactions may possibly be noted in different patients in the same study or in the same patient on different occasions, all in response to the same unintended process. All therapies that have a specific effect in all probability have an unintended reaction that will enhance or retard the specific effect.

The unintended effects that relate to any psychotherapeutic technique depend upon (1) the milieu; (2) the patient; (3) the psychotherapist; (4) the initial status of the patient prior to the onset of treatment;[2,3] and (5) psychobiologic rhythms. One or more of these factors may stand out, depending in part upon the type of psychotherapeutic procedure used. Various factors appear to pertain equally to the environment and the patient on the one hand, or to the patient and the therapist on the other hand, and it may be difficult at times to differentiate between these sources. Expectancy, suggestibility, dependency, and motivation are often so interrelated as to defy specific delineation at this time. A patient's expectancies in psychotherapy depend in part upon his earlier experiences with physicians and his images of them.[4] In a broader vein, the patient's experiences with authoritative persons, in general, color his anticipation as to his relationship with a therapist.[5] This is important because a patient who is positively oriented toward a therapist and to psychotherapy, and who expects that the therapy will be successful, will undergo the greatest change in personality structure.[6] Unsophisticated, superstitious, and suggestible patients are prone to develop positive placebo effects. These patients manifest marked "magical thinking" in which there are strong unconscious desires for a protective parental surrogate. These infantile expectancies for dependency gratification may significantly contribute to a positive placebo effect early in therapy. However, if these infantile expectancies are not gratified, a negative placebo effect may intervene as treatment progresses.

This pattern holds for hypochondriacal patients who, while they are prone to manifest positive placebo effects initially, very readily shift to a negative placebo reaction if their expectations for symptomatic relief are not rapidly met. Positive placebo reactions in schizophrenic patients are very fickle and are subject to rapid fluctuation. Sociopaths have a very low degree of expectation and are prone to develop negative placebo reactions. Positive placebo effects are very uncommon in patients with conversion hysteria. On the other hand, individuals who manifest a marked degree of overt anxiety are prone to demonstrate a positive placebo reaction. This parallels the finding that patients with marked overt anxiety respond more effectively to treatment than do patients who demonstrate very little or no overt anxiety.[7] There is a level of anxiety at which the patient can free-associate most readily; I have referred to this as the "communication zone," the quantitative range of which differs for each patient.[8] It is in this "communication zone" that the greatest degree of improvement occurs. Within certain limits it has been found that the greater the patient's need for the relief of distress, the greater the expectancy for such relief.[4,6]

Patients have four types of expectancies: (1) of certain effects from *treatment* in general; (2) that the *therapist* will be the main source of relief; (3) that the *technique* will be the main source of aid; and (4) the patient's belief in *himself* as the main source of help. Only the last of these expectancies appears to be directly related to subsequent improvement.[9] If a patient views psychotherapy as a very superficial process

605

prior to the onset of treatment, he will not anticipate intensive far-reaching changes as a result of this technique. This points up the need to create a realistic framework within which the patient's range of therapeutic expectancies can fit.[10]

At first glance the literature dealing with expected and perceived improvement in psychotherapy as they pertain to the patient's expectancies would appear to be contradictory. Some authors have maintained that the effects of treatment are partially dependent upon the potentiation and activation of a patient's favorable expectancies with regard to improvement.[11,12] On the other hand, others have found no statistically significant relationships between expected and actual patient improvement.[13] Still another author found that the expectation of a patient's improvement held by the psychotherapist had more potent influence on these criteria than did the patient's own expectation.[14] Goldstein, in a recent review of the literature, helps clarify this apparent confusion.[15] The explanations with regard to the relationship between patient's expectancies and actual improvement have been gained from level of aspiration research which indicates a reality-unreality dimension of goal-setting behavior. It was found that moderate expectation of improvement in psychotherapy appears to be the most realistic of the range of possible patient prognostic expectancies, whereas extreme expectations are associated with unrealistic aspiration setting.

The patient's conceptualization of psychotherapy itself determines the role he expects to play and the role he expects the therapist to play in return. Kelly found that the patient's initial view will effect his behavior during treatment most markedly in the early interviews.[10] Some patients consider that psychotherapy is an end in itself and not a means to an end, or that it is a means of changing circumstances; others assume that if they are "good" patients, they would be rewarded by relief from their psychic distress. Entering treatment is taken by some as proof that they are indeed ill. Still other patients expect a specific "healthy state of mind" to be layed out for them.

In situations where the role and behavior expectancies of the patient and psychotherapist are very dissimilar, the therapeutic relationship is placed under great stress. Therefore, congruity of patient and therapist role behavior expectancy is of prime importance for effective treatment.[16-18]

The patient's previous conceptualization as to the "proper" role of a somatically ill individual seriously affects his total relationship with a psychiatrist. Parsons has found that the nonpsychiatric medical patient is traditionally expected to be passive dependent, to seek help, and to be helpless to a major degree, not to judge his doctor's expertness and to delegate ultimate responsibility for his care to another person, usually a relative.[19] In general medicine the good patient is one who wants to be told what to do.[20]

This attitude is diametrically opposite to the role expected of the psychiatric patient whose failure to take the initiative is considered by the therapist as evidence of unfulfilled dependency needs. Dependency and submissiveness, considered so essential in the medical patient, are deemed undesirable behavior patterns in the psychiatric patient. In keeping with this idea, the psychiatrist confronts a dependent "medically oriented" patient with his "excessive" dependency needs which he often equates with magical thinking. Therefore, in psychiatric patients there can be great conflict between the psychiatrist's expectations of what his role should be and his own previously learned medical sick role. This type of incongruity in itself can block effective treatment.

Psychiatric patients are not a homogeneous group in the appraisal of their sick roles.[21] Those in a state hospital setting see their role as paralleling the expected role of a nonpsychiatric medical patient, namely that they expect to be passive and to be helpless to a great degree. Indeed, the state hospital patient is often in conflict with his psychiatrist in this regard in that he has greater dependency expectations than his psychiatrist deems appropriate.

This problem parallels difficulties experienced by psychiatrists in private practice who in their dealings with patients referred by nonpsychiatric colleagues often expect these patients to be more independent and active in treatment than the patients consider to be appropriate. Therefore, both the state hospital patient and patients referred by nonpsychiatric physicians seen in private practice initially feel that the psychiatrist should be doing more for him, while at the same time the psychiatrist may feel that the patient is resisting. One of the most important and often one of the most difficult tasks that the psychotherapist has to perform with this type of patient is the modification of his more traditional, dependent, medical role expectancy. The earlier this conceptualization is altered, the smoother will be the course of psychotherapy.

The more dependent expectancy patterns seen in state hospital patients may be related in great measure to their socioeconomic backgrounds. Individuals from the lower economic groups tend to assume a more passive, submissive role. This is an aspect of a style of life that is commonly noted from early childhood in this segment of the population with regard to authority figures. Psychiatric outpatients, particularly those seen in private practice, often enter psychotherapy with a different

607

concept of role behavior. They consider their role on a level of greater equality and independence, and as being less bound to the authority of the psychiatrist.[21] This is more in keeping with the psychiatrist's point of view. In contrast with the state hospital patients, most of the patients seen in private practice come from a higher economic and educational group. This appears to account, in part, for the greater congruency noted in the patient-therapist role behavior expectancies in private psychotherapeutic practice.

Social class is related to a patient's concept of his sick role, just as it is related to the choice of doctor and the type of treatment selected.[21,22] As one learns to be a good citizen, one learns early what his sick role is supposed to be.[23] Apfelbaum evaluated patients' expectancies with regard to the personality and behavior of prospective psychotherapists and then compared therapeutic results with these expectations.[24] He divided patients into three "expectancy types": (1) Nurturant—patients who have infantile expectancies for which the therapist would be a complete parental substitute; (2) model—patients who expect a mature, diplomatic, permissive, neutral listener; (3) critic—patients who expect the psychotherapist to be a critical and analytic individual who will demand that they assume many responsibilities. In correlating these types of transference with therapeutic results, he found that the patients with "nurturant expectancy" had the greatest degree of psychopathology, as one might expect, while the "model expectancy" patients had the least degree of psychopathology. In keeping with the Law of Initial Value, but surprising from the standpoint of clinical prognosis, patient improvement as measured on the MMPI test and therapist ratings was the greatest with the "nurturant expectancy" patients.

In the United States, our culture is socioeconomically polyphasic, in contrast to that found in the communist countries such as the Soviet Union. For example, in the United States at one end of the social structure are men and women who are completely dependent upon themselves for their financial stability. These patients expect to return to an individualistically oriented milieu and to the particular type of adaptive struggle that is characteristic of this milieu. The various psychoanalytic and psychoanalytically oriented psychotherapies emphasize the individual patient's awareness of himself, those factors that stress the "I" and "me" and "mine," and are therefore uniquely suited for individualistically oriented patients.

In contrast to this socioeconomic group, at the other end of the spectrum in the United States is the large mass of the population whose adaptation to their lives depends upon a collective type of security. They are in several groups: (1) groups employed by large corporations; (2) groups of workers in industry, belonging to craft and industrial unions; (3) groups of persons employed by the local, state, and federal government. Their prepsychotherapeutic role in life and the type of adaptive struggle which they expect to have with their environment after the completion of treatment is far different from that described for the individual entrepreneur or self-employed professional man. This affects the role they expect to play in psychotherapy. In some of these patients psychoanalytic types of psychotherapy have stimulated the patient's self-awareness and self-preoccupations to the point that the could not effectively adjust to their collectively oriented socioeconomic milieu.[23] At the same time, however, most of these patients did not have sufficient intellectual ability or ego strength to advance in their milieu, nor did they have the ability to leave this group and function competitively in private business. These patients originally entered treatment anticipating that they would play a role that would prepare them to adapt to their socioeconomic milieu, but as a result of the very technique of psychotherapy some found it more difficult to function in their culture.

To be optimally effective, psychotherapeutic concepts and techniques must anticipate and then be adapted to a given socioeconomic and sociopolitical milieu. Instead, in general, patients have been adjusted to traditional theories and techniques. Most patients seen in psychotherapy return to the same socioeconomic and sociophilosophical background from which they came prior to treatment. They correctly anticipate returning to the same adaptive struggle with their milieu and expect that they will be specifically helped in this direction, and the type of therapy they receive should prepare them for the realistic environmental challenges they must face.

The factors that have been discussed in this paper with regard to patient expectancies are but a few that are of importance and that have been investigated. For example, the so-called "spontaneous remissions" and "transference cures" are related in great measure to this problem. However, the general findings dealing with all unintended aspects relating to the psychotherapies are of immense importance if treatment is to acquire a more scientific basis.

REFERENCES

1. LESSE, S.: Placebo reactions and spontaneous rhythms—their effects on the results of psychotherapy. Am. J. Psychother. 18 (Supplement #1): 99, 1964.
2. ——: Placebo reactions and spontaneous rhythms in psychotherapy. Arch. Gen. Psychiat. 10:497, 1964.

3. WILDER, J.: Basal levels and the paradoxic reaction in the evaluation of psychotherapy. Am. J. Psychother. 18 (Supplement 1): 89, 1964.
4. FRANK, J. D.: Dynamics of the psychotherapeutic relationship. Psychiatry 22:17, 1959.
5. SNYDER, W. U., AND SNYDER, B. J.: The Psychotherapy Relationship. New York, Macmillan, 1961.
6. LIPKIN, S.: Clients' feelings and attitudes in relation to the outcome of client centered therapy. Psychol. Monogr. 68:No. 376, 1954.
7. LESSE, S.: Anxiety and its relationship to the Law of Initial Value. Seventh International Conference of the Society for the Study of Biologic Rhythms. Panminerva Medica 1960.
8. ——: Psychotherapy in combination with psychotropic drugs. Presented at the American College of Neuropsychopharmacology Conference, October 24, 1964, Washington, D.C.
9. CARTWRIGHT, D. S., AND CARTWRIGHT, R. D.: Faith and improvement in psychotherapy. J. Counsel. Psychol. 5:174, 1958.
10. KELLY, G. A.: The Psychology of Personal Constructs. New York, Norton, 1955.
11. FRANK, J. D., GLIEDMAN, L. H., IMBER, S. D., STONE, A. R., AND NASH, E. H.: Patient's expectancies and relearning as factors determining improvement in psychotherapy. Arch. Neurol. & Psychiat. 77:283, 1957.
12. CHANCE, J. E.: Personality differences and level of aspiration. J. Consult. Psychol. 24:111, 1960.
13. BRADY, J. P., RESNIKOFF, M., AND ZELLER, W. W.: The relationship of expectation of improvement to actual improvement of hospitalized psychiatric patients, J. Nerv. Ment. Dis. 130:41, 1960.
14. GOLDSTEIN, A. P.: Therapist and client expectation of personality change in psychotherapy. J. Counsel. Psychol. 7:180, 1960.
15. ——: Therapist-Patient Expectancies in Psychotherapy. New York, Macmillan, 1962.
16. TOLMAN, E. C.: A theoretical analysis of the relations between sociology and psychology. J. Abnorm, Soc. Psychol. 47:291, 1952.
17. GROSS, N., MASON, W. S., AND MCEACHERN, A. W.: Explorations in Role Analysis: Studies of the School Superintendency Role. New York, Wiley & Sons, 1958.
18. LENNARD, H. S., AND BERNSTEIN, A.: The Anatomy of Psychotherapy. New York, Columbia U. Press, 1960.
19. PARSONS, T.: The Social System. Glencoe, Ill., Free Press, 1951.
20. SOBEL, R.: Role conflict or resistance: A new look at certain phases of psychotherapy. Am. J. Psychother. 18:25, 1964.
21. SOBEL, R., AND INGALLS, A.: Resistance to treatment-explorations of the patient's sick role. Am. J. Psychother. 18:562, 1964.
22. OVERALL, B., AND ARONSON, H.: Expectations of psychotherapy in patients of lower socioeconomic class. Am. J. Orthopsychiat. 33:421, 1963.
23. LESSE, S.: The relationships between socioeconomic and sociopolitical practices and psychotherapeutic techniques. Am. J. Psychother. 18:574, 1964.
24. APFELBAUM, B.: Dimensions of Transference in Psychotherapy. Berkeley, Calif., U. of California Press, 1958.

The Timeless Therapeutic Trinity

by JULES H. MASSERMAN, M.D.

I N THIS FINAL CHAPTER I shall endeavor to review, as clearly and suc-
cinctly as possible, those residues of reified reflections in library, clinic
and laboratory—and at the editorial desk—with which I have filled three-
score years of a full and perhaps only partly futile life. I cannot hope
that the triplicate product of these tripartite experiences is any parallel to
Einstein's tri-termed $E = mc^2$, other than that my formulation as to the
interrelationships of the causes, phenomena, and control of behavior also
consists of but a trio of interdigitating concepts, each again triply divisible,
to wit:

First, that man has only three ultimate (Ur) sources of concern: 1) his
physical health and longevity; 2) his social securities; and 3) his vital,
existential significance.

Second, that whenever these primary Ur-anxieties become manifest in
excessive and disabling somatic and behavioral aberrations, man seeks a
corresponding triad of therapies designed: 1) to restore his physical well-
being, 2) to recultivate his social alliances, and 3) to reconstitute his faith
in life's meaning and values.

Third, that these statements can be validated by recourse to the triune
epistemologic sources of all sciences: 1) the historical, 2) the comparative,
and 3) the experimental. Let us explore each heuristically in this order.

I. HISTORICAL APPROACHES TO THE ESSENTIALS OF THERAPY

Physical

Since his origins as *homo sapiens,* man has tried to mitigate his fears
of his inimical universe through his sciences and technologies. In two of
the most important of these—medicine and surgery—he has sought to find
means to cure his ills and restore his skills by empiric medicaments ranging from herbs and minerals to the first specific use of quinine for malaria
in 1820, and various procedures from the ancient binding of fractures to

611

the modern embedding of plastic hearts. Psychiatry, too, as a branch of medicine, has always employed pharmacologic, surgical and other modes of relieving man's material fears and their somatic reflections and, fortunately, is once again intensely developing this important rubric of therapy.

Social

Scientific and technical advances, nevertheless, have repeatedly proved inadequate for man's quest for security, inasmuch as:

a) expanding knowledge revealed mysteries and challenges ever beyond man's puny powers, however much he learned and applied; and,

b) each man realized that the tools his neighbors developed could be as or more lethal than his own.

Ergo, man learned to seek ever more inclusive human comradeship ranging from parental ties and familial loyalties through allegiances to the clan, tribe, city and state to their present limits in highly uncertain international alliances. Within all of these aggregations, specially selected men were given specific trusts and tasks toward enhancing group welfare: kings* and constables for internal government, soldiers for collective security (which of course included external conquest), and medicine men who, as proto-physicians, treated illness and, as proto-psychiatrists, corrected excessive deviations from locally accepted norms of conduct—a reintegration of medical and community function that, fortunately, is also being revived in modern psychiatry.

Mystical

But these irregular and sometimes inchoate strivings, even when combined with man's pyramiding technical knowledge and skills, have never yet been enough to allay a third and even broader concern, since no cabal of human scientists, however large or learned, has ever been able to control the heavens, secure the future, explain the nature or meaning of life, or mitigate the inadmissibility of death. Man has therefore always erected transcendent cosmic systems presumably within his ken, and operated by supernatural beings whom he could conveniently control either directly or through special mediators here on earth. Designated as such were priests and medicine men who, in their temples and sanatoria, were thus wishfully charged with this third task: not only to minister to the physical and social needs of men, but also to influence in their favor the mystical goals and gods of the universe.

---

*Our term "king" (German *Koenig*), head of state, is derived from Anglo-Saxon *cyning,* head of kin (Perry).

It would obviously require too long a series of ponderous tomes to cite in detail the threefold treatment of these triple trepidations of man throughout history, but perhaps a brief recall of how, with both conscious and intuitive skill, each aspect of the therapeutic trinity was intuitively invoked during one enlightened period—for example, in the Asklepiad sanatoria of ancient Greece—may serve to illustrate the general thesis. In brief, the methods employed in these classically effective mental health centers (named after the son of Apollo, the handsome, wise and good god of music, mind and medicine and thereby the very image of every psychiatrist) mitigated man's Ur-anxieties as follows:

First, by Restoring Physical Well-being: After the patient had left his contentious home and travelled to one of the sanatoria in the salubrious environs of Cos, Memphis or Knidos, he was welcomed not by a clerk or social worker but by no less a parent-surrogate than the Head Priest or Priestess, who then further cheered and reassured him by conducting him past piles of discarded crutches and bronze plaques bearing testimonials from grateful ex-patients. Immediate attention was then concentrated on restoring the patient's strength and tranquility through rest in pleasant surroundings, nourishing and appetizing diets, relaxing baths and massages, and the carefully measured administration of nepenthics—drugs that resembled modern ataractics in that they apparently soothed both the patient and the doctor. Indeed, the Greek word *therapeien* itself meant service, just as later the Latin *curare,* to care for, gave rise to our term "cure."

Second, by Recultivating Human Relationships: In accordance with this objective, equal effort was expended in counteracting the patient's Ur-anxiety of Social Isolation as follows:

1. Dyadic Confidence in the Physician: Then as now, the patient was encouraged to relate to his therapist:

a) As a kindly and protective parental figure who provided a source of security and comfort.

b) As a learned and experienced teacher, whose wise counsels for more restrained and balanced, and therefore healthier and happier, modes of life could be followed on rational and practical grounds (e.g., as in the various Stoic schools).

c) As a more intimate mentor interested in the supplicant's individual difficulties in function and conduct (his "present illness") and willing to explore their relationship to his past experiences (psychiatric history), their meanings and values (symbolisms) and their derived expressions in deviated goals, values and actions (retrospective analysis), in order that the intellectual understandings ("verbal insights") so derived would be applied ("worked through") to more satisfying, lasting and useful (e-motional—moving, or better, operational) personal and social adaptations. Socrates required his students to resolve their own perplexities in group discussions under his mentorship, Plato explained

613

the unconscious significance of dreams and fantasies, and Aristophanes, in his delightful comedy "The Clouds," pictured the distraught Strepsiades instructed to lie on a couch, express his every thought in free-association and thus clarify and dispel his obsessive fantasy about controlling the phases of the moon so that his monthly bills would not fall due. Less passively, Soranus records the cure of a case of "hysteria" in a virginal bride by a form of direct action (i.e., "lighting the torch of Hymen") that would shock a libidophilic Freudian.

d) Finally, the needful dependence of the patient on the physician (transference) that was so cultivated also led to an avid acceptance by the patient of the efficacy of the physician's quasi-scientific, quasi-mystical remedies, some of which were covertly punitive for, and thereby comfortingly expiative of, social and religious transgressions implicit in the patient's illness—a term related to Anglo-Saxon *yfel,* evil. Among these were not only a vast variety of unpleasant purgings, bleedings, coolings, roastings and broilings, but even more direct physical and surgical interferences with cerebral function, such as the Egyptian practice of trephining the skull and incising the cortex or, as described by Pliny the Elder, subjecting the patient to convulsive therapy by discharging electric eels through his head. We read of Hippocrates' condemnations of the ignorance and superstition inherent in many of these "false remedies" but this alone proves how widely practiced, then as now, they must have been.

2) Group Therapies. But the patient's social rehabilitation was not left to such partial and intermediate transactions with the physician alone; concurrently, his essential group relationships and skills were also recultivated through the following modalities:

The use of Music, which provided esthetic expression and encouraged group belongingness through feelings of conjoint rhythm, harmony and counterpoint.

Calisthenics and Dancing, which afforded similar possibilities of reorientative interaction and communion.

Competitive Athletics, not only for the joy of healthy action but for public recognition through nondestructive competition and reward.

Poetry and Dramatics: Here the esthetic psychiatrist (and there should be no other) may well reflect: What writings better explore and epitomize basic human relationship than the Homeric epics or the plays of Euripides, Aeschylus or Aristophanes? And what dramatizations of these legends can offer the beholder, either as witness or participant, more varied identifications, vivid experiences or vicarious solutions of his own interpersonal problems? The Greeks cherished these tragedies and comedies for their deep human empathy and ageless significance, endlessly varied their themes and were personally involved as actors, chorus or affectively moved audience—and thus explored in essence the basic interactions utilized in modern forms of group therapy.

Social Reintegration: This offered a transition between a passive dependence on the sanatorium to a growing recognition of the advantage of a return to the community and service for the common good.

Third, Metaphysical: Finally, the Greeks in their wisdom recognized a third human Ur-necessity of a Belief in some Inscrutable but Transcendent Order—and, parenthetically, demanded that Socrates pay the ultimate penalty for threatening man's trust in the existence of beneficent Celestial Beings. To capitalize on this ultimate faith, the Asklepiad sanatoria, like many hospitals today, were built and operated by one or another religious cult which added the following powerful factors to therapy:

a) A "divinely revealed" doctrine in which all believers could feel an exclusively self-elevating bond of fellowship.

b) A comforting ritual which, through its symbolization of human needs and longings, included such exquisitely gratifying procedures as:

1) The symbolic eating and drinking of the parent-god's body in the forms of mystically potentiating food and wine (as exemplified in the ancient worship of Melitta and Mithra).

2) The temple hymns, sung and played in the simple, repetitive, hypnotic cadences of a mother's lullaby—and often resulting in a "temple sleep."* Such regressive trances could be then varied with Dionysian orgies of food, drink and sexual indulgences to be triply enjoyed, since they also honored one's permissive and accommodating gods.

3) The "anointing" or "laying on of hands" to cure an injured bodily part—a direct reminiscence of the soothing parental stroking of an injured child, as ever since exemplified in the healing powers of the King's Touch, exploited in the seventeenth century by Greatrakes the Stroaker, and still sought by the emotionally immature and physically deprived avid of massage and chiropractic.

4) Implied likewise was the supreme promise of all religions—or, for that matter, of all "scientific" systems: the conquest, through life eternal, of man's most grim and implacable enemy: death itself.

5) Finally and even more profoundly, the physician-priest mediated an ethereal Promise of the *Spiritual*—a concept as fundamental to *aspiring* existence as is our first breath of air or *spiritus*. Every human is indeed variously *inspired,* acquires an *esprit de corps,* peoples his fantasies with *sprites,* occasionally becomes *desperate* and *despairs,* and finally *expires* so that his immutable *spirit* can begin life anew. And here, too, the physician-priest functions in knowing the Spiritual World, purveying professed contrition and remorse to the Spirits of our Fathers, and requiring only a gratifying small penance with which to avoid the posthumous horrors of searing exile from the Heavenly Progenitor and His Family. In the interim, the temple then and now furnished a divinely protected sanctuary from earthly stresses and problems, much as Lourdes is a haven of comfort and healing today.

These, then, were the ancient—and are the perennial—practices that embody what physicians have intuitively known for centuries: that although no man can ever be certain of his health, friends or philosophy,

---

*Two thousand years later, Mesmer was to extol the mystic powers of "animal magnetism" and, through Charcot and Janet, influence Freud; in contrast, Bernheim was to warn, "It is a wise hypnotist that knows who is hypnotizing whom."

the illusions of security in each of these spheres are essential to his welfare; and that all methods of medical-psychiatric therapy are effective only insofar as they restore physical well-being, foster more amicable interpersonal relationships, and help the patient amend his beliefs so as to render them more generally acceptable and useful.

II. The Comparative Approach to the Essentials of Therapy

To supplement this historical survey, it would require still another five-foot shelf to review the current and equally illuminating anthropologic, ethnic, and trans-cultural studies of Gillin, Margolin, Lambo, Kiev and Leighton, or to cite Ziferstein's and my own comparisons of Soviet and American techniques, or to acknowledge the contributions of other socio-psychiatrists with sufficient breadth of interest and objectivity to investigate the vast variety of therapeutic practices throughout the world; moreover, it would take an integrative genius to demonstrate that, despite their deceptive diversity, nearly all of these fall into the familiar rubrics of physical, social and metaphysical readaptation. However, even if we do not go so far afield, perhaps a parochial re-examination of the various modes of therapy in our own culture, from colonic lavage to Christian Science, may demonstrate a similar threefold efficacy. This, of course, requires a harrowing willingness to concede that seemingly disparate concepts and cults are comparable to the one we personally cherish—a challenge that few of us are willing to accept. Nevertheless, playing the role of a pre-henbane Socrates in a peripatetic dialogue with my psychiatric residents and analytic trainees, I have sometimes proposed some outrageous postulate such as: Resolved, that electroshock therapy and psychoanalysis are essentially more alike than different in their basic therapeutic actions and effects. In the past, though not so much recently, this usually evoked a storm of protest that as a duly anointed psychoanalyst* as well as a certified neuropsychiatrist, I should know that the two methods were manifestly incomparably different, in that: a) EST is "physical," "enforced," "impersonal," "stereotyped," "rigidly conducted," "suppressive," "antimnemonic," "intellectually impairing," etc., whereas, in diametric contrast, b) psychoanalysis is "psychologic," "voluntary," "exquisitely interpersonal," "flexible," "evocative," "restorative of memory," and "designed to develop to the full the patient's cognitive and adaptive capacities" through "insight."

At this juncture, I occasionally pointed out that the last assertion directly begged the question since, in the historical and comparative contexts in

---

*It has been my rueful observation that, as not infrequently misapplied, orthodox analytic therapy may result in a reversal of Freud's aphorism, to wit: "Where Ego was, there shall Id be."

which I had posed the question, "insight" itself could be defined only as that transiently ecstatic state in which patient and therapist temporarily shared the same illusions as to the cause and cure of either's difficulties. With this additional goad, some of my residents began to explore subtler dimensions of therapeutically operative similarities between electroshock and analysis, and came up with the following disconcerting symmetries:

Physical parameters: Both methods offer an escape from the mundane stresses of external reality onto a sensorially isolated bed or couch provided by society and protected by a parental surrogate for about the same average number of recumbent hours.

Both methods serve to disorganize current patterns of deviant behavior: EST by direct cerebral diaschises followed by reorganization; analysis by semantic and symbolic dissociations and alterations of concept and reaction.

Interpersonal influences: In both methods, the patient selects (whether "voluntarily" or by equivalent "external" pressure) *the method of therapy and the therapist* he regards as most suitable for his needs.

In both methods, the therapist sympathetically accepts the patient as more or less helpless and "ill," is convinced of the special validity of his own therapeutic theories and the efficacy of his techniques—*and thus rounds out an operationally effective folie a dieux.*

Social Parameters: Both methods entail covert physical, economic, social and other penalties for the persistence of disapproved conduct: in EST, more incarceration, exclusion of visitors, post-shock headaches, and other adverse sanctions; in analysis, more time, more expense, more patronizingly disillusioning "interpretations," plus the onus of having an "unanalysable (i.e., permanently rejected) character disorder." *Conversely, there are desirable reacceptances and rewards for progressively more comforting behavior* (the "patient compliance" of Ehrenwald): e.g., the therapist's favor, expanding privileges, renewed familial hegemony and finally, membership in Recovery, Inc. after "successful" EST; and after analysis—at least until recently—acceptance in the sophisticated elite of the "thoroughly analyzed" at cocktail parties, or, in the case of Institute trainees, ecstatic admission to, and referrals from, the local Psychoanalytic Society.

Mystical: Finally, in both cases, patient and therapist join in an essentially worshipful belief that either Cerletti or Freud brought providentially inspired salvation to ailing mortals, attainable through respectively prescribed rituals of suffering, expiation, enlightenment and the reacquisition of metaphysiologic grace. Any agnostic who, at national meetings, has attended the Section on Electro-Convulsive Therapy or—usually at another hotel at a discretely noncommunicative distance—a Seminar of Psycho-

617

analytic Theory and Therapy, will unmistakably have experienced the devotional aura as well as the scientific import of both proceedings.

Similar operational parallels can, of course, be constructed, say, between vitamin therapy and "non-directive" counseling or between *Dauerschlaff* and psychodrama. Such comparisons should, of course, never obscure the specific attributes and special clinical applicabilities of each method, but within the bounds of reductionist sophistry, objective, operational analysis may help clarify the universal factors of therapy we have been considering, viz: to help the patient realize that his formerly cherished modes of conduct in the three spheres of physical, social and philosophic adaptation are no longer either necessary or profitable, and to learn, by exploration and personal experience, that new ones will prove more personally pleasurable, socially advantageous and existentially compatible.

III. Experimental Validations of the Essentials of Therapy

This brings us to our final heuristic resource: the experimental approach. In the words of Adolf Meyer, every friend and patient can be studied as a ready-made "experiment of nature," but for more adequate controls and precise analysis, animal research becomes necessary. I have elsewhere[10] rather extensively reviewed the rationale, the fascinating ethologic evidence and the experimental studies of many other investigators in this field; here, we can only in outline form summarize the basic premises as to "normal" conduct and the methods of inducing and reversing deviant behavior that have emerged from our own studies. The four "Biodynamic Principles" thus evolved, in briefest statement, are these:

Principle 1: Motivation. The behavior of all organisms is actuated by physiologic needs, and therefore varies with their intensity, duration and balance.

Principle 2: Perception and Response. Organisms conceive of, and interact with, their milieu not in terms of an absolute "external reality," but in accordance with their individual genetic capacities, rates of maturation, and unique experiences.

Principle 3: Range of Normal Adaptation. In higher organisms, these factors make possible many techniques of adaptation, which in turn render the organism capable of meeting stress and frustration and maintaining an adequate level of satisfaction by a) employing new methods of coping with difficulties when the ones formerly employed prove ineffective, or b) by modifying old goals or substituting new ones when the old become unattainable.

Principle 4: Neurotigenesis. However, when physical inadequacies, environmental stresses, or motivational-adaptational conflicts exceed the organism's innate or acquired capacities, internal tension (anxiety) mounts, neurophysiologic (psychosomatic) dysfunctions occur, and the organism develops over-generalized patterns of avoidance (phobias), ritualized behavior (obsessions and compulsions), regressive, hyperactive, aggressive or other deviant interorganismic transactions ("sociopathy"), or bizarrely "dereistic" (hallucinatory, delusional) responses corresponding to those in human neuroses and psychoses.

Experimental Conflict: As indicated in Principle IV, marked and persistent deviations of behavior were induced by stressing individual animals between mutually incompatible patterns of survival: as, for instance, requiring a monkey to secure food after a conditional signal from a box which might unexpectedly contain a toy snake—an object as symbolically dangerous to the monkey as a live one, harmless or not, would be. In this connection we further amended Freudian doctrine by demonstrating that "fear" in the sense of threat of injury need not be involved at all; i.e., equally serious and lasting aberrations of behavior could be induced by facing the animal with difficult choices among mutually exclusive satisfactions—situations that parallel the disruptive effects of prolonged indecisions in human affairs.* Either form of conflict produced physiologic and mimetic manifestations of anxiety, spreading inhibitions, generalizing phobias, stereotyped rituals, "psychosomatic" dysfunctions, impaired social interactions and other persistent regressions and deviations of conduct.

Constitutional Influences: Animals closest to man showed symptoms most nearly resembling those in human neuroses and psychoses, but in each case the "neurotic" syndrome depended less on the "specificity" of the conflict (which could be held constant) than on the constitutional predisposition of the animal. For example, under similar stresses spider monkeys reverted to infantile dependencies or catatonic immobility, cebus developed various "psychosomatic" disturbances including functional paralysis, or preferred hallucinatory satisfactions such as chewing and swallowing purely imaginary meals while avoiding real food to the point of self-starvation.

Methods of Therapy: Since we induced experimental neuroses in animals not only to study their causes and variations but primarily to search for the principles of therapy, this portion of our work was accorded most time and effort. After the trial of scores of procedures, only nine general methods—

---

*Applying this principle on an international scale, the economist M. F. Millikan asked "How much freedom of choice can people not used to many degrees of freedom take without psychologic strain that threatens the stability of the system?" And answered, "My hunch . . . is that a good deal of the instability . . . in the underdeveloped world may [thus] result."

significantly parallel to those used with human patients—proved to be most effective in ameliorating neurotic or psychotic symptoms. Again in bare summary, these techniques could once more be marshalled under "physical", "social" and—if the term be used in a broadly operational sense—"mystical" subheads as follows:

1. Physical Methods: These included

a) The satisfaction of one or more of the opposed biologic needs that induced the impasse by facilitating the achievement of one or another goal, such as hunger or thirst *vs.* sex, or exploratory drives *vs.* evasion of injury—conflicts of motivation that often induce adaptational difficulties in humans.

b) Removal from the laboratory to a less stressful environment; by human analogy, a better home, job or climate—or even an occasional "vacation" from the cumulative strains of daily living.

c) The provision of opportunities for the re-utilization of neurotically inhibited skills: in the cat, making available another device for obtaining food; in the human, inducing a crashed, unhurt, but temporarily phobic fighter pilot to fly a second plane immediately, and thus dispel his mounting anxiety over his threatened loss of essential mastery over his milieu.

d) The preventive administration of various drugs such as alcohol that blunted perceptions of impending trauma or gave the animal later surcease by dampening excessively intense, complex, or prolonged residual responses to conflict. Some neurotic animals which experienced such effects from the ingestion of alcohol sought out the drug if made available and became avid alcoholic addicts until their neurosis was relieved by other means—thereby extending the human analogue.

e) The use of electroconvulsive or other methods of producing sufficient cerebral anoxia and diaschisis to disrupt undesirable patterns of behavior, provided they were relatively recently induced and thereby more dissoluble than those more deeply established and engrammed—again in direct analogy to clinical EST; and lastly,

f) The employment of surgical or electrocoagulative techniques to produce neurologic lesions and consequent disorganizations of aberrant behavior similar to those produced by human lobotomies or thalamotomies.

2. 'Social' Methods: These, in turn comprised:

a) Environmental. The resolution of the motivational conflict through progressive exposure to neurotically feared situations, always keeping the animal's reactions within its re-adaptive potentials—a method that may be employed clinically in the so-called "behavior therapy" of obsessive-phobic

620

patients, provided they possess sufficient flexibility and fortitude ("ego strength").

b) *Dyadic*. The retraining of the animal by carefully *individualized* care and guidance, the experimenter acting as a "personal therapist" who helps the subject re-explore early experiential conflicts and dispel their neuro-tigenic effects; or, as in psychoanalysis, helping the patient recall early traumatic events and re-evaluating their residues in the here and now by "corrective emotional experiences" vis-a-vis the therapist and elsewhere in a physically, socially and philosophically re-evaluated world.

c) The provision of a therapeutic association with a corrective coterie of well-adapted ('normal') conspecifics, in peer-pedagogic parallel to sending a "problem child" to a "good school", i.e., where children behave in the manner desired.

3. Mystical Connotations:

Finally, if this term be extended to its full meaning of behavior trustingly based on faith in the unprovable, then a dog's unreasoning confidence in its master's magical prowess and devotion to its interests may also be extended to the therapeutic techniques 2 a) and c) as described under "Environmental" and "Social" above.

CLINICAL SUMMARY

If, then, all of the historical, comparative and experimental data here briefly surveyed where to be integrated and interpreted, our three essential principles of therapy could be clinically derived as follows:

To begin with, we must discard our cold armor of aloof "professional dignity," and accept each patient not as a diagnostic "challenge," or a recipient of "specific therapy for the organic pathology" (a repulsive solecism)—and least of all as only another research datum—but as *a troubled human being seeking comfort and guidance as well as relief from physical suffering.* It is, of course, imperative that, whether we regard the patient's complaints as primarily "organic" or "psychogenic," bodily discomfort and dysfunction are to be relieved by every medical and surgical means available including, when indicated, carefully prescribed sedatives and hypnotics temporarily useful to dull painful memories, relieve apprehension and quiet agitation;* however, in nearly all medical and surgical specialties we recognize that such surcease, usually of mixed suggestive and

---

*Parenthetically, in my own research studies and in my clinical experience, I have found that the barbiturates, bromides, aldehydes and other well-tested drugs, when wisely used, are often preferable to many of the widely promoted but dubious "ataractics" and "tranquilizers."

pharmacologic origin, is merely the first stage of therapy. As soon as the patient's tensions and anxieties have abated sufficiently to make him more accessible and cooperative, we must strive to re-evoke his initiative, restore his lost skills, and encourage him to regain the confidence and self-respect that can come only from useful accomplishment.

But since no man is an "Island intire of its Selfe," the wise physician, whatever his specialty, has a broader task: to recognize that his patient may be deeply concerned about sexual, marital, occupational and other problems that may also seriously affect his physical and social well-being. This involves an exploration, varying in depth and duration but always discerning and tactful, of the attitudes and values the patient derived from his past experiences, his present goals and tribulations, his successful (normal), socially ineffective (neurotic), or bizarrely unrealistic (psychotic) conduct, the ways in which these patterns relieve or exacerbate his current difficulties, and whether they are accessible to various other methods of medico-psychiatric therapy. It is customary at this juncture for the psychiatrist to warn his colleagues in other fields off his supposedly esoteric preserves; instead, let me confess that it has been my gratifying experience that in most cases any intelligent, sensitive physician (or other well-trained professional under medical guidance when required) can conduct the essential psychotherapy required. In essence, this will consist of using gentle reasoning, personal guidance and progressive social explorations to help the patient correct his past misconceptions and prejudices, abandon infantile or childlike patterns of behavior that have long since lost their effectiveness, revise his goals and values, and adopt a more realistic, productive and lastingly rewarding ("mature") style of life. In this skillfully directed re-education (good psychotherapy, despite a recent fad to the contrary, is about as "nondirective" as good surgery) the enlightened cooperation of his family, friends, employer and others may, in triadic or group transactions, be utilized to the full. By such means the patient's second Ur-defense will be strengthened by renewed communal solidarity and security—a *sine qua non* of dyadic and rehabilitative therapy.

Lastly, and to mitigate the third, or existential Ur-anxiety, the patient's religious, philosophic or other convictions, instead of being deprecated or undermined, should be respected and strengthened insofar as they furnish him with what each of us requires: a belief in life's purpose, meaning and value. In this fundamental sense, medicine, being a humanitarian science, can never be in conflict with philosophy or religion, since all three seem to be designed by a beneficient providence to preserve, cheer and comfort man and thereby constitute a trinity to be respected by any physician deeply concerned with man's health and sanity. Indeed, with respect to these key terms, it is of historic-philologic significance that the term *sanatos* implied to the ancients the indissolubility of physical and mental functions (*mens sanis in corpora sano*); so also, our more "modern" word "health" can be traced to the Anglo-Saxon *hāl* or *hōl*, from which are derived not only physical *haleness* and *healing*, but the greeting, *"Hail, friend!,"* and the concepts *wholeness* and *holiness*. Once again, Greek, Roman and Gaul have bequeathed to us, in the rich heritage of a syncretic language in which "reality" and "illusion" merge, their recognition of the indissoluble trinity of physical, social and philosophic components of medical and psychiatric therapy.

REFERENCES

1. GILLIN, J.: Cross-cultural aspects of socio-cultural therapy. Estudios Anthropologios. Manuel Samio, Mexico D. 1956.
2. KIEV, A. (Ed.): Magic, Faith and Healing. New York, The Free Press of Glencoe, 1964.
3. LAMBO, T. A.: Patterns of psychiatric care in developing African countries. Ibid., pp. 443-453.
4. LEIGHTON, A. H.: My Name is Legion. New York, Basic Books, 1958.
5. MARGOLIN, S. G.: On some principles of therapy. Am. J. Psychiat., 114:1087-1094, 1958.
6. MASSERMAN, J. H.: Battlements and bridges in the East: a liaison with Soviet psychiatry. Am. J. Psychiat. 117:4-18, 1959.
7. MASSERMAN, J. H.: Contemporary psychotherapies: a review. Arch. Gen Psychiat. 10:461-464, 1962.
8. MASSERMAN, J. H.: The sphere of psychiatry. In: Current Psychiatric Therapies, Vol. V, Masserman, J. H., Ed. New York, Grune & Stratton, 1964, pp. 280-303.
9. MASSERMAN, J. H.: Practice of Dynamic Psychiatry. Philadelphia, W. B. Saunders, 1955.
10. MASSERMAN, J. H.: The biodynamic roots of psychoanalysis. In: Frontiers of Psychoanalysis. Marmor, J., Ed. New York, Basic Books, In press.
11. MASSERMAN, J. H.: Psychotherapeutic progress in Latin America. In: Progress in Psychotherapy. Vol. III. Masserman, J. H., and Moreno, J. L., Eds., New York. Grune & Stratton, 1963, pp. 282-310.
12. MILLIKAN, M. F.: Problems of underdevelopment: an economic view. Am. J. Psychiat. 22:1393, 1966.
13. PERRY, V. W.: Lord of the Four Quarters. New York, Braziller, 1966, p. 10.
14. ZIFERSTEIN, I.: Therapeutic methods in the Soviet Union. In: Science and Psychoanalysis. Vol. IX, Masserman, J. H., Ed. New York, Grune & Stratton, 1966, pp. 291-295.

INDEX OF SUBJECTS

626

627

Methadone, 292
Methaqualone, 262
Methyprylon, 262
Midtown Manhattan Project, 322
Milontin, 61
Miltown, 262
Mind-tapping, 573, 590
Modeling, 177
Mongolism, 41

Nalorphine, 285
Naloxone, 285-286
  addiction, 285
  effects, 286
National Training Laboratories, 386
Negativism, 73
New York State Psychiatric Institute, 41
Nicotinic acid, 258
Night hospitals, 515, 516
Notec, 262
Nursing, 557, 562

Occupational therapy, 474
Odyssey House, 296
Office of Economic Opportunity, 496
Omnipotence, 295
Opiates, withdrawal, 294
Opportunity for failure, 473
Overnight therapy, 384
Oxazepan, 262

Panic, 434, 436
Paraldehyde, 262
Paramethadione, 61
Parole, for sex offenders, 222
Pentazocine, 293
Perception
  disorganization of, 237
  reorganization of, 239
Perphenazine, 255
Personality, existential, 134
Perversion, 212
Pharmacotherapy, 251
Phenothiazines, 61
Phenurone, 62
Phenylketonuria, 40
Phobias, 144
  thanatophobia, 336
Physician-patient privilege, 580, 589
Placebo, 150
  definition of, 604, 605
  indications for usage, 605
Placidyl, 262
Preoedipal stages, 113
Primidone, 62

Privilege
  and communication, 551, 571, 578, 588
  legal, 552
Psychoanalysis
  in children, 72
  negative therapeutic reaction to, 115
  present trends in, 113
  and therapeutic management, 115
Psychosexual development, 125
Psychosexuality and criminal law, 582, 586
Psychosurgery, 244
Psychotherapy, 269
  art in, 597
  and aversion therapy, 205
  biphasic, 599
  choice of therapist in, 354
  and chronic schizophrenia, 237
  and countertransference, 602
  and dependency, 607
  direct analysis in, 125
  and drugs, 48
  emotional understanding in, 599
  family group, 348
  group, 193
  joint sessions in, 354
  for male homosexuals, 193
  marital, 353
  and material secrecy, 551, 571
  for mother and child, 519
  in schizophrenia, 245
  and schools, 601
  and transference, 598
  and transvestism, 203
  values in, 102
  for youthful offenders, 101
Punishment, 143

Rauwolfia, alkaloids, 52
Reality testing, 107
Regression, 330, 517
Rehabilitation, 471, 514
  and game playing clients, 475
Relaxation, degree of, 148
Release of confidence, 575, 584, 591
REM, 269
Resistance, 220
Responsibility, 139
Resocialization, 221
Rivalries, familial, 359
Role, validation of, 470

Schizophrenia
  and art, 160
  catatonic, 471
  compensation progress in, 239

INDEX OF NAMES

632

633

634

635

636

637

Wheatley, D., 260, 261
Whillock, F. A., 214
Whisnant, C. L., 264, 269
White, B., 257
Wikler, A., 264, 269, 281, 282, 290, 296,
    308
Wilder, J., 610
Wilkinson, R. H., 548
Willis, S. H., 547
Wineman, D., 109
Wing, J. K., 80, 533
Winick, C., 373
Winnicott, D. W., 118
Witenberg, E. G., 374
Wittenborn, J. R., 296
Wittenborn, S., 296
Wittkower, E. D., 414
Wolberg, L. R., *163,* 168, 169, 172
Wolf, A., 367, 374
Wolf, M. M., 80
Wolf, S., 150, 155
Wolff, K., 334
Woloshin, A., 471

Wolpe, J., 147
Woolfson, G., 260
Wright, B. A., 78
Wright, Helen, 344
Wulff, M. H., 265, 269
Wunderlich, R. C., 402, 407

Yablonsky, L., 308
Yalom, I. D., 389, 394, 395
Yarrow, L. J., 526

Zabransky, F., 260
Zaks, A., *281,* 290
Zaslow, R. W., 75, 76, 77, 78, 79
Zaslow, S. L., 247
Zeller, W. W., 610
Ziferstein, I., 616, 623
Zim, A., 394
Zimet, C., 399
Zinberg, N. W., 334
Zung, W. E. K., 236
Zunin, L. M., *140*
Zwerling, I., 460